The Crystalline Lens System: Its Embryology, Anatomy, Physiological Chemistry, Physiology, Pathology, Diseases, Treatment, Operations and After-Changes with a Consideration of Aphakia

Louis Stricker

THIS BOOK IS DEDICATED

TO THE MEMORY OF

OTTO BECKER.

The Inspiration of this Work is the Fruit of His Labor.

TABLE OF CONTENTS.

THE CRYSTALLINE LENS SYSTEM.

INTRODUCTION—GENERAL CONSIDERATION.

PART I.

THE NORMAL LENS SYSTEM.

CHAPTER I.

THE DEVELOPMENT OF THE LENS SYSTEM.

CHAPTER II.

THE GROWTH OF THE LENS SYSTEM.

CHAPTER III.

THE PHYSIOLOGICAL RETROGRESSION OF THE LENS AND ITS ELEMENTS.

CHAPTER IV.

THE MANNER IN WHICH THE NORMAL AND PATHOLOGICAL LENS-SYSTEM IS NOURISHED.

The direction and course of the Nutritive Stream in the Lens.
The Physical changes which take place in the lens with increasing age. (The increase and reduction in volume).
The Chemistry of the Lens and its surrounding fluids. (The chemically demonstrable difference which exist between the nucleus of the senile noncloudy and the senile cataractous Lens).

PART II.

THE PATHOLOGICAL LENS SYSTEM.

CHAPTER I.

THE PATHOLOGY OF THE ZONULA OF ZINN.

Atrophy, Hypertrophy, Dissolution, Anomalies of Formation. Solution of Continuity.

CHAPTER II.

THE PATHOLOGICAL CHANGES IN THE LENS. LENTICULAR CATARACT.

Senile Cataract.
Cataract formation in Youthful Lenses.

CHAPTER III.

THE PATHOLOGICAL CHANGES IN THE INTRACAPSULAR CELLS—CAPSULAR CATARACT.

The degenerative changes.
The new cellular formations which develop from the intracapsular cells.
    a. Regenerative New Cellular Formations.
    b. The processes and products of Atrophic New Cellular Formations.
    1. Epithelial covering of the posterior capsule.
    2. Wedl's Vescicular Cells.
    3. Capsular Cataracts. (*a*) Capsular Cicatrices.
                    (*b*) True capsular Cataract.
    4. Enclosure of foreign substances.
    5. Formation of Pus in the Lens.

CHAPTER III.

MALFORMATIONS OF THE LENS SYSTEM IN CONSEQUENCE OF
UNSYMMETRICAL DEVELOPMENT OF THE ZONULA
FIBRES.

Coloboma Lentis.
Ectopia Lentis.

CHAPTER IV.

ACQUIRED ANOMALIES OF POSITION NOT DUE TO MALFOR-
MATIONS. LUXATIO LENTIS.

Spontaneous Luxation.   1. Normal Lens. *"Synchisis corporis vitrei."*
                               2. Cataractous Lenses.
Traumatic Luxation.   *a.* 1. Causation.
                               2. (*Sympathetic Opthalmia.*)
                               3. Symptoms.
                         b. Subluxation.
                         c. Total Luxation.
                         d. Freely Moveable Lenses (Results of Luxation).
Secondary Luxation.

CHAPTER V.

MALFORMATION OF THE LENS WITHOUT DEMONSTRATABLE
PATHOLOGICAL CHANGES IN OTHER PORTIONS OF THE
EYE.

Indented or Notched Lens.
Lenticonus-Krystaloconus. *a.* Anterior.
                           b. Posterior.

CHAPTER VI.

PARTIAL CATARACTS.

A. Axial Cataracts. (Cataracta Axialis).
    1. Cataracta Centralis. Congenital central lens cataract.
    2. Cataracta Polaris Anterior. Cataracta polaris pyramidalis.
        a. Congenita.
        b. Acquisita.
        c. Cataracta Capsularis Anterior.
    3. Cataracta Polaris Posterior. *Vera.*
    4. Cataracta Fusiformis—Spindle Cataract.
B. Zonular Cataract—Lamellar.—Cataracta Zonularis.
C. Various forms of congenital partial cataracts.
        a. Cataracta Punctata.
        b. Cataracta Stellata.

CHAPTER VII.

COMPLICATED CATARACTS. CATARACTA ACCRETA. CATARACTA COMPLICATA.

Casuistik.

Calcifications of the Lens. Cataracta calcarea.

Ossification of the Lens. Cataracta ossea.

Perforation of the capsule of the lens as the result of the traction of cyclitic bands.

CHAPTER VIII.

CATARACT DUE TO DISEASE OF ONE EYE WITHOUT THE PRESENCE OF ABNORMAL ADHESIONS.

Cataracta mollis ex chorioiditide.

CHAPTER IX.

CONSTITUTIONAL CATARACT.

A. Cataracta polaris posterior (Retinitis pigmentosa).

B. Cataracta Chorioidealis.

C. Total congenital cataract on both Eyes. Causes of cataracts of sudden development.

D. Total acquired cataract on both Eyes.

a. Cataracta mollis juvenum.

b. Cataracta Diabetica.

1. Casuistik.

2. Manner of Development.

3. Aetiology.

E. Cataracta senilis praematura. Cataracta nuclearis.

Cataracta punctata (see Chapter VI).

F. Cataracta Senilis—Senile Cataract. Aetiology.

Chronic Nephritis.

Carotidis Atheroma.

G. Cataracta Hypermatura. 1. a. Cataracta hypermatura reducta.

2. b. Cataracta hypermatura fluida.

H. Cataracta Nigra.

CHAPTER X.

CATARACTA CAPSULARIS. SIMPLEX—COMPLICATA.

CHAPTER XI.

PATHOLOGICAL CONDITIONS IN ORIGINALLY NORMALLY FORMED LENSES PRODUCED BY EXTERNAL FORCE.

CATARACTA TRAUMATICA.

By Blunt Force. a. Cataracta ex Contusione.

b. Traumatic Luxations, tears in the zonula and rupture of the capsule.

By Puncture or Incision. c. Unintentional (accidental injuries). Cataracta Traumatica.

d. Intentional (operative secondary cataracts).

PART IV.

THE THERAPY OF THE DISEASES OF THE LENS.

CHAPTER I.

THE MEDICINAL TREATMENT.

CHAPTER II.

THE OPERATIVE TREATMENT.

The Purpose.

Dislocatio cataractae:	Depression.	Definition.
		Historical Review.
Extractio cataractae.	Extraction.	Definition purpose.
		Historical Review.
Discissio cataractae.	Discission.	Definition and purpose.
		Historical Review.

Suction.

CHAPTER III.

THE PROCEDURES AND CHANGES WHICH TAKE PLACE IN AN EYE DURING AND AFTER A CATARACT OPERATION.

Introduction.

Reclination. The difference in the nature of the injury produced by keratonyxis and scleronyxis.

The difference in the reaction following reclination.

The anatomical examination of eyes on which reclination had been practised.

Discission. The manner in which an eye is injured by discission, and its sequelae.

The value of these methods.

Extraction. An analysis of the essential points of a Cataract Extraction.

a. The Flap Extraction (Daviel).

b. Peripheral Linear Extraction (Von Graefe).

c. Modern Scleral Flap Ext. d. Corneal Flap Ext.

The advantages vs. the disadvantages of an Iridectomy.

The size of the incision.

Description of the steps of a cataract extraction.

The Linear Extraction for soft and membranous cataract.

The capsular forceps.

The changes which take place during the extraction.

Mishaps liable to occur during the operation.

Irrigation of the anterior chamber.

The results of clinical observation of the corneal wound.

The abnormal conditions which may develop during the processes of healing.

The processes of healing with incomplete results.

Cataracta complicata.

The position of the various forms of corneal incision.

The irregular healing of wounds.

The secondary cataracts—complicated.

Cyclitis. Detachment of the vitreous, ciliary body, retina.

Glaucoma.

The After Treatment. The artificial ripening of cataract.

The preparatory treatment.

Use of atropine and eserine.

Care of the conjunctiva.

The principles of after treatment.

Mental derangements after extraction.

When to discharge the patient from the physician's care.

When to prescribe cataract glasses.

Secondary operations.

The treatment of recent injuries.

The treatment of traumatic and secondary cataract.

The therapy of luxation of the lens.

PART V.

THE APHAKIC EYE.

The definition and diagnosis of aphakia.

The optical system in aphakia. Aphakic hyperopia.

Emmetropic aphakia—the emmetropic aphakic eye.

Myopic and hyperopic aphakia.

The average values of the emmetropic eye.

Conditions between aphakic hyperopia, length of the optic axis, also prior to the operation.

Accommodation in the aphakic eye.

Degree of vision in aphakia.

Causes for the diminution of the acuity of vision in aphakic astygmatism as a result of the operation.

The apparent and the real acuity of vision in aphakia.

Artificial accommodation in the aphakic eye.

The selection of spherical glasses.

The cylindrical correction.

The influence which glasses exert on the vision of the aphakic eye.

A few of the peculiarities of the aphakic eye. Erythropsia.

Binocular vision in aphakia.

INTRODUCTION.

At the time this work was first contemplated, the intention was to make a translation of *Otto Becker's Pathologie und Therapie des Linsen-sytems," Graefe-Saemisch Handbuch, Vol. V.* 1877, but as the work progressed it became evident that many of the ideas therein expressed were not in accord with the teachings of modern pathology. The introduction of more delicate and accurate methods for pursuing microscopical investigations, the use of the refracting opthalmoscope, the introduction of cocaine, the application of antisepsis, later of asepsis to eye surgery, have all added their share to the elucidation of this subject. No one who has carefully read Becker's great classic on the Crystalline Lens could possibly fail to be impressed with the keenness of his observation and the clearness and simplicity of his style. His historical references are so accurate, and his clinical pictures so vivid and concise, that up to the present time they have not been excelled. In 1883 he supplemented this work by another classic, *"Zur Anatomie der Gesunden und Kranken Linse,*[1] the results of further histological and pathological investigation. These two great classics, which to the great majority of the English-speaking opthalmologists are as a sealed book, together with a most careful and critical review of all that has been published on this and kindred subjects since that time, form the basis of this work.

---

[1] Unter mitwirkung von Dr. J. R. DaGama Pinto und Dr. H. Schafer. Weisbaden, 1883.

GENERAL CONSIDERATION.

In taking up the study of the *Crystalline Lens System*, one can not properly consider the Crystalline Lens without at the same time studying its suspensory ligament, *The Zonula of Zinn (Ligamentum Suspensorium Lentis)*. By means of this ligament the lens is suspended, supported and retained in its proper relation to the remaining structures of the eye. The great importance of this system of fibrillae can only be fully realized after a careful study of its congenital malformations, its condition both in health and disease, and its physiological relation to the lens.

The Zonula of Zinn is the anatomical medium by means of which the ciliary muscle and the lens, which are not in direct contact, are brought together. Without a perfect and regular development of this structure, perfect power of accommodation can not exist. The proper centering of the lens in its relation to the cornea, likewise in how far the axis of the lens and the cornea coincide, will be dependent on the above fact. The visual axis is greatly influenced by the position of the lens in the eye.

The lens system is an integral portion of the so-called refracting media of the eye, and since the index of refraction of the aqueous humour in front of it, and the vitreous humour behind it, are both nearly equal to that of distilled water, and less than that of the lens; hence even in a physical sense, the Crystalline Lens is a lens.[1] It differs from the ordinary lens independent of any asymmetry of its surface in that, in the first place, it is not a homogeneous body, but consists of concentric lamellae which are most closely packed near the center, and in the second place has the ability of changing its form under influence of the ciliary body. As a result of contraction of this muscle, the lens becomes thicker, the radii of both its surfaces, and in all probability the equatorial diameter also becomes less. During this change the posterior pole keeps its position, whereas the anterior pole, as can be proven, nears the cornea. The power of accommodation is dependent on this ability of the lens to change its form.

Our more advanced methods of making a functional examination enable us to demonstrate changes of a histological nature, the senile included, even before they can be recognized by the microscope. This is fully considered in works on Accommodation and Refraction. In the interest of

---

1 Helmholtz's Physiological Optic, p. 63.

undisturbed function of the lens system, considering only the physical side of the subject, it is necessary that the index of refraction, and the elasticity of each individual fibre should remain unchanged, for as is demonstrated by even the slightest senile or other pathological change, they become matters of the very greatest importance, not equaled by like changes in any other tissue of the body. As regards their transparency, the elements of the lens, likewise those of the cornea, have following every pathological change a cloudiness, hence functional disturbances.

In order that the lens may perform its functions normally, it is necessary that it should be transparent, that its separate parts should be movable one upon the other; that each lamella should have a different index of refraction regularly increasing toward the center of the lens; that the surface of the lens should have an almost spherical curvature, and be almost centered in the corneal axis, and that the lens in its entirety be freely movable, and be in no pathological manner adherent to neighboring structures, more particularly the iris.

The lens is an epithelial structure. It consists of the ordinary epithelial cells, and so-called lens fibres, which are simply epithelial cells which have taken on an extraordinary development and become elongated. Externally the lens is covered by a structureless membrane, the lens capsule, which encloses it completely.

Notwithstanding its apparently simply construction, the study of its more minute structure, and the various processes which take place in the lens, has been connected with the very greatest difficulties. This was dependent not only on the proper recognition of the nature, and the function of the individual elements of the lens, but here more than in any other structure of the body was the difficulty encountered, of understanding the manner in which the individual lens fibres are laid down and connected with neighboring fibres. Only after the embryology of the lens had been studied, was a definite and clear idea of its architecture and histological structure understood. The proper understanding of the wonderful regularity in the arrangement, and the peculiar manner in which the fibres are adherent to each other, has only been attained by a study of the development and growth of the foetal lens. The importance of this knowledge will become apparent at once, when it is known that a departure from this regular development, even the slightest interference with this absolute connection between the individual fibres, is followed by an interference with the function of the lens as a transparent body which refracts the light in an absolutely regular manner.

Every departure from the normal is to be sought in an interference with the normal development of the lens, or in an anomalous growth, as the result of an abnormal nutrition, or conditions which persist in consequence of an interrupted physiological progression. Hence the study of the development, progression and growth of the human lens are not only of scientific interest, but are of the very greatest practical importance.

The study of the embryology will elucidate many of the seemingly difficult to understand malformations and anomalies of position and attachment, and aid us in fixing the most probable time of the development of certain congenital pathological conditions.

The lens being fully developed, we shall follow it through its period of physiological growth and retrogression, note the changes which the individual fibres, as well as the lens, as a whole, undergoes. Further, the mode of entrance and exit of the nutritive fluids into the lens. Lastly, consider the chemistry of the lens and its surrounding fluids. It has been hoped, and not without good cause, that the investigation of the mode of nutrition and chemistry of the lens, and the chemistry of its surrounding fluids, would throw some light on the aetiology of cataract—more especially the constitutional forms such as occur in Bright's Disease and Diabetes.

The pathological processes which play a part in the pathology of the lens are, on the one hand, those of proliferation and degeneration of its *intracapsular cells*; on the other, sclerosis, separation and softening of the *fibres of the lens,* together with all the secondary changes which follow these conditions. The lens may secondarily be affected either as a result of disease of other structures in the eye, or as the result of inequalities in the development of the Zonula of Zinn, or as the result of pathological conditions of the same.

As a result of these pathological changes the full functions of the lens are modified in the following manner:

1. The single lamellae gradually become changed into a homogeneous mass (*Senile Sclerosis*). The refracting power of the lens is reduced and the far point is removed from the eye, *Acquired Hypermetropia* (*H. Acquisita*).

2. The moveableness of the separate elements and lamellae against each other is gradually diminished and finally abolished, at the same time the ability of the lens, as a whole, to change its shape, becomes gradually reduced and finally abolished (*Senile Sclerosis*). The near point gradually becomes removed from the eye, and, as a consequence, the amplitude of accommodation more restricted, until finally there is an entire loss of accommodation (*Presbyopia*).

3. Though its form remains unchanged, the lens suffers in its trans-

parency. As a result, there is a general diminution in the ability to see accurately, until finally only a quantitative difference can be distinguished on throwing light into the eye. This condition is recognized as *cataract*, and is the most generally recognized pathological condition of the lens.

The various diseases and pathological conditions of the crystalline lens system, the causation and clinical description of the same, *the malformations associated with anomalies of the hyaloid artery or the vascular capsule of the lens*, those due to *unsymmetrical development of the Zonula fibres (Ectopia Lentis)*; likewise *the acquired anomalies of position not due to malformations; (Luxatio Lentis)* also the *independent malformations of the lens* will be successively taken up, all of which, as will be seen, excepting the congenital, and the traumatic, are the result of nutritive disturbances. *An altered chemical constitution of the nutritive supply is the initial step toward the formation of cataract.*

The formation of a nucleus is a perfectly physiological process, and no sharp line of demarcation, either histological or in point of development, exixst between the nucleus (*Nucleus Lentis*) and the cortex of the lens (*Substantia Corticalis*). An interference with the regular sclerosis of the nucleus has been said to be the initial cause of the development of senile cataract. *The chemically altered fluid which fills the interspaces between lamellae gives rise to an abnormal interchange between this chemically altered fluid and contents of the lens fibres. This in its turn leads to an altered condition of the cortex, the expression of which is an altered refractive condition and loss of transparency which we designate as cataract.*

These changes once having set in, it is apparent how useless all attempts at restitution by therapeutic measures must be.

The various methods of removing the interference with sight (cataract) will be successively discussed. It would be useless to consider in detail all the minute changes which the various operators have introduced; only such will be considered as have a general bearing on the subject, and which illustrate the fundamental principles on which the various methods are based.

In no department of surgery does the personal equation of the operator play so prominent a role as in the extraction of cataract. The eyeball being a globe, the moment it is incised the relative position of its various structures is changed, and the intraocular pressure is altered. Further, since the successful extraction of a cataract in and of itself, does not insure a successful restoration of sight, the study of all those processes which take place during the period of healing, and subsequent thereto, likewise are of the very greatest importance. Hence, a definite understanding of all these conditions is essential to the proper management of the individual case.

Finally the subject of aphakia will be considered.

THE NORMAL LENS SYSTEM.

PART I.

CHAPTER I.

THE DEVELOPMENT OF THE LENS.

"To-day all investigators agree that the first disposition to the formation of the lens consists in a thickening of the ectoderm. This original
group of cells undergoes an invagination; later on these cells are cut off and
a hollow vesicle is formed. *Kolliker* accepts this mode of development for
the cuttle fish. *Remak* and *Barkau* for the frog. *Huschke, Remak, Henle*
and *His* for the chick, and *Kessler* and *Kolliker* for mammals."

"His[1] accepts this involution of an open vesicle in the formation of
the lens in the human embryo, and so illustrates it. Kessler agrees with
him, having had the opportunity of examining a human embryo expelled
three weeks after the last menstruation, and with a loup he observed in
this the funnel shaped involution. Bambeke[2] states that in an embryo in
the fourth week, which he examined, he found the lens still connected with
the cuticular epiblast, by a short, thick, pedicle' which showed a funnel
shaped opening. Ritter[3] declares that in a five weeks embryo which he
examined, the pedicle had no lumen, and the lens seemed to contain a
small hollow space." *The first period of development of the lens is completed with the closure of this vesicle.*

The time when this occurs has been but partially determined. According to *Kolliker*,[4] in the chick the lens vesicle is cut off by the third day,
and this is in accordance with an illustration by Kessler of a hatching egg
of three days and seven hours. *Kolliker* (p. 634) observed in a rabbit a

---

1 Anatomie menschlicher Embryonem, Leipsig Bd. I mit Atlas. 1880. Bd. II,
1882, page 49, Bk. I.

2 Contribution a la historie du developpement de l'oeil humain. Gand, 1879.

3 Zweiter Beitrag zur Histogenese des Auges. p. 145.

4 Entwickelungsgeschichte des Menschen und hoheren thiere Leipsig, 1879,
p. 632.

thickening of the cuticular plate on the tenth day, and by the twelfth day the vesicle had already been cut off. *His* fixes the age of a human embryo 22 mm. in length, and in which the optic vesicle was not even recognizable at from twelve to fourteen days, the age of one 7-7.5 mm. in length at four weeks. He illustrates one 4 mm. in length in which there is a thickening of the Epiblast, even before the primary optic vesicle could be discerned. Surely from the above we could not be far from wrong in attributing to an embryo 4 mm. in length an age of about three weeks. This would bring . *the completion of the first period about in the FOURTH WEEK.* Bambeke and Kessler's observations quoted above agree with this, likewise with those of Kolliker. (P. 637). But, as Becker states, it is well to bear in mind the fact that the processes of development may go on more quickly in one individual than in another, hence exact statements as to the age of Human Embryoes can not be determined according to certain fixed laws.

During this period of development, the eye is devoid of the so-called "form-giving coverings," especially the cornea and sclera.[5]

THE SECOND PERIOD OF DEVELOPMENT OF THE LENS. In its further development, the cells at the proximal wall grow in a distal direction, in man is a saggital direction, pushing in between each other, so that on meridional section they appear to be arranged in rows. The cells in the centre grow more rapidly, hence are larger than those at the sides. Since the nuclei of all the fibre cells are found in the anterior fifth, they will form a convex zone which is almost parallel to the anterior wall of the Lens. Meanwhile, the cells at the anterior wall arrange themselves in a single layer, but show no signs of growing lengthwise. These distal cells assume the appearance of Epithelial cells.

Kessler gives the following description for the chick:—

"Even before the lens is cut off, signs of growth begin to manifest themselves, more especially in the median (proximal) portion of the lens germ, corresponding to the region of the subsequent capsule. Simultaneously, with a general increase in the enlargement of the organ, the cells arrange themselves closely together, and each individual cell increases in size and volume. They assume spindle shapes, and their sharp points force their way in between the neighboring lamellae. Meanwhile, the cells of the inner lamellae grow more rapidly backward, those at the sides more anteriorly, while those nearer the axis of the organ grow more rapidly than any of the others. Every individual cell reaches the posterior limit of the lens (the capsule of the lens), whereas

5 See Ritter, p. 82, p. 147.

anteriorly, to the distal cell wall, and thus the hollow space disappears up to a just appreciable space, which on cross section can be recognized only by its sharp contour."

"This gradual transition of distal into epithelial cells, and of the proximal into fibre cells, primarily occurs posterior to the Equator of the lens, but this process gradually extends more anteriorly until the Equator is reached. This takes place in various animals in a two-fold manner. Either the cells of the anterior wall become narrower and higher, assuming more the character of cylinder cells slanting somewhat backward and curving around those more anteriorly situated, so that the concavity of the curve faces forward, and thus gradually merging in the direction of the proximal fibres, or there are forced in between the distal epithelium and the proximal fibre cells, also between proximal fibres and the proximal wall, a circle of fibre like cells, of at first increasing and finally decreasing lengths, those posteriorly gradually merging with the proximal fibres, in a manner analagous to the previous method. This latter method is true of birds and several reptiles, the former of the remaining vertebrates, and especially does it apply to man. *THIS SECOND PERIOD IS COMPLETED* when both distal and proximal cells have arranged themselves in a single row, and the hollow space which had existed at the beginning of this period has been entirely obliterated by the growth of the proximal fibres."

Undoubtedly this same process which Kessler has described for the chick also occurs in man, and all the illustrations which Arnold has given us for the calf, and Kolliker of the rabbit, are of exactly the same character.

"Owing to pathological conditions in the human lens, which will later on demand our attention, a number of observations which Kessler made on the embryoes of the Lacerta and the sheep, must be here shortly mentioned. Whereas at one stage in the development of the lens in the chick, the nuclei of the proximal cells are arranged anteriorly in a regular convex zone, in the Lacerta they are irregularly arranged along the entire wall of the lens. The cells nearest to the equator, those most peripherically situated, are the first to become elongated, and in their growth make a semi-circular sweep, whereas those more centrally located in part assume a spindle form; others appear irregularly distended, and tumescent. In a number of sections of the lens of the sheep, Kessler did not observe, as in other sections of the lens of the same stage of development, the lens fibres growing lengthwise toward the distal surface; but he found a portion even of the longest fibres making very sharp curves towards the lower surface, and even here they seemed elongated and extending toward the dorso-proximal fibres. Kessler does not state whether this is to be looked upon as the first indication of the formation of seams. This observation is cited to demonstrate the fact that irregularities in the development of the lens have been observed during the second period of development."

, The proximal fibres have been observed to elongate in the embryo of a Triton 3.5 mm. in length and the hollow space entirely filled up in on? 4.5 mm. in length. In the chick, this stage is completed on the fourth day. (Kessler). This hollow space was found still present in the embryo of a calf 3 cm. in length, but entirely filled out in one 4 cm. long, hence the time required for this process to be completed is equal to that which an embryo requires to grow from 1.5 cm. to 4 cm. (Arnold Kwetzky). In the rabbit this process begins on the thirteenth day and is completed on the eighteenth day, possibly a little sooner. (Kolliker). The time has not been exactly determined for man, but undoubtedly takes place during the *second month of foetal life.*

THE THIRD PERIOD OF DEVELOPMENT OF THE LENS is principally occupied in the multiplication of the cellular elements, lens cells as well as lens fibres. The former increase by direct cell division, and are distributed over the entire distal wall; the latter by means of the growth of the epithelial cells, which lie along the Equator and somewhat behind it, into lens fibres. This successive transition of the equatorial epithelial cells into the outer layers of nucleated lens fibres can be demonstrated in all Vertebrates, and this alone is sufficient proof to demonstrate the fact, that these new lens fibres are derived from the Epithelial cells and further that in the growing lens, the identity of epithelial-like and fibre-like cells is to be maintained.

At the close of the second period of development, the lens has attained the form from which it takes its name, as the result of the growth of fibres in an axial direction, these assume a slight curvature with the concavity toward the edge of the lens, in contradistinction to those which, developing later on, do so meridionally. From now on, owing to the development of new fibres, at the Aequator, these embryonal fibres are gradually pushed away from the line of contact with the anterior epithelium, and the posterior wall of the capsule, (Henle), even at this time, the shortest; hence the youngest fibres continue to make a curve with the concavity outward. But as soon as they have made their way into the capillary space between the anterior ends of the distally growing embryonal fibres, and the distal epithelium, and posteriorly between the posterior ends of the embryonal fibres, and the posterior capsule, they take on a curvature with the concavity toward the axis of the lens. The more this condition progresses, the more the fibres of the second period are pushed away from the capsule and the epithelium, and finally they form the centre of the complete organ, which is concentrically surrounded by the fibres of the third period.

THE STRUCTURE OF THE LENS can only be understood, if we will bear in mind the fact, that all the fibres take their origin from the whorl located along the aequator, and that its growth is not a limited one. As far as is known, in the embryonal lens of no mammal does a full-grown fibre encompass one-half of the circumference of the lens. In most animals this is less than one-half.

The simplest structure is found in the globular lenses of some fishes, amphibia and reptiles, such as the "stock-fish," triton, salamander, frog and lizard. In these animals the fibres of each lamella go from pole to pole, each fibre encircles one-half of the lens, each two form a complete circle. Their arrangement presupposes that the fibres are broader at the Aequator and become more pointed toward the pole, so as to form a point; or, speaking more correctly, come together in a circle of irregular limits. This has been proven by H. Muller [6] to be the case in the Lacerta, and has been substantiated by Kessler, Leukart, Sernoff and Babuchin.

In a large proportion of fishes, amphibia and a few animals (delphin, rabbit, squirrel) the lens fibres of one sheath regularly meet each other anteriorly and posteriorly in a short seam (a segment of a circle) and the directions of these cut each other at right angles. If at the anterior pole, this line lies horizontally, at the posterior it lies vertically. At the same time it becomes impossible for the fibres to entirely surround one-half of the lens. For instance, if a fibre begins anteriorly at the end of the seam, it will end as it proceeds meridionally backward, posteriorly about the middle of the seam, hence in the axis of the lens at the posterior pole. In doing this, the fibres describe a curve anteriorly and one posteriorly in order to gain a point of attachment to the seam. Hence every fibre describes a double curve. The fibres of each layer, however, possess about the same length. In several fishes, such as torpedo, a sort of intermediate step be-tween these two types has been observed, all the fibres coming together at the posterior pole, whereas anteriorly they come together in a straight seam. In most mammalia the fibres of each sheath meet each other so as to form a regular three-rayed star figure, the central point of which lies at the pole and the rays of this star, corresponding to the seams, forming with each other angles of 120 degrees. The levels of these rays do not lie in the same plane anteriorly and posteriorly, but are turned from each other at an angle of 60 degrees, so that each ray of the anterior surface falls within the open angle of the posterior. Even in this form of arrangement,

6 Gesammelte und hinterlassene Schriften herausgeg, von Otto Becker. 1872. Bd. I, p. 74.

in order that the fibres may attach themselves to the seam or ray, they make two slight curves in opposite directions. However, all the fibres in one lamella are of equal length. We know absolutely nothing as to the cause of these various types. Woinow [7] has studied the manner of the manner of the formation of this seam for the second type, and the third type can be understood from Arnold's illustrations. Possibly, the above-quoted observations of Kessler concerning the lens of the sheep belongs to this category.

If after the close of the second period of development new fibres are only developed in the Aequatorial region, a stage comes on, in which these fibres force their way along the inner surface of the capsule toward the axis, without, however, reaching those which are making their way in from the opposite side. As a consequence, the fibres of the second period are detached from the capsule, pressed toward the centre of the lens, and these growing fibres come together behind them. Hence for a time, on meridional section, one will find a triangular space, filled with tissue fluid; this space, as a result of the continued growth of young fibres, becomes filled up by these, and in very thin sections can only be recognized as the line at which the fibres meet each other.[a]

It is especially interesting to note that Kolliker was able to show this three-rayed lens star present in a five months' human embryo. The presence of the three-rayed star, on the anterior and posterior surface of the lens, simply signifies that at least the first layers of lens fibres which have taken their origin along the Aequatorial region, have attained their full growth, the fibres of the one side anteriorly and posteriorly, touching those coming from the opposite direction.

Hence the third period of development lasts from about the middle of the second month up to such a time, which for man has not yet been exactly determined, but which, however, at the very latest falls within the first half of the period of foetal life.

At this time not all, but only those which form the first layers of lens fibres, have attained their full length. The fibres extending from aequator to seam, both on the anterior and posterior surfaces of the lens, are arranged

---

[7] Uber die enstehung der bipolaren anordung der linsen-fasern. Wiener Sitzungsberichte, 1869). Bd. LX, 2 Abth., p. 151.

[a] These observations have been beautifully illustrated by Arnold. (Beitrage zur entwickelungsgeschichte des Auges. Heidleberg, 1874. Die Kittsubstance der Endothelien. Virchow Arch. Bd. LXVI. p. 77.) His figures 13 and 14 correspond exactly with figures 3 of Woinow. Figure 15 shows a similar proceedure for the anterior half. In figures 18 and 19 the three-rayed star is already present.

like the tiles on a roof, so that the broad ends of the fibres form an uninterrupted mosaic at the inner surface of the posterior capsule and the anterior epithelium.

Only those fibres which are some distance removed from the surface reach to the seam. These seams or rays are therefore simply the optical expression of imaginary lines along which the ends of the lens fibres touch each other. And on meridional sections, they can be followed almost to the centre of the lens; never, however, along a straight line. The nearer we get to the centre, the smaller is the encompassed space. As a necessary result it follows, that though all the fibres in a single layer are of equal length, in the various layers from without inward, their length regularly diminishes. Each fibre is developed from an epithelial cell at the equatorial region. As the cell elongates, the nucleus, which was originally near the centre of the cell, gradually moves farther and farther away from the capsular end, until, finally, as the posterior end of the fibre grows to excess, the nucleus again comes to lie in the anterior third of the fibre. Hence, on meridional section the nuclei of all the fibres, in their various stages of growth, present a very beautiful picture, the optical expression of all the nuclei being a double curve, this being another mode of demonstrating the natural curve which the lens fibres describe. In the beginning, the concavity of the curve faces anteriorly, and finally the convexity is almost parallel with the surface of the lens. Since this curve is not an absolutely regular one, Becker [8] suggested that the name "Kernbogen" *NUCLEAR CURVE*, would be better than that adopted by H. Meyer, *KERN ZONE, NUCLEAR ZONE.* [9]

Kölliker was the first to recognize this gradual transition of the epithelial cells into lens fibres, and Von Becker [10] gave to the picture which these cells and their nuclei present on meridional section the name which it has since retained, "Linsenwirbel"—*Lenswhorl.*

THE DEVELOPMENT OF THE CAPSULE OF THE LENS has given rise to endless discussion, and the importance of this subject will become more apparent when the subject of capsular ciatrices and capsular cataract comes under consideration. One group of observers, *Remak,*

8 Uber den Wirbel und den Kernbogen in der Menschlichen Linse. Arch. f. Augenheilkunde, Bd. XII. 1, 1883.

9 Beitrag zu der Streitfrage uber die Entstehung der Linsen fasern. Muller's Arch., 1851, p. 202.

10 Untersuchungen uber den Bau der Linse bei den Menschen un den Wirbelthieren. Ach. fur Opth. IX, 1873.

Babuchin, Sernoff, Lieberkuhn and *Arnold*, contend that the capsule is of *Mesodermic* origin, the same from which the vascular covering of the lens is derived; the other group, more especially *Kessler*,[11] *Kolliker, Fr. Kriebel*[12] and *Rubatel*[13] look upon it as an excretive product of the cells of the lens vesicle, hence of *ECTODERMIC* origin. *Schirmer*,[14] as the result of his histological and more especially his chemical investigations of fresh capsules, capsular cicatrices and capsular cataracts, joined the adherents of the later view, namely, that they are not to be looked upon as of connective tissue origin. Availing himself of Ewald and Kuhne's discovery, that the capsule of the lens, as well as structureless membranes, are easily digested by means of trpsin, acids and alkaline solutions, whereas connective tissue remains totally undigested, he finally concluded "that there is a large preponderance of proof in favor of the view, that both the capsule and its pathological formations are derived from the same source, being products of the Epithelium of the Capsule."

Babuchin,[15] in examining Sernoff's preparations, claims to have seen nuclei in the capsule of the lens, in the embryo of a chick. Berger[16] states that he made similar observations in the human embryo. But Schirmer, basing his views on his histo-chemical investigations, logically questions the accuracy of their observations.

Kessler claims to have seen the capsule present at the close of the Second Period of Development, as does also Arnold. The latter, however, at the same time leaves the question undecided, as to how the formative cells, at the posterior capsule, which at that time have already become elongated into lens fibres, could produce an exudative substance to form the posterior capsule. Kessler tried in vain to prove that the capsule was formed simultaneously with the lens vesicle. Becker[17] took a position between the two, and states that he believes the structure of the capsule of the lens to be a complex one, and that it is only important to prove its presence at the beginning of the Third Period. "For without this closed

---

11 Zur Entwickelung des Auge der Wirbelthiere, Leipsig, 1877.

12 Zur Entwickellung des Glaskorpers. Arch. fur Anatomie and Physiologie. Ant. Abth., 5 and 6 Heft., 1886.

13 Recherches sur le developpement du cristallin. Geneve. 1885. Referate Hirschberg's Centralblatt. 1885. p. 255.

14 Histologische und Histochemische untersuchungen uber Kapselnarbe und Kapsel Cataract nebst bemerkungen uber das physiologische Wachsthum und die Structure der vodern Linsenkapsel Graefe Arch., Vol. XXXV. Bd. I. 1889.

15 Stricker's Handbuch der Gewebslehre. Leipsig. 1872. p. 10. 90.

16 Bemerkungen uber die Linsen Kapsel. Hirschberg's Centralblatt fur Prakt Angenheil. 1882.

17 Anatomie und Pathologie, etc., p. 24.

elastic mèmbrane, which holds the entire contents of the lens together and which offers the slight resistance to the young lens fibres which push their way in between the proximal fibres on the one hand, and the capsule and its epithelium on the other, one could not comprehend the regularity both in the form and arrangement of the lens fibres which we so much admire." Schirmer, however, contends that the capsule is developed at the time when the epithelium is still present along the posterior capsule, hence during the First Period of Development and at the same time, when as a result of the elongation of the proximal cells, their power to form capsular substance is not entirely lost. He even attributes to the young cells as they develop along the equator a similar power, though to a less degree. In a series of calf embryoes which he examined he found but a very slight difference in thickness between the anterior and posterior capsule, and states that the difference only becomes apparent later on, when the posterior remains thinner than the anterior. He asserts that the posterior lens fibres continue to produce capsular substance even in extra-uterine life. All the evidence at the present day indicates the *Cuticular (Ectodermic)* origin of the lens capsule, and that it begins to form with the very first period of development of the lens.

The question of the development of the Zonula of Zinn is even at the present day, a matter of doubt. The view, however, is generally accepted that it is derived from the Vitreous and of Mesodermic origin.

Julius Arnold,[18] reviewing all the literature on the subject, shows us that quite a diversity of opinions existed, and even at the present day they have not been entirely set aside. *One* set of observers, among them *Zinn*, (Desc. anat oculi humain), from whom this structure takes its name; *Maitre Jean* (Trait des maladies de Loeil), *St. Yres* (Trait des maladies de yeux), *Bonhomme*, (Cephalotomie), *Cassebohm*, (Method sec.), and *Petit* (Mem. St. Acad. 1726) contended that the zonula was derived from the limiting membrane of the vitreous, which at the orra serrata split up into two leaves which attached themselves to the anterior and posterior capsule of the lens. A second contingent, among them *Ferrein, Palluci* and *Salomon*, considered the zonula as a continuation of the retina. A third, among them *Rudolphi, Dollinger, Hesselbach* and *Weber*, considered the zonula as entirely independent formation.

Henle (Eingeweid lehre 1866) joined in the views of the first group with this difference, that though he looked upon the zonula as derived from the hyaloid, he considered the latter a continuation of the limitans interna retina. Lieber-kuhn (Uber das Auge der Wirbelthieren. Marburg

---

18 Graefe Saemisch Handbuch. Vol. I, p. 305, 1874.

1872), however, proved that the hyaloid had nothing to do with the retina, and that it is the limiting membrane of the vitreous, hence derived from the mesoderm. *Schwalbe* [19] coincides with Lieber-kuhn as to the origin of the zonula from the vitreous. He does not accept a splitting of the hyaloid at the orra serrata, but contends that a thickening takes place at the orra serrata, and that the entire membrane extends forward to form the anterior wall of Petit's Canal, the posterior wall being due to a thickening of the vitreous. A. Hannover [20] offered a still more complicated view, stating that after the splitting into two leaves, the anterior again split into two leaves, one extending over the ciliary body and its processes and then going over to the anterior surface of the lens, whereas the posterior of the first two together with the posterior of the original division should form a second canal posterior to Petit's Canal known as Hannover's Canal.

Arnold gives us the following explanation: "At an early period of foetal development, the lens is imbedded in a delicate tissue derived from the mesoderm, which is pushed in between the lens and the secondary ocular vesicle. This tissue gives off processes which, spreading around the lens, gain its anterior surface. Later this tissue goes to form the choroid, processus ciliare and the iris. That portion posterior to the lens forms the vitreous, the part anteriorly forms the membrano-capsulo-pupillaris. The portion along the equator forms the zonula. At a certain time no more intimate connection than this exists between vitreous and retina, or between zonula and the ciliary portion. Later on, a more intimate connection is established between zonula and ciliary body." He concludes that the limiting membrane of the vitreous, as also the portion from which later on the zonula is developed, are totally independent of the retina in their origin and that the zonula is simply a "peculiarly arranged and specialized part of the vitreous," originally solid in its construction and of mesodermic origin. This, he states, "does not preclude the possibility of softening or fluidity of the intercellular cement substance so as to permit the formation of fibrillae, as we see them in the posterior part of the zonula." Merkel (Die Zonula Ciliaris Leipsig, 1870) was the first to doubt the existence of Petit's Canal, and that the zonula was a continuous membrane. He looked upon this space as the result of the elements of the zonula.

Czermak [21] investigated this subject very carefully, and his views agree with those expressed by Gerlach, (Beitrag zur normalen anatomie des Auges.

[19] Graefe Saemisch Handbuch, Vol. I, p. 458.
[20] Entdeckung des Bau des Glaskorpers. Muller's Arch., 1845.
[21] Zur Zonula Frage-Graef Arch., Vol. XXXI, Bd. I. p. 74-134, 1885.

Leipsig, 1880), who believed that the zonula consisted of a system of meridionally placed fibres, which take their origin from the ciliary body and the orbicularis ciliaris, and that they are independent of the vitreous body, and he further denies the existence of Petits Canal. Later investigators, Schoen [22] and Topolanski,[23] agree almost *in toto* with Czermak. As the result of his investigations, Czermak states that in early foetal life, the space between ciliary body and lens is filled up by a large number of foetal cells, which arrange themselves in rows, leaving spaces between them. These cells elongate, forming fine threads or fibrillae arranged meridionally, hence the zonula is not a membranous structure, but a complicated system of fibres from the beginning. In a six and one-half month foetus he found the entire posterior chamber occupied by the zonula, and a condition present never seen in a fully developed eye, namely, pencils of these rays of fibrillae extending from the peripheric portion of the iris and the most anterior part of the ciliary body. Later on, as the result of rarefaction, these fibres are restricted to the posterior portion of the posterior chamber, and the pupillary membrane disappears at the same time. He looks upon the zonula as of *mesodermic* origin, derived from the portion of the embryonal vitreous which fills up the space destined to become the posterior chamber, and that this tissue is "modified both physically and chemically so as to serve its function."

Others again, as Abey [24] and Kuhnt and Berger,[25] return to the view that the zonula is a membrane, the fibrillae Berger considered as fibrillae which support the membrane.

Finally, E. Treacher Collins,[26] as the result of the examination of an eye, enucleated from an infant three months old under the supposition that it contained a new growth, and which was found to contain a persistent hyaloid and exhibited fibres of the suspensory ligament in all stages of their development, and the subsequent examination of several foetal eyes, formulated the following idea as to the development of the zonula.

"For a long time the primitive lens remains in contact at its sides with the portion of the secondary ocular vesicle destined subsequently to become

[22] Zonula und Grenzehaut des Glaskorpers. Graefe's Arch., Vol. XXXII, B. 2, p. 149, 1886.

[23] Uber den Bau der Zonula und Umgebung nebst bemerkungen uber das Albinotische Auge. Graefe's Arch., Vol. XXXVIII, B. 1, 1891.

[24] Der Canalis Petit und der Zonula Zinnii beim Mensch und bei Wirbelthieren. Graefe Arch., Vol. XXXVIII, B. I, 1882.

[25] Beitrag zur Anatomie der Zonula Zinnii Arch. fur Opth. XXVIII, B. II, 1882.

[26] On the development and abnormalities of the Zonula of Zinn. The Royal London Opth. Hospital Reports. Vol. XIII, Vol. I, p. 81.

the ciliary body. The lens becomes encircled by what is termed its fibro-vascular sheath, derived in part from the central artery of the vitreous and in part from the vessels growing in between the lens and the cornea. The portion of the inner layer of the secondary optic vesicle still in contact with the lens—that is, the pars ciliaris retinae—acquires adhesions to this sheath. Then, as the eyeball enlarges, it does so at a greater rate than the lens, so that a portion of the ciliary body which was in contact with the lens grows away from it and the adhesions which have formed between them become stretched, and the cells forming them much elongated, until only fibres with nuclei lying on them can be distinguished, and ultimately the nuclei go, leaving only the delicate fibres of the suspensory ligament as we see them in the adult eye."

As a result of the tension of these elongating fibres, the antero posterior diameter of the originally almost globular lens takes on its lenticular form. He also suggests that this mode of development may throw light on some of the congenital abnormalities.

Collins, however, raises the whole question again, when he states that he was unable to definitely determine whether the cells which form these fibres are derived from the fibro-vascular sheath of the lens, hence *mesoblastic*, or from the cells of the inner layer of the secondary optic vesicle which form the pars ciliaris retinae, hence Epiblastic, or n part form one or in part the connective tissue class, hence of mesoblastic origin.

CHAPTER II.

THE GROWTH OF THE LENS.

In contradistinction to its period of foetal development, the growth of the lens may be said to begin at the time when the first lamellae of lens fibres which take their origin at the Equator, completely surround the proximal fibres which, as we have seen, grow in an axial direction and form the original nucleus, *the lens body of the second period*, and press them away from the distal epithelium and the posterior capsule. From this time, up to birth, this production of fibres, which one after the other elongate to reach a seam, goes on. During this period, the lens is almost globular, but owing to the presence of many fibres which have not attained their full length, all of which cross the equator, the equatorial diameter must be somewhat greater than the axial. Since the human lens at birth shows the same star figure as does a five months' foetus, *the first period of growth extends from about the middle, to the close of foetal life.*

The Second or Extrauterine period of growth is essentially a continuation of the first period, with this difference, namely, a diametrically opposite process begins, which we will designate as one of *PHYSIOLOGICAL RETROGRESSION*. These diametrically opposite conditions divide the extra-uterine period into two great periods, one of extra-uterine growth, up to its complete development: the other, that of retrogression together with the changes incident to a reduction in volume.

How great the increase in volume is, may be judged by the following: The weight of a lens taken from a foetus in which the total ocular axis measured 15 mm. was 0.07 grammes, (Becker), whereas, at birth, in an eye having an ocular axis of 17 mm. the lens weighed 0.10 grammes, (Becker), and Sappey estimates the average weight of an adult lens at 0.218 grm. This increase in volume is accompanied by a very natural increase in the equatorial diameter of from 5 mm. to 10 mm., whereas the saggital diameter, the axis of the lens according to Sappey, remains almost unchanged, 4 to 4.5 mm. The lens of the human foetus and of the new-born child is almost globular, whereas in an adult the surface has a much sharper curvature.

In the following table the absolute weight agrees exactly with the statements of Sappey. Weight and volume (with but one exception) increase steadily with age. The specific gravity varies slightly from the average. The extremes, however, bear no close relationship to the age.

Some slight doubt is cast on the accuracy of these results, because the lenses had been in Muller's fluid for various periods, some for several years; and further, because the number of examinations is not large enough. All the lenses were obtained post mortem.

No.	Age.	Absolute Weight. Gr.	Volume. Cu. Ctm.	Specific Gravity.
1	Foetus.	0.070	. . . . .	. . . . .
2	At Birth.	0.10	. . . . .	. . . . .
3	20 yrs.	0.18	0.155	1.16129
4	20 "	0.185	0.159	1.16352
5	22 "	0.215	0.177	1.13158
6	40 "	0.190	0.153	1.24248
7	49 "	0.225	0.194	1.15979
8	49 "	0 240	0.198	1.21212
9	54 "	0.245	0.214	1.14486
10	54 "	0.245	0.214	1.14486
11	60 "	0.251	0.217	1.15668
	Average . . .	0.219	0.198	1.16946

Priesthey Smith[1] has verified all Becker's statements, at the same

---

[1] Oph. Society, 1883, p. 79, reprinted in his monograph, "The Pathology and Treatment of Glaucoma," 1891.

time avoiding his sources of error, since all the eyes which he used were removed one hour after death, and at once immersed in vitreous fluid, in order to prevent gain or loss in bulk. He states (Page 84), "156 eyes were removed from dead subjects in nearly equal numbers, to the six decades of life between 20 and 80 years, and a smaller number between 80 and 90. Each lens was accurately weighed, and then measured as to its volume by means of a special apparatus devised for the purpose. In most cases the linear dimensions were measured. The specific gravity was calculated in each case from weight and volume. The crystalline lens, so long as it is healthy, increases in weight and volume throughout the whole of life. During the 40 years, between 25th and 65th year, it adds about one-third to its weight, one-third to its volume, and one-tenth to its diameter. The specific gravity seems to vary little in the individual cases, but shows no decided changes with the advance of life. (Page 89.) In many text-books the dimensions of the Crystalline Lens are incorrectly stated. Thus in Graefe's Saemisch Handbuch, Vol. I, p. 43-45, the antero-posterior diameter of the lens is given as 3.7 mm. This is too small, even for a young adult, and for the middle and advanced adult life it is much too small in elderly people. I have found the lens measuring 6 to even 6.5 mm. in diameter."

PAGE 174. AVERAGES.

AGE IN YRS.	A WEIGHT IN MGR.	B VOLUME IN CUB. MM.	C SPEC. GRAV.	D DIAMETER.
20–29	174	168	1067	8.67
30–39	192	177	1085	8.96
40–49	204	188	1085	9.09
50–59	221	205	1078	9.44
60–69	240	225	1067	9.49
70–79	(245)	(227)	(1079)	9.64
80–89	(266)	(244)	(1090)	9.62

NOTE.—Above the age of 69, the number of transparent lenses examined was much smaller than in the earlier decades. The averages are given in brackets, and must be taken as less certain than those belonging to the earlier periods.

Bernhard Dub.[2] examined a series of lenses ranging from the ninth month up to twelve years. All his measurements were made with a Zeiss millimeter scale under the microscope. As will be seen from the table, though the equatorial diameter is not exactly proportionate to the age, it shows, nevertheless, that the lens increases in size as age advances.

2 Beitrag zur Kenntniss der Cataracta Zonularis. Graef Arch.,Vol. XXXVII, Vol. 4, 1891.

No.	Age.	Length of Body.	Equatorial Diameter. mm.				Sagittal Diameter. mm.			
			Size.	Maxim.	Min.	Average.	Size.	Maxim.	Min.	Average.
1	10 mths.	52	6.8	. . .	. . .	. . .	2.2	. . .	. . .	. . .
2	11 "	50	8.0	8.0	6.8	7.46	2.4	2.8	2.2	2.46
3	11 "	60	7.6	. . .	. . .	. . .	2.8	. . .	. . .	. . .
4	12 "	62	7.8	. . .	. . .	. . .	2.6	. . .	. . .	. . .
5	12 "	66	6.9	. . .	. . .	. . .	2.5	. . .	. . .	. . .
6	13 "	62	7.6	. . .	. . .	. . .	2.5	. . .	. . .	. . .
7	13 "	74	8.0	. . .	. . .	. . .	2.6	. . .	. . .	. . .
8	1¼ yrs.	84	8 0	. . .	. . .	. . .	2.9	. . .	. . .	. . .
9	1¼ "	64	8.1	. . .	. . .	. . .	2.6	. . .	. . .	. . .
10	1¼ "	62	8.0	. . .	. . .	. . .	2.8	. . .	. . .	. . .
11	1½ "	82	8.0	. . .	. . .	. . .	2.6	. . .	. . .	. . .
12	1½ "	70	8.1	. . .	. . .	. . .	2.5	. . .	. . .	. . .
13	1½ "	65	8.3	8.3	6.9	7.87	2.6	2.9	2.2	2.57
14	1½ "	64	7.5	. . .	. . .	. . .	2.2	. . .	. . .	. . .
15	1½ "	68	8.0	. . .	. . .	. . .	2.4	. . .	. . .	. . .
16	1½ "	74	8.2	. . .	. . .	. . .	2.6	. . .	. . .	. . .
17	1½ "	76	7.4	. . .	. . .	. . .	2.6	. . .	. . .	. . .
18	1½ "	74	7.8	. . .	. . .	. . .	2.5	. . .	. . .	. . .
19	1¾ "	62	7.8	. . .	. . .	. . .	2.8	. . .	. . .	. . .
20	1¾ "	72	8.1	. . .	. . .	. . .	2.6	. . .	. . .	. . .
21	1¾ "	71	8.1	. . .	. . .	. . .	2.6	. . .	. . .	. . .
22	1¾ "	66	7.9	. . .	. . .	. . .	2 4	. . .	. . .	. . .
23	2 "	76	8.2	. . .	. . .	. . .	2.6	. . .	. . .	. . .
24	2 "	82	8.4	. . .	. . .	. . .	2.5	. . .	. . .	. . .
25	2 "	78	7.9	8.4	7.9	8.2	2.8	3.0	2.5	2.72
26	2¼ "	68	8.3	. . .	. . .	. . .	3.0	. . .	. . .	. . .
27	3 "	70	8.6	. . .	. . .	. . .	2.8	. . .	. . .	. . .
28	3½ "	86	8.6	8.6	8.2	8.46	2.9	2.9	2.8	2.83
29	3½ "	80	8.2	. . .	. . .	. . .	2.8	. . .	. . .	. . .
30	4 "	84	7.8	. . .	. . .	. . .	3.1	. . .	. . .	. . .
31	5½ "	100	8.4	. . .	. . .	. . .	3.2	. . .	. . .	. . .
32	7 "	85	8.2	. . .	. . .	. . .	2.9	. . .	. . .	. . .
33	12 "	129	8.8	. . .	. . .	. . .	3.4	. . .	. . .	. . .

Finally, Treacher Collins [3] examined a series of foetal eyes from the fourth to the ninth month. This table also shows that the axial or transverse diameter of the lens, which at the fourth month is only a little more than the antero-posterior, in the adult is nearly three times as much. Also, that in adult life the antero-posterior diameter is somewhat less than in foetal life.

	Age.	No. of Eyes Examined.	Diameter of Eyeball.			Diameter of Lens.	
			Antero Posterior.	Lateral.	Vertical.	Antero Posterior.	Equatorial or Transverse.
Foetal Life.	4 mths.	3	8.1 mm.	7.8 mm.	7 5 mm.	2.8 mm.	3.3 mm.
	5 "	1	11.75 "	11.5 "	10.5 "	3.5 "	4. "
	6 "	4	12.50 "	12.0 "	11.1 "	3.8 "	4.5 "
	7 "	8	14.30 "	13.2 "	12.6 "	4. "	5. "
	9 "	3	16.75 "	16. "	15.8 "	4.8 "	5.55 "
	Adult.	Merkel.	24.3 "	23.6 "	23.4 "	3.7 "	9.00 "

Thus, if we arrange a table from the foregoing, showing the growth of the equatorial and axial diameter of the lens from the early period of

[3] Abnormalities of the Zonula of Zinn. The Royal London Opth. Hospital Reports, Vol. XIII, p. 86, 1893.

foetal life up to the extreme age, it at once becomes evident how extremely rapid the growth of the lens is in intrauterine life, as compared with the extrauterine. Further, that in earliest life the lens is almost globular, but as life advances becomes flatter.

			EQUATORIAL DIAMETER.	ANTERO POSTERIOR DIAMETER.
COLLINS.	FOETAL LIFE.	4th month,	3.8 mm.	2.8 mm.
		5th "	4.0 "	3.5 "
		6th "	4.5 "	3 8 "
		7th "	5.0 "	4.1 "
		9th "	5.7 "	4.2 "
DUB.	AFTER BIRTH.	9th to 12th "	7.46 "	2 46 "
		1 to 2 years,	7.87 "	2.57 "
		2 to 3 "	8.2 "	2.72 "
		3 to 4 "	8.46 "	2.83 "
		4 to 5 "	7.8 "	3.1 "
		5 to 6 "	8.4 "	3.2 "
		7 "	8.2 "	2.9 "
		12 "	8.8 "	3.6 "
PRIESTLY SMITH.	AFTER BIRTH.	20 to 29 "	8.67 "	
		30 to 39 "	8.90 "	
		40 to 49 "	9.09 "	
		50 to 59 "	9.44 "	
		60 to 69 "	9.49 "	
		70 to 79 "	9.64 "	
		80 to 89 "	9.62 "	

The following average measurements for the lens in the new born are quoted in a recent publication by E. V. Hippel (Uber das Auge des Neugeborenen. Graef Arch.. Vol. XLV, Part II, p. 293, 1898):

	ANTERO POSTERIOR.	EQUATORIAL DIAMETER.
V. Yager,	4.5142	6.8528
Huschke,	5.18	6.76
Sommering,	4.2864	5.188
Krause,	4.512–4.737	6.768—7.219
Merkel & Orr,	5.0	9.6. For both Ant. and Post. Surface. Radius of Curv-
Dieckman,	5.1	6.29 [ature, 3.3 mm.
Treacher Collins,	4 3	5.75
E. V. Hippel,	{ 3.76 { 4.00	6.00. (Two absolutely fresh Eyes.) 6.5

As we have seen on page 23, the tri-star figure is accepted as the type at birth, with the star on the posterior surface of the lens turned at 60 degrees to the one on the anterior surface. But in its further development after birth, a more complicated figure is formed by the formation of secondary rays. Near the pole, each primary ray divides into two rays forming equal angles of 60 degrees, or each ray divides into three rays, thus forming equal angles of 40 degrees, or four rays, forming angles of 30 degrees. But, as Becker states, (Anatomie, p. 27), "This does not exhaust the variety of types," and he further (p. 28) draws attention to the fact, that the star figure on the anterior and posterior surfaces are not of the same type, hence all the fibres in a lamella are not of equal length, as we found them where there is the single tri-star. He claims to have seen the only case (in a girl twenty years of age) in which the type on the anterior and posterior surface was the same. According to Kolliker,[4] in these complicated star figures, it becomes more difficult to understand the arrangement of the fibres, since the fibres, as they attach themselves to the seam, are bowed in opposite directions, so that their arrangement reminds one of a feather, at times forming a perfect vortex ("*vortices lentis*"). Thus it happens that the peripheral fibres of the fully formed lens only lie for a short distance in a single plane.

Dr. Percy Friedenberg,[5] as the result of his investigations, (with Zehender-Westien corneal loup; also with lenses removed from the eye and treated with Nitrate of Silver, 1:500 or 1:100), claims that these schematic figures have no basis in fact, that he has found four, five, six and seven pointed primary rays, and secondary rays could be counted up to almost any limit of visibility, making the total of rays twenty or more. The figure at the pole is rarely that of a true star, as the angles between the adjacent rays are usually unequal; besides this, the rays do not issue from the pole or from a point which corresponds to it approximately, but usually start from a sutural line running through the pole. In most cases this line is vertical, but not at all infrequently oblique. The number of rays in the various quadrants is not the same, being greatest in the upper, next in the lower, then the temporal quadrant, the nasal always being the least. He found in mammals that the lens star corresponds to that of man.

The function of the Eye, or, more properly speaking, the influence of light on the eye, begins at birth. This is not exactly true of several isolated cases of mammals, as the rabbit and the marsupia. At this time the anterior segment of the eye finds itself in contact with a different medium. As long as the external surface of the cornea is in contact with the Amniotic fluid, there is scarcely an anterior chamber. This is only formed after the corneal epithelium is covered by a capillary film, whereas the endothelial layer continues after, as before, to border on the increasing quantity of the Aqueous. This is in accordance with the fact, that in animals which live in the water, especially in fishes, there is scarcely an anterior chamber.[6]

---

[4] Handbuch der Gewebslehre, 1867, p. 693.

[5] Then Lens-star figure in Man and the Vertebrates. Archives of Ophthalmology, April, 1895.

[6] Leukart R. Organologie des Auges. Graef Saemisch. Bd. II, p. 145, 1876, p. 259.

"In many of these animals the lens touches the Cornea, so that the anterior chamber is practically reduced to a narrow space restricted to the periphery. In these cases the Cornea is very flat. Water, Cornea and Aqueous have the same index of refraction." Hence in animals which live exclusively in the water, we find that the refraction of light is mainly dependent on the lens, in contradistinction to animals which live in the air. And in accordance with this fact, the lens is found to be almost globular. Here, then, conditions purpose, effect and result mutually equalize each other. In the new-born infant ocular inspection is often sufficient to demonstrate that there is scarcely an anterior chamber. Owing to the gradual accumulation of the aqueous, the lens is not only pressed backward, but its general contour is changed. This increased filling out of the anterior chamber has likewise a lateral extension, especially toward the less resistant posterior chamber. By this means the Zonula is drawn tense, and the lens is compressed in a saggital direction.[7] From now on, contraction of the Ciliary Muscle causes relaxation of the Zonula, and as a result the lens returns to its more globular form, as it existed during foetal life.

At birth the lens assumes various changes in its shape, dependent on accommodative effort. These changes can not be entirely set aside, even in foetal life, since aside from the changes in the "Electrical Conditions" of the Oculo-Motorius, which must be followed by contraction of the Ciliary Muscle, the converging movements of the eyes are associated with accommodative efforts, even in utero. Though, as far as we know, accommodative efforts do not take place during the first few days or even weeks of extra-uterine life, nevertheless the action of light on the retina must lead to a contraction of the ciliary muscle.

As regards the length of lens fibres, there appears to be a very material difference between this and the foregoing period of growth. In all that has previously been said; in the foetal lens, all the individual fibres of each concentric lamella were of equal length. In each succeeding lamella the individual fibres must be longer than in the preceding, if the rays of the lens star increase in length and each fibre occupies relatively the same position, as its corresponding fibre in the layer beneath. This gradual increase in length extends to the close of the first period of growth, as long as the simple tri-star figure continues. Robinsky[8] has beautifully described this condition. He estimates that a fibre which starts exactly at the pole anteriorly, attaches itself posteriorly exactly at a point where the anterior

---

[7] For a different explanation see Collin's Theory, p. 30.

[8] Untersuchungen zur Kentniss der Laage und Anordnung der Augen linsenfasren. Centrab. f. d. med. Wiss, 1882, No. 27.

and middle third of the corresponding radius meet. The succeeding fibres on the anterior surface are all successively removed one fibre's breadth from the pole, and on the posterior surface along the corresponding radius, all the fibres reach one fibre's breadth successively nearer to the pole, so that finally the fibre which finds its point of attachment on the anterior surface at the junction of the anterior and middle third extends posteriorly to the pole." According to Robinski, a fibre taken from the most external lamella of the lens of a new-born infant measures 5.5 mm. Measurements of the lens fibres of adults, as compared with the increase in the size of the equatorial diameter of the lens, did not show a relative increase in size, and, aside from this, they varied greatly (2.74''' to 4.06''') 7.17 to 10.64 mm. Hence the fibres are neither of equal length, nor can they reach from one pole to the junction of the outer and middle third of the corresponding radius of the opposite side. Direct observation has shown that they end in the outer third of the corresponding radius. The length of the fibres vary in each lamella, and this variation is all the greater, the more complicated the star figure.

If one will make a sketch of both the anterior and posterior surface of the adult lens, showing the lens star, one will see that if the number of rays is the same on both surfaces, all the fibres will be of equal length, just as in foetal life. But if this complicated type is different on the two sides, as a necessity the fibres must vary greatly in length. Since, with the single exception mentioned above, this latter type is the one always met with, the fibres of a single lamella in a human lens, and which develop in extrauterine life, will not only be shorter, as compared to the portion of the lens which they encompass, but they will no longer possess an equal length as compared with each other, as they did in foetal life. This inequality in the length of the lens fibres is to be looked upon as the cause of the great increase in the radii which go to make up the star figure and the production of the variety of types seen on both surfaces.

In lieu of a more plausible explanation of this unequal growth of the lens fibres in extra-uterine life, one might be permitted to seek it, in the functional activity of the lens, and in its uninterrupted formation.

The position of the nuclei of these fibres is dependent on the above described irregularities in the length and the laying down of the new-formed lens fibres. In embryonal lenses, even in the new-born, the Nuclear Zone of nuclei form a convex curve on section. This is not the case in older lenses. Von Becker[9] drew attention to the fact, that at first the fibres

[9] Untersuchungen uber den Bau der Linse bei den Menschen und den Wirbelthieren. Arch. f. Opth., Bd. IX, 1873, p. 10.

grow only at their anterior extremity, as one is justified in concluding from the position of the nuclei, soon, however, the posterior extremity also grows. Thus it happens that in the beginning the nuclei form a limited, and later on, a somewhat broader curve, which is open anteriorly and which then merges into the larger anteriorly convex curve. According to Von Becker, from now on, the growth of both ends of the fibre is almost equal. Since the proportion of each fibre which is on the anterior and posterior surface is dependent on the arrangement of the radii, or, more properly speaking, on the part which each separate fibre plays in the formation of these radii, therefore their nuclei must also occupy a variety of positions, depending on the above circumstances. Though the general law, that the nuclei are always found in the posterior portion of the anterior half of the fibres, is almost universally accepted, on section the curve formed by all the nuclei which form the Meyer's nuclear zone will always be found in the outer portion and with the concavity of the curve turned toward the anterior surface of the lens. Whether this curve will in certain portions of the lens extend anteriorly, or more toward the centre, or even backward, will depend on the variety and even the condition of the rays of the lens star. Von Becker very properly concludes, that one should not picture to one's self this nuclear zone as though it passed through the equatorial plane of the lens, as though it were a diaphragm, but rather as though it were a sheet attached at the periphery and which extended through the substance of the lens, in a wavy manner and equidistant from the radii of the lens star. If we can thus explain certain departures in the position of the nuclei, as we find them in very thin sections, aside from these, we do meet with well-preserved nuclei in the deeper layers, dispersed in the most irregular manner. This rule, therefore, has its exceptions.

In very thin sections of the lens one may observe still other abnormalities. Henle (Zur Anatomie der Krystallinæ Gottingen, 1878) has pointed out one which is of great importance, namely, that the lamellae do not increase regularly in thickness, as we go from without inward. Such a condition indicates that the growth of the lens is not a perfectly regular and continuous one, but that it is influenced by the same fluctuations in the general nutrition of the body, as are other organs, as per example, the skin, the hair, more especially the nails, on which, subsequent to a long-continued fever, one can observe a line of demarcation. There can hardly exist a doubt but that during the time in which a child is well nourished, the lens fibres grow rapidly, become broader and more succulent; whereas, in anaemic children, the growth is interfered with or possibly totally arrested. Such an irregular interference with the growth of the lens fibres will manifest itself by the irregular manner in which the nuclei of the youngest fibres follow one another. At times they follow each other in a regular curve, then again their curve is interrupted by one or more nuclei lying far removed from it.

A host of the older observers have stated, that in the lens star is to be found a partially homogenous, partly finely granular substance which separates the fibres as they come to meet each other from opposite sides. Bowman (Lectures on the Eye, London, 1849) described in lenses depending on their construction, one, two, three or more tri-stars with their points directed toward the centre. He considered these non-fibrous planes "central planes." Kolilker (p. 711) found but little of this substance where the lenses had been hardened in chromic acid and the fibres were well-preserved. Babuchin and Sernoff assert that the fibres are in direct contact (p. 1086, Babuchin. Die Linse). Von Becker set up the hypothesis that these central planes were in direct connection with a system of inter-fibrillar spaces, which he supposed had some bearing on the accommodative act. Otto Becker agrees with Babuchin and Sernoff, but denies the existence of these "central planes" and inter-fibrillary spaces. These spaces are lenticular in shape and filled with a finely granular substance. Their exact nature is not quite clear, but Otto Becker suggests that they "are due to irregularities in the exact coaption of the one lamella over the other." Hence these spaces are partly congenital and are to be looked upon as having been present during life. It is possible that these interspaces stand in some causative relation to some forms of congenital punctate Cataracts or to acquired Cataracts which first manifest themselves as punctate.

THE MANNER IN WHICH THE LENS FIBRES ADHERE TO THE EPITHELIUM AND TO THE POSTERIOR CAPSULE. Just as we found that there is nothing other than the so-called ordinary tissue fluid of the body occupying the spaces between the ends of the fibres as they come together to form the lens star, so, likewise, this same fluid exists between the fibres laterally and between the successive layers; likewise it is found between the anterior capsule and the epithlium and between the fibres and the inner surface of the posterior capsule. Nevertheless, at all the above-mentioned situations we find a demonstratable amount of organic material, which during life is fluid or soft and which after death in the hardened state may, or may not be demonstratable by the use of various methods of staining. This substance is the source of those prettily arranged shallow depressions seen on the inner surface of the posterior capsule of the lens, which have been so frequently the subject of discussion. Henle looked upon them as due to coagulated albumen. (Anatomie, p. 680). In his Pathologie and Therapie, page 165, Becker expresses himself that "these ledges are hyaline deposits due to the coagulation of albuminous fluid which becomes changed into these Morgagni's globules. Seen on the flat, they look very much like the cells of a honeycomb, but they are not regularly six-sided, and show differences in size. This coagulation may occur during life as well as after death." But at that time he had the erroneous idea that the ends of the fibres could not cause similar pictures. (P. 166). Deutschman [10] expressed himself that there is constantly a sub-capsular layer of albuminous fluid present between capsule and lens substance. Finally, Henle so modified his original statement as to admit a connection between the protruding ledges and the narrow splits which are bounded by the blunt edges of the fibres. He says, "They divide the inner surface of the posterior capsule into veritable fields, the dimensions of which equal the diameters of the fibres." Kolliker gives the same explanation in his microscopical Anatomy, Vol. II., page 707. It is more than likely that these ledges become permanent after death, the albuminous tissue fluid coagulating as a result of the cooling off of the body, or they are possibly artificially produced when the eye is placed in the hardening fluid. This appears to be all the more probable since these structures are found more frequently and to a greater extent at the posterior capsules of young animals in which the posterior capsule is still in direct contact with the ends of the fibres.

Although Becker acknowledges the correctness of this view for a certain proportion of cases, he does not consider the matter as definitely settled. He says, "I am still of the opinion that the coagulation of the so-called Morgagni's globules is the cause of the impressions and the formation of these ledges. These depressions are always nearly circular, and at times some of them are still found occupied by these Morgagni's globules. These globules vary greatly in size. In some specimens they are very large, and one can observe how they are just beginning to loosen up. Finally, I have never observed both formations in the same preparation. To a degree they seem to exclude each other, the former being observed more especially in the fresh eyes of the young, the latter being exclusively found in cadaveric eyes. This is explained by the fact, that in eyes in which this Morgagni's fluid accumulates between lens and capsule, the lens fibres are no longer in contact with the inner surface of the capsule, and hence can no longer give rise to these depressions. In the cadaver the albuminous fluid which accumulates between the epithelium and the lens, the occur-

10 Zur regeneration des Humour Aqueous. Arch. Opth., Bd. XXVI, p. 121 and p. 99.

rence of which has given rise to the false teaching that this is to be looked upon as Humour Morgagni, also leaves behind it, when it coagulates, depressions of an analogous character on the inner surface of the Epithelium. These figures are often mistaken for Wedl's Vesicular Cells."

THE FORMATION OF NEW LENS FIBRES. As has already been indicated, on page 22, the lamellae of the lens are developed by the formation of new lens fibres along the equator. As these new fibres develop, they gradually press those already formed away from the surface.

As long ago as 1851, Herman Meyer,[11] in order to uphold this view, drew attention to the changes which the nuclei of the fibres undergo as they gradually become removed from the surface, and he considered this as an indication of the gradual death of the nuclei. An incidental utterance of H. Muller [12] makes it probable that he also believed that the new fibres are found at the whorl. Kolliker (p. 731) believed that cellular division took place along the Equator, thus constantly replacing the cells which had been changed into fibres, and Von Becker claimed that he observed this cellular division going on along the same line. Frey [13] even mentions nuclear division in the lens fibres of an eight months' human foetus. Whereas, Sernoff, Iwanoff and Arnold did not observe these karyokinetic figures, Henle attempted to explain the assertions of Kolliker and Von Becker, who claim to have seen conglomerations of small cells along the epithelial border, by demonstrating that this appearance of a number of layers of small cells was due simply to the close packing of the cells which had become elongated into fibres, and the swellings at the points where the nuclei lay, were located at various heights so that the fibres could accommodate their positions to each other. To this general description, Becker adds, "that in the calf embryo, as in young pigs, he found a broad zone, in which the nuclei were smaller, closer together, almost touching each other, and taking the analine and haemotoxylin stains with avidity. The nuclei which in the center of the anterior capsule of the ox are perfectly round and have a diameter of 0.0047 mm., whereas the cells themselves have an average diameter of 0.0067 mm., at the Equator have a diameter of 0.0025 mm., with a diameter of cell equal to 0.0029 mm. At the same time the nuceli increase in height from 0.0047 to 0.009 mm., and the cells elongate from 0.0067 to 0.0174 mm. One can easily understand that such a change in shape will be very apparent where the long axis of the nucleus is exactly

11 Beitrag zur der Streit frage uber die Entstehung der Linsen-fasern. Muller's Arch., 1851, p. 202.

12 Gesamelte und Hinter lassene Schriften herausgegeben von Otto Becker, 1872, Bd. I.

13 Handbuch der Histologie und Histochemi, 2 Auf., p. 287.

perpendicular to the surface of the capsule. From all that has been said, it seems to be highly probable, that these peculiar pictures stand in close relation to the nuclear and cellular increase, and that the large cells are to be looked upon as "mother cells." Becker also coincides with Henle's views, namely, that there are no so-called *Formative Cells* (Von Becker) along the Equatorial Zone.

When Henle (Zur Anatomie der Krystallinse, 1878) published his Monograph, he left the question as to how the new fibres are formed on the surface of the capsule, an open one, but since that time, he has published some successful studies which have elucidated this subject. In a thesis styled "Zur Entwickelungsgeschichte der Krystallinse und zur Theilung des Zellkerns,[14] he recites his observations on the larvae of Frogs and Tritons, in which he found cells interspersed between those at rest, and often at a considerable distance from the place at which the cells become elongated into fibres undergoing karyokinetic changes. He states: "In the lenses of these animals, as in all other globular lenses, the epithelium extends beyond the Equator on to the posterior surface. Along the Equator the cells still have their polygonal shape, as on the anterior surface; then follow a number of rows of elliptical, almost quadrilateral, cells; next to these, as long as the lens continues to grow, rows of longer cells, which run parallel to the fibres, and so arranged as to lap over each other, like the tiles on a roof. In the polygonal cells, which lie near the region of the equator, one observes these karyokinetic changes going on. At times these changes are noted singly, then in numbers; but I could not find that their number stood in any relation to the age of the larvae. Neither are the cells nearest the Equator always the ones in which the changes are farthest advanced. One finds cells undergoing division dispersed everywhere, and it is absolutely impossible to state, what it is in the individual case, which gives the initiative to these changes." Henle finally states that he never observed these changes in a fully developed frog (without a tail and with feet). It was not until after "indirect nuclear division" had been fully proven by Strassburger for the plant cell, by Fleming for the animal cell, by Arnold for pathological cells, that the subject of how the cells of the lens capsule increase, both in the normal and pathological conditions, could be definitely settled. It was then shown that these nuclear changes are pretty evenly distributed over the entire surface of the capsule. They are, however, only demonstrable when the specimen is hardened in Fleming's Solution.

There were two possibilities as to where these karyokinetic changes take place; either, as Muller thought, they occur near the Equator along

14 Arch. fur Mikr. Anat., Bd. XX, p. 418.

the lens whorl, or the increase takes place all over the anterior capsule, thus gradually forcing all the epithelial cells toward the Equator. Henle and Becker believed in this latter mode of increase. Henle says: "Just as according to Ebert, the posterior epithelium (?) of the cornea grows over the surface, not as the result of the addition of cells at the edges, but by the interposition of new cells over the entire surface, as the result of karyokinesis, the cells push themselves in between the old ones."

The observations of Eberth and Leber are of especial interest, owing to the great importance which this subject of the movements of the epithelial cells across the surface of the capsule bears to a proper explanation and understanding of the pathological processes. (Capsular Cataract, etc.) Eberth [15] has shown that where there is regeneration of the corneal epithelium, this proliferation is not confined to the edge of the defect, but occurs at a considerable distance from this spot, and in cells interspersed between those at rest. Leber [16] has shown that during the healing of capsular wounds the karyokinetic figures develop in a zone which is at a considerable distance from the defect. Between small cells, with small nuclei, others are found which are considerably larger and clearer, showing all the various stages of karyokinesis. In the embryoes of calves and children, Becker found these karyokinetic figures all over the capsule, without a special activity being noticeable in any particular zone. Such an increase of cells presumes that these new cells force their way in between those already formed; the latter are compelled to change their position, and in a centrifugal direction, that is, from the pole towards the Equator. Thus it has been shown by direct observation that the cells multiply over the growing capsule, and that they change their position over the surface of the capsule, and it is also very probable that the entire epithelium in turn replaces those cells which are changed into lens fibres.

THE CAPSULE OF THE LENS.—It is generally conceded that the capsule of the lens grows during extra-uterine life. According to Ritter,[17] in the new born, the capsule of the lens at the anterior pole measures 0.012 mm. in the thickness, whereas in the adult it measures 0.016 mm., at the equator, 0.005 to 0.007 mm., and at the posterior pole, 0.0075 to 0.008. As has already been indicated on page 26, to Schirmer (reference on page 26), who proved that the capsule of the lens is an excretory product of the epithelium of the lens, are we indebted for the most

---

15 Uber Kern und Zelltheilung. Virchow's Arch., LXVII, p. 523-525.

16 Zur pathologie der linse Zehenders Klin Monats blatt. beilag heft, p. 33, 1878.

17 Anat. du cristallin—Wecker Traite des Maladies des yeux, 2d Ed. II, p. 3.

modern and generally accepted views regarding this structure. In the course of his investigations on Capsular Cicatrices, Schirmer observed that the new formed vitreous lamella behind the cicatrix increased in thickness with the age of the capsule, and to a degree equal to that of the surrounding true capsule. At the same time the everted edges of the ruptured capsule appeared continuously to decrease in thickness. This, he concluded, must be a physiological process.

In order to gain more accurate data as to the rapidity of both this increase in thickness, and the diminution in thickness of the outer lamellae, he measured all the cicatrices produced in his experiments on animals, also the new lamellae. He estimates Julia Sinclair's (Experimentelle Untersuchungen zur Genese der erworbenen Kapsel cataract. Inaug. Diss Zurich, 1876) measurements as undoubtedly too large. The anterior capsule equals 0.022—0.030; whereas his own measurement of normal capsules of small rabbits at anterior pole equal 0.0075 —0.009 mm., and in a large rabbit 6½ years old, equals 0.018 mm. In the following table the relative thickness of capsules is taken as one, and though some slight errors may exist, the general results can not be entirely ignored. They show that the thickness of the new lamellae steadily increases with the age of the cicatrix, whereas the old lamellae steadily grows thinner. Further, the increase is greater in the beginning than later on, and similarly, the old lamellae diminish more rapidly in the beginning than later on.

AGE OF THE CICATRIX.	ENTIRE CAPSULE.	ABSOLUTE THICKNESS.		RELATIVE THICKNESS.	
		LAMELLAE.		LAMELLAR.	
		OLD.	NEW.	OLD.	NEW.
		Punctured with a Discision Needle.		Punctured with a Discision Needle.	
4 weeks.	0.028	0.026 mm.	0.002 mm.	0.93 mm.	0.07 mm.
9 "	0.0094	0.0177 "	0.0017 "	0.82 "	0.18 "
		Punctured with a Knife.		Punctured with a Knife.	
10 "	0.0188	0.0155 mm.	0.0033 mm.	0.82 mm.	0.18 mm.
4½ months.	0.012	0.009 "	0.002 "	0.75 "	0.25 "
6 "	0.0094	0.0064 "	0.003 "	0.69 "	0.32 "
7½ "	0.0113	0.0066 "	0.0047 "	0.59 "	0.41 "
8½ "	0.0197	0.0117 "	0.008 "	0.60 "	0.40 "
10½ "	0.013	0.0065 "	0.0065 "	0.50 "	0.50 "
3 years.	0.0345	0.0075 "	0.030 "	0.20 "	0.80 "
8 "	0.043	0.008 "	0.035 "	0.19 "	0.81 "

Schirmer says: "Either the anterior surface of the capsule undergoes a steady resorption, or it undergoes a steady shrinkage; hence, every capsular lamella which is excreted within a certain length of time, in its turn, with advancing age, becomes thinner." The first supposition requires that within a certain period of time, a certain quantity of capsular substance should be restored, and in a continuous and regular manner, until finally it in turn entirely disappears; but this can not be proven. The theory of shrinkage has in its favor the fact that in the beginning this is greater than later on, and also that the new is produced more rapidly at the beginning, always presupposing that the energy of the epithelium to produce capsular substance remains the same."

Changes in the physical properties accompany the above changes, as evidenced by the edges of the injured capsule rolling up outwardly. Even where free movement is guaranteed by suspension in an indifferent fluid, the same eversion takes place. This same fact was proven where fine sections of fresh capsule, obtained by the freezing microtome, were exposed to the digestive process. In both alkaline and acid solutions the capsule invariably turned up outwardly, and it was impossible to be mistaken, the epithelium being an accurate guide. During this process of digestion, he observed (under high powers of the microscope) exceedingly fine and closely arranged striations, running parallel to the surface, in the beginning confined to the innermost portion of the capsule. Gradually minute interspaces began to develop in the inner lamella, due to separation of the minute lamellae, and this process gradually extended more anteriorly. After a time these interspaces grew so coarse as to give the impression of a veritable network, and thus slowly the inner layers were digested before the outer were affected by the digestive power of the trpysin. Similar pictures were obtained by placing the capsule in nitric acid, and then heating wth permanganate of potash or lime water. This also will explain the figures which Robinski [18] observed on surface preparations treated with nitric acd, and which he described as "L'Capsule Corpuscles," and as analogous to those found in the cornea.

E. Berger [19] demonstrated the lamellar construction of the lens capsule before this time by a different method. He satisfied himself by "teasing" the capsule, and by maceration in permanganate of potash, that the torn edges are not like straight lines, but zig-zag or step-like. He observed that we must distinguish at least three lamellae, although many sections led him to believe that there were more. Schirmer states that he got his best results after macerating for several days in a one-tenth per cent. solution, or in a ten per cent. NaCl solution. He succeeded in this way in demonstrating at least five lamellae, and does not coincide with Berger's view that the outer lamella is a zonular lamella. He says: "Certainly the zonular fibres are only attached to the outer lamella, since they can be followed for

18 Untersuchungen uber die Augen linsenkapsel. Berliner Klin. Wochenschrift, 1886, Bd. No. 12, p. 71.

19 Bemerkungen uber die Linsen Kapsel Hirschberg's Centralblatt fur Prak. Augenh., 1882. Beitrage zur Anatomie der Zonula Zinni. Graefe Arch., 1882, Vol. XXVIII. Alth. 2. p. 28.

a certain distance into the substance of the capsule; but this is not a reason for looking upon it as something essentially different from the other lamellae, and it does not seem justifiable to attribute to it a different structure. Even Becker [20] states that "he never succeeded in determining by a striation the exact point at which the the zonula fibres are inserted into the capsule." "Hence, if we must abandon this view, the other two lamellae can demand no further consideration as preformed structures." Schirmer looks upon the maceration experiments as pointing to the same conclusions as the digestive experiments; namely, "that these delicate lines indicate a previous solution of continuity, or that the epithelium, as the result of some external influence, has suffered a serious interference in its excretory power, of which these lines are an expression, and that these lines move more anteriorly the longer the time since the injury. Disturbances, as per example a wound, the formation of a capsular cataract or a widespread degeneration of the epithelium in consequence of a contusion, lead to an irregularity in the disposition of the excretory substance, the optical expression of which, on cross section, is fine lines. The older a lamella of capsular substance becomes, the more these irregularities sink in the background, and the entire capsular substance forms a compact mass, and it is only after long reaction by the above method that these striations are disclosed. This explanation excludes the assumption of a chemically different lamellar cement substance."

Schirmer does not attempt to give the causes for these irregularities in the life of the epithelium, but suggests that it is a continuous process, repeating itself innumerable times, like the alteration of day and night, or sleeping and waking. He says he has observed not less than seventy-five lines in the inner fifth.

The capsule also has the property of elasticity. Even Becker drew attention to this, in cases of luxated lenses, stating "where the equatorial diameter of the lens is reduced, no folds appear." As the lens grows, the capsule, which originally encompassed a smaller space, increases in size by expansion, and adapts itself to a greater surface. Even after the lens has attained its full size, the individual capsular lamellae as they are pushed forward expand, since the outer surface of the capsule is greater than the inner. This curling up outwardly of the capsule is an expression of difference in the elasticity of the various lamellae.

The chemical conditions of the posterior capsule are similar to those of the anterior.

Schirmer reports an interesting case, in which a piece of the anterior capsule

---

20 Anatomie, p. 43.

was extracted three years before the examination. In this lens he found a wound of the posterior capsule, which the conditions present led him to believe was an old one, dating back to the time of the operation. Here he found no sign of new formed posterior capsule, nor had cicatricial tissue formed, there being no epithelium covering posteriorly.

At the present day the *Zonula of Zinn* is generally conceded to consist of a system of meridianally placed fibres, which take their origin in the vitreous lamellae, which cover the pars ciliaris, the ciliary body and its processes, as far forward as to where these latter go over to form the root of the iris. The fibres are made up of innumerable, very fine and exceedingly delicate fibrillae, which are interlaced in the most complex manner, and it is this intricate structure which forms the suspensory ligament of the lens. It is no longer looked upon as a membranous formation, consisting of two plates enclosing "Petit's Canal;" hence, this latter has lost its identity, and is now looked upon as a part of the posterior chamber. Henle [21] believed that these fibres were held together by a cement substance, which could not be demonstrated after death. But as Czermak has so aptly remarked, the interspaces between the fibres are everywhere much wider than the thickness of the fibres, and further, no sign of a membrane has ever been observed under the microscope; therefore, he considers this a network and not a membrane. Secondly, if the fibres were held together by a cement substance, does it not seem strange that it should disappear so completely, especially since cement substances everywhere else in the body are acted upon entirely different by hardening fluids; as, per example, the neuralgia which becomes hardened?

Czermak (page 28) has done more to elucidate this subject than any other investigator.[22] He describes the origin and insertion, in substance, as follows: "The delicate fibrillae take their origin in the vitreous lamellae, and run together like pencils of rays to form coarser fibres; these in their turn form bands, and in their course, as they proceed toward the capsule of the lens, they give off to and take up fibrillae from neighboring bands, so that the bands do not grow smaller. The points of origin and insertion vary. They begin to develop posteriorly about 1.5 mm. from the orra serrata, and as they proceed forward they form acute angles, the convexity of the course facing anteriorly; but before the fibres reach the ciliary body they begin to split up again, some of the fibrillae inserting themselves again into the vitreous lamellae of the orbiculus ciliaris; others proceed onward, insert themselves into the vitreous lamellae covering the ciliary body; others

21 Handbuch der Anatomie, 1866.
22 Zur Zonula frage Graefe Arch., Vol. XXXI, B. I, 1885.

again go to the ciliary processes, while the majority pass onward to the capsule of the lens. At the same time fibrillae originate along all these respective parts, each in its turn sending out fibrillae to neighboring parts and to the main bands, which are on their way to the capsule of the lens. This explains why it is that on meridianal section one sees fibres crossing in all directions. He has divided these fibrillae into three groups:"

First. Those which spring from the orbiculus ciliaris and from the ciliary body and extend to the anterior and posterior capsule of the lens, the *Orbiculo and Cilio Capsular Fibres.*"

"*Second.* Those fibres which spring from the orbicularis ciliaris and again become inserted more anteriorly; others again which insert themselves into ciliary processes, the *Orbiculo Ciliary Fibres.*"

"*Third.* Those which spring from the interspaces between the ciliary processes on their way to join others, and those which extend from one ciliary process to another, the *Inter and Intra Ciliary Fibres.*"

Hence, each of the coarser fibres contain fine processes from each of the other varieties, more especially of the first two, whereas the former give off the fibrillae to neighboring bundles. Thus a most intricate and perfect network is formed. As the fibres approach the lens, they again split up into the very finest fibrillae, which are gradually lost as they become merged in the outer lamellae of the capsule. A partial crossing of fibres takes place, some of the most anteriorly situated giving off fibrillae which go to the posterior surface of the lens, and vice versa. The fibres have peculiar sharp contours, are smooth, and appear like hyaline or glass threads."

Not alone do these fibres form a suspensory ligament, by means of which the lens is supported in its proper position and relation to neighboring parts, but owing to its peculiar construction, it exerts an equal degree of tension in all directions. This network of fibres is the intermediate member which permits of the proper increase or reduction of tension during the act of accommodation.

CHAPTER III.

THE PHYSIOLOGICAL RETROGRESSION OF THE LENS AND ITS ELEMENTS.

The phenomena and changes which take place during the physiological retrogression of the lens, are not restricted to any special period. Strictly speaking, they begin as early as the third period of foetal life, and undoubtedly can be demonstrated as soon as physiological growth begins. They take place in the cells as well as in the fibres. They are subject to the same

laws, as are the epithelial cells of the skin and mucous membranes, which
likewise, in intrauterine life, lose their nuclei, are cast off and are found
in the vernix caseosa and amniotic fluid. In the lens, however, since the
capsule is a closed sac, the cells are not cast off, but quite the contrary, the
young growing fibres press the older ones toward the center. There they
are subjected to various physical and chemical changes, which lead to the
formation of a nucleus and the cortex.

As soon as the intelligence of the child is sufficiently developed to
permit of making the proper experiments, it can be shown that there is a
gradual decrease in the accommodation, which is a functional proof, that
a process of hardening is going on in the center of the lens, which influences the power of the lens.

These changes in the lens are of a chemical, physical and morphological nature.

The MORPHOLOGICAL changes have been the subject of the most
exhaustive studies, and have been most beautifully described in the so
often quoted monograph of Henle. His examinations have been made
amongst all the various classes of vertebrates. In reptiles and birds and
most fishes he found that the fibres gradually diminish in width. In other
classes he found that the width of the fibres gradually diminish from without inward, but this process does not proceed as regularly as in birds; and
aside from this there is frequently a reduction in the number of fibres, owing to the gradual merging together of entire rows. In his observations
on the lenses of man and many animals, Henle observed [1] that the fibres
could be divided into three groups. "Whereas, as a rule, the fibres diminished in size towards the center, there is pushed in between an outer and
an inner layer of prismatic fibres, a layer of ribbon-like cells, so that at some
distance from the periphery, the thickness of the fibres is considerably and
rapidly reduced, and then again as they approach the center again increased." Henle looks upon this as a constant condition found in the lens
of man, and states that "it is not the result of an irregular growth, but
due to subsequent alteration in the full grown fibres." But he gives no
reason for such a regular condition. Not only the width and thickness of
the fibres diminish, but the edges appear serrated. If we were to peel off
layer after layer of an adult lens, until it were reduced to foetal size, one
would expect to find all the fibres resembling those which are on the surface
of a foetal lens; this, however, is not the case. Even in the foetal lens one
meets with the same successive changes as observed in the mature lens.

According to Henle, these serrated edges fit into those of neighboring

[1] Zur Anatomie der Krystalline, p. 39. Gottingen, 1878.

cells and these serve to hold the individual layers together. He supposes that these serrations are outgrowths from the fibres. Becker suggests that this is rather an evidence of the death of the cell corresponding to similar changes in the cells of the Rete Malphighi of the skin and in the corneal epithelium, in which the younger cells rarely or never show any signs of serration. This seems to indicate that these serrations are due to shrinkage. It has been proven that as we proceed towards the centre, the cells diminish both in width and in thickness, hence what would appear more natural than that these serrated edges are the result of shrinkage of the fibres.

DEATH OF THE NUCLEI OF THE LENS FIBRES. As has already been stated, as the cells elongate along the equator, the nuclei also gradually change their shape from the circular to the eliptical. They become longer and flatter, so that it does not become necessary to assume an increase in the volume of the nuclei. The form and size remains about the same in all grown fibres. They all show the karyokinetic changes when preserved in the proper fluids. As we proceed towards the centre, the structures begin to fail. The chromatic substance runs together into one or more clumps, until finally it entirely disappears. Until the fibre has attained its full length the nucleus retains its life-like appearance. *But as soon as a fibre extends from one radius of the star figure to another, the nucleus begins to show signs of death.* This can be observed in the lens of the new-born infant, and is true of every period of life.

THE PHYSICAL CHANGES which the individual fibres undergo with increasing age, consist of an increasing hardness and yellowish color, and an increasing index of refraction. The hardness becomes manifest by the resistance offered to pressure when a specimen is under the cover glass. The yellow color becomes evident when a number of lamellae are superimposed one upon the other. All these changes are due to the giving up of water, leading to greater dryness and friability of the inner layers, partly however, also as a result of chemical conditions of the older fibres.

That there is a chemical difference between the inner and the outer portions of the lens seems to be attested by a fact which, though known for a long time and frequently discussed, has been variously accounted for; namely, that in the lenses of all vertebrates and young animals which during life have been perfectly transparent, immediately after death, as soon as the animal becomes cold, the inner portion of the lens becomes cloudy. Michel [2] drew attention to the fact and showed that the cloudiness in the

---

2 "Uber naturliche und kunstliche Linsentrubungen?" Festschrift zur Feier des 300 Yahrigen Bestehen der Julius Maximilius Universitate zur Wurzburg, 1882.

centre of the lens of cats, pigs, and calves would disappear again if they were warmed up to 15 to 20 degrees C. This could be repeated as often as desired, and each time the lens would clear up again. This cloudiness is produced by the presence of innumerable roundish, highly refracting droplets in the central portions of the lens, and is not in any way connected with the decomposition of the contents of the lens, such as is produced by freezing (*l. c.*, p. 62). In these experiments there can not arise any question as to the separation of the water from the albumin. These droplets become less numerous as we go from within outward. Treated with alcohol and ether, their number becomes less, and they are reduced in size. Hence it appears that they must consist of a fatty substance, which has a very low melting point, though it is impossible to state anything more definite at this time. The interest which the appearance of these bodies at a low temperature arouses is due less to their presence than to the fact that they occur in the inner lamallae of the lens, that their number varies in different species of animals, and that their deposit ceases a few months after birth. From this it follows that in the chemical formation of the lens, especially in the older layers of the same, very pronounced changes take place. Since, according to Kuhne and Laptschinsky, the amount of fat is greater in the old than in the young, hence it can not be due to a quantitive but rather to a *qualitative change.*

Various authorities have drawn attention to the fact, that these described changes in the lens keep pace with the physical and morphological changes which take place from the center toward periphery. Some of the peculiarities of the peripheric lamellae are in accord with this. From year to year the nuclei in the nuclear zone become less numerous; the nuclear zone comes less near to the axis, its curvature grows less; in other words, the number of smooth, non-changed lens fibres which reach to the lens star, grows less year after year.

In the capsular epithelium the changes due to the age are less marked. Innumerable measurements have shown that the diameter of the base of the epithelial cells remains almost the same during life, at least as long as they retain their shape. Not so, however, with the height of the cells. Beginning at a point corresponding to the pole, the base of the cell gradually grows less, whereas at the beginning of the whorl the cell is about three times as high as it is wide. In course of time the height of the cell at the pole, as well as along the equatorial region, gradually diminishes, and sections taken from very old people show the height of the cell to be that of the nucleus, whereas the protoplasm between the nuclei is shrunken to an almost immeasurable thickness. In some sections some of the nuclei are found wanting and some cells are entirely wanting. Nothing could be more wonderful than the regularity with which the perfectly circular, 0.005 mm. in diameter nuclei are found in the epithelium dispersed over the capsule of young lenses.

Examinations of unstained specimens show beautifully the nuclear figures at rest; whereas stained with Haemotoxylin and Eosin, these figures show less distinctly; with Alum Carmin they are somewhat more distinct. The outlines of the cells are likewise more distinct in the unstained sections. The protoplasmic bodies touch and limit each other, as most exact hexagonal figures. In some exceptional cases the contours of the cell bodies take the stain as do the nuclei, reminding one of Arnold's "indigo-carmin ledges." When the staining is done rapidly with a concentrated Haemotoxylin solution, some of the nuclei take on a darker, more pronounced stain than others. These always are a measureable trifle longer than the paler nuclei, or they show a tendency to form star figures. Frequently the nuclei, in the vicinity of one of these darker cells, form a circle around it, or the dark nucleus appears as the head of a spiral which is formed on succeeding 10-15 nuclei. As a result of this arrangement the surface of the capsule covered with the epithelium assumes a perfectly regular, almost life-like appearance. It is more than probable that these nuclei, which take the stain more deeply, were just about to undergo nuclear division at the time the sections were placed in Muller's fluid.

As we approach the equator the nuclei grow smaller, are packed closer together, take the stain more deeply than the surface preparations. In older individuals nearing the fortieth year, the picture changes, in so far that the deeply stained cells grow less in number, as do also these peculiar circles and spiral figures. From now on the distinctly stained nuclei and cells grow less and less, but never entirely disappear. In extreme old age it often happens that on pieces of capsule the epithelium is found wanting for certain distances; here undoubtedly either the epithelium remained adherent to the lens or dropped off during the manipulations incident to staining, dehydrating, etc. Where capsules hardened in Muller's fluid are shaken in water, whole sections of capsular epithelium may be detached, and here frequently the capsule shows the impressions where the cells were adherent. This is due probably to the cement substance of the epithelial cells. Deutschman's subcapular layer, which has remained adherent to the capsule.

Again, here and there, cells are found wanting or changed into Vesicular Cells. At times they form veritable nests. It is remarkable how little coloring matter is taken up by the nuclei of the cells and by the capsule, irrespective of age. Nevertheless, the nuclei take up the stain in a more regular manner than do these distended cells. If these latter are to be looked upon as dying or dead cells, then we must accept a second variety of death of the nucleus. In other sections, at times one finds large numbers of nuclei just about to die, just as noted in the lens fibres. Again, one notes cells of the capsular epithelium which are still perfect in contour, showing nuclei greatly reduced in volume, and which take the stain deeply, as noted in fibres in which the nuclei are just about to disappear.

CHAPTER IV.

THE PHYSIOLOGY OF THE LENS SYSTEM.

THE MANNER OF ITS NOURISHMENT IN HEALTH AND DISEASE.

THE DIRECTION AND COURSE OF THE NUTRITIVE STREAM IN THE LENS. The lens is enclosed in a structureless membrane, which under normal conditions, is not permeable to formed elements. Until near the close of embryonal life, a vascular membrane is closely applied to this structureless capsule. Beyond a doubt, the vessels of this membrane serve, during the developmental period, to supply the nutritive material to this hyperplasia and increasing growth of the cells and the fibres within this capsule. After the degeneration of this vascular capsule, we are confronted by the peculiar condition, namely, that the lens is only indirectly, by means of the zonula fibres, held in connection with the firm portions of the eye. And, further, since the zonula fibres contain neither nerves, blood vessels nor lymph-channels, the lens must receive its nutritive supply either from the aqueous or vitreous, possibly from both. These media likewise possess neither nerves nor blood vessels. It is just possible that the iris stands in relation to this interchange of fluids, since the pupillary edge is merely separated from the anterior capsule by a capillary layer of fluid.

Such being the conditions, the question to be determined was, along which lines does the nutritive fluid gain entrance to the lens? In his Pathologie and Therapie, p. 257, Becker expressed his belief that "the nutritive stream gained entrance in the equatorial region, between the two leaves of the zonula, because probably along this line, under normal circumstances, the new formation of cells and positively the growth of fibres "progressed most actively." Deutschman [1] investigated this subject more closely. He gave a rabbit one grm. of pot. iodide in solution and three hours later killed the rabbit. The lens, enclosed in its capsule, was placed in a palladium-chloride solution and was proven to be impregnated with the pot. iodide and most intensely along the sub-capsular albuminous layer of the posterior capsule, as well as along its entire equator, to a less degree

---

[1] Cataracts Senilis, 1879. Graefe Arch., Bd. XXV, 2, p. 212.

the sub-capsular layer under the anterior capsule, but disclosed no sign of impregnation in the nucleus or anterior corticalis. Here should be incidentally mentioned that he [2] also observed that if he opened the lymph sac in salt-water frogs and in this lymph sac placed crystals of chlor natrium, the cataract which resulted was due to the extraction of water. Hence Deutschman considered it as very probable that the nutritive stream entered along Petit's Canal. Ulrich [3] arrived at the same conclusion as the result of the following experiments. He injected ferro-cyanide of potash sub-cutaneously and subsequently placed the eyes in a solution of chloride of iron alcohol. He states: "The line along which the ferro-cyanide of potash gained entrance to the lens could only be detected by the stain along the line of the equator; the posterior capsule of the lens remained unstained. The experiments which *Schoeler* and *Uhthoff* made according to Ehrlich's methods [4] by using fluorescin, led them to even a more advanced conclusion, stating, "Under physiological conditions (by sub-cutaneous injection) the fluid reached the equator of the lens, exclusively through Petit's Canal. Never, however, does the fluid go directly through the vitreous to the lens. Further, the colored fluid which has once been taken up by the lens is never given off again through the vitreous."

Samelsohn came to a positive opinion as to the line along which the interchange of tissue fluids occurs, by observing the changes which took place in three lenses, in each of which a minute spicule of iron had become impacted in the lens. In all of these he observed that the particles of rust always changed their position in the same manner. In summing up his conclusions, he states,[5] "It appears that the principal direction of fluids is directed from behind forward and on reaching Petit's Canal becomes 'dammed up' (Ulrich) along this line; it also gains entrance to the lens along the line of the equator. From here on it traverses the entire lens centripetally and comes together again at the anterior pole; from here it again goes out centrifugally toward the insertion of the Zonula fibres, where it leaves the lens and enters the posterior chamber."

Along the line where the nutritive fluid is supposed to leave the lens,' Samelsohn assumes the presence of special pores in the capsule, which offer

---

[2] Deutschman—Untersuchungen zur Pathogenese der Cataract. Arch. f. Ophtbal., Bd. XXIII, p. 117.

[3] Uber die Ernahrung des Auges Graefe's Arch., Bd. XXVI, 3, p. 33-82.

[4] Das Fluorescin in seiner Bedeutung fur den Flussigkeitswechsel des Auges. Yahresber der Scholerischen Augen Klinik, 1881.

[5] Zur Flussig-keitsstromung in der Linse. Zehenders Monatsbl., Bd. XIX, p. 282.

the least possible hindrance to the escape of the used fluid which, however, are not sufficiently wide to permit the passage of formed elements. The pores are the same as those which Morano [6] believes he saw, but which no one else up to the present time has seen.

Uhlrich's ("Stauungs theorie") "damming back" theory,[7] on which Samelsohn bases his statements, reads as follows: "The most intense blue color of the vitreous (and in fact the most intense in the entire globe which can be attained by the use of sub-cutaneous injections of ferrocyanide of potash) develops in the region of the equator of the lens. The filtration of tissue fluid out of the vitreous proceeds from the vitreous border into Petit's Canal and on reaching its anterior wall it again meets with a detaining filter, the free portion of the Zonula of Zinn, which likewise shows a blue discoloration. As a natural result of the placing of two parallel filters in the region of the equator of the lens, there must naturally follow a damming back of the streams of fluid. This detention is more favorable to the nutrition of the lens, since it takes place at the equator, where the space is very limited, and, further, since the iris, which will receive further consideration later on, acts as a third parallel filter." Without going any further into Uhlrich's views concerning the individuality of the posterior chamber as compared with the anterior, and his views concerning the passage of fluid through the iris from behind, forward, it is nevertheless proper to refer to the investigations of Deutschman,[8] in which he states "that in a certain sense, or under certain conditions, the iris acts as a protective organ to the periphery of the anterior surface of the lens."

In all that has so far been stated, attention has only been drawn to those experiments in which coloring matter was given the animal, either per os or subcutaneously. Only these seem to possess demonstratable proof. But this is not the only reason [9] why Knies' investigations have not been cited before this. In his critical studies relative to the Nutrition of the Eye [10] he arrives at anatomical conclusions, with which Becker does not agree. Knies states (page 340*): A form of cataract which begins in the Equator shows to us as a necessity that there is an affectation of a portion of the Uveal tract, which is situated anteriorly to the Orra Serrata and posterior to the anterior lamellae of the Zonula of Zinn, namely, of the pars ciliaris choroideae and the processes ciliares,

---

6 Interno agli atomi dell end othalio della capsula del cristallino Atti dell assoclar. Ottal Ital Rianione di Napoli, Settembre, 1879, p. 61.

7 Uber die Ernabrung des Auges. Graefe's Arch., Bd. XXVI, 3, p. 41.

8 Die Veranderungen der Linse in Eiterproceesen im Auge. Arch. f. Opth., Bd. XXVI, 1, p. 144.

9 Becker says, page 92.

10 Arch. F. Augenheil-kunde, Bd. VII, p. 320.

This is true of the ordinary senile cataract, and at the bottom of page 341 he says: "Let us consider the lens and ciliary processes as far as the nutrition physiologically is concerned as a single organ, etc." These ciliary processes, however, are external and anterior to the Zonula Zinii, and the latter is between the ciliary processes and the equator of the lens, which even Knies concedes to be the line of entrance for the nutritive stream of the lens. The ciliary processes form the secretory organ for the aqueous humor, and, as it appears, have nothing whatever to do with the nutrition of the lens, or at most only secondarily.

Becker, in his essay on the nuclear zone of the lens, drew attention to a heretofore not mentioned condition of the lens capsule of youthful individuals, which he tries to bring in connection with the entrance of nutritive fluid. He states: "The capsule is materially thickened at a particular point which lies posterior to the Equator." I have formerly observed a similar thickening of the capsule in secondary cataracts, which I also attributed to this swelling, and which I have attempted to bring in connection with the rapid increase in the size of the cells during the formation of the Crystalline Pearl. This would seem to indicate that the abnormal conditions which had resulted from an operation had caused an especially active nutritive stream to pass through the capsule, and thus cause the capsule to swell up. It is possible that analogous changes could occur in uninjured, rapidly-growing lenses, but as to whether this change takes place during life must remain an unanswered question. Assuming this to be a post mortem swelling, occurring after the specimen has been placed in hardening fluid, this observation would not be without interest, since one is justified in concluding that a different condition existed in the capsule at this point, even during life. "This point of thickening," he states with great certainty, "is posterior to the posterior limit of Petit's canal." How long after birth this peculiarity of the capsule of the lens persists, and whether it is in any way connected with the retrogressive formations of the vascular capsules of the lens, I can not state, owing to lack of available material. It was still perceptible in the capsule of a seven-weeks' old child.

Even in fully developed cataracts one may demonstrate the existence of a nutritive stream. This was proven long ago by the beautiful experiments of Bence Jones [11]. In a number of experiments on animals to whom a large variety of substances were given via the digestive tract and by subcutaneous injection, at a later date he demonstrated beyond a doubt their presence in the lens. Likewise, in a number of experiments on human beings and animals, which were given carbonate of lithia, in a few minutes this could be found in every part of the body, but it required thirty to thirty-two minutes before it appeared in the lens. Cataract patients to

---

11 Proceedings of the Royal Institute of Great Britain. Vol. IV, Part VI, No. 42, October.

whom 20 grammes of lithia was given in water, and who were later operated on by Bowman and Critchett, the lithia was found in every part of the lens, when the extraction was done two and a half to three hours after the ingestion of the lithia water. After four days lithia was still found in all parts of the lens; after five days it began gradually to disappear, and after seven days it was scarcely possible to demonstrate a trace of lithia in the extracted lens.

The attempt has been made to prove by this and a few negative experiments, that the interchange of nutritive fluid is an exceedingly slow one. Ulrich has, as it appears with perfect right, drawn attention to the fact that this conclusion is not justifiable, if one will only stop to compare the nutritive conditions of the non-vascular lens with other vascular tissues.

Schlosser [12] looked upon the spindle-shaped interspaces around the nucleus of the lens as a veritable system of lymph channels. His investigations were all made where pathological conditions were present, and, as we shall see further on, these splits are a pathological production and therefore invalidate his conclusions. He states, "In the normal lens these perinuclear spaces are few and very narrow, whereas in cataractous lenses they are widely dilated." "The spaces," he says," follow the direction of the fibres." He bases his conclusion on the above-quoted views of Samelsohn, stating "that the nutritive stream enters the lens along the equator, thence proceeds to the center of the posterior cortical substance and to the posterior star figure and reaching the peri-nuclear canals, flow toward the anterior star figure, finally converging toward a circular area beneath the anterior capsule," which he considers the line of exit.

At the time the Naphthalin experiments were first practiced, it was hoped that they, by the pathological processes which followed in the lens, would shed some light on this still interesting question, but this hope has not been realized. A large number of investigations were made by *Bouchard* and *Charrin*,[13] *Pannas*,[13a] *Dor*,[14] *C. Hess*,[14a] *Magnus*,[14b] *Kollinski*,[15] and Prof. Hugo Magnus.[15a] The last named concluded that the

[12] Uber die Lymphbalmen der Linse. Munchener Med. Wochenschrift, No. 7, 1889.

[13] La semanie medicalle, 1886, No. 52.

[13a] Etudes sur la nutrition de l'oeil dapres des experiences faites avec la flourescine et le Napthalin Arch. Opth., 1887, Mars Avril.

[14] Bulletins et memories de la societe Francaise d Opth, 1887, p. 150.

[14a] Berichte uber 19th Versamlung der Opth. Gesel. Heidelberg, 1887.

[14b] Therapeutische Monalschrift, October, 1887.

[15] Zur lehre von der Wirking des Naphalins auf das Auge und uber den Sogenanten Napthalin staar. Graefe Arch., XXXV, B. 2, 1889.

[15a] Experimentelle Studien uber die Ernahrung der Krystalline und uber Cataract Bildung.

nutrition of the lens could be interfered with as the result of interference with the circulation of nutritive fluids in the lens or by changes in the chemical condition of the nutritive fluids of the lens. He concludes "(1) that the nutritive processes go on more actively and in a more complete manner in the posterior half of the lens. (2) A zone posterior to the equator and running parallel to this, appears to take up a greater nutritive stream. (3) A zone anterior to the equator of the lens and running parallel to this also appears to take up nutritive fluid, but to a less degree. (4) The posterior pole likewise takes up a nutritive stream, which is still less than the two just mentioned. (5) Nutritive fluid does not appear to be taken up at the anterior pole. (6) The equator of the lens itself does not take up a separate nutritive stream, but is dependent on the two zones anterior and posterior and removed from it. (7) The manner in which the nutritive fluids escape from the lens is still unknown."

THE PHYSICAL CHANGES which the lens undergoes as the individual advances in age, and under pathological conditions, affects its *volume* and *weight*, its *hardness* and *dryness*, its *colorlessness*, its *transparency*, and its *index of refraction*.

The gradual increase in *weight* and *volume* is a necessary result, due to the continuous formation of new fibres at the equator, which, under normal circumstances, is scarcely ever interrupted, even up to advanced age. This is beautifully illustrated in Priestly Smith's table on page 31. The exception to this rule he found in lenses which began to show even slight cataractous cloudiness. Having weighed these with especial care, he found that at the beginning of the process the cataractous lenses had a reduced volume (and weight) as compared with non-cataractous lenses of the same age. Therefore, we are indebted to Priestly Smith for the valuable knowledge relative to the study of the cataract, namely, that *a reduction of volume precedes the formation of cataract*.

Owing to the giving off of water from its innermost lamellae, and which process gradually progresses toward the periphery, the lens becomes *dryer and harder* from within outward. Nucleus and cortex are principally differentiated by this difference in hardness.

Loss of *colorlessness* accompanies the above changes. As early as the twentieth year, the yellowish tinge begins to manifest itself. This change continues gradually to increase as long as the lens remains transparent, but this progress is not always an equally progressive one. We must either assume that this discoloration is not of the same intensity in all cases, or that the chemical changes are of a different character in different individuals. Whereas, at times we meet with very aged individuals whose lenses show but a very slight yellowish discoloration, we, on the other hand, meet with the so-called *Cataract Nigra,* in which the color of the lens is so dark and its transparency so far impaired, that vision is reduced to the greatest degree, so that one is forced to remove this *non-cataractous lens* by operative procedure..

It would scarcely seem necessary to state, that during the formation of cataract the transparency of the lens is greatly interfered with. *Every opacity of the lens system is called a Grey Cataract. In Senile Cataract, the initial opacities are due to chemical changes in the stagment fluids which occupies the interspaces; the fibres secondarily become cloudy due to chemical decomposition and the mechanical disintegration.* In the soft cataracts of the young and in most consecutive cataracts, we find that after the taking up of aqueous inside of the capsule, the first opacities in the lens fibres are due to the formation of vacuoles.

The hyperplasia of capsular epithelium is perfectly transparent in the beginning (Knies). It is only later on, after the structure becomes organized, that it loses its transparency. In all probability the large vesicular cells (yet to be considered) occur in transparent lenses. They only lead to opacities, when they undergo hyaline (or colloid) degeneration, which does occur very soon.

According to all former assumption, *the change in the index of refraction of the lens* was explained in the following manner: As age advanced, instead of there being a steady increase, from periphery to centre, there is a gradual decrease, and the lens is gradually merged into a homogenous body having the index of refraction of the nucleus. After Helmholtz had shown that a homogenous transparent body having the form of the crystalline body and possessing the index of refraction of its nucleus (hence the very greatest which the normal lens possesses) will have a much smaller total index of refraction than the combination of the various lamellae of the youthful lenses, each of which possesses a different index of refraction, the attempt was made [16] to explain the gradual transition of the emmetropic eye to the hypermetropic, as age advances, as due to the gradual transition of the lens into a more homogenous body. But Becker states that he has not been able to find an experimental demonstration of the fact that the difference in the index of refraction of the individual lamellae of the lens is less. Priestly Smith [17] gives a different explanation of this reduction of refraction in the aged. He states: "The continuous growth of the lens sufficed to explain the acquired hypermetropia of old age, without assuming that the lens changed its form.

---

[16] Donders—Anomalies of Refraction and Accommodation. 1866.
[17] Growth of the Lens. Med. Times and Gaette. January 20, 1883.

This subject has recently been investigated by L. Heine.[a] He used the eyes of human corpses, in which the refractive conditions were determined by skiasopy before death. Subsequently, he found that the radius of curvature of the anterior surface of the lens had not changed; but, on severing all the zonular fibres, the radius of curvature at the anterior pole was increased to such a degree, that the radius in the latter condition was to the former as 6 to 10. Similar experiments in old people did not show an increase in the radius of curvature. In the eye of a corpse the radius of curvature at the anterior pole of the lens is 13 to 14 mm., whereas, after severing all the zonular fibres, the radius is reduced to 8-10 mm.

In determining the *index of refraction* of the lens, an Abbe's refractometre was used; and the estimates were based on Matthiessen's [18] general formula, that the *total* index of refraction of a lens, consisting of equally centric lamellae, is as much greater than the index of the centre of its nucleus, as the difference between the latter and the index of its cortical substance. In other words, the total index of refraction is obtained by finding the index of the substance at the anterior pole; also of the nucleus; and adding the difference between the two to that of the nucleus. The index of refraction found in the lens held tense by zonula fibres was looked upon as the *non*-accommodating lens; whereas, with all fibres cut, this was considered as the accommodating lens.

The index of refraction of substance obtained at anterior pole......1.390—1.395
The index of refraction of isolated accommodating lens...........1.380—1.385
The index of nucleus..1.408—1.410

Estimated from these figures:

The index of refraction of entire lens during act of accommodation..1.435—1.440
The index of refraction of entire lens at rest...................1.425—1.430

As long as the zonula is held tense, an albuminous body is found at the anterior pole of the lens, which has a lower index of refraction. This produces an increase in the total index of refraction. As a result, during the act of accommodation, the refractive condition is in part covered (1-2 D). The change in the contour of the lens is, nevertheless, the main factor in producing an altered refractive condition.

It was noted that the older the individual, the higher the index of refraction at the anterior pole—the values gradually increasing from 1.395 to 1.405. The index of the nucleus likewise increases, but not to such a

[a] Beitrage zur Physiologie und Pathologie der Linse. Graefe Arch., Vol. XLVI, Part 3, p. 525. 1898.

[18] Zehender, Matthiesen and Jacobson. Uber die Brechungscoefficient Kataractoser Linsen substanz. Zehender's Klin. Monatsbl., Bd. XV, p. 237-311. Zehender's Klin Monalsblatter, Bd. XVII, p. 307.

degree, (at most, 0.005). Therefore, the total index of the senile lens is much less than in the youthful lens. The values of senile lens range from 1.415 to 1.425—and hence it must appear evident that this reduced index of refraction causes the hyperopia of old age. No doubt the general increase in thickness of the lens may compensate for this, within certain limits.

The following is a Schematic table of the average total indices of refraction:

Senile hyperopia.. 1.415

Presbyopia, depending on the age and thickness of lens.............1.420—1.425

Youthful lenses... 1.430

Lenses during act of accommodation............................ 1.440

N. B.—In the schematic eye a change of one in the second decimal place changes the total index of refraction 1½ D (equals ½ mm. difference in optic axis).

In cataractous lenses the index of refraction is nearly always found increased. This may be due to various causes: First, the anterior pole may disclose an abnormally low index; this would increase the total index. Second, the nucleus may be very markedly sclerosed, and thus the index may be increased. Third, both conditions may be combined. In the first group belongs, possibly, the mature cataract, the Morgagni's and soft cataracts in which the nucleus is sclerosed; in the second group are found mature cataracts and certain forms of diabetic cataracts, in which irregular sclerosis and softening has not as yet destroyed the structure of the lens. Thus can be explained the clinical observation, that at times during the incipient stages of cataract formation, myopia develops.

THE CHEMISTRY OF THE LENS AND THE FLUID MEDIA WHICH SURROUND IT.

With the exception of the increase in weight and volume of the transparent lens, all the above-described changes are dependent on the chemical changes which take place in the lens. These in their turn will be largely dependent on the constitution of the nutritive supply which is obtained from the vitreous.

That very marked chemical differences exist between the lens of the young and those advancing in age has already been pointed out, (on page 51), on the evidence of anatomical proof.

Our knowledge of the chemical constitution of the crystalline lens is inseparable from the name of Berzelius. In the ox's lens he found an albuminous substance like his globulin, which he named *Krystalline*. It appears that human lenses were not submitted to a quantitative analysis.

According to Kuhne,[20] the lens contains water 60 per cent., albuminous material 37.5 per cent., fat and traces of cholesterine 2 per cent., and ashes at most 0.5 per cent. Later analyses are from the laboratories of Hoppe Seyler. Laptschinsky,[21] as the average of the analysis of four calves' lenses, gives the following: Water 63.51 per cent., albuminous material 34.93 per cent., lecithin 0.23 per cent., cholesterine 0.22 per cent., fat 0.29 per cent., soluble salts 0.53 per cent., insoluble salts 0.29 per cent.

Whereas Kuhne, like Simon, Alex. Schmidt, Lieberkuhn and Vintschgau, states that, after careful trituration in sand, extraction in water and filtration, he obtained a faint opalescent fluid, in which he found at least three albuminous bodies, globulin, kali albumin, and serum albumen, *Laptschinsky* obtained no precipitate from the clear filtrate of the precipitated globulin which he dissolved in a weak acid, whereas the solution became cloudy at 55 degrees and at 70 degrees showed a flaky coagulate. Therefore, according to the latter, the lens does not contain a potassium albuminate, but merely a globulin (24.68 per cent.) and serum albumen (10.31 per cent.). Cahn [22] triturated fresh animal lenses (according to Hammarsten's method) with crystallized magnesium sulphate and afterwards washed this out with a saturated soda magnesium solution, during which process more of the albuminous substance was taken up by the solution. From this he concluded that the entire lens was made up of a globuline. He adds: "Whether or not this is a single one is yet to be determined." Prof. Michel and Henry Wagner [23] investigated this subject again. They concluded that at least in the pig's eye, also in the ox's eye, we find *lento-globuline* and *lento-albumine*. To digress here for a moment. Michel [24] has made some very interesting experiments relative to the temperature within the eye-ball, and with special reference to its action on the crystalline lens. With a peculiarly constructed electrical thermo element he made a series of investigations in the eyes of rabbits. The temperature in the rectum was 38.5 degrees C., the average in the anterior chamber was 31.9 degrees C., and in the middle of the vitreous 36.1 degrees, which he also considers to be the average temperature in the centre of the lens. In the anterior chamber the temperature fell several tenths of a degree, when the point of the instrument was brought close to the cornea, whereas it rose proportionately as it approached the iris, almost attaining the tem-

20 Physiological Chemie, p. 404. Leipsig, 1868.

21 Ein Beitrag zur Chemie des Linsengewbes. Pflugers Arch., Bd. XIII,p.631.

22 Zur Physiol. and Pathol. Chemie des Auges, Strassburg, 1881, p. 17.

23 Physiologische Chemische Untersuchungen des Auges. Prof. Met. D. W. Graef Arch., XXXII, Book 2, p. 155, 1886.

24 Die Temperature Topographie des Auges. Graefe Arch., Vol. XXXII, B. 2. 1886.

perature in the vitreous. Again, in the vitreous the temperature increased as the instrument neared the coats of the eye, and attained the body temperature when they were touched. The temperature increased 2.3 degrees when the lids were closed and on the application of an ice bag the temperature fell 13 to 15 degrees C. in the course of one and a half minutes. The relatively low temperature of the anterior chamber may be due to the rapid dissipation of heat by the cornea; also due to the fact that the blood vessels are relatively far removed. This latter cause may also explain the low temperature in the centre of the vitreous. From a physiological standpoint these temperature conditions appear to be especially important, since undoubtedly they exert a very decided influence on the albuminous bodies in the eye, *especially in the lens.* Michel gives the following experiment. If a small ice bag is laid on the eye of a cat, a total cloudiness of the lens will follow in a short time, which will again disappear shortly after the ice bag is removed.

It would hardly seem necessary to remind one of the therapeutic value of the above experiments, which show the rapid changes in the temperature due to closure of the lid, or the application of an ice bag.

Laptschinsky found that the amount of the cholesterine varies greatly, ranging from 0.06 per cent to 0.49 per cent. He also found that the normal transparent lens contains lecithin.

Our interest is especially directed toward discovering the differences in the quantities of water, albuminous material, also lecithin, found in the *senile non-cataractous* and in the *senile cataractous lenses.*

Water. Deutschman [25] demonstrated for the *non*-cataractous lens, that which up to this time had been accepted, but which never had been experimentally proven, by weighing human lenses removed from the body shortly after death, and then permitting them to dry out completely, and in this way he succeeded in demonstrating as a fact, that though there is a general increase as age advances, there is a diminution both absolute as well as relative to the weight of the entire lens (from 70.8 to 64.6 per cent.) of the amount of *water contained,* whereas the amount of *dry constituents increases.* Naturally, there were differences in the weight of the different lenses, as well as in the relation between the amount of water and the dry constituents of the lens. The weight of five senile cataracts, four of which had been extracted by H. Pagenctacher, and the fifth was a cataracta incipiens and had been taken from a corpse, showed (p. 216) that the *senile cataractous lens contained considerably more water* (76.23 per cent. as opposed to 69.06 per cent.) *than the non-cloudy senile and that they were poorer*

---

[25] Cataracta Senilis, 1879. Graefe Arch., Bd. XXV, 2, p. 214.

in solid constituents, especially the albuminous products. Both features were less developed in C. incipiens.

Jacobson's statements [26] are at variance with these, who found just the opposite, namely, that *cataractous lenses contain less water* (63.45 per cent. as opposed to 73.6 per cent.) than the normal. This, however, is due to the fact that Jacobson made his estimates from lenses which had been extracted without their capsules, and hence there can be no doubt but that a part of the watery cortical substance remained behind in the eye. Unfortunately, Deutschman failed to state how his lenses were preserved while being transported from Wiesbaden to Goettingen in order to protect them against alterations in their watery constituents. Both Priestly Smith and J. Treacher Collins [27] agree with Jacobson. The latter examined six fresh eyes one hour after enucleation; also ten cataractous lenses, with following results:—

	FRESH EYES, 10-64 yrs.		10 CATARACTOUS LENSES, 46-80 yrs.	
Average Total Weight,	0.204		0.118	
Water,	0.1446 =	71 per cent.,	0.078 =	65 per cent.
Solid Constituents,	0.059 =	29 "	0.040 =	35 "
Ashes,	0.0013 =	0.6 "	0.0014 =	1.57 "

Collins states: "The weight of the cataractous lens is far below that of the normal." The cataractous lens is not to be looked upon as the result of excessive changes due to age, but rather the result of nutritive disturbances of an entirely different nature, *chemical, not morphological.*

Albuminous Substances. Cahn [28] analyzed cataracts which had been extracted by Laquer without their capsules and been subsequently preserved in alcohol, and he has compared his results with those of Laptschinsky which the latter made in normal calves' lenses. Since these are the only quantitive estimates of human lenses, they are quoted here and will be referred to again later on:—

100 PARTS OF SOLID CONSTITUENTS CONTAIN	IN CATARACTS.		IN NORMAL OX LENSES.
	I.	II.	
Albumen,	81.48	85.87	94.71
Cholesterine,	6.22	4.55	0.62
Lecithin,	4.52	0.808	0.63
Fat,	. . .	1.19	0.79
Alcoholic Extract,	0.83	1.45	0.71
Watery Extract,	3.94	2.76	1.52
Soluable } Salts,	1.81	2.41	1.36
Insoluable }	1.14	1.45	0.46

26 Uber die Brechungs-coefficienten und uber die Chemische Beschaffenheit Kataraktoeser Linsensubstanz. Zehender's Klin. Monatsblatt. Bd. XVII, p. 307.

27 The Composition of the Human Lens in Health and in Cataract, etc. Opthalmic Review, November, 1880.

28 Zur Physiol. and Pathol. Chemie des Auges. Strassburg, p. 18. 1881.

According to the two analyses, the average absolute decrease of albumen equals 0.95 to 0.84 per cent.

Cahn, however, also had the opportunity of analyzing a number of freshly extracted senile cataracts. He preserved them in quite a concentrated sol. of common salt until he had a sufficient number, and then utilized them to determine the amount of albuminous material in senile cataracts by comparing the results of that which is insoluble in water and CO, to that which is soluble. *The absolute amount of albuminous material soluble in water and CO was found to be diminished.* Both the soluble and the insoluble albumines were then dried, and the average analysis of the two analyses showed that the proportion of the soluble to the insoluble albumines was to that of the normal ox lens as 24, 62: 10, 31; that is, as 2.38: 1 is to 15.09: 1. Now, since as we have seen all albuminous substances which are present in the normal lens are *globuline*, and that the apparent incomplete elimination of serum albumen is dependent on the abnormal quantities of water and CO, Cahn draws the conclusion from this fact, that *where cataracts are treated with water and CO, a much greater portion of albuminous substance is eliminated, and that during life a portion of the albuminous substance has been so modified as to have become insoluble. It is not difficult to assume that this very circumstance adds to the cataractous cloudiness.*

Cahn does not decide what this modification is. Becker,[29] reasoning by analogy, expresses the belief that since the lens, like the skin and hair, is derived from the ectoderm, keratine might be found in the nucleus of the senile or cataractous lens. Knies, by means of Kuhne's digestive method, proved that this assumption is not true.[30] He also examined senile cataracts which had been extracted without their capsules; hence, essentially their nuclei. The result was a fluid which gave all the reactions of peptone, and did not in any way differ from a peptone fluid which resulted from digestion of albumen. According to Knies, the substance of the nucleus of cataract is albuminous in its nature, though it did show certain difference in its chemical relation to other albuminous substances. This digestive method has in other ways proven its importance to the anatomy and chemistry of the lens.[31] By this means it has been shown that since the capsule of the lens, like Descemet's membrane, can be completely di-

---

29 Pathologie Therapie. p. 169.

30 Knies Zur Chemie der Alters veranderungen der Linse. Untersuch a. d. Physiol. Inst. d. Univ. Heidelberg, Bl. 2, p. 114.

31 Kuhne and Ewald die verdauung als Histologische Methode. Verhand der Naturhistor Med. Verein in Heidelberg. Bd. 1.

gested, it is not an elastic membrane. It seems to coincide very much with the cement substance of the lens. In fact, the entire lens may be digested, leaving but a slight residue.

Cholesterine and Fat. The various authorities seem to coincide as to the amount of cholesterine in cataractous lenses. Kuhne [32] found in senile (human) lenses which had assumed an amber color a greater amount of fat and cholesterine than in the normal lenses. Laptschinsky (cited above, page 639) could only reiterate this statement as to the amount of fat found in cases of amber colored lenses in oxen. It is however questionable whether we can consider the lenses of slaughtered animals as senile, in the sense which we consider lenses in old people suffering from senile cataract.

We are indebted to Jacobson for the most thorough investigations concerning the amount of cholesterine contained in the human lens during the various periods of life. This analysis was made at the instigation of Zehender and Matthieson. He found (cited above, page 315) that the lens of a new born infant does not contain any cholesterine, and in the lens of a young woman of 20 years, he found but slight traces. He was the first to draw attention to this increase in the cataractous lens (page 313). Though he had to make a partial retraction in a latter publication (2d paper cited, page 309), he nevertheless states: "*In young individuals, as a class, the amount of cholesterine is much less than in individuals more advanced in life, and, as a whole, cataractous lenses are richer in cholesterine than normally transparent lenses.* Jacobson (p. 308) found in 64 lenses taken from individuals under 60 years of age, that 2.11 per cent. of the dry substance consisted of cholesterine, and in 27 *transparent* lenses taken from individuals over 60 years of age, 2.36 per cent., and in 86 cataracts taken from individuals over 60 years of age, 2.68 per cent. Both of the analyses of Cahn are in accord with these figures. As compared with the 0.62 per cent. cholesterine (100 parts of solid substance) in the normal cortical substance, he found in the centre of the cataract 5.38 per cent. cholesterine Jacobson was further able to show that the nucleus of the cataract contains three times as much cholesterine as the cataract substance. *Therefore, he considers it as probable that cholesterine is not a foreign substance, which is carried to the lens by the nutritive fluid, but that it is rather the result of a change in the albuminous substance contained in the lens.*

Lecithin. Laptschinsky found lecithin in the cortical substance of the normal lens, as did also Cahn in both his analyses, and in the last very much increased in quantity. He does not attempt to draw any conclusions from this.

---

[32] **Physiologische Chemie**, 1868, p. 400.

If we now briefly make a resume of the above, we find that *Deutschman*
inferred from the reduction of the absolute quantity of dried cortical substance in cataracts, an absolute reduction of the albuminous substance in
cataract; *Jacobson* states that a portion of the albumen has been changed
into cholesterine, whereas *Cahn*, as the result of his chemical investigations
of non-cataractous lenses and senile human lenses, states that in cataract
there is a reduction of albuminous material, partly changed into an insoluble substance, with at the same time formation of cholesterine (and lecithin, increase of the extractive and anorganic substances). Though Cahn
states that he is not able to draw any conclusion from his results concerning the cataractous process, Becker draws this very important conclusion,
that "*though all agree as to the physical condition, there has nevertheless been
proven that there are demonstratable chemical differences between the nucleus
of the non-cloudy and the nucleus of the cataractous senile lens.*"

A substance which has been occasionally noted in the lens, and which
does not occur under normal conditions, is *sugar*. Its presence in the lens
in cases of diabetic cataract has attracted the greatest attention. Its presence here has been utilized as the basis on which to build a theory for the
development of this particular form of cataract. There may be various
reasons why its presence is not a constant one, which will be touched on
again. In order to avoid doubts which might arise in the minds of
the reader as to the accuracy with which these tests were made, Prof. Kuhne
kindly permitted the publication of the methods pursued in his laboratory.

On March 9, 1881, Kuhne examined for Becker a cataract, which the latter
had just extracted. His letter reads as follows: "The cataractous mass which
I received on March 9th was rubbed up minutely in water heated to the boiling
point, sufficient acetic acid added to give it a weak acid reaction, filtered while
still hot, and the filtrate washed in boiling water, and the clear filtrate dried
over a water bath. The colorless firm residue was then boiled with absolute
alcohol, and this filtered after cooling left nothing to be reduced. After this
mass, which was insoluble in alcohol, had been further extracted in ether, this
was dissolved in a few drops of water, to which were added a few drops of
over-proof alcohol; this was heated; after cooling filtered, and the residue left
on the filter after evaporation was taken up anew in water, and used in making
Trommer's test. In order to be able to recognize even the faintest reduction, to
the solution to which caustic soda had been added, just sufficient sulphate of
copper solution was added to give the faintest trace of blue color to the solution.
On placing the test tube in water, having a temperature of 80 degrees C., the
color rapidly disappeared, and a reddish color developed. Each time, on cooling, a new quantity of the sulphate of copper solution was added, until the blue
color was retained on heating. In the meanwhile, there had been such a rich
deposit of reddish crystals of oxide of copper, that it was possible to determine

that there was a very considerable quantity of sugar in the lens. The insolubility of the reduced body in absolute alcohol, and the rapid appearance of the reduction at a temperature below 85 degrees C., were all guarantees of the identity of this substance with *diabetic sugar*.

The second cataract was extracted from this same individual March 29, 1881, and examined by Dr. Mays. His report reads as follows: "The lens was placed in boiling water, and thus reduced in size. After this solution had been made weakly acid by the addition of acetic acid, and then allowed to boil for a while longer, it was filtered; the filtrate strongly compressed, and alcohol added. During the compression a small exudate had formed, so that it became necessary to filter once more. The filtrate was next evaporated to dryness, and the residue was taken off in water. With this solution the Trommer's tests were made. After the solution had been made alkaline by the addition of caustic soda solution, there was added just a sufficient quantity of a dilute sulphate of copper solution, to give the slightest perceptible shade of blue. The color disappeared on heating in a water bath, without, however, at once causing a noticeable deposit. After the addition of several more drops of the sulphate of copper solution, the fluid retained its color in the water bath. After the fluid had stood during the dinner hour, a quantity of the fluid was drawn from the bottom of the test tube by means of a pipette, and examined under the microscope. The presence of a few, but not to be mistaken crystals of the oxide of copper, proved that the reduction had taken place, from which one is justified in declaring that sugar was present." Kuhne added the following remarks: "According to the reduction test the quantity of sugar appears to be less than in the cataract which I examined on March 9, 1881. Since this difference does not appear to be in the amount of oxide of copper which was reduced, since this was not estimated, but lies in the precipitated oxide, this may also depend on the presence of substances which keep the oxide of copper in suspension in alkaline solutions. Such disturbing additions were more certainly excluded in the method of examination pursued in the first lens; the second method, though simpler, is not to be recommended, because it offers us a less quantity of material with which to make an investigation.

In order to decide this question, whether the lens or a cataract does contain a substance which, on the addition of an alkaline solution would give the oxide of copper reduction, Kuhne was kind enough to examine (for Becker) five senile cataracts and one traumatic cataract, all taken from *non-diabetic* patients, just as they chanced to follow each other in operations at the clinic. Such a supposition seemed verified, for Kuhne found that the watery extract free of albumen, taken from the lens of a rabbit, had the property of discoloring the copper solution on making the Trommer's test, and at times minute crystals of the oxide of copper were seen under the microscope. The results of Kuhne's examination was as follows: The lenses were triturated in water, and after the addition of a trace of acetic acid, were boiled. The filtrate was evaporated to complete dryness, and the remains were taken up in alcohol (1). That which the alcohol left insoluble was taken up in 80 per cent. alcohol (2). And the third insoluble remainder was taken up in water (3). 1 and 2 were evaporated and changed to a watery solution, and in the reduction test gave a negative result, as did also 3. All three portions were next just turned perceptible blue by the addition of hydrate of soda and sulphate of copper solution, and heated over a water bath for a considerable length of time at a temperature of 100 degrees C, during which the color did not change. Later on the color was made decidedly blue by addition of more Cu, and then thoroughly heated over a flame; but at the end of twenty-four hours none of these tests showed a precipitate in which the oxide of copper could be detected microscopically. *These lenses, therefore, did not contain any sugar, and in fact, nothing which could be reduced.*

Armaignac [33] observed in a cataracta nigra, small, globular granules, which he considered *haematoidin.* The only spectroscopical analysis so far reported was made by Gillet de Grandmont.[33a] He extracted a very large black cataract. The fundus disclosed a general chorio retinitis. The spectroscopic examination proved that the black color was due to liver pigment. The occurrence of the fundus disease explains the pathogenesis of the form of cataract. Pykalt believed the color was due to the choroidal pigment, for dilute sulphuric acid easily dissolved the pigment of the blood, and he made similar observtions when he treated sections of cataracta nigra with dilute sulphuric acid. H. Meyer stated that he believed there were two forms of cataracta nigra, one due to the taking up of the pigment of the blood, the other due to the general sclerosis.

Vitreous and Aqueous. For reasons explained on pages 53 and 54, analysis of the vitreous and aqueous assume great importance, especially so owing to their relation to the pathological conditions of the lens. It is a matter of regret that we possess but few analyses of sufficient accuracy. The investigations of Cahn (l. c., p. 14) have settled this question beyond a doubt. The humor aqueous has a somewhat strong alkaline reaction, and has a specific gravity of 1.009. It does not contain any mucin, but a globulin and serum albumen. The former simulates blood serum as to the point at which it coagulates. The aqueous has this qualitative difference, "that in cooking the faintly acid solution, the albumen becomes slightly flaky and is precipitated, leaving a clear fluid; whereas, the vitreous always remain cloudy, and only gives a clear filtrate with great difficulty, a condi-

---

[33] Note sur la cataracte noire—Journal de Med. de Bordeaux, Bd. IX, p. 357.
[33a] Extraction de Cataracte Noire. Society d Opth. d Paris, April, 1893.

tion which Lohmeyer emphasized and which Deutschman misinterpreted, supposing this to be due to larger quantity of albumen. All quantitative estimates coincide. The average of six estimates showed the vitreous to contain 0.0738 per cent. of albumen; the aqueous, 0.081 per cent.; hence, a somewhat greater amount. An analysis made with a larger quantity of vitreous (280 cc.) showed the albumen equal to 0.0907 per cent. Lohmeyer found it to be 0.053; Deutschman, 0.12—0.113 per cent. The following is Cahn's complete analysis:

	HUMOR VITREOUS.	HUMOR AQUEOUS.
Albumen, ...	0.074	0.082
Remaining Organic Substances,	0.071	0.148
Ashes, ...	0.971	0.998
Water, ...	98.884	98.777
INORGANIC SUBSTANCES.		
K_2SO_4, ...	8.74	5.99
K cl, ...	5.57	2.92
Na cl, . . : .	74.43	78.11
$PO_4H Na_2$, . . .	1.82	1.99
$(PO_4)_2Ca_3$, . . .	0.44	0.62
$(PO_4)_2Mg_3$, . . .	0.22	0.40
Na_2Co_3, . . .	12.67	8.72

"According to this the watery fluids of the eye are very similar to the cerebro-spinal fluid, and the transudates which are weakest in albumen."

The material from which these analyses were made was taken from animals. In older analyses made by Berzelius and Kletzinsky, the aqueous used was taken from human eyes, but none has been made from the vitreous. One should judge, that since the index of refraction of both fluids is the same under normal conditions, any abnormal addition leading to a changed constitution of the one or the other of the two fluids ought to be demonstratable.

Fleischer [34] fixed the indices of refraction by means of Abbe's refractometer. The value for distilled water (Line D, 18 per cent.) being 1.3340, he found that of the aqueous equal to 1.3373, and of the vitreous equal to 1.3369; hence, somewhat less.

Notwithstanding the difficulty of making estimates with Abbe's Refractometer of the small quantities of aqueous or vitreous which can be obtained from man, we can nevertheless determine to a degree the index of refraction of the fluids, and gain comparatively accurate knowledge, as to whether the fluids are normal in their constitution, or whether they contain abnormal substances. For example: The index of refraction of a three-quarter per cent. Na. Cl solution, 1.3356; whereas that of water equals 1.3340. (Line D. 18 degrees

[34] Neue Bestimmungen der Brechungs exponenten der Durchsichtigen Flüssigeh Medien des Auges Inaug. Dissert, 1872.

C.) Egg albumen, 0.110 per cent. in a three-quarter per cent. Na. Cl solution equals 1.3365; egg albumen, 0.165 per cent. equals 1.3368; 0.33 per cent., 1.3370 0.5 per cent., 1.3373, etc. If the anterior chamber of a normal eye is punctured, a fluid will be obtained showing an index of refraction equal to 1.3362. If the anterior chamber is punctured again, ten minutes later it will be found 1.3389. *From experiments made on animals, it is a well known fact, that with each success-ive puncture, the albuminous portion of the aqueous increases.* The vitreous of an intensely icteric patient, taken but a few hours after death, had an index of re-fraction equal to 1.3379, whereas, on boiling, it showed but a slight opalescence.

If we will now hold fast to the fact that both aqueous and vitreous are poor in albumen, and that the amount of organic as well as inorganic con-stituents scarcely differ from each other; hence, any addition of substances which are normally present, or any other substances which do not occur in them under normal circumstances, will lead to the following important conclusion concerning the nutrition of the lens: *In general any increase or abnormal contents in the vitreous, be they organic or inorganic, will cause abnormal nutritive conditions in the lens, and like conditions occurring in the aqueous are the result of an interference with the proper interchange of fluids in the lens.*

Lohmeyer [35] succeeded in demonstrating the presence of sugar in vit-reous, taken from two human beings who had died of diabetes. The acid reaction of the fluid media (lactic acid) of the eye, which he claimed he had found, and which he also claimed passed through the lens, Leber [36] was not able to find in the aqueous taken up with a pipette from the con-junctiva during a cataract extraction done on a diabetic patient. Hence, Leber assumed that the acid reaction which Lohmeyer obtained, was due to post mortem change. Deutschman [37] proved the presence of sugar in the aqueous and vitreous of the corpse of a diabetic, which did not contain a cataract, and whose lens did not contain sugar. The aqueous was highly alkaline, and contained 0.5 per cent, the vitreous 0.36 per cent of sugar.

We know as yet absolutely nothing concerning a change or increase in the amount of albumen in the vitreous in cases of senile cataract.

The first analysis relative to the amount of albumen in the aqueous, in cases of senile cataract, are to be found in Edward Yager's work, "Uber die Einstellung des dioptr. Apparatus, eat." (p. 142) and were made by Kletzinsky. The aqueous was taken from the living eye by puncture of

---

[35] Beitrag zur Histologie und Aetiologie der erworbenen Linsenstaare. Zeit-schrift. f. rat Medicin N. F., Bd. V, p. 99, 1854.

[36] Uber die Erkrankung des Auges bei der Diabetes Mellitus Arch. fur Opth., Bd. XXI, 3.

[37] Zur Regeneration des Homor Agueous. Arch. f. Opthal., Bd. 26, p. 99.

the cornea. Notwithstanding the slight quantity which he could obtain (0.2—0.5 gr.), Kletzinsky estimated the amount of albumen in a normal eye to be 0.0456 per cent., and that of three cataractous eyes to be 0.3618 0.0764 and 0.0899 per cent. Hence, the cataractous eyes showed a great increase of albumen over that found in the normal eye. Leber (l. c., p. 301) found a very considerable increase of the albumen (on heating a thick precipitate occurred), together with a 1 pro mille of sugar, in a patient who had diabetic cataract, removed two and one-half hours after death. This observation incited Deutschman to examine the aqueous in senile cataracts for albumen. He found during the process of ripening of senile cataract a greater amount of albumen in the aqueous than under normal conditions; hence, he coincided with the Yager-Kletzinsky statement. In a case of acute nephritis, with exceptionally excessive albuminuria, the lens being transparent, no increase of albumen could be found in the eye. From this together with several other investigations, Deutschman concluded that *the increase of albumen which is found in the aqueous in cases of cataract, is derived from the lens, but that the cataract is not due to an inceased amount of albumen in the humor aqueous.*

Aside from the fact whether the tests made by Kletzinsky, with such small quantities, and the so-called optical tests of Deutschman, are of sufficient accuracy to give definite results, which could be of service in determining this important question as to the causes of cataract, they nevertheless coincide fully with those with which we are acquainted, concerning the direction of the nutritive stream in the lens. Hence, we can understand the reason for the constant presence of a greater amount of albumen in the aqueous, in cases of advanced senile cataract, which must have been derived from the lens, and passed out by diffusion.

One could account for the presence of sugar in the lens and aqueous by a similar mode of reasoning.

PART II.

THE PATHOLOGICAL LENS SYSTEM.

CHAPTER I.

THE PATHOLOGY OF THE ZONULA OF ZINN.

Even at the present day but little is known concerning the pathological anatomy of the zonula of zinn, on the normal integrity and development of which the lens is so prominently dependent, not only for its proper
position, but also for its ability to properly perform its function during the
act of accommodation. It might also be compared to the hairspring of a
watch.

Becker [1] states that at times there is such a complete *atrophy* of the
zonula fibres that one can not recognize a trace of its fibrous construction.
This may lead to a spontaneous detachment of the lens in its capsule, partial or complete. This condition in all probability agrees with one described by Wedl and Bock [2] as *senescence of the zonula*. They describe the
zonula fibres as taut, apparently closely packed together, and easily torn
from their attachment on the application of a certain degree of force. When
detached they are tense and friable. This condition is taken advantage of
when the lens is extracted in its capsule (Pagenstecher's operation).

Again, Becker states [3] that it is not at all uncommon in cases of disorganized eyes, more particularly in cases where cataract has developed, to
find a marked *increase* of the zonula fibres. These, he states, may be observed in the fresh as well as in hardened specimens, as *cloudy*, thickened
fibres, adherent to the ciliary body and the capsule of the lens. Wedl and
Bock (p. 77) state that in cataractous eyes the connective tissue corpuscles,
which are normally present at the time, are greatly increased, and lead to
a cloudiness of the zonula. In the great majority of disorganized eyes,
such as phthisical bulbi, those which have suffered from iridocyclitic processes, the inflammatory products fill up the posterior chamber, and the
zonula fibres likewise become immersed in the exudate. Later on these
inflammatory products organize; tense bands develop, and as they undergo
cicatrical contraction lead to dislocation of the lens, even to detachment of

---

[1] Pathologie and Therapie. Graefe Saemisch Vol. p. 161, No. 11.
[2] Pathologische Anatomie des Auges. Wien, 1886. p. 177.
[3] Pathologie and Therapie, p. 162.

the entire ciliary body. No doubt at times these bands have been mistaken for thickened zonular fibres. More as the result of clinical observation than of anatomical examination it has been observed, that in cases of *synchisis corporis vitrei*, the zonular fibres are also affected, loose their consistence, and are totally dissolved. This is evidenced in cases of spontaneous luxation of the lens, where at the beginning there is iridodonesis, with the lens still properly centered. Later on, due to the continuous movements of the eyeball, and consequent oscillation of the lens, as a natural result of the continuous tension, the zonula fibres finally rupture. Owing to the intimate genetic relation existing between the zonula fibres and the vitreous (as pointed out on page 27), one might assume that the same causative agent which leads to the pathological destruction of the vitreous, or its chemical decomposition, acts exactly in the same manner on the zonular fibres.

Solution of continuity can always occur as the result of the application of mechanical force, but the manner of its production may be brought about in various ways. Two causes have already been cited above. Traction which the shrinking capsular cataract exerts on the zonula, or the dragging which it experiences where the aqueous is suddenly evacuated, due to a corneal rupture, the result, either of a trauma or operative proceedure, may produce this disaster, the lens moving anteriorly a distance equal to its axial diameter. More frequently, however, the zonula does not rupture at once, but the lens remains adherent at the point where the perforation occurred; and it is only after the anterior chamber is re-established, and the aqueous accumulated, that the zonula tears. Ectatic processes, hydropthalmus, cornea; globosa, staphyloma intercalare; in fact, all forms of staphylomata of the anterior segment of the globe, lead to partial or entire rupture of the zonula, due to the continually increasing tension exerted on the zonula fibres by the gradual distension of the anterior segment of the globe. Where the eye is struck by a blunt force and suddenly flattened out, and assumes again its normal shape, not infrequently the lens is found luxated, and this is only possible where there is at least a partial tear of the zonula. The same result is noted of a contusion, and as is well known; this latter condition most frequently occurs in the region of the ciliary body. Lastly, the zonula may be torn by a foreign body penetrating it alone, or at the same time involving neighborly structures as ciliary body and lens, without necessarily leading to loss of either aqueous or vitreous.

Certain anatomical anomalies of the eyeball are associated with *anomalies in the formation of the zonula.* In all the varieties of colobomata (coloboma of iris, ciliary body, choroid, and retina), supposed to be due to late closure of the ocular fissure, one finds, as one would naturally expect to find, a failure of perfect development of the zonula fibres, especially along the line where the closure took place, and in these places the lens follows the tension from above. Treacher Collins (see page 29) explains cases of coloboma lentis as due to want of proper adhesion between the ciliary portion of the retina and capsule of the lens at a very early period of development, before the expansion of the eyeball begins. Ectopia lentis, he explains in a similar manner, as due to a lack of development of the zonula fibres. He further states: "If, as a result of persistence of the hyaloid artery, the fibro vascular sheath around the lens persists and becomes thickened, it may occur that the lens be forced forward between iris and ciliary processes, without leading to adhesions laterally; as a result, there will be no traction and no *zonular fibres*, simply an epithelial deposit on the posterior capsule, and the lens then assumes an almost globular form."

CHAPTER II.

THE PATHOLOGICAL CHANGES IN THE LENS.

LENTICULAR CATARACT.

"During the present century the pathological anatomy of the lens has been the subject of a great many, and in part very accurate, publications. Hundreds of years ago, owing to the extreme importance which opacities of the lens bear to those so afflicted, the operations for cataract awakened an interest which was not alone confined to the physician. Hence, it is easy to understand why every effort has been made to clear up, by accurate anatomical investigation, the cause of cataract." It is only since the early part of the last century that we know that grey cataract has its seat in the lens, and it is only during the past fifty years that we know anything at all concerning its histological structure. The past twenty-five years have been ripe with a succession of publications, more especially the past fifteen years, owing to the refinement in the technique in the preparation of specimens and in our possession of better microscopes; and as a result, our knowledge of the pathology of the lens has gradually been placed on a solid foundation. And at this point it seems no more than just and proper to again draw attention to the great efforts made in this direction by Otto Becker, whose masterly descriptions are the basis of the following:

"The impetus to study the pathological anatomy of the lens was given by Malgaigne, and corresponds with the time when histology in general was undergoing revision by Schwan. Malgaigne contended (1840), and based his contentions on post mortem examinations, that there was no such thing as a capsular cataract; that is, that there existed no true cloudiness of the capsule *per se.* This statement aroused extraordinary interest, and thereupon Cunier, the publisher of 'The Annales de Oculistic,' took occasion to offer a prize for the best essay on this subject. This was very learnedly and scientifically answered by two young German physicians, Horing and Stricker. Especially in the work of Horing do we find the correct ideas regarding the formation of the lens, and in this he was far in advance of his contemporaries. Both declared against Malgaigne; but it appears that both sides misunderstood each other. It is not necessary at the present day to draw attention to the fact that at the time Malgaigne was making his investigations, a large proportion of the cases of cataract dependent on cloudiness of the cortex, were considered as capsular cataracts. In looking over the clinical histories of that time, one frequently finds the statement made, that after reclination the capsular cataract which remained in the pupil was gradually absorbed. As that which we today designate as capsular cataract is not affected by the aqueous humor, and as one does not wish to doubt the correctness of their observations, the cloudiness which remained in the pupillary area must have been remains of cortical substance. Therefore, Malgaigne was correct when he contended that that, which at that time was called capsular cataract, was situated in the cortical substance and *not* in the capsule."

SENILE CATARACT.

It seems advisable, in taking up the study of the pathology of the lens, to begin with the study of *senile cataract.* Because of its frequency we have better opportunity for making clinical observations, which can be verified by anatomical examination. Senile cataract also offers us the opportunity of studying all those changes which are characteristic of other varieties of cataract, which manifest themselves here in varying degrees of intensity. The pathological changes may be considered under two general groups. First, those of *degeneration* or *retrogressive metamorphosis and of new cellular formation;* second, those of *regeneration,* the so-called *atrophic cellular hyperplasias.*

Becker states:[1] "In senile cataract one must assume that where the sclerosing process does not proceed in an absolutely regular and continuous manner, so as finally to lead to the formation of a *cataracta nigra,* the complete saturation with nutritive fluid is interfered with, and thus leads to a loosening up of the lamella immediately adjacent to the nucleus. Besides this there is a mechanical cause for this loosening up of the lamellae. Owing

---

1 Pathologie and Therapie. Section 30, p. 182.

to the compact condition, and hence reduced volume of the nucleus, there necessarily follows a certain amount of traction on the more peripheral portions of the lens. Those portions of the cortex in the region of the anterior and posterior pole and the capsule, since they are not fixed by the zonula, can give to this traction. But in the equatorial region the conditions are different. To begin with, here the connection between the lamellae is less intimate, since it is here that the youngest lens fibres are found. Then again the zonula fixes the capsule, and prevents the equatorial portion of the lens from becoming further removed from the ciliary body, and approaching the axis of the eye. Hence, it can not be such a matter of surprise that in senile cataract, the equatorial portion of the lens is the first to suffer a loosening up and separation of its cortical lamellae (*gerontoxon lentis*), and that this is subsequently followed by a true cloudiness of the lens fibres, and a molecular disintegration (*cataract formation*).

Foerster[2] appears to have been under the impression that "the first indication of a cataract *always* makes its first appearance around the nucleus of the lens, as a result of interference with the gradual sclerosis," and states "that a very delicate but sharply defined line of demarcation can be observed along the equatorial line of the nucleus, which at times may even be observed with the naked eye or use of a loup after the lens has been extracted."

Since the introduction of the refracting opthalmoscope for diagnostic purposes by Hirschberg[3] and Magnus,[4] it has been successfully demonstrated that it is possible to study the development of cataract from its very incipiency. This has not only given us the means for making an early diagnosis, but has assisted us in formulating a theory as to the cause of its development. By starting with a -|- 6 D lens, and gradually increasing its strength, one can successfully focus the entire thickness of the crystalline lens, and by this means note the minutest changes. In this manner Magnus conducted 166 examinations, and was enabled to observe the very first delicate changes which lead up to the development of senile cataract. Generally speaking, he observed two types of development. In 92.77 per cent. of the cases which he examined, the first signs developed along the equatorial line of the lens; that is, in a zone running parallel to the anterior and posterior surfaces, Ammon's so-called *gerontoxon lentis*. The second type in which the changes are rapidly developed, form about 7.23 per cent of the

---

2 Becker's Anatomie, p. 52.

3 Centralblatt fur Prakt Augenheilkunde. 1886, p. 333; 1888, p. 360; 1889, p. 330.

4 Pathologisch Anatomische Studien uber die Anfange des Altersstaares. Graefe's Arch., Vol. XXXV, B. 3, 1889.

cases, and disclose the first signs along the *equator of the nucleus of the lens.* Thus Magnus was enabled to differentiate five varieties of interspaces, as manifestations of developing cataract at a time when the lens was apparently perfectly normal. *"First;* pear-shaped interspaces arranged concentrically around the equator. *Second,* large spindle-shaped interspaces, in all probability outgrowths of the pear-shaped. *Third,* small spindle-shaped interspaces which at an early stage are found throughout the lens. *Fourth,* small and large globules dispersed through all the lamellae. *Fifth,* fine dust-like opacities which occur at an early stage throughout the cloudy zone. In the beginning the interspaces appear perfectly transparent, like capillary tubes filled with clear fluid; later on, they appear as though covered by a delicate veil; then the cloudiness becomes more saturated and the contours more sharply defined, until finally they coalesce with neighboring interspaces. These cloudy interspaces extend either uniformly toward the centre or they sit as radii on the equator." As the cataractous process goes on, they coalesce, forming band-like processes, which surround the equator of the lens, or they extend inward toward the centre of the axis of the lens as prismatic sectors. As has been stated above, Becker looked upon these interspaces as the result of interference with the otherwise regularly progressing sclerosis of the lens, and as a result a less intimate and regular connection between the individual lamellae; the first demonstrable sign of an interference with the formation of a nucleus. In these interspaces the tissue fluid stagnates, undergoes chemical changes and leads to degenerative processes in the lens fibres themselves. "The originally normal fluid which has an index of refraction equal to that of the formative elements of the lens, after a time stagnates in these spaces, and thus leads to abnormal processes of diffusion between itself and the contents of the lens fibres. As a result, it withdraws from the lens fibres a part of their contents and give up a part of its own. This leads to disturbance of nutrition, which in turn leads to an alteration in the chemical constitution of the tissue fluid and the lens fibres, and these changes are manifested by a change in the index of refraction of both the stagnant fluid and the lens fibres."[5]

Priestly Smith, in a paper read before the Opthal Society,[6] expressed a similar opinion, stating: "In the tabulated results the relation of senility to the development of cataract comes out clearly. Lenses which showed any opacity were distinguished from others and were found when tabulated to be, on the average, smaller than transparent lenses of the same age. As this difference was present even when the opacities were very slight, it

---

5 Becker At. P., p. 58.
6 Med. Times and Gazette, January 20, 1883.

seemed likely that a period of diminished rate of growth preceded the formation of the opacities of senile cataract and were in most cases limited to the equatorial zone, where the capsule and the cortical layers of the lens were subjected to the traction of the suspensory ligament." Thus he supports Becker's conclusions quoted above.

By the recognition of this heretofore overlooked factor, namely, that those *lenses in which senile cataract has begun to develop have a lesser volume than lenses of the same age which are free from opacities*, we certainly have advanced greatly in our understanding of the genesis of senile cataract. Hence the splitting and fissuring of the cortical substance will be followed by a degree of shrinkage, greater than the physiological retrogressive process.

The sclerosing process proceeds differently in different individuals. It may go on uninterruptedly to extreme old age. Becker states that he observed a yellow nucleus and clear cortical substance with vision equal to 6-9 in an individual ninety-four years of age. In other cases the lens is changed into a dry, hard brown mass up to the very capsule, which, without any cloudiness appearing in the pupillary area, absorbs so much light as to materially impair vision. (Cataracta nigra.) Again, the process is arrested when it reaches certain peripheric lamellae, the nucleus separates from the cortex, and the latter disintegrates, the products of which when they have reached their greatest degree, absorb so much light that simply quantitative perception remains. (*Cataracta senilis matura*). The sclerosed nucleus suffers no further change except in cases where the condition remains for a long time; the outer lamellae may then become softened and melt away. As the cataractous process goes on, the volume of the lens increases, and the more rapidly, the more cloudiness develops. After the cortical cloudiness is complete and attains its greatest volume, the volume again becomes lessened and the cataractous mass begins to thicken. The taking up is followed by the giving off, of water. In the course of this reduction, a stage is reached in which the volume of the lens equals that of a senile lens. (Arlt's "Stage of Ripeness.") This is followed by the stage of over-ripeness characterized by a reduction in the volume of the lens, and the appearance of whitish, punctate and striated opaque spots on the inner surface of the anterior capsule and by the disappearance of the hitherto recognizable radial arrangement of the lens fibres.

For the further retrogressive metamorphosis, we are forced to assume entirely different changes in the lens. Either the cortical substance becomes more and more thickened, accompanied by the formation of capsular cataract, or the cortex gradually becomes a fluid pasty mass, in which is found an abundance of cholesterine and chalky deposits, and in which the nucleus finally sinks to the bottom (*Cataracta Morgagni*).

On microscopical examination, these splits and interspaces are found to be filled with coagulated albuminous globules. Innumerable direct observations have settled this as an unassailable fact, and this has been especially demonstrated in lenses which, during life, had shown signs of *cataracta incipiens,* and have conclusively proven, that it is these formations which are the cause of the first opacities in the cortex of incipient cataract. These are the so-called "*Morgagni's globules,*" and have long ago been observed in posterior cortical cataract. It must, however, remain an undecided question as to whether this fluid coagulates into globules during life, or whether this is simply the result of a cooling off of the body after death, or due to the action of the hardening fluid, or due to both the latter. Due to the influence of the changed fluid in these interspaces, the fibres undergo a variety of changes, all the various degrees of which can be observed without any difficulty under the microscope, beginning with the punctate molecular cloudiness of the fibres up to highly refracting droplets, from the irregularly serrated borders of the fibres up to the transverse striations; from the tumesence to the gradual transition into cylindrical tubes. The first stage of disintegration, the dislocation of the lamellae one against the other, the breaking down, disintegration and total destruction of the individual fibres, the formation of albuminous globules, molecular pasty masses, calcareous granules, fat, cholesterine crystals, can all be observed under a low power of the microscope.

If a nucleus has formed, the cataract as a rule must develop in those portions of the lens which are not yet sclerosed. The older the individual at the time the cataract begins to form, the larger, generally speaking, will be the nucleus which is surrounded by the cataractous mass; whereas the younger the individual at the time the cataract begins to form, the easier will it be for the entire lens to become cataractous. But no sharp line between nucleus and cortex can be drawn, estimated by the age; it is an exceedingly rare occurrence to find the centre of a lens undergoing cataractous changes after a nucleus has once formed. In those cases where the centre of the lens is first attacked, it is still an undecided question whether the cataractous process had been preceded by the formation of a nucleus, or whether it had occurred as a result of the failure of a nucleus to properly form.

CATARACT IN YOUTHFUL LENSES.

The causation of the spontaneous development of soft cataracts in youthful individuals is still wrapped in the deepest darkness. Anatomical investigations are entirely wanting, and our knowledge is therefore entirely restricted to the results of clinical investigation. The only case which Becker was enabled to examine anatomically was obtained from a diabetic patient, a girl nineteen years of age. It is a well-settled fact that a developing diabetic soft cataract of a youthful individual differs in no way in its appearance from any other soft cataract of youth. The lens is tumescent, shows the well-known pearly grey, radially-arranged silky opacities which aid us in recognizing the arrangement of the lens fibres around the anterior pole; between these are the dark striations which are to be looked upon as the interspaces filled with the transparent fluid. *The traumatic cataract* has exactly the same appearance when it occurs in a youthful individual. Examination of such traumatic cataracts and the diabetic cataract has shown that they have this in common, that the interspaces and splits are especially pronounced and numerous, between the lamellae and the fibres, and that they are undoubtedly the cause of the opacities. It is worthy of special emphasis that the dark striations between the silky striations which seem to be due to splits, on anatomical examination of traumatic cataracts were found in reality to be due to splits. It is further worthy of note, that if one takes a lens denuded of its capsule and exposes it to the air until it is perfectly dry, it will split up similarly into small sectors. Robinski[7] makes mention of the same fact. Hence, in the development of soft cataract of youthful individuals, we are likewise dealing with a splitting up of the lens, and in these cases the peripheric lamellae are first attacked, the more centrally located, later on. Here the cloudiness of the lens, as it appears to the one making the examination, as well as the impermeability to light in the eye so affected, is caused by the difference in the index of refraction of the lamellae as they are superimposed one over the other. Undoubtedly the individual lens fibres, and the lamellae composed of these, possess a greater index of refraction than the fluid which has accumulated between them. Though it be true that the fluid which accumulates in the interspaces in incipient senile cataract is simply tissue fluid which is normally present, but in increased quantity, it is equally true that in the soft cataracts of youthful individuals the fluid which occupies these interspaces has from the very beginning gained entrance in an abnormal way, namely, by diffusion, from without into the capsule sac. This seems to be attested by the fact, that the substance which occupies these interspaces has an index of refraction about equal to that of the aqueous. In traumatic cataracts the source of this fluid is

---

7 Augen Linsen Staare der Menschen und der Wirbelthiere Centralblatt f. d. Med. Wiss., 1877, Nos. 3 and 4.

evident. It enters through the wound in the capsule. Subsequently, streams of diffusion between the fluid which has entered and the contents of the lens fibres, as well as between the lens and the aqueous through the capsule will take part. This hypothesis seems necessary because at times we find the capsule closes again, and still the opacities increase.

From the very beginning we have assumed streams of diffusion to explain the development of diabetic cataract.

Even in the consecutive cataracts of youthful individuals, the appearance is exactly that of the foregoing. Under such circumstances there develops, even in very advanced old age, as the result of the rapid taking up of water, a cataract with a soft cortex, and it appears that it may even soften up a sclerosed nucleus. In these cases, no other explanation seems possible than that the addition of a pathologically changed nutritive fluid has led to this splitting up. The taking up of water, the stage of tumesence in the soft cataract, just as in the senile cataract, is to be looked upon as the second stage of the formation of cataract.

The subsequent changes are almost identical with those of senile cataract; only that we find appearing in the fibres of youthful individuals, especially after discission or a trauma, the well-known and frequently described *vacuoles* in large numbers. The wavy contours of the tumescent peripheric fibres are very striking. Finally, the entire lens seems to take part in the cataractous degeneration, there being no hard nucleus. It seems much easier for calcareous deposits to take place in this final stage than in cataracts occurring in old age.

CHAPTER III.

THE PATHOLOGICAL CHANGES IN THE INTRACAPSULAR CELLS.

CAPSULAR CATARACT.

A. THE DEGENERATIVE CHANGES.

The degenerative processes are sharply differentiated from the phenomena of physiological retrogression already described. If one may be permitted to so express himself, the latter consists of an atrophy of the nuclei and cells, whereas we are here dealing with a metamorphosis beginning in the nucleus, then affecting the entire cell; as a result the cells become changed into a pathological substance, the chemical nature of which has not been as yet fully determined.

H. Muller, in his first essay on this subject,[1a] describes two kinds of deposits on the inner surface of the anterior capsule. He states, "Some of these extend over the surface and seem in profile as striations which are easily differentiated from the capsule; for a certain distance they may show a regular degree of thickness. On the other hand, they may form plaques, with no evident connection with one another. Either they are adherent by a broad flat base, or they form globules or tenpin-like structures, which show great similarity to the papillae of the descemetis or the isolated "Drusen" (warty, hyaline excrescences) of the vitreous lamellae of the choroid." The substance which forms these structures is very much like the capsule itself is transparent, and refracts the light. Again, it may not show such a perfectly regular, homogenous structure, but show yellowish lighter and darker spots, even granular masses.

This latter form of deposit, which Muller has described as bearing such a close similarity to the Drusen of the choroid, Becker states, he was enabled to study from its very incipiency. The cataract was preserved five weeks in a 45 per cent. solution of alcohol, the capsule was stained with haemotoxylin, and a portion was then imbedded and cut; the larger portion was put up in glycerine. The specimen having grown pale in course of time, it was stained again with haemotoxylin and eosin, and then put up in Canada balsam. This specimen showed long stretches of well preserved epithelium and beautiful nuclei, nearly all the nuclei being at rest. At other places the nuclei show that they are undergoing most peculiar changes, without showing any particular changes as to size or form, they show that they are all more or less advanced in undergoing a change into a homogenous, reddish brown, highly refracting substance, so that but one portion has taken up the blue coloring matter. Due to this change, the chromatic substance is gradually pushed into a very narrow peripheral zone. The contours of the cells are, however, well defined and distinctly seen. When the nucleus has undergone a complete change, owing to the taking up of material from without, it becomes enlarged, but for a considerable time it retains its globular form. The protoplasmic portion of the cells gradually disappears, since the globular, glassy (hyaline) masses which fill out the nuclei touch each other, and finally melt into one mass, thus forming the "Drusig" (hyaline) figures, which assume the most characteristic forms, and frequently extend over large areas. In these globular, at times flattened "Drusen," I have found stained nuclei enclosed. In all cases they are surrounded at their edges by nuclei, showing evidences of karyokinesis. Sometimes the nuclei are smaller, then again larger, and can be plainly seen to surround these excrescences.

This capsule showed these formations in all their various stages, beginning

---

1a Untersuchungen uber die Glashute des Auges, etc.; und Uber die Anatomische Verhaltnisse des Kapselstaars. Wurzburger Sitzungsberichte, 1856, p. 254.

with the isolated nuclei just beginning to show changes up to the complicated formations 1.5 mm. in length, 1 mm. in width, and 0.5 mm. in height. At times this colloid (?) substance is covered with stained nuclei; again but a few are scattered around the base and edges; again, the interior of the hyaline mass is perfectly free, with but a few nuclei scattered around the edges.

It is not often that one has the opportunity of observing, as in the above specimen, so distinctly, through all its stages of development, the development of these hyaline masses out of the nuclei of the epithelium. There is, however, scarcely a capsule, covering a senile cataract which has existed for any length of time, on which one can not discover various stages in the development of these hyaline excrescences.

The frequency of this anatomical condition corresponds to the round, white, light reflecting spots frequently observed on the inner surface of the anterior capsule, in over-ripe cataracts, mention of which was made above.

B. NEW CELLULAR FORMATIONS WHICH DEVELOP FROM THE INTRACAPSULAR CELLS.

a. REGENERATIVE NEW CELLULAR FORMATION.

In close proximity to the above-described hyaline excrescences (Drusen), one always finds a greater or less number of nuclei which take the stain with avidity, are small, and show karyokinetic figures. Not infrequently one finds perfect nests of these nuclei. On focusing these very carefully, one discovers that they are no longer in the same niveau as the capsular epithelium, but seem to ascend on the sides of these excrescences. In cases in which these Drusen are very extensive on the inner surface of the capsule, these new-formed cells often take on great dimensions. They not only completely cover these excrescences on their inner surface, but they seem to project into its very substance. *However, it still remains a question, whether these excrescences, surrounded as they are by strands of cells, are not from their very beginning formed from other cells which these enclose. Thus one form of capsular cataract is described.*

b. THE PROCESSES AND PRODUCTS OF ATROPHIC NEW CELLULAR FORMATIONS.

Aside from the above-described cellular new formations around the hyaline excrescences, Becker states that he was successful in finding on the inner surface of every senile cataract which he examined, *new cellular formations.* As they have exceptionally been observed in lenses which showed no cloudiness, they can not be looked upon either as the cause of cataract formation, or as one of its sequences. He rather suggests that the same cause which, during the senile sclerosis, is active in producing the lenticular cataract, likewise induces this new cellular formation. He further makes the emphatic statement, that *all new formations of cells within the uninjured capsule always take their origin from the cellular elements which are normally present, that is, from the capsular epithelium in its more restricted sense, further from the cells along the whorl, and possibly from those cells which have become changed into fibres.* As a result of this active hyperphasia, we meet with an *epithelial covering on the inner surface of the posterior capsule*; also, *large vesicular cells* which are frequently located both in the anterior and posterior cortical substance; also, *nests of these* are at times found *in the equatorial region*, which greatly simulate the hyaline excresences spoken of above, as well as the *true capsular cataracts.*

There are various methods of proving that there is a hyperphasia of the epithelium during the formation of cataract. Nuclear fission is undoubted evidence. During the whole of life, the size and form of the nuclei of a normal human capsular epithelium show an astonishing regularity. A surface view shows them to be circular and with a diameter of 0.005 mm., and equally far removed on all sides from the borders of the protoplasm. Therefore, when in a case of cataract we find a portion of the epithelium of absolutely normal size, form and position, and again in other places find the size of the cells, their form and their nuclei materially changed from the normal, this of itself is evidence of a hyperphasia, a pathological new formation, even when the cells are found where epithelium is normally found and when arranged as a single layer.

a. EPITHELIAL COVERING OF THE POSTERIOR CAPSULE.

When epithelial cells are found at places where under normal conditions they are absent, there can be no doubt, but that we are dealing with a new cellular formation. Even H. Muller observed, that at times in cataractous lenses a layer of epithelium clothed the inner surface of the posterior capsule. Iwanoff, Gayet, Becker and others verified this statement years ago.

H. Muller (cited above, p. 269) states, "There appears also to be a hyperphasia of cells, as I have several times found a layer of irregular cells on the posterior capsule." He refers to this again in his following publications (pp. 264, 266, 277, 283). Iwanoff studied this condition of the epithelium in eyes which had been enucleated on account of disease. He states,[1] "The cells which are most sensitive and earliest affected by

---

1 Beitrag zur Path. Anatomie des Hernhaut und Linsen Epithel. Pagenstechers Klin Beobachtungen, Bd. III, p. 126.

irritation are the formative cells of the lens." Every time one of the above diseased conditions begins to act, the lens swells and the *formative* cells are affected. The product of these formative cells is normally epithelial cells arranged on the inner surface of the anterior capsule, as new lens fibres and as *epithelium on the posterior capsule.* This new-formed epithelium seldom has the attributes of normal epithelium. In most cases it appears more swollen, the nuclei easily undergo fission, and in fact appears to possess but little viability(?). The epithelium on the posterior capsule easily undergoes degeneration, (colloid, mucoid), hence one so often sees these large, transparent, variously shaped vesicles, containing a nucleus which has been pushed to one side."

H. Muller made all his investigations on cataractous lenses. Hence it is of interest to note that he likewise drew attention to the rapid disintegration of the nuclei of these new-formed epithelial cells, and he likewise looks upon the equatorial zone as their source of origin. Gayet [2] likewise investigated the question. He believed that as a result of the formation of these vesicular cells, which are altered epithelial cells, the neighboring normal epithelial cells are pushed aside, and as a result are found along the posterior capsule.

Becker states that he is satisfied that "the epithelial covering of the posterior capsule is derived from the surface growth of the anterior epithelium. This, however, can only begin to act when the lens whorl, as such, has ceased to exist." He denies the existence of the so-called *formative* cells in the sense in which von Becker used them: he states, however, that "the pathological production of new cells takes place, nevertheless, from that region where normally the growth and regeneration of the epithelium takes place. The cells, however, as they are forced backward, are not changed into lens fibres through the medium of the lens whorl, since either the lens whorl no longer exists, or since the mechanical conditions themselves are changed. As a result, the cells are pushed past the position of the whorl, far backward, and thus to a greater or less extent cover the inner surface of the posterior capsule. On this account, changes along the lens whorl in cataracts are of great importance. In fact, it seems that whenever a cataract has advanced to any degree, the connection between the whorl and the capsule, also with the youngest fibres, is loosened up."

The mechanical conditions are changed insofar, that the new cells need no longer overcome so much pressure, and thus can push and force themselves on the one hand in between the epithelium and the posterior

---

[2] Sur un Point d'Histologie de la Cataracte Capsulaire. Lyon Medic., XXXIII. p. 15.

capsule, and the lens fibres, on the other hand, relatively speaking, without any hindrance whatever, and under much less pressure, hence they develop into the large vesicular cells directly to be described, or, as epithelial cells, permit themselves to push backward to the posterior capsule. In complicated cataracts one can often accurately follow the direction which they take.

As compared with the epithelial cells on the posterior capsule which disclose departures from the normal, we frequently meet with vesicular cells in the region of the whorl.

There can be no doubt but that these new cells again produce cells. Not only are these large vesicular cells formed, but in rare cases, structures which are identical with the so-called capsular cataracts of the anterior capsule. Both the pseudo-epithelium on the posterior capsule, as well as those vesicular cells along the equator, show the presence of elongated nuclei poorly stained, the karyokinetic changes very indistinct and the cells very much enlarged. Becker expresses the belief that these cells may reproduce other cells, but at the same time acknowledges that he never observed karyokinetic changes in the nuclei of the pseudo-epithelium nor in the vesicular cells.

b. WEDL'S VESICULAR CELLS.

BLASCHENFORMIGEN ZELLEN. These cellular vesicles, which were first described by Wedl and later by Iwanoff, Knies and others, have a twofold origin. They are either products of the posterior capsule, or the cells at the whorl which have undergone enormous distension, or they are developed from the fully-developed lens fibres, due to a very peculiar change in the contents of the fibre around the nucleus. These cells are never found wanting in examination of senile cataracts, especially in the diabetic and congenital cataracts.

Neither Wedl, Iwanoff, Knies nor Becker offer an explanation as to their origin. The only one who has decided their origin is Gaylet.[3] He believes that during the formation of a capsular cataract he has discovered similar changes to those which H. Leloir[4] has described as occurring in the rete malpigi during the formation of smallpox pustules.

"Around the nucleus of the cell there is developed a white zone, which gradually enlarges at the expense of the protoplasm of the cell, at the same time pressing the nucleus to one side, and thus materially enlarging the cell. Thus

[3] Sur un Point d'Histologie de la Cataracte Capsulaire. Lyon Med. XXXIII, p. 15.
[4] Contribution a l'etude Formation des Pustules et des Vesicules sur la peu et les Muqueuses. Arch. d Physiologie Normal et Pathologie, 1880, p. 307.

the cell becomes changed into a vesicle. In which the nucleus atrophies, and gradually undergoes a fatty degeneration. These greatly enlarged vesicular cells, owing to pressure against each other, assume polyhedral shapes. and press those cells which have not undergone such a change into characteristic angular shapes; they then become granular, and finally disappear. This vesicular degeneration of the epithelial cells necessarily leads to a surface enlargement of the entire epithelial layer, and according to Gayet explains the cause for the spreading of the epithelium to the posterior capsule."

Becker denies that he has ever noted such changes during the formation of these vesicular cells, and states that we do not as yet possess a satisfactory explanation of this peculiar change. Is this hyaline or colloid, or is it a peculiar hydropsie of the individual cells?

The vesicular changes are most easily studied along the equatorial line of secondary cataracts, and in all probability a study of their development here will aid us in clearing up the processes which form the basis of this change. Since the days of Vrolick and Sommering we know that after a reclination or extraction the cells along the lens whorl remain in the capsule. After the operation the production of cells springs up anew. However, the mechanical conditions being changed, these cells become flat, and on cross section are no longer six-sided lens fibres. but assume irregular polyhedral shapes, similar to the vesicular cells found in cataracts within uninjured capsules. The pressure being removed, the lens fibres along the equatorial region, those which have remained dormant for years, become active again, and now being developed under a reduced pressure. do not form fibres, but assume polyhedral shapes. Becker describes a second mode of development. A peculiar change of the protoplasm around the nucleus occurs in the cells at the equator. It becomes thickened, more highly refractive, involves either the entire thickness of the fibre, or leaves a portion of the substance of the fibre to one side, and thus seems to become constructed at first into an elliptical, finally into a globular disk. All this time the nucleus appears to be at rest. Notwithstanding the great difference which exists regarding the mode of development of the vesicular cells, the question must still remain an unanswered one. as to whether they possess anything more in common than their form. Concerning the relation of these cells to cataract formation, these differences are of but little moment, since the cells developed according to the second method are very few.

The large cells are especially prone to degeneration. Their nuclei show all the evidences of a gradual death. The borders of the cells become indistinct and the contents of neighboring cells run together, forming a homogenous mass. Iwanoff designated this change as colloid or mucoid.

Since the occurrence of mucin in the capsule sac has not been proven and since this changed product does not give the reaction of colloid material, both names are improper. Becker states that it would be more correct to speak of them as hydropsical cells. The supposition that the disintegration of the vesicular cells aids in bringing about the fluidity in cases of cataracta Morgagni has much in its favor.

Becker's view, that all capsular cataracts are the result of a hyperplasia of the capsular epithelium, is today accepted. He believed (Anatomy, p. 76) that the hyaline processes of the newly developed cells in some manner softened up the capsule, worked their way in between the layers (?) of thé capsule, thus splitting it, and that the capsular cataract then developed in this space.

As long ago as 1858, H. Muller drew attention to the great similarity between capsular cataracts and connective tissue, and up to within a few years this formed one of the nicest questions in the whole range of the study of ocular pathology. General pathology teaches that connective tissue structures must be formed from cells of the mesoderm, and hence can not be derived from the ectoderm. Manfredi [4] attempted to overcome the difficulties in the way, by declaring that a capsular cataract could only form after an injury to the capsule, and where it had been made possible for cells of the mesoderm—that is, connective tissue cells—to gain entrance, and thus further produce connective tissue cells; and thus he positively asserts that capsular cataracts is a connective tissue structure. Leber [5] bases his utterances on examination made on capsular cataracts experimentally produced. He expressly states, that he excluded all elements which might have entered from without. Notwithstanding this, he designates the tissue of a "true" or "genuine" capsular cataract as *connective, tissue-like,* and states that he verified to his own satisfaction "that from a tissue which originates from the ectoderm, hence which is a true epithelial tissue, a substance can be produced which has the structure of connective tissue." Becker struck the proper chord, when he pointed out, that this question would eventually be settled as the result of chemical investigation.

The question presents different features when there has been a solution of continuity of the capsule. Here one can not so easily exclude the entrance of foreign elements. Nevertheless, as the result of two series of

---

4 "Discussion sur la Cataracte Capsulaire." Compte rendu du Congres Periodique Internat. d Opthal. de Milan, 1881.

5 "Zur Pathol. der Linse." Zehender's Klin. Monatsblatt. Beilageheft, p. 33. Verh. der Heidelberg Gesell, 1878.

experimental investigations pursued under the direction of Prof. Leber, R. Wengler,[5a] and R. Schuchard,[5b] the position was taken that capsular circatrices are due to a hyperphasia of capsular epithelium, whereas in a later work by C. Schlosser[5c] the old view is asserted that the cicatrix is of connective tissue origin. He states that the capsular cicatrix is made up of connective tissue fibres, the only portion which is of epithelial origin being the layer of epithelial cells and the structureless membrane which separates the cicatrix from the lens proper. But he ignores entirely the question, from whence these connective tissue cells may come. This whole subject has finally been most scientifically investigated by Otto Schirmer.[6] He first studied the formation of artificially produced capsular cicatrices in rabbits' eyes.

CAPSULAR CICATRICES.

Immediately upon rupturing the capsule, the aqueous acts on the lens fibres, causes them to swell up, and unless the rupture is very great, the opening is soon plugged up by a thin, fibrinous covering which clothes the point where the defect in the capsule exists. Examinations made during the first few days show present in this fibrinous exudate two kinds of nuclei; first, degenerated forms of epithelial and lens fibre nuclei, and second, a few leucocytes. Schirmer states that he found a fully formed cicatrix as early as the third day. He looks upon this regenerative process as the result of a hyperphasia of the capsular epithelium because: First, the defect heals from the margin; second, the cicatrix gradually goes over the normal capsule; third, because at the beginning the cicatrix has a peculiar structure consisting of spindle cells without the presence of an intercellular substance; fourth, because of the possibility of demonstrating all the gradual, intermediate steps between epithelial and spindle cells; fifth, the epithelial appearance of the nuclei in the cicatrix; sixth, the lack of pigment; and, finally, seventh, because of the relatively small number of cells found in the fibrinous membrane which have a different appearance from the general mass of cells found in the cicatrix."

Following the formation of the cicatrix, the fibrinous veil on the surface is absorbed by the aqueous, and no doubt the cells which it encloses are destroyed at the same time. In the course of the next few weeks this

---

[5a] Uber die Heilungs Vorgange nach Verletzungen der Vodern Linsenkapsel. Inaug. Dissert, Goettingen, 1874.

[5b] "Zur Path. Anatomie der Discission." Inaug. Dissert, Goettingen, 1878.

[5c] Experimentelle Studie uber Traumatische Cataract. Munchen, 1887.

[6] "Histologische und Histochemische Untersuchungen uber das Physiologische Wachsthum und die Structure der Vodern Linsenkapsel." Otto Schirmer, Graef Arch., XXXV. B. 1, 1889.

cicatrix gives one the impression of becoming smaller. About the middle of the first month, one observes that the epithelium gradually extends as a single layer over the inner surface of the cicatrix, until it finally entirely covers in the cicatrix. At once the epithelium begins to excrete a vitreous lamella of new capsular substance, which gradually increases in thickness, and in every case this new-formed substance can be followed for a certain distance on to the old capsule. In the beginning we are dealing with spindle cells, later they are imbedded in a hyaline substance which the spindle cells excrete.[7] In course of time the nuclei all disappear and there is left a homogenous cicatrical tissue, covered by a layer of epithelial cells and the vitreous lamella, and with this stage, the process of the formation of a capsular cicatrix is completed. As a rule, the injury causes a minute, circumscript area of disintegration of lens tissue, surrounded by transparent lens substance, and as the new lens fibres develop and increase in length and extend toward the anterior pole, they force their way between the cicatrix and the mass of detritus, so that a "cavity of detritus" is formed which is gradually forced toward the centre of the lens.

TRUE CAPSULAR CATARACT.

Here there has never been a rupture of the capsule, hence there can be no question as to the origin of the new structure, it being the result entirely of the hyperplasia of epithelial cells. It is immaterial whether this be a congenital formation; that is, developed during foetal life; whether it develop during childhood, be the result of a blenorrhoea neonatorum or otherwise caused corneal perforation, a primary cataract formation, or secondary to senile cataract, or whether it be a partial phenomenon of a *cataracta consecutiva* or the principal portion of a *cataracta secundaria* (still to be considered) or of a traumatic cataract (as has been demonstrated above), *all are the result of a hyperphasia of the capsular epithelium.*

Becker states (Anatomie, p. 75). "Depending on some cause as yet unknown to us, this hyperplasia may at once undergo a retrogressive metamorphosis, and as a result of a repetition of the original process lead to the formation of a capsular cataract of a greater or less thickness." The original hyperplasia of epithelial cells may be looked upon as the *first stage*. Next, these cells elongate and take on spindle shapes, *not connective tissue*), and imbed themselves in a peculiar hyaline substance which they themselves excrete, and this forms the *second stage*. This is followed by a surface growth across this new formation of the normal capsular epi-

[7] Leber—"Zur Pathologie der Linse." Bericht der 11th Opth. Gesellshaft, Heidelberg, 1878.

thelium, the *third stage*, and finally this normal epithelium excretes a hyaline substance, exactly like the true capsular substance, the *fourth stage*. If the causative factor continues, a second capsular cataract may develop from this epithelial layer, etc. Becker tried hard to prove that the membrane which covers the capsular cataract is derived from a splitting of the true capsule. Schirmer, however, showed that this theory is not tenable, because, first, "this is an excretion of the capsular epithelium; secondly, why should it be possible for cells to get in between the layers and split the vitreous lamellae from within, when it has been shown to be an impossibility to do so from without? Further, these splits could only be followed as fine lines, but no one ever observed a veritable separation, nor has anyone ever recorded the observation of the beginning of such a split." The fact that one seldom finds the capsular cataract completely covered with epithelium is possibly due to the growth of the cataract. The age of the patient may play an important role, for Schirmer noted that in senile cataracts the epithelial covering of the capsular cataract is not so complete as in the complicated cases which occur most frequently in younger individuals.

The structure of the true capsular cataract bears a striking likeness to connective tissue. Teased specimens morphologically were shown to have the same structure as the capsular cicatrices.

Schirmer, using Ewald and Kuhne's digestive method (referred to on page 26) as his main stay, chemically tested capsular cicatrices and capsular cataracts and found them both to consist of identical tissue, which does *not* give the same reaction as connective tissue. Both gave the same reaction as the capsule, a not inconsiderable proof that the capsule, as well as its pathological formations, are derived from the same source, namely, *products of the epithelium of the anterior capsule.*

Schirmer, using a very simple apparatus, made his experiments in the following manner: Two small dishes, one a little larger than the other, were placed on top of each other, so as to form a wet chamber. A third smaller one was placed inside of these, and this latter was covered with a glass slide. During the experiments just sufficient fluid (salicylic acid solution, 0.5 per cent.) was placed in the wet chamber so as just to touch the glass slide. The digestive process was either carried on in the small dish, or more frequently on the glass slide. In the latter method, the cover glass was supported on the one side by a piece of glass fastened to the slide, thus forming a triangular chamber, in which the object to be tested was placed, and here it could likewise be observed under high powers of the microscope. The digestive solution was made from the extract of the pancreas of the calf, to which was added five times its weight of a 0.5 per cent. solution of salicylic acid, and then kept for several hours at 40 degrees C., and after this had cooled it was filtered.

He first verified Kuhne's experiments, and also found that connective tissue is *not* digestable; but that it is easily digestable if previously acidulated, and then heated to 70 degrees. Control experiments were made at the same time with normal capsular substance. Normal capsules of pigs' and rabbits' lenses were easily digested in from five to six hours. Allowing them to remain in alcohol for eight days did not alter this power, whereas, if allowed to remain for several months, the tissues were decidedly more resistent, and always left a flaky mass behind. If the sections were imbedded in celloidin, they could be left for days in the digestive fluid without being acted on. Since alcohol and ether did not delay the digestion, one must assume that the celloidin penetrated the tissue and made it indigestable. If the capsule was previously treated with 1 per cent. osmic acid solution, then washed out in water, the capsule became more resistant, and all the more so the longer the capsule had remained in the osmic acid.

Capsular cicatrices and capsular cataracts gave identically the same reaction to trypsin as did the normal capsule.

The Boiling Experiment.—It is well known that boiling will lead to a solution of fibrillae, and on cooling lead to the formation of a jelly. According to Arnold and Ritter,[8] after boiling for several hours, a solution does take place, but no jelly forms on cooling. One centimeter of water is sufficient to dissolve the anterior capsule. Capsular cataracts and capsular cicatrices showed the same properties, but did not form a jelly on cooling. Thin pieces of connective tissue allowed to swell up in a 1 per cent. solution of sulphuric acid; here the fibrillae dissolve in water at 40 degrees C., and the flocculi which remain consists of elastic tissues and cells. The capsule, capsular cicatrices and capsular cataracts do not dissolve in similar treatment.

The slight resistance of the capsule to strong acids is well known, especially to nitric acid, which in but moderative concentration, can bring about solution. The same is true of capsular cicatrices and capsular cataracts. The reaction is especially characteristic as compared with elastic tissue.

Schirmer's conclusions, which are generally accepted today, are as follows:

"*First.* Capsular cataracts and capsular cicatrices develop from the anterior capsular epithelium without the aid of other tissues.

"*Second.* Both are a tissue *sui generis*, morphologically like connective tissue, chemically differing from this, but both capsular cicatrices and cataracts are alike.

"*Third.* Chemically, aside from the cells, both are identical with the capsular substance. Morphologically, both forms of capsular cataracts

---

8 Die Linse und das Strahlen Platchen. Graef Saemisch Handbuch, Bd. 1, S. 288 and 216, 1874.

consist of elongated ('band-like') cells, which are imbedded in a vitreous-like substance. The latter is a product of the former.

"*Fourth.* The pigment which is at times found in the cicatrix is derived from the iris, and is largely carried there by the leucocytes.

"*Fifth.* The delicate vitreous lamella which is found in the older capsular cicatrix and capsular cataracts is excreted by the epithelial covering, which in such cases is always found between the cicatrix and the cells. This lamella grows with the age of the cicatrix.

"*Sixth.* If this lamella can be followed into the capsule adjacent to the cicatrix or capsular cataract, one will note that this is not a split in the original capsule, but that this capsular substance is likewise newly formed. The line of demarcation between the old and the new capsular substance is the optical expression of an interference with the regular and continuous excretion by the capsular epithelium."

Foreign substances enclosed in the capsular cicatrices and cataracts, Becker states,[9] "with the exception of calcareous concretions, and rarely observed cholesterine crystals and very peculiar highly refracting masses, which for want of a better name he designated as colloid, no other substances are found. These are to be looked upon as the result of disintegration and precipitation, and of chemical decomposition in the already formed cataracts, hence formed *in situ.*"

"It is worthy of especial mention that the calcareous deposits are always around the cellular elements in the intercellular spaces in the form of amorphous granules, but at times they form veritable deposits even to actual formation of stalactites as H. Muller expresses it. This expression, however, may only be correct as far as the form goes, for stalactites are always crystalline structures and I have never seen calcareous crystals in the lens." (Becker, p. 77).

As long ago as 1838, Muller stated that the capsule formed an absolute barrier against the entrance of foreign elements. Becker likewise contended that as long as the capsule remained intact it formed an absolute barrier against the entrance of any foreign body. At one time it was supposed that the capsule of the lens possessed stomata, (Morana), then again it was supposed that the white blood corpuscles could pass through the capsule by diapedesis. Deutschman [10] quotes Floriani [11] as expressing himself in favor of the endogenous formation of pus. Deutschman, however, de-

9 Anatomie, p. 77.

10 "Die Veranderungen in der Linse bei Eiterprocessen im Auge." Arch. f. Opth., Bd. XXVI, 1, p. 134.

11 Studio Experimentelle Sulla Inflammatione del Cristallino. Anna di Ottal, 1871, p. 145-189.

nies this, and, like Julie Sinclair,[11a] he explicitly states that the entrance of pus is always preceded by destruction of the capsule. Since the lens is an epithelial structure, the pus cells must come from without. In cases where there had been an injury to the capsule, their presence was easily explained, but it has been known for a long time that there are cases of spontaneous purulent inflammation in which the presence of the pus cells could not be so easily explained. The question to be decided was, did the cells wander through the capsule by diapedesis, or was the capsule first destroyed as the result of a "melting away" of the tissue?

In his experimental investigations, Deutschman (quoted as above) demonstrated that a local perforation and softening of the capsule did occur, and that entrance to the pus cells was thus given, and he concluded that before this occurred not a single pus cell could enter, though the lens be imbedded in pus. Both Leber [12] and Wagenman [13] corroborated these investigations. Leber states: "Aside from the larger holes, numerous microscopical perforations are observed, in which solitary or groups of cells are found, and between these cocci." Wagenman suggested that it appeared as though the cocci first entered the capsule, and that the pus cells then followed. Otherwise, he states, it would be difficult to explain why these perforations should occur in circumscribed areas, rather than attack the entire surface of the capsule to an equal degree. Thus there still remained to be explained, what it is that produces this softening and "melting down" of the capsule. This Leber has done in his exhaustive, critical and experimental work, "Die Entstehung der Entzundung und der Wirkung der Entzundung erregenden Schadlichkeiten," Leipsig, 1891; and he has made it the subject of special observation and criticism in the 38th chapter, "Purulent softening and 'melting down' of tissues." He states (p. 528) that "a purulent exudate free of microbes contains an *enzym* which has a fluidifying effect on fibrin, gellatin and dead animal tissue; that *this enzym is produced by the leucocytes*, but acts independently of them on surrounding tissues. In purulent inflammations this *enzym* is the principal factor in dissolving fibrin and animal tissues, and also in preventing the coagulation of fibrin. The prevention of coagulation is due to the fact that the fibrinogen in the exudate or the already coagulated fibrin is converted into a non-coaguble pepton-like substance by the action of the

11a Experimentelle Untersuchungen ur Genese der Erworbenen Kapsel Cataract. Inaug. Dissert, 1876.

12 Bericht uber die XX Vers. d'Opth. Gessel, 1889. Zehender's M., B. 1, XXVII, Beilagh Heft., 8-45.

13 "Uber die von Operationsnarben und Vernarbten Iris vorfallen augehende Glaskorper eiterung." Von Graef Arch., XXXV, 4, S. 140-144, 1889.

enzym produced by the pus cells." He further expresses the belief that the solution of organic substances taken up in the cells, which Metschnikoff designates as intracellular digestion, is possibly due to the action of the same enzym as the above-described, in the extracellular processes of solution. Leber uses the expression *histolyse* to designate this purulent softening and melting down of tissue. This he ascribes to chemical changes similar in their action to the processes of digestion. The changes, he contends, are essentially chemical in their nature and dependent on the action of a ferment. "Chemical, not mechanical forces have the power of converting firm organic substances into the fluid state, and the microscopical examination of tissues undergoing purulent infiltration demonstrates that its elements are undergoing a chemical change." Numerous investigators contend that the enzym is produced by the micro-organisms, but Leber contends that though the microbes may take part in hastening the disintegration of tissues, the essentially active principle is derived from the leucocytes.

Though the subject is not as yet absolutely settled, nor as yet fully explained, we may nevertheless look upon this ferment, this enzym, as the essential factor, which, acting on the capsule, digests it and thus prepares the way for the pus cells to gain entrance into the lens.

CHAPTER IV.

THE GENERAL PATHOLOGY AND PATHOGENESIS OF THE LENS.

I.

THE PROGRESSIVE CHANGES IN THE LENS.

Becker states, "In all the non-traumatic cataracts which he examined he observed a new cellular formation, exceeding the normal, which was derived from the capsular epithelium." Exceptionally, he observed this condition in the lenses of individuals, which during life had shown no signs of cataract. If we will now consider this as the most important fact so far settled, the duty remains to discover the cause, which incites this hyperplasia of capsular cells during the formation of a cataract. As we have seen, this abnormal cellular production discloses itself, first, as a hyperphasia of the capsular epithelium, which is added to the formation of hyaline excrescences; second, as a hyperphasia of the capsular epithelium, leading finally to the formation of a capsular cataract; third, in the formation of large vesicular cells; fourth, in the formation of an epithelial-like covering which clothes the inner surface of the posterior capsule. All varieties of new cellular formations are observed in the different forms of grey cataract, though in various degrees and under various conditions. *It is a remarkable fact, however, that entirely different causes within and outside of the lens lead to similar formations.*

1. CAUSES OF THE ABNORMAL NEW CELLULAR FORMATIONS IN SENILE CATARACT.

In the early chapters of this work, special stress was laid on the pressure which the closed lens capsule exerts on the form and size of the individual lens fibres, as well as on the entire architecture of the lens. As age advances, the lens gradually becomes more rigid and the capsule less elastic, and in consequence of the increasing pressure, this at first impedes and gradually leads to entire cessation of increase in its volume. After the pressure reaches a certain degree, the cells lose their power of undergoing cell division.

The degree of intracapsular pressure is dependent on the relation which two processes bear to each other, during the entire period of growth of the lens. These are the *actual processes of physiological growth*; as seen in the increase of the capsular epithelium, the formation of new lens fibres, and the resulting increase of surface space of the capsule and the total increase in the volume of the lens; and subsequently *the physiological retrogression* of the lens fibres, which as soon as they have reached the rays of the star figure of the lens and have completed their growth, begin to undergo retrograde changes in all three dimensions. The first process produces an increase in volume, whereas the second produces a reduction in volume. As age advances, the phenomena of growth become less active, whereas those of retrogression become more apparent, the more the elements are affected. From this it must follow, generally speaking, that a period will be reached, when both processes, relative to their influence on the lens, will be evenly balanced.

Priestly Smith, basing his statement on a series of weighings, found that under normal conditions this period is only reached in very advanced life. Up to the ninetieth year, he always found a number of lenses which showed a steady increase both in weight and volume. This is in accord with the anatomical examinations, also with the steady and gradual decrease in the width of accommodation. The former, as well as the latter, indicate that there must be a true balance between these two antagonistic processes, though in fact this is only reached in very extreme age.

Priestly Smith also found a less number of senile lenses, as compared with other lenses taken from individuals of the same age which were more or less cataractous, or differently expressed, he found that *all cloudy lenses, even those which were but partially cloudy had a reduced volume.*

After that which has been said in a previous chapter, *we can only seek for this cause of reduction in volume in the chemical conditions of the nucleus of the cataract as compared with that of the non-cloudy lens.* (Page 67.)

The capsule and its adherent peripheric lamellae as far as the elasticity of the capsule and its connection with the zonula will permit, will follow the gradual decreasing volume of the lens. But this naturally also has its limit. If this is once reached, the intracapsular pressure begins to fall, and with this, one of these causes which limited the production of new cells within the capsule begins to be limited, and finally abolished.

As we have seen, *there are always a number of epithelial cells which, notwithstanding the changes of physiological retrogression, still retain their viability and power of proliferation.*

But with the reduction of the pressure, the laws of formation are changed, and the formative process becomes perverse. At the equator, conditions develop similar to those observed subsequent to a cataract operation, where the so-called "crystalline pearl" of Sommering develops in the pockets of the capsule. Here the cells along the whorl increase in size, forming large, irregularly shaped vesicular cells. Along the anterior capsule, the new-formed cells do not push themselves in between the older and force these more toward the equator, but the young cells are either forced inward and swell up, forming large vesicles, or they undergo hyperplasia, forming a capsular cataract. Finally, after destroying the whorl and loosening up the fibres from the posterior capsule, these new-formed cells are pushed over the posterior capsule, thus forming a sort of epithelial covering for the same. Notwithstanding the great morphological difference, vesicular cells may secondarily be developed from these cells; also true capsular cataracts.

Bécker [1] drew attention to the peculiar circumstance that in the formation of Sommering's crystalline pearl, the *secondary cataract* was formed from the epithelial cells derived from the whorl. These cells, after having remained almost totally inactive for many years, suddenly undergo active reproduction again. One might almost suppose that the impetus to the regeneration is due to the entrance of foreign elements, which gain entrance after the capsule is opened. *The absence of proper relations of pressure,* is certainly one of the causes of the hyperplasia of cells and the formation of a secondary cataract.

---

1 "Krystalwulst." Zehender's Klin. Monatsblatter. 1875. p. 445.

The contents of the lens capsule can never be made up of cells other than epithelial cells, except when the capsule has been ruptured.

The secondary cataracts may be divided into two classes: *First*, the simple secondary cataract, in which the cataract is the result of a hyperplasia of the epithelial cells which line the anterior capsule. *This is a true epithelial structure.*

Second, the acute and inflammatory secondary cataract is one, which, per example, follows an iritis in which anterior synechia form, large numbers of leucocytes are thrown out, fibrin is formed on the capsule; this gradually undergoes a formative process, and as a result a membrane is formed on the external surface of the anterior capsule. *This is a connective tissue formation.*

2. THE CAUSES OF THE NORMAL NEW CELLULAR FORMATIONS IN CONSECUTIVE CATARACTS.

As consecutive cataract, we designate every variety of cataract which can be diagnosticated both clinically and anatomically as a disease of the eye, and which, with a certain degree of regularity, occurs as a complication of some general disease process of the body, and which has also been shown to occur as a complication of disease in other portions of the eye. Hence all cataracts occurring in both eyes of an individual due to constitutional diseases (diatheses), also all total cataracts due to chronic or acute diseases of an eye, and all partial cataracts which occur subsequent to the local action of a disease of the eye, belong to this category.

All of these diseased conditions lead to an abnormal production of cells inside of the capsule.

A. CONSTITUTIONAL CATARACT.

a. CATARACTA DIABETICA.

Of all the cataracts said to follow a diathesis, the one said to occur during diabetes mellitus has been most positively determined. By the demonstration of the fact, that sugar is present in the vitreous and in the lens, the abnormal condition of the nutritive supply to the lens has been proven. The formation of the vesicular cells which have been observed in diabetic cataract can only be ascribed to this abnormal nutritive supply. However, since, in all cases of diabetic cataract, a large increase in the volume of the lens has been observed clinically, and since it has been shown this is due to the taking up of water, it would be possible for this unusual condition to lead to a softening and swelling up of the capsule and also to a passing reduction of the intracapsular pressure. We would then have as favorable conditions for the hyperplasia of cells, a reduction of hindrance to growth, and an increased amount and abnormal constitution of the nutritive fluids. At the same time, attention is drawn to the fact, that a large part of the fluid contained within the capsule does not enter with the nutritive supply in the physiological way, but by diffusion through both the anterior and posterior capsule.

b. CATARACTA CHORIOIDEALIS.

The total cataracts which occur subsequent to disease of the posterior segment of the eyeball are especially prone, as Iwanoff[2] noted, to the formation of enormous intracapsular hyperplasias, both in those cases in which the lens is surrounded by the fluid media, as well as in those in which abnormal connections have been formed as the result of detachment of the retina, intraocular tumors, cyclitic, iridocyclitic or iritic bands of new-formed tissue, or as the result of simple iritic adhesions.

Since the final result of all these cells is the same in all the above-named conditions, it might be correct to seek the cause in a pathologically changed nutritive material, which is carried to the lens and which is the real cause of the hyperplasia of the cells. In cases of extensive adhesions, interference with the exchange and the giving off of products of decomposition must likewise be considered. Contact with the capsule may lead to softening and thus permit of an abnormal entrance of nutritive fluid, and thus lead to a hyperplasia of the intracapsular epithelium. Often but a few days are requisite for the entire posterior capsule to become covered on its inner surface with a layer of epithelium.

c. CONSECUTIVE PARTIAL CATARACT.

ANTERIOR POLAR CATARACT.

For the present let us ignore the congenital forms of anterior axial cataract. In the acquired form of anterior polar cataract, the conditions are such, that following a perforation of the cornea and evacuation of the aqueous, the pupillary portion of the anterior capsule comes in contact with the surface of the ulceration. A relatively short time is sufficient to arouse the cells lying at this point inside the capsule to undergo a hyperplasia. The localized extent of this new formation permits us to conclude that this has resulted from a localized cause. Further, it is certain that at this point, we are dealing with a nutritive flow which is both abnormal in its direction, and in its constitution. There can be hardly a doubt, but

---

[2] "Beitrag zur Pathologischen Anatomie des Hornhaut und Linsenepithels." Pagenstecher's Klin. Beobachtungen, Bd. III, p. 126.

that the contact with the pathological secretion of an ulcer, softens the capsule in a circumscribed area, (Muller), that it becomes less resistant and places the cells on its inner surface in a condition of reduced pressure. The change of form which the capsule assumes, in the formation of a *cataracta pyramidalis* seems to be favorable to this theory. However, the increased and pathological condition of the nutritive fluid will surely take a greater part in the cause of this hyperplasia, than the reduction of tension. Further, one must not forget that this form of cataract is most frequently seen in youthful individuals, in whom undoubtedly the cells more easily divide and increase.

Those cases of pathological hyperplasia of the intracapsular cells which develop after corneal ulcers and chronic inflammatory processes of the whole eye, especially in its posterior segment, if they lead to capsular cataracts which can be diagnosed, are known as *inflammatory*, in contradistinction to the *non-inflammatory*, which develop in senile cataract during the stage of over-ripeness. After the identity of both had been anatomically established, Becker attempted to characterize the hyperplasia, as the result in part of an "atrophic hyperplasia" partly due to an increased nutritive supply.

At the present day we are in a position to recognize the fact that both conditions are identical, though incited by a variety of different causes. In the more restricted sense, we can not today look upon the acquired anterior capsular cataract as an inflammatory hyperplasia or new cellular formation. If, for clinical reason, it may appear desirable to retain the expression, *"inflammatory capsular cloudiness,"* or *"inflammatory capsular cataract,"* it should only be used in the sense, that there are capsular cataracts, the formation of which are due to inflammatory processes occurring in other parts of the eye.

REGENERATIVE CELLULAR HYPERPLASIA. On page 84, a form of capsular epithelium was briefly referred to, which must once more be briefly reconsidered. In the neighborhood of the hyaline excrescences, the epithelium almost invariably show a great tendency to divide and increase. Here the principle of "atrophic hyperplasia" can not be applied, because the increase is confined to a limited area, in the immediate neighborhood of the hyaline excrescences. For this very reason it seems most probable that this is a regenerative process. As the result of the colloid metamorphosis, a part of the epithelium having been lost, the effort to reproduce this, leads to cellular fission and increase. Another fact which demands an explanation is the *localized growth* of the capsular cataract. We have seen that it most frequently begins in the centre of the anterior capsule; at times it covers large surface areas, and in exceptional cases the entire capsule. Undoubtedly, this is in some manner influenced by the direction of the stream of normal and pathological nutritive fluid. Exceptionally, the capsule is from 1 to 2 mm. in thickness, whereas, under normal conditions it is not over $\frac{1}{10}$ mm. The abnormally large and thick capsular cataracts are nearly always found in the consecutive and complicated cataracts.

Certain varieties of shrunken cataracts, which appear to be congenital or acquired during early life, consist simply of a thickened capsular cataract enclosed in a folded capsule. Here there has been a very active hyperplasia of the intracapsular cells; the new formation of cells, however, has not been sufficient to fill the entire space enclosed by the capsule, but has rather exhausted itself before going so far.

To explain this fact one, might be permitted to quote a remark made by Ziegler.[3] He draws attention to the fact that, just as in the fermentation of alcohol, the increase of the yeast plant ceases, when the amount of alcohol has reached a certain quantity; similarly, the increase of both connective tissue and epithelium become restricted in their formative powers by their own products. For the former, it is the formation of an intercellular substance; for the latter, it is the intimate relation, brought about by the cement substance, which restricts the further growth. *Vice versa*, the solution of the intercellular substance, and the loosening up of the epithelium can again start up this hyperplasia. If we will now apply this idea to capsular cataract, one would say, that it is the *change of the body of the cell into a dense, thick, intercellular substance*, which there acts as the limiting factor. This explains the reason, why it is that we fail to find the evidence of the cellular hyperplasia which has taken place, in fully formed capsular cataracts or in the congenital membranous cataracts. In this is also to be found the reason, that *one never finds a hyperplasia of cells which becomes greater than the size of the lens, and why it is that there are no tumors of the lens.*

II.

RETROGRESSIVE CHANGES.

a.

THE LENS FIBRES. While studying the sclerosis of the lens and the formation of a nucleus, we noted changes which we designated as those of *simple atrophy.* Owing to the present state of our knowledge, the chemical changes, which take place in the lamella which surround the nucleus, are not definitely known. The most we can say is, that this is

[3] Lehrbuch der Algemeinen und Speciellen Path. Anat. und Pathogenese, 1882, 2 Auft., 1 Thiel, p. 124.

partly a fatty metamorphosis, inasmuch as cholesterine and margarin (?) crystals are found.

Knies described this cataractous disintegration of the lens-fibres, as changes which he compares to those of so-called *"cloudy swelling."* (Virchow). Becker points to the fact that even Knies drew attention to the fact, that nothing positive is known concerning the resorption of albuminous cloudy lens fibres and the coincident clearing up of the cloudiness. Likewise, the idea that the formation of a cataract is a parenchymatous inflammatory process can not be looked upon as a "happy thought," since, in order to prove this, its nourishing vessels would of necessity be involved, an experiment which even Knies admits he could not carry out.

b.

As we have seen, the *intracapsular cells* may show signs which can be ascribed to atrophy. An almost constant accompaniment of the over-ripe senile cataracts, is the change in the nuclei of the cells which have been designated as the products of colloid metamorphosis. Finally, the so-called vesicular cells which develop both from the preformed epithelium of the posterior capsule, are in all probability to be looked upon as *hydropsical cells.*

All cells which are found within an uninjured capsule, both the cells which are normally present on the anterior capsule, more especially all new-formed cells, possess to a high degree, the common tendency of undergoing soon and quickly retrogressive change. Thus one constantly finds in the tissue of a capsular cataract a portion of the cells from which the structure is formed, imbedded in a colloid mass. Finally, a deposit of lime salts is at times found in the tissue of a capsular cataract, which is known as a *petrifaction,* a condition similarly noted in other tissues.

All the assumptions, excepting possibly the last, are wanting in chemical proof. Thus it still remains an open question whether this is really a colloid metamorphosis or a hyaline degeneration.

But, assuming that our assumptions are true, it certainly must seem astounding, that such a variety of known changes, both progressive and retrogressive, can take place within an uninjured closed capsule. But only as long as one fails to recognize the fact, that all these processes are likewise observed in other epithelial structures, as the result of a disturbed nutrition, hence one would expect, since the lens is a pure epithelial structure, to find them here with a certain degree of regularity.

PART III.

ANOMALIES OF TRANSPARENCY.

In the following section the various forms of cloudiness of the lens will be considered. Since departures from the normal, both in size and form of the lens, occur but seldom congenitally, whereas, when acquired, are always accompanied by cloudiness of the substance of the lens, hence it will be unnecessary to devote a special section to their consideration, but they will be considered together with the opacities of the lens.

CHAPTER I.

THE GREY CATARACT.

DEFINITION. Every opacity of the lens system is called a grey cataract or "staar."[1]

SYNONYMS. Glaucoma, glaucosis, glaucosies; hypochyma, hypochysis; suffusio, s. aquae, aquae descensus; catarrhacta, cataracta; cataracte; cataract; cataratta, star or staar.

"The expressions, 'staar' and 'cataract' were in common use at the time Brisseau and Maitre Jean conclusively proved, that the cause of the interference with sight, which for hundreds of years previously had been removed by depression, was not due to a new-formed membrane in the pupil, which the cataract was supposed to be, but that it was due to a cloudiness of the lens. Although in ancient times a diseased cloudiness of the lens had been known, and called *glaucoma*, one was nevertheless justified in retaining the name 'cataract' for the new conception of the disease, as the possibility of restoring vision by operative interference still remained as a mark of difference between *glaucoma* and *cataract*."

"The arguments used against Brisseau by the French Academy were essentially those of Galen. The latter's medical knowledge, however, was but that, as it had been developed since the time of Hippocrates."

"In Greek literature are found the following expressions: $\gamma\lambda\alpha\acute{\upsilon}\chi\acute{\omega}\sigma\iota\varepsilon\varsigma$ ($\gamma\lambda\alpha\acute{\upsilon}\chi\acute{\omega}\sigma\iota\varsigma$) or $\gamma\lambda\alpha\acute{\upsilon}\chi\chi\omega\nu\alpha$ and $\acute{\upsilon}\pi\acute{o}\chi\upsilon\mu\alpha$ or $\acute{\upsilon}\pi\acute{o}\chi\upsilon\sigma\iota\varsigma$. Of these expressions, the Latin writers only retained *glaucoma*; they translated, however, $\acute{\upsilon}\pi\acute{o}\chi\upsilon\sigma\iota\varsigma$ as 'suffusio.'"

---

[1] There is no English translation for the word Staar other than Cataract. Its derivation will be considered further on.

"It is difficult to determine at the present day, which forms of disease the ancients designated by these names, owing to their great lack of anatomical knowledge and sufficiently accurate methods of examination, which but in recent years have been perfected to such a degree as to admit of a proper understanding of the various forms of this disease.[2] It is very probable, however, that every disease leading to a discoloration of the pupil received the same name, at one time being designated as *glaucoma*, at another as *hypochysis*. Then differentiations began to be made, but having no accurate anatomical basis, were but poorly kept apart. Gradually they became accustomed to speak of 'suffusio' where an iritis, pupillary membrane and primary cloudiness of the lens existed, which, however, was looked upon as a *new-formed membrane*, but they designated every conceivable form of complicated cataract as *glaucoma*, aside from the disease, glaucoma, as we understand it today."

"The only expression known to Hippocrates was γλαυχώσιες. This is evident from Aphorism, XXXI., 3, in which he enumerates the diseases of the aged, and uses the word γλαυχώσιες to designate cataract, and with the occurrence of which he must have been very familiar. Celsius, however, quite contrary to the above, uses the word 'suffusio,' and thus shows that he located the disease in a place other than in the lens; rather in front of it, 'qua parte pupilla est, locus vacuus est.'[3] At the same time, Plinius used both expressions successively without defining them. He, however, suggests, from his very rich therapeutic treasures, different remedies for each, so that one is led to believe that he looked upon them as two separate and distinct diseases.[4] Oribasius has saved for us, the opinion of Rufus, who lived some time after Plinius: 'Glaucoma humoris glacialis, i. e. crystallini qui ex proprio colore in glaucum convertatur et mutetur, morbum esse putavertunt, suffusionem vero esse effusionem humorum inter uveam et crystalloidem tunicam concrementium,' and he adds, that all cases of glaucoma are incurable, but that ὑπόχυμα is; but strictly speaking, not every case.[5] We find that Galen expressed the same opinion. According to Kuhn's translation,[6] Galen says, 'Suffusio est concretio aquosi humoris quae visum magis minusve impedit. Differt suffusio a glaucomate tum quod suffusio concretio sil dilute humoris, glaucoma vero naturalium mutatio humorum in caesium colorem, tum quod glaucomate haud prorsus in suffusione aliquantulum cernant.' "

---

[2] Von Graefe Glaucoma, 1858.

[3] Lib. VII, cap. 7, 18.

[4] His. Nat., XXVIII, 8; XXIV, 6; and XXXII, 4.

[5] Morgagni, l. c. Synops. Libr. VIII, cap. 47, p. 130, ed. Stephen.

[6] Vol. XIX, S. f. Med. 363 Lips, 1830, p. 438.

"One may say, that these words give a comprehensive account of the knowledge which the medical world possessed on the subject up to the beginning of the eighteenth century."

"According to the Latin translation by Emerius, the teaching of the physician and philosopher, Leo, who lived about 800 B. C., (p. 146), reads as follows: 'Suffusio (ὑπόχυσις) est cum inter membranum uviformam et corneam humor pituitosus et crassus quasi returbidus coagulatus est et pupillam obfuscat nec sernere sinit: qui hoc morbo laborant initio culices vident. Curator vero punctione, non principio sed postquam aliquamdiu perstiterit.' A few lines below he says: 'Glaucosis est ubi crystallinus humor veluti coagulatus est et albidior factus et visum impedit: fit autem semper in senibus malumque sanari nequit.'"

"About the year 1150, the Salernian Physician Matteus Platearius speaks of *cataract* as one of the diseases of the eye, and defines it as follows: 'Cataracte visus inter conjunctivam et corneam tunica nascuntur et uveam tunicam subalbidam reddunt.' Four hundred years later, we find the celebrated Ambrose Pare, the first physician who wrote in French, speaking of a 'suffusio,' 'cataracta' or 'coulisse,' a 'concretion d'humeur' placed between cornea and lens; and this, along with glaucoma, heteroglautis, leucoma, aygrias and acatastasia crystalloidous; the last of these was already being spoken of as a luxation of the lens."

"Not that during all these years the correct view had not time and again been expounded. In 1673 Werner Wolfing of Hamburg, Professor at Jena,[7] is said to have shown that the cloudiness in the pupil, which is amenable to operative interference, has its seat in the lens. In Gassendi[8] one finds the following: 'Since Lasnier[9] has shown that an animal without a lens can see, it is not necessary to seek for further proof to demonstrate that the power of vision does not depend on the lens.' He has shown that the cataract is not a membrane between uvea and lens, which can be torn away with a needle and depressed into the depths of the eye, but that it is the crystalline body itself, which is shrunken, is separated from the ciliary processes, and is depressed into the vitreous. The celebrated Franz Quarre, as Morgagni tried to prove, expressed the same opinion even before Lasnier. The great physist, Mariotte;[10] also Jacques Rohault[11] and Borrelli[12] were of the same opinion as the above-named investigators. Rohault says: "Que

---

7 Dissert Anat. Lib., b. c., p. 73.
8 Physic III, Lib. 7, D. B., 1660.
9 Remy D. Paris, 1650.
10 Nouvelles decouvertes touchant la vue Paris. 1668.
11 Tractus Physics I, cap. 35.
12 Historiore et observations medico-physicae, IV, Paris, 1657.

la cataracta n'est pas une taye qui se forme del humeur cristalline, comme on la cru long temps, mais bien une alteration de cette humeur me me qui a enteirement perdu sa transparence.' According to Heister, in 1707. the great Boerhaven taught the same idea in his clinic, before he had read the writings of Brisseau and Meister Antonius, but these few voices were but little heeded by their contemporaries. To the two last-mentioned gentlemen fell the task of overcoming the opposition of the Paris Academy of Medicine, and of gradually introducing to the medical profession at large the correct solution of this question."

"On the 6th of April, 1705, in the hospital at Doornick, Brisseau operated on the eye of a soldier who had died of the flux, and who had a simple ripe cataract. He made a depression, and after he had removed the membrane, which he held it to be, and the pupil was black again, he dissected the eye, and found that the opaque lens was not in its proper position, but that it was depressed into the vitreous. On the 17th of November of the same year, he reported his observation to the Academy. The Academy, however, totally ignored his announcement, and one of the members—Duverney—advised him to keep his discovery to himself, and not to make himself the laughing-stock of the Academy. Brisseau's silent resolve was, further investigation, on which to base his opinion. In 1707 he operated a hard cataract; this split into pieces, and thus he was convinced that it could not be a membrane, but must have its seat in the lens.

"Maitre Jean [13] tells us that he had arrived at the same conclusion as early as 1682. Later on, he examined the eyes of a corpse, which were cataractous, and saw plainly that the cloudiness was in the lens."

"One of the greatest learned men of his time, who took up the new teaching in a positive manner, and who with untiring efforts defended it against many disbelievers, even after the French Academy had given in, was Prof. Lorenz Heister, Professor at Altdorf and Helmstedt. In his 'Tractus de Cataracta glaucomate et amaurosi,' Altdorf, 1812, he writes, "duo industrii galii post-multa experimenta sedem cataractae exhumore aqueo penitus in humorem crystallinum transtulerunt.' "

"The discussions of the French Academy from 1705 to 1708, caused by Brisseau and Maitre Jean, show the views of the corporate body of medicine of that time. At that time, cataract was held to be a small, somewhat thickened membrane situated in the pupil, and which had formed in the aqueous humour, and which could, by means of a needle, be successfully rolled up and depressed into the depths of the eye. Even at that time, glaucoma was held to be an opacity of the lens, said to be incurable, in contra-

---

13 Traite des Maladies de l'oeil Troyes, 1707.

distinction to cataract. At first the Academy took a stand on the authority of Galen, then again it held an opposite view, that an eye without a lens could not see; then they permitted Littre to appear before the Academy and demonstrate an *iritic membrane* as a true cataract. Finally, however, it entered upon the road of investigation itself, in that the Academy had eyes dissected before it, which had been operated on for cataract by Mery. Naturally, since it was impossible to be otherwise, these investigations finally demonstrated the truth of the fact which had been so hotly contested. In the year 1808, the Academy began its acknowledgement with the following memorable words:

"La verite commence a se decouvrir sur la question des Cataractes," and a few lines further down continues: "M. Brisseau, medecin de Tournai et M. Antoine, tous deux inventeurs en meme temps ou plutot restaurateurs, sans le scavoir, du nouveau sisteme de feu M. Rohault, qui confondoit le Glaucoma et la Cataracte, soutenoient et par una suite de ce sisteme el par des experiences dont ils etaient convaincus, que l'on peut voir sans cristallin, c'est a dire, sans ce qui a toujours passe pour le principal instrument de la vision. Quelque etrange que soit ce Paradoxe, l'Academie en avoit des l'annee precedente apperçu la possibilite, mais enfin il est devenu un fait constant l'Academie a vu un Cristallin que lon avoit tire a un Pretre en presence de Mery et elle a vu ce meme Pretre lire du meme oeil avec une forte loupe ces gros Cataractes, que les Imprimeurs appellent Parangon." [14]

"The proceedings of the Academy during the years 1705-1708 are in other respects very important to opthalmology. They contain the views, concerning the new teachings, contained in a series of optical studies by De la Hire, father and son, by whom it was shown that the aqueous and vitreous humour have the same index of refraction, and in which for the first time the dioptric conditions of the aphakic eye were properly presented."

"Though the new ideas were accepted by the Academy in the most enthusiastic manner and were taken up by the learned world of France and the neighboring countries, those were not wanting who violently opposed them. The most stubborn opponent was Woolhouse, an English physician resident in Paris. The many discussions between him and Heister are, even at the present day, worthy of being read. Later on, the conception of cataract was changed by Gunz, (Schnitzlein, praes Gunz, diss de suffussionis natura et curatione), who describes as cataract every dark body situated between cornea and vitreous, which impeded vision, or it was said that cataract was every cloudiness between cornea and vitreous, (Macken-

---

14 Hist. de l'Acad. Royale des Sciences, Annee, 1708, p. 39.

zie), until finally Velpeau [15] defined cataract as "une opacite contre nature dun des millieux transparence de l'oeil, que traversent habiluellement des rayons lumineux pour arriver a la retine.' Other authoritis, like Wardrop, went a step further and defined every perceptible disease in the pupil which disturbed vision as a cataract, and used as synonyms the following expressions: *Cataracta nigra, gutta serena, black cataract* and *amaurosis.*"

"Beyond all doubt, the word 'cataracta' is of Greek origin, $\varkappa\alpha\tau\alpha\rho\rho\acute{\eta}\gamma\nu\mu\iota$ ($\varkappa\alpha\tau\alpha\rho\rho\acute{\alpha}\sigma\sigma\omega$), and hence was often written 'catarrhacta.' It was never used by the ancients to describe a disease of the eye. The first time it is found used in the literature of this subject, is in the above given definition by the Salernian physician, Platerius, 1150,[16] and here it is used to express the same idea as suffusio or hypochysis. In Mackenzie's work,[17] the opinion is expressed that ,the Arabs—who, as is well known, in scientific affairs, especially medical, depended entirely on the teachings of Galen —found this expression, $\ddot{\upsilon}\pi\sigma\chi\upsilon\sigma\iota\varsigma$, and translated it literally, and then later on, when the Salernian translated the works of Albulcasis and Avicenna into Latin, this expression, which had come into general use, was retained, and thus *the new word 'cataract' was coined*. In the translation of Albulcasis by Gerard de Cremona, (1114), the subject of the twenty-third chapter reads, 'De cura aquae quae descendit in oculo vel cataracta.' The time when the passage was written corresponds about to the time of Platearius, and the original sense in which the word 'cataract' was used was to convey the idea of 'a flowing down of water,' 'a water fall.' As a matter of fact, in Avicenna,[18] the Arabic expression given for grey cataract is 'nuzul el ma,' which, literally translated, also means, 'a flowing down of water.' There can, therefore, be no doubt but that Mackenzie's idea is the correct one. This is all the more striking, since *the literal meaning of the word,* used to designate the grey cataract *became the accepted view of the nature of the disease* by later authorities. Thus, Ambrose Parre, (born in 1517), translating the word 'cataract' into French, uses the word *'coulisse,'* or *'curtain,'* and he declares, 'C'est en effet du sens de cloture de *coulisse* qui ferme, que la mot cataracte a passe au sens d'opacite du cristallin.' Antonie Furetiere (1690) gives the same definition in his 'Dictionaire Universal;' he however quotes Parre. This proof is all the more important, since Parre was looked upon as the first doctor who wrote in French. Only after the decree of King Francis I., 1522 and 1529, and the edicts of Villers-Cot-

---

[15] Clinique Chirurg., 1840, p. 517.

[16] Hirsch Klin. Monatsblatter, 1869, p. 284. Practica, I, II and VII, ed. Lugd. Bat., 1525, fol. 239. DiRienzi Collect Salernit Napoli, 1853, Tom. II, p. 146.

[17] Ed. von Warlomont und Testclin. II, p. 300.

[18] Lib. III, Faun III, Tract IV, Cap. 18.

terets (1539) was the court compelled to carry on its proceedings in the French language. As is well known, Calvin originally wrote his 'Institutio religionio Christianae' in Latin; and first in 1536, when filled with hatred against the language of the Pope and its traditions, and when he found himself compelled to turn to the people, he concluded to translate his principal work into his native tongue. As a like proceeding does not occur in all scientific writings up to this time, Ambrose Parre, who wrote in the forties of the sixteenth century, is therefore to be presumed was the first to have the written, '*cataracta,*' *as a French word.* So far had the etymology of the word been lost, that the Academy, in its discussions with Brisseau, did not hesitate to state as a fact, that the word 'cataract' meant a membrane before the pupil, and used this as an argument against the new teaching. 'Les cataractes des yeux ont este ainsi appellees dun mot Grec qui signifie une Porte gu'on laisse tomber de haut en bas comme une Sarrasine, el en effet ce sont des especes de Ports, gui ferment l'oeil aux rayons de la lumiere.[19] To quote but a single passage from the literature of foreign countries, taken from the writings of Laurentius Heisterus, (31, p 1), 'Vulgo autem el notiori inter medicos vocabule *cataracta* vocatur, quae vox, teste Livio (XXVII., 28) portas pendulas et recidentes, quae ad ingressum urbium, praecipue munitarum, conspiciuntur, significat, quibus recidentibus vel demissis liber prohibetur transitus et vernaculo sermone *Fall Gattern* appellantur. Notat etiam cataracta pessulum vel obicem, quo porta obfirmi solet. Belgae quoque cataractas vocant robustissimas illas valvas, quibus aquarum irruentium vim cohibent, ne plus, quam par est, aquae in oppida veb campos influat, et ab iis vernacula sua *Sluysen* nonimatur.' "

"It is evident that this erroneous idea was evolved after the word 'cataract' had come into use, and the historical development of the word had been entirely forgotten. The true meaning of the word 'trapdoor' or 'sluiceway,' as used by the ancients, had become entirely changed to that of a *waterfall,* this coinciding more nearly with the prevailing idea as to the anatomical conditions of a cataract."

"The German word 'staar,' likewise the compound word 'staar-blind,' are very old. In the Keronishe Glossen of the eighth century one finds the following: 'Hyerna bestia staraplint (Reichenauer Ausgabe; hyaena stara bestia plint) cujus pupillae lapideae sunt des seha augono stani sint.' This passage is copied in Graft's Diutiska, I., 239.[20] Weigand [21] says, 'Als

19 Hist. del Acad. Roy des Sc., 1706. p. 12.
20 See also Graft's Althoch Deutscher Sprachschatz. III. S., 263.
21 Deutsches Worterbuch. 1L S., 779.

Wurzelverbum ist aufzustellen ein goth. stairan, ahd, steran unbeweglich stehen, woven ahd, staren, mhd, starn = die Augen unbeweglich auf etwas richtet, starren.' *Therefore, 'staar' signifies, a staring look.* I have not been able to discover, where it was that the word first came into use." `

"Since the word 'staar' was originally used to denote a symptom of an eye disease, namely, the staring look, one can easily see how gradually it began to be used to designate various diseases of the eye. As we began to discern differences, it began to be used in connection with other words to designate the variety as the grey, the black, etc., and these expressions are in use at the present day. They were, however, in former times a great variety of other forms in use, which have since been set aside. Thus George Bartisch of Koenigsbruck, citizen, oculist and Surgeon to the King's City of Dresden, in his work on opthalmology, published in 1583, speaks of the green, the white, the yellow and the blue 'staar.' At the present day the word 'staar' used alone, without the prefix 'grey,' will be synonymous with cataract, meaning a cloudiness of the lens.

"The knowledge of the original meaning of the word, seems gradually to have been lost, both by the physician and the general public. This very same Bartisch writes, (l. c., p. 42), 'I have not been able to discover, why this is called "staar," or where the word originated. The word is so well known and in such common use, that it is equally often used by citizen or farmer, the educated or ignorant. For whether they speak of, see, or hear of a blind person, they know of nothing further to say than that it must be a "staar," and they say —"*he is staar-blind.*" ' In his very next statement, however, he says, "that it is no wonder that the word "staar" has been used to designate a disease of the eye, since there are other infirmities, defects, and ills of man which have been named after animals and other things, such as krebs, lupus, carfunkel and ranula." On the next page, he goes on to state, that there are people who imagine that this defect is due to the starling, a bird, for if we eat it frequently, or drink from the same water of which the bird has partaken, or in which it has taken a bath, (we become staar-blind)(?) This, however, is a superstition and a false delusion. Luther spelled the word 'starr'; Bartisch, as we have seen, 'star.' In Andersen,[22] I find, 'Im mhd bedeutet star, also subst sturnus, als adj rigidus, di nach gewohnlicher Schreibweise im mhd *staar* und *starr*. Seit dem aber das ahd staraplint statt durch starr-blind, wie es hatte lauten sollen (vgl austarren, stieren) viel mehr durch staar-blind weidergegeben wurde und ein subst, staar (augenstarre hin zugetreten ist, gerieth man spater auf dem gedanken den vogelnahmen stahr zu

---

22 Deutsche Orthographie, S., p. 18.

schrieben. Leicht ist es einzusehen, dass, wofern nicht, was unstreitig das einfachste ware, die mhd, form fur beide worter verbleiben kann, mindestens das eine der verbaldehung lieber eintriethe, weil da durch der zúsammenhang mit starr desto deutlicher hervortrete.' This also answers Stricker's question (Star or starr?).[23] The work of Lichtman mentioned by him (Nuremburg, 1720), contains the above-given passage of Bartisch."

"Later on, the word 'staar,' was used with an entirely different meaning, (though seldom so applied), to signify the pupil ('augenstern'), as per example, by Baggensen and Matthison. The word 'augenstern' could be used to signify a pupil containing a 'star,' or cataractous formation, but not in the opposite sense. Though one does meet with the expression in Rabener's work, (IV., 36), 'I have a star (stern—a star in the firmament) on the one eye," this does not give us a clue to the derivation of the word, nor is this suggestive that the word is derived from 'stern,' (a star in the firmament), or even derived from the English word 'star,' (a derivation which has been hinted at). Opposed to all this, is the fact that the English, as well as the French and Italians, have for a long time never used any other term for 'staar' than *cataract*.'

CATARACTA VERA AND SPURIA. Several authors differentiate between true and false cataracts. In cataracta spuria we find a deposit on the anterior surface of the anterior capsule, be this a pigmented exudate following an iritis, or an organized tissue, the result of an inflammatory deposit. (See page 99). After a corneal perforation, if the lens comes in contact with the corneal surface, and subsequently on closure of the perforation, the lens on returning to its normal position, may take with it some of the cicatrical tissue adherent to the anterior capsule, *cataracta capsularis anterior spuria*. Exudates due to iritis may almost fill the anterior chamber without leaving a permanent trace on the anterior capsule of the lens. More frequently an organized membrane remains partly adherent to the iris and partly to the capsule of the lens. These adhesions are not to be classed as *cataracta spuria*. Still, they are an etiological factor in the development of true cataract.

"THE VARIOUS FORMS OF TRUE CATARACTS. Anatomically considered, true cataracts are divided into capsular and lenticular, *cataracta capsularis* and *cataracta lenticularis*. The latter is again divided into cortical and nuclear, *cataracta lenticularis corticalis* and *cataracta lenticularis nuclearis*. If both nucleus and cortex are cloudy, one speaks of *cataracta lenticularis totalis*; if there is both capsular and lenticular cata-

---

[23] Walter von Ammon, Journal fur Chirurgie und Augenheilkunde Neue Folge, Bd. VI. 1847.

ract, this is designated as *cataracta capsulo-lenticularis*. Where the cloudiness is in the axis of the lens, one speaks of a central cataract, or *cataracta centralis*; a better name, however, is axial cataract, *cataracta axialis*. Depending on the part of the axis in which the cloudiness is located, one differentiates between a *cataracta centralis lenticularis*, the seat of the cloudiness being in the centre of the lens, from a *cataracta centralis anterior or posterior*. Here again a separation ought to be made between *cataracta centralis capsularis anterior and posterior* and *cataracta corticalis anterior and posterior*. Equatorial and meridional cataracts are also spoken of."

"At times we meet with opacities of the lens which are partial; then again, others which are complete. But since every complete opacity must at the time of its development have been partial, the name *partial cataract* has been applied to those cases which clinical experience has proven to remain stationary during the whole of life, or at least during a great many years. On this account, the following expressions, *cataracta partialis* and *cataracta stationare*; also, *cataracta totalis* and *cataracta progressiva* have come into use."

"The former are often the result of errors in the original formation, hence congenital. There are, however, congenital cataracts which are not partial, *cataracta congenita* and *acquisita*."

"The grey cataract may develop at any time of life. It is, however, more frequently met with in children and the aged, than in people in the middle period of life—*cataracta juvenum* and *cataracta senilis*. Cataracts occurring in children are usually classed with the *cataracta congenita*."

This separation is of practical value, since the consistency of the cataract to a large degree depends on the age of the individual. Cataracts of the young as a rule are soft; in the aged they are either hard or of a mixed consistency; in the latter, where the nucleus is hard and the cortex soft—*cataracta mollis, dura* and *mixta*. The extremes of these varieties are called *cataracta fluida, cataracta lactea, cataracta lapida, calcarea, ossea* and *cataracta Morgagni*. Some of these expressions will be met with again, when we come to consider and divide forms of cataract due to the products of chemical disintegration, or new formation—*cataracta gypsea, calcarea, ossea, putrida ichorem tenens*."

"Though there are good grounds for considering eyes in which cataract develops, as otherwise diseased, still in most cases, aside from the cataract one is not able to discover any special disease. In these cases the cloudiness develops primarily. There are, however, certain diseases of the eye to which frequently or at certain stages the grey cataract is secondarily added; this form, together with all cataracts which are due to constitutional diseases or diatheses are today designated as *consecutive cataracts*.

(See page 99). This avoids the confusion which formerly existed, since formerly the consecutive cataracts were designated as secondary—together with the 'nach'staar,' the cataract which develops subsequent to a cataract extraction, and which today are considered as true *cataracta secundaria.*"

"The conception of the *complicated cataracts* is somewhat more general. Every consecutive cataract is also a complicated one, since it is a complication of the underlying causes which have led to the formation of a cataract. The cataract may, however, develop, without depending on any general disease, in an eye which is diseased and in such a manner as to influence the result of an operation or the probability of a cure. In such a case we are dealing with a complicated cataract, which, however, is truly a primary formation, *cataracta complicata.* Thus, in consequence of glaucoma, a cataract may develop, *cataracta glaucomatosa;* and this, though a secondary cataract, would also be a complicated one. Where glaucoma develops in an eye previously, simultaneously, or after the grey cataract has developed, independently of the cataract. This should be designated as *cataracta in oculo glaucomate affecto,* and ought to be considered as a primary cataract, but *complicated.*"

"The stages of the development of cataract become of especial importance, owing to the choosing of the proper time for operation. Hence we are compelled to designate the various stages, *cataracta incipiens, nondum matura, maturesence, matura* and *hypermatura.* At times the volume of the cataract is dependent on the stage of its development. A very rapidly developing cataract has a larger volume than the normal *cataracta tumescens;* whereas, an over-ripe cataract frequently has a much smaller volume. This shrinkage often reaches a high degree when the cataract is a congenital one, or develops during the first years of life, or after an injury, especially when the lens becomes loosened from its zonular attachment. In cases where the anterior and posterior capsule almost touch each other, the cataract has received the name, *cataracta membranacea.* If the folded capsule covers a small, hardened, shrunken remains of a lens, simulating in its appearance a pea in its covering, which had been picked before it was ripe and then dried, one then speaks of a *cataracta arido siliquata.*"

"Depending on their color, some special varieties have been called *cataracta lactea;* also, black-grey cataract, known as *cataracta nigra.* In the diagnosis of the consistency of a cataract, the color plays an important role.

"If a cataract, no matter what its variety may be, is complicated by posterior synechia, which bind it to the iris, it is known as *cataracta accreta.* If, however, the zonula is partially or completely ruptured, so that the cataract is movable, we speak of this as a *cataracta tremula, natalis,* or *natans."*

"After it had been recognized that the seat of cataract is in the lens, it did not take long until a great variety of forms and classifications were made. Laperone and Morand were the first to differentiate between *lenticular* and *capsular cataracts,* and drew especial attention to the fact that the latter was not a deposit in the pupil, but an opacity of the capsule. St. Yves was the first to point out the fact that the cataract may be a congenital anomaly. He likewise was the first to classify as special varieties 'the milk' and 'the pus' cataracts. On 'milk cataract,' which he looked upon as a 'tumor cysticus,' we received a special dissertation by Roscius (1740). The following year, Morgagni (l. c., VI. 90) denied that the lens possessed any blood-vessels, and asserted that cataract was due to a lack and an improper nutritive supply. This nutritive fluid was named, after him, *liquor Morgagni;* and his view for many years exerted an important influence on the classifications of cataract. He considered the capsule as a second seat of cataract. According to his view, the lens was always secondarily affected. J. G. Gunz (7-11) says the cataract may have a three-fold seat."

"He speaks of *spuriae,* when the cataract is seated in the aqueous, *verae* when in the lens, *mixtae* when it has its seat in both. The *verae* he divided into lens and capsular cataracts. The latter are either anterior *adversae* or posterior *aversae.* The capsular cataracts he called *cataracta compositae crystallinae.* Peter Guerin was the first to separate the primary from the secondary cataract, and was the first to mention the *cataracta traumatica.* Jean Janin, whose anatomical investigations are today of value, was the first to show that the lens is neither a continuation of the hyaloid nor of the retina. He drew a sharp line of distinction between the capsular and lenticular cataracts, and declared that Maitre Jean's pus cataract is a *cataracta Morgagniana.* According to their stage of development, he separated cataracts into *cataracta incipiens* and *cataracta completa.* He designated as ripe, the cataract which had become loosened from its connection, so that 'a sinking down' had followed. He also considered very fully the subjects of the operation for, and the development of, secondary cataracts. Finally, he was the first to give an accurate description of *cataracta nigra.* A. G. Richter (1773) separated cataracts into gelatinous, milky, (*purulenta, cataracta cystica autorum*), caseous, horny, and those of stony consistency. To G. A. Schmidt are we indebted for formulating our first conception of *cataracta natalis,* (the cataracta tremula—Richter), *cataracta pyramidata, cataracta capsularis arida siliquata,* the *cataracta capsularis cum bursa ichoremcontinente, cataracta trabecularis* and *arboresences.* Beer (1817) again took up the old classification of Gunz, of the true and false cataracts, and the latter he divided into a number of special varieties. This brought discredit to his work in later years. Still, one should not forget, that the clinical pictures which he portrayed are a positive masterpiece, so that even at the present day his first chapter is worthy of careful study. With but few exceptions, his clinical pictures are as true today as when they were written."

"The important differences between lenticular and capsular cataracts was vigorously opposed by Malgaigne, and he had many adherents to his belief. He denied the existence of capsular cataract, and based his opinion on twenty-five dissections of cataractous lenses. The outcome of this long discussion finally led to a different anatomical definition of capsular cataract, so that one might more readily recognize it during life. Malgaigne was correct when he asserted that that, which up to that time had been called a capsular cataract, was in fact a cortical cataract. This is further evidenced by the clinical records of that time, for the capsular cataract of that time was often said to have been completely absorbed after the operation. We, however, know today that the capsular cataract remains entirely unchanged by the action of the aqueous humor."

"The expression 'liquor Morgagni' is an obsolete expression for the tissue fluids found between the individual lens fibres. If this expression is retained, one more form of cataract must be enumerated, *cataracta stellata.* The form *cataracta Morgagni* is due to an entirely different cause."

THE DIAGNOSTIC FEATURES OF CATARACT. "Nearly all those characteristics which aid us in making the finer distinctions between the various forms of cataract can be observed by the eye, or be determined by visible peculiarities, such as their consistence. Therefore, the diagnosis of grey cataract is pre-eminently an objective one. However, the vastly improved methods of examination which have come into vogue have greatly facilitated this work. By this, I mean the oblique or focal illumination, the easy and convenient use of the alkaloid of belladonna, sulphate of atropine; also, homatropine, and at a still later day, of cocaine, and the refracting opthalmoscope." The opthalmoscope dates back to the year 1851, whereas atropine is older, Himly having spoken of it in 1806. (289, p. 35). Cocaine was introduced into opthalmology by Koller in 1882. The present state of the completeness of diagnosis, has been attained as the result of the impetus given by Helmholz to Von Graefe and Liebreich,[21] and at a still later day to Hirschberg, Magnus, Schoen and others. The

---

[24] Arch. f. Opth., I, 2, p. 351.

combined use of a mydriatic and the refracting opthalmoscope have raised the diagnosis of cataract, to a positive position, as a result of the objective examination of the eye.

"If, by means of a lens of short focal length, one concentrates the light from a lamp, on the pupil of an eye dilated by a mydriatic, one sees nothing of the parenchyma of the lens, if the individual is young. Under certain conditions, one does see the reflected images of the light on both surfaces of the lens—but nothing more. However, even in children, if one accurately concentrates the point of a bundle of rays exactly in the centre of the pupil, one may get a very faint greyish reflex, which moves simultaneously with the movement of the lens. This grey reflex, however, never becomes so pronounced, as its analogous phenomenon when practiced on the transparent cornea.

In older individuals, as early as the twentieth year, the anterior surface of the lens discloses a faint silky gloss. That this does not originate in the capsule, but in the most superficial layers of the lens, is evident, notwithstanding the fact that it seems to be in the same plane with the edge of the pupil, because one simultaneously sees the radiating striae, also the anterior lens star and its wedge-shaped spaces. About the thirtieth year, often not until near the fortieth year, one observes in the depth of the lens a faint, and increasing with years, a gradually increasing yellowish reflex, the sure sign of the formation of the senile nucleus. As age advances, the silken gloss increases and the anatomical arrangement of the lens fibres becomes more distinctly perceptible, and the yellowish reflex becomes a more distinct red. In exceptional cases, perhaps where the equatorial diameter of the lens is abnormally small or where the base of the cornea is very large, one will observe, when the pupil has been dilated *ad maximum*, that the edge of the lens is reflected as a yellow ring. In very exceptional cases, one can perceive at the equator of the lens fine radiating lines, which extend beyond the edge of the lens, and these must be looked upon as the insertion of the zonula fibres. In cases of congenital and acquired coloboma of the iris one can often see the edge of the lens, but even then the zonula fibres are but rarely seen. In advanced age there appears, however, beside the equatorial marked contour, somewhat inward from this, a second concentric grey cloudiness (gerontoxon lentis), without, however, on this account an actual cloudiness being present.

In the aged, as is well known, the pupil no longer has the pure black color, as it exists in children. The more dilated the pupil, the more noticeable this becomes. As a result, in an eye under the influence of a mydriatic, one observes, even with the naked eye, (more distinctly, however, by focal illumination and especially frequent in myopic eyes), the nucleus of the lens encased in a globular, cloudy opacity, with a gradually fading, washed-out periphery, whereas the zone more toward the equator appears darker; that is, is more transparent.

The warning can not be too emphatically stated, to beware of making a diagnosis of cloudiness of the lens, and of cataract, when such reflexes are present. *The diagnosis is only then permissable when examination with the opthalmoscope discloses non-transparent spots or opacities, in the same places where these reflexes were observed on focal illumination.*

In making the examination by means of the opthalmoscope, the rays reflected from the fundus are the important ones, not the incident rays. By means of the mirror, an illuminated field is created behind the lens, in front of which field, the entirely transparent medium, the lens, seems to float. If the lens system is likewise clear, aside from the possible reflexes on the surface of the lens, one does not become aware of its presence. If, however, there are portions which are not fully permeable to light, these portions will appear in front of the illuminated background, as non-illuminated, hence dark or black spots, since they obstruct the returning light. Therefore, only then, after those centrally located grey, cloudy masses which appear on focal illumination, likewise appear as dark spots on opthalmoscopic examination, is one justified in making a diagnosis of cataract. Frequently this is not the case. However, such a nuclear cloudiness often differentiates itself in such a manner, that one can see, in the middle of the dilated pupil, at a perceptible distance from the pupillary plane, a dark-red globular body. But one can easily observe, on moving the mirror, that the contours change their position, so that this phenomenon can also be accepted as a sign of total reflection, by means of which the non-homogenous, strongly light-reflecting nucleus has separated itself from the cortical substance.

According to Schweigger, (1309, a. p., 26), by means of focal illumination and the opthalmoscope, one can determine (in myopes) if there is an abnormal increase in the index of refraction of the nucleus of the lens. Conducting such an examination with the naked eye, using the ordinary daylight, (more so, however, by focal illumination), the nucleus of such an eye reflects more light than does a normal eye. On making an opthalmoscopic examination with a plane mirror, the nucleus is easily differentiated from the cortex. This is most easily observed, if by making slight movements with the mirror one tries to get around the nucleus. This change is frequently one of the partial phenomenon of myopia; it does, however, also occur during the initial stage of so-called nuclear cataract.

Whereas, on focal illumination, the edge of the lens appears as a fatty or glistening, golden ring, on use of reflected light, it appears as an equally broad, dark, band-like ring. The incident rays of light are met near the equator by the rays of light reflected from the fundus as they pass from the lens into the aqueous humor, and are totally reflected in a narrow zone. This, at times glistening, at times black ring, grows broader during the act of accommodation; also, in cases in which the zonula is torn. In this way, a partial tearing of the zonula can be diagnosticated.[25] Only twice was Becker able to see these folds and the insertion of the zonula fibres with the opthalmoscope.

F. Dimmer,[26] states that "the light from the fundus is reflected in such a manner by the edge of the lens that it can not be observed by the investigator as he looks through the little hole in his opthalmoscopic mirror. This edge, however, becomes light red as soon as the observer's eye is brought in such a position as to permit the reflected light to enter the pupil of the observer. Then, however, only the edge appears red. In the normal lens the same conditions may be observed, only that the dark edge is narrower. In luxated lenses, which assume a more globular form, the reflection of light along the edge must be greater. He also considers the phenomenon of reflection of light along the edge of the lens, by *focal illumination*. He differs from all authorities, and states that this reflex is only visible when the lens is in its normal position, (not even when there is a large defect in the iris). This he concludes is due to total reflection of light on the posterior surface of the lens.

In the alternating use of focal and direct illumination with a dilated pupil, we have at our command the absolute means of finding every; in fact, the minutest opacities of the lens; of recognizing and demonstrating them. Only then does the opthalmoscope lose its value to diagnosticate cataract when the cloudiness has become so dense and advanced to such a degree as to prevent the light being reflected from the depths of the fundus, hence no longer giving a red reflex. On illuminating the pupil with the opthalmoscope, the mirror now acts just as it does on focal illumination. In such cases, however, the presence of cataract is no longer a mooted question. The more accurate diagnosis as to the quality of the cataract depends on the focal illumination.

The following statements of Becker are especially interesting and of historical value, since they were made before the *refracting opthalmoscope* had come into use, by means of which instrument, as has been pointed out on page 77, it has become possible to detect, one might almost say, micro-

---

[25] A study for making the edge of the lens visible, see "Function der Ciliarfortsatze," Wien. Med. Yahr. b. 1863, S. 165.

[26] Graefe Arch., Vol. XXXVIII, B. 4, 1892. "Beitrag zur Opthalmoscope."

scopical changes in the lens, long before they begin to make themselves a
source of discomfort and annoyance to those so affected. With this instrument, it is possible to study the development of cataract from its very incipiency and, one might say, to focus every lamella of the lens. Becker
says, "In the examination of partial and incomplete cataract formations,
the opthalmoscope is especially valuable. Here it serves, not only to give
a more intense illumination, but acts as a magnifying glass. To accomplish
this, a myope must approach the eye to the distance of his near point, the
emmetrope and hyperope must make himself a myope by adding a convex
glass to his opthalmoscope. Very advantageous in such cases is the
method suggested by Mauthner, Liebreich and Becker, by the direct method,
placing a strong convex glass between the mirror and the eye, as near as
possible to the latter. Himly [27] attempted to accomplish the same end and
proposed putting a pair of "cataract glasses" on the cataract patient and
then making the examination by a bright illumination. Such an examination can almost be considered a microscopical one. True, by this method,
one has not been able to discover any new facts, but the ability to decide
the relative position of the cloudy portions to each other has been made
very much easier. By bringing a two-inch (20 D.) lens as close as possible
to the cornea, one can easily approach the posterior pole of the lens. This
method will become still more prevalent in examinations of secondary cataracts, cataracta accreta, capsular cataracts, and posterior polar cataracts.
Thus we see that though they did not possess the valuable instrument
(refracting opthalmoscope), they were already on the right road to its development.

The opthalmoscope also aids us in differentiating between cloudiness
in the lens and other media of the eye. Macula corneae can be recognized
by focal illumination, but when vitreous opacities are present, the opthalmoscope at once demonstrates its great value.

If the eye is held perfectly still and the fundus illuminated by the
mirror, all those opacities which lie in the line of the returning rays of
light will appear as shadows on an illuminated background, and at the
same time will appear to be removed a certain distance from the edge of
the pupil. Thus all opacities on the cornea, in the lens or vitreous, which
lie in the line of the axis of vision will cover each other. If, however, the
observer moves his head and the mirror slowly to one side, the various
opacities lying at different depths will not only shift their relative positions
and distance to each other, but they will also do this in their relation to
the edge of the pupil. Only those opacities which lie exactly in the plane

---

[27] J. B. Fleury, Diss. Sur la Cataracte. Paris.

of the pupil do not change their distance from the edge of the pupil. Since, where the topographical relations are normal, the anterior capsule of the lens occupies this position, this relation gives us a positive means of recognizing anterior central capsular cataract; also, deposits on the anterior capsule. On rotating the mirror, those opacities most anteriorly situated seem to move in an opposite direction, whereas those farthest back seem to go in the same direction as the edge or rim of the mirror. The further they are removed from the iris, the more rapid appear to be the changes in position. Opacities in the vitreous seem to reach the edge of the illuminated area much more rapidly than do opacities in the lens, and likewise disappear more rapidly behind the iris. If the observer remains quiet, and the examined eye is moved, all the phenomenon take place in an exactly opposite direction. The diagnosis gains in certainty because vitreous opacities are but seldom fixed, and as a rule they move about, even after the eye has been brought to rest. Hence it is always necessary to examine by both methods.[28] 'In exceptional cases, it may become necessary to prove that the lens is present in the pupillary area. For this purpose, we avail ourselves of the images reflected on the surface of the lens. The appearance of but one of the images is sufficient to demonstrate positively the presence of the lens. Before the invention of the opthalmoscope, and before its methods of use had been perfected, the examination by focal illumination and the study of the images reflected on the lens were of the very greatest value. This method was introduced into opthalmology by the Parisian oculist, Sanson, and the small reflected images were named after him and their discoverer, Purkinje, the Purkinje-Sanson pictures. Even today, this method will conclusively decide whether a cloudiness near the posterior capsule is in front of or behind it. If there be an opacity of the lens, the light being placed in a certain position, the reflected image will either disappear entirely or become more or less indistinct at the point corresponding to this opacity. If, however, this opacity is in the vitreous instead of in the lens, the reflected image will not only be present in the posterior capsule, but in some instances it will become even more distinct and stand out more clearly.

In diagnosing diffuse opacities of the lens, these reflected images become valuable. Whereas the picture on the anterior capsule can be made visible everywhere, that on the posterior capsule will appear blurred, ("washed out"), or entirely hidden. Mauthner (l. c., p. 148) observed a most peculiar condition of this picture, it appearing to him blood-red. This peculiar color determines the presence of a diffuse cloudiness of the lens.

28 Liebrich, l. c., 486. Mauthner, c. p., 153.

A faint reddish hue is almost always present, even when the picture is but slightly blurred. This is due, as is well known, to the influence which cloudy media exert on mixed rays of light; the same reason causes the setting sun to appear red. Ignorance of this fact has more than once led to the diagnosis of the presence of blood or blood coloring matter in the lens. Reuti [29] passingly makes this remark, to which I desire to call attention. He says, (speaking of the lens capsule as a permeable membrane which permits endosmosis), "This explains the reason, why at times the lens takes on a red color when the coloring matter is present in the vitreous and aqueous.

Case. " An aged nurse was struck with a whip in the right eye by her mistress. The slight injury to the lid healed readily. Though externally the eye appeared normal, the woman declared that she could see nothing with that eye, and the family not believing her, she brought suit for damages. The pupil was round, black and reacted to light. As a result, the doctors who examined her at the trial, stated that the woman's declaration was untrue. She then applied at the clinic of Prof. Yaeger, and the examination revealed the fact that no light was reflected from the fundus. The Purkinje-Sanson pictures, however, proved that the lens was present in its proper place. Projection of light was retained in all directions, fingers, however, could not be counted. The retina must, therefore, have been everywhere adherent to the choroid, and the disturbance of vision must necessarily have been due to a large amount of blood in the vitreous."

Liebreich's corneal microscope is also useful, especially in examining the anterior portion of the lens. By this method one is able to differentiate much more easily than by focal illumination, anterior cortical cataract, capsular cataracts and deposits on the anterior layer of the capsule. In examinations of secondary cataracts and cases of occlusion of the pupil after cataract operations, this instrument is of service and may be of great value more especially in determining with certainty, whether or not new-formed vessels are present in this secondary cataract. If a binocular microscope is used, the very important point, (namely, the decision as to the seat and position of the opacity) is made much easier.

The application of the same principle in a simple manner, consists in the use of a lens, while practicing focal illumination. This method was also recommended by Mauthner (l. c., p. 136). One can use as a corneal loup, a simple convex lens, such as every doctor carries in his vest pocket. For clinical demonstration, the binocular lens should certainly be preferred to an ordinary reading glass. Owing to the stereoscopic distortion, the differences in depth stand out very distinctly.

[29] Haudworterbuch der Physiologie, III. 2. S., 235.

The examination by the above-mentioned methods gives such great and positive assistance in determining with certainty the presence of opacites in the crystalline lens, that the examination by ordinary daylight without the aid of optical appliances has, with right, been relegated to the past. It is true that one may recognize not only the mature or nearly total cataract, with the naked eye, but even at times the partial cataract. It is also true that a trained eye can not overlook the central capsular cataract, a central lens cataract or other forms which are apparent. But one can not warn too often against making a diagnosis with the naked eye, of cataract in every case of discernible opacity back of the pupil in old people. A very apparent and perceptible grey color of the lens may be due to senile sclerosis of the lens.

The presence of cholesterine in the lens gives it a most peculiar appearance. Even with the naked eye, one at once recognizes the fine glistening points. Where a large number of these crystals are present, on focal illumination they may take on a stary appearance. As a rule, they give no evidence of movements. However, if the cortex has become fluid, they can be seen to move about. The presence of these crystals always signifies that not only a retrogressive metamorphosis has set in, but that it is already somewhat advanced. Consequently, they are only found in over-ripe cataracts. They develop more frequently, however, in the soft cataracts of youth.

A most interesting case is described by Van Graefe,[30] in which the nucleus was totally transparent, and the cortical substance between the individual conglomerations of crystals seemed to be but slightly affected, as though they had been breathed on. Though light was reflected from the fundus, it was very difficult to gain a distinct view of the fundus. In the other eye this woman, who was 73 years of age, had a Cataracta Morgagni.

"THE SUBJECTIVE SYMPTOMS which are caused by grey cataracts are, generally speaking, those due to disturbance of vision. Before the invention of the opthalmoscope, by subjective symptoms alone, cataracta incipiens was recognized, or rather concluded to be present. Among the older works on the eye—and I will mention one, which is just on the border-line of the new era of opthalmology, 'The Pathology of the Human Eye,' by Dalrymple, 1852—the consideration of the subjective symptoms is given a strikingly large amount of space. The differential diagnosis between beginning optic atrophy, glaucoma and cataract up to 1852 knew no aids other than the most ingenious use of the subjective symptoms." Today the inability to recognize a beginning cataract is confined only to those

---

[30] Arch. f. Opth., 17, p. 323.

who do not know how to use the opthalmoscope in a methodical manner. However, even today a knowledge of the objective symptoms is a valuable adjunct. They teach us how to recognize with a great degree of certainty, even without an examination, the cause of the complaint with which the patient comes. By these alone it is possible, when a mature total cataract is present, to decide if a complication is present or not."

"According to Arlt, (l. c., p. 277), a portion of the disturbances of vision which must follow where a lens is affected with a partial cataract can be studied by the following experiments. He uses a lens having a focal length of two inches and fastens on this, globules and striae of wax, of different sizes and form, some on the anterior, some on the posterior surface, some in the region of the pole, some on the edges. By cementing together two plano-convex lenses between which has been placed a circular piece of paper, either partially transparent or totally dense, leaving a greater or less wide transparent margin around the periphery, the nuclear cataract can be imitated. At the same time, by holding in front of this diaphragms of various sizes, one can demonstrate the influence of a wide or a narrow pupil. The image of a window or a lamp, thrown up by a lens treated in this manner, can be caught in the room on a white paper screen. Such experiments become very elegant, when a camera obscura is used, or an apparatus such as is used by me (Becker) in demonstrating, the anomalies of refraction." By means of a water trough placed between the lens and a ground-glass plate, the influence of such opacities on the form and direction of these deflected bundles of rays can be very prettily shown. By the combination of two plano-convex glasses, between which various thicknesses of paper have been fastened and then cemented together with Canada balsam, one possesses a splendid means of demonstrating the influence of total cataract on vision. More especially the fact, that in cases of total cataract the power of projection of light is retained by the retina, is worthy of experimental demonstration in the clinic before the students. Generally speaking, the disturbance of vision dependent on grey cataract, at first interfere with the accuracy of distinguishing objects at a distance; gradually this is also lost for near, until finally objects can no longer be recognized by their contours, without ever at any time sensation to light or the appreciation of color being lost. This is true of partial as well as of total cataracts. Nevertheless, disturbances of vision in both forms deserve a separate consideration."

"PARTIAL CATARACTS, when small or located in the periphery, have such unimportant influence on the eye, that the individual does not feel necessitated to have the eye examined. Such stationary opacities at times are accidentally met with. If such stationary opacities are larger, they cause an unsymmetrical refraction of the rays of light in the transparent portions of the lens and can give rise to lenticular astygmatism. Opacities situated directly in the axis of the lens, often congenital, need not necessarily give rise to disturbances of vision. In and of themselves, they only cause a less amount of light to take part in the formation of the retinal images; consequently, they only influence the brightness of the image. The sharp outline of the retinal image is influenced, when the opacity in the lens is not sharply defined or is not perfectly opaque, so that the diffuse light shed on the retina makes the image appear as though covered by a veil. This also occurs frequently where there is an anterior central capsular cataract, and this always occurs where there is a posterior polar cataract, and the capsule has lost its convexity and become wrinkled. Very large axial cataracts can greatly disturb vision, because they may totally block the pupillary area. If experience teaches us that the axial cataract is frequently associated with nystagmus and very reduced vision, it is not to be assumed, as is shown by Reute, that this condition of nystagmus is the result of the axial cataract, but the cause of both the cataract and the nystagmus is to be sought in the lack of development in size."

"Zonular cataract is deserving of especial mention. Such eyes are myopic, and have reduced vision. The myopia is due in part to the fact, that only those rays of light come together to form the retinal image which pass through the edge of the lens; partially due to the eye strain developed while looking at near objects."

"During the earliest years of life, such patients see best, for though the zonular cataract remains stationary, it will become more compact as long as the individual continues to grow. If the lamella in which the opacity is located is very thin, even if this be not continuous, the patient will see by means of the rays of light which pass through the cataract. The more the light is cut off by the zonular cataract, the more the patient will be dependent on the light which passes through the periphery of the lens. He will therefore see better when the pupil is dilated. If the zonular cataract progresses, the effect will be exactly the same as though there were a total cataract."

TOTAL CATARACT. Philip von Walter (l. c., p. 48) claims to have observed that just previous to the development of the cloudiness in the lens, the features of the patient are especially clear and sharply defined. Later authorities have not been able to verify this observation; however, all agree with him in another observation, namely, that during the formation of a cataract many eyes which formerly were not, become myopic. Scarpa [31] supposed that this was due to the fact, that in cataracta incipiens

---

[31] Traite Practiquqe des Maladies des Yeux. Paris, 1802, II.

the lens becomes more convex. Where the development is a rapid one, (therefore, generally speaking, in cases of soft cataract), there is a marked convexity of the anterior surface of the lens; this, however, occurs at a time when vision has become greatly reduced, so that the question of myopia is no longer to be considered. Arlt has assigned a better reason (l. c., p. II., 278). According to him, myopia only occurs then, when the opacities are of such a size, and in such a position, as to prevent the passage of rays of light through the axis and adjacent parts of the lens, so that only those rays which pass through the periphery of the lens are brought to a focus. The condition of the lens influences the character of the image produced on the retina, in that it is poorly illuminated, is faint and indistinct, and, all things being equal, not so far away from the lens. This also explains why it is, that every cataract which originates in the centre of the lens interferes with the proper perception and differentiation of distant objects.

However, one should not overlook the fact, that a portion of this myopia is only apparent. The fact is undoubtedly true, that in incipient cataract objects of a certain size must be brought closer, in order to be recognized. Here we are dealing with a condition similar to that observed in amblyopia, and as is especially noted in high degrees of hyperopia.

On bringing an object close to the eye, especially when the pupil is movable, the circles of dispersion do not grow as fast as the size of the image; even though it be not so distinct, one does see comparatively good under such circumstances, when an object is brought very near to the eye. It is a well-known fact, that for this very reason, as late as the fifties, high degrees of hyperopia were mistaken for myopia. (Stellwag and Von Graefe). That a large percentage of the cases under consideration were hyperopic, and not myopic, is apparent from the fact, that vision can be improved by the use of a moderately strong convex lens, just at the time that a cataract is developing. Donders. (l. c., p. 190), however, draws attention to the fact, that where there is a reduction of vision, the wearing of a convex glass is seldom of any benefit, and in those cases where a beginning cataract is the cause of the disturbance of vision, he advises especial care, owing to the frequency of complications.

For the more recent views on this subject, see (Chapter IV., Part I., page 60) the considerations concerning "*The change in the index of refraction of the lens.*"

"In cases of cataract, the power of accommodation is always reduced, or entirely wanting. This is not entirely dependent on the fact, that the power of accommodation is always reduced in the aged in whom cataract most frequently develops, for this same fact is almost invariably noted when there is a partial or stationary cataract. This has more especially been found to be the case in zonular cataract, having verified this years ago in a series of examinations conducted by Prof. Schulek and myself. (Becker). Even young individuals who have zonular cataracts and apparently otherwise strong and healthy, do not show more than one-twentieth of the normal amount of accommodation. They are myopes, though slightly. In just such cases, Arlt's explanation would seem to be the correct one."

"If the opacity begins in the centre of the lens; or, as one is wont to say, in the nucleus, the patient will see less, and be unable to differentiate objects, if he looks toward the light. If, however, he places himself at the side of, or even turns his back toward the light, he will see better. This is due to the fact, that the light causes the pupil to contract, hence the rays of light fall directly on the centre of the lens, just where the opacity is greatest, whereas, when the eye is turned away from the source of light, the pupil is dilated and the rays of light fall on the transparent edge of the lens."

"The case is entirely different, where the opacity starts in the periphery of the lens. In this case, the patient sees better when there is a narrow pupil and in a bright light, and worse when the pupil is dilated, always presuming that the opacity has not advanced as far as the centre of the lens."

"The foregoing paragraphs are taken verbatim from the work of J. A. Schmidt,[32] published in 1831. This is true, and hence the oft-repeated advice to use atropine where there is a beginning cataract is not always a successful practice. It is not at all an infrequent occurrence, to observe, that where the pupil is dilated in order to allow more light to enter the eye, vision becomes more indistinct, and the patient is blended. It can easily be proven, that the dilated pupil is the cause, since by simply placing a diaphragm in front of such an eye, sight will be restored to its former degree, and even, in some cases, improved."

"According to the investigation of Listing,[33] there are met with in the lens, four varieties of entoptic, recognizable and distinct objects which are constantly present: Pearl spots, dark spots, faint striations, and dark lines. Often the two first mentioned are in all probability dependent on cellular formations on the posterior surface of the anterior capsule; the faint striations are mostly confined to an area corresponding to the anterior lens star. The dark lines are supposed to be dependent on a thickening of the capsule (?). Therefore, in a patient in whom we suspect incipient cataract, where by means of a diaphragm we have brought these objects into

[32] Von Ammon's Zeitschrift, I, p. 345.
[33] Beitrag zur Physiol. Optik., 1845.

view, we are enabled to decide whether or not pathological opacities are present in the lens. The patient, without the slightest hesitation, can draw these opacities on a piece of paper for you. By having this done repeatedly, one can accurately determine every increase and change of form which these opacities undergo. An increase nearly always is accompanied by a proportionate optometric reduction in vision."

"It is not without interest to note, that, 800 A. D., the philosopher and physician, Leo,[34] makes mention of the fact that at times, during incipient cataract, *mouches volantes* appear. Chapter XXXIII. reads as follows: περι ὑποχύσεως: οι δέ τοιοῦτοι κατ ἄρχάς βλέπουσι κωγώπια initio culices vident.

"The diaphragm becomes useful in another way in diagnosticating a beginning cataract. If a nuclear cataract is present and the pupil is not dilated, the diaphragm will materially diminish vision, its action being similar to that of a very narrow pupil. In cases of cortical cataract, vision can often be markedly increased by experimentally moving the diaphragm about, until the suitable area is found. In such a case, the light passes between two cloudy portions, through a transparent part of the lens to the retina."

"According to the investigations of Von Helmholtz, (l. c., p. 141), the polyopia monocularis, which occurs in all normal eyes, is due to the fact, that one may imagine the lens made up of a number of sectores, which vary slightly in their index of refraction and hence lead to slight lateral displacements of the various images against each other. Monocular polyopia was also studied by Thomas Young.[35] He looked upon them as a part of the entoptic phenomena due to irregularities in the lens. Helmholtz satisfied himself, by experimenting on his own eye, that certain light and dark striations which belonged to the entoptic pictures of the lens, gradually became merged in the light and dark spots and striations of the star figure of monocular polyopia, when he gradually increased the distance of the diaphragm from the eye. In beginning cataract we also find objective recognizable irregularities of the lens, hence it should not be a matter of surprise, if this polyopia became more conspicuous. Not infrequently the very first subjective symptom of beginning cataract is this phenomenon of monocular polyopia. By the general term, 'optical irregularities,' Helmholtz fails to make himself clear as to whether he really means irregularities in the conditions of the dioptic system; which, however, is most probably the case. Such irregularities of refraction exist in the lens from youth, but owing to the power to accommodate accurately these slight differences,

[34] Anecdota Medica Graeco ed Ermirius Lugd. Bat., 1840, p. 146.
[35] Phil. Trans., 1801, 1 pl. VI, p. 40.

scarcely make themselves noticeable; but with increasing age and the gradual diminution of the width of accommodation they become more apparent, and when cataract begins they become not only more numerous, but the inequalities become more apparent. Frequently this phenomenon is due to the reflexes caused by the opthalmoscopic mirror. Not infrequently the real cloudiness of the lens is preceded by a stage in which the lens, so to speak, is fractured. By the use of focal illumination, these fissures and splits in the lens reflect the light and appear as true cloudy places, very similar to etchings on glass. When the light is thrown into the eye in certain directions, the same phenomena are seen, whereas from a somewhat different position of the head they disappear entirely. Such reflecting surfaces in the lens must of necessity be followed by a very prominent polyopia."

These cases were classed as cases of irregular astygmatism due to this fracturing of the lens; they, however, did not know that such a fracturing of the lens is always the forerunner of the formation of cataract.

Becker relates a most brilliant example, in an individual employed as a lamplighter in a princely palace. The patient stated that in the evening when he would light the side brackets and the central chandelier, he would see thousands of lights, which confused and frightened him to such an extent that he began to imagine that he was bewitched. After this condition had increased for a certain length of time, it gradually decreased again; in the meantime, the cataract continued to develop, vision gradually being reduced.

Due to a particular arrangement of the veils, this can also lead to a prismatic deflection of the rays of light as they pass through the lens. On this account, occasionally even large objects appear distorted, bent out of position, or slanting. That such a formation of prisms does exist in the lens, is attested by the fact, that in a certain percentage of patients in whom cataract is developing, the complaint is made that the light is separating into its colors.

Aside from this, the cloudy striations dissipate the light, in that they act like corneal opacities. Totally non-transparent, partial opacities of the lens cause disturbances of sight, depending on their position and in proportion to their size. Isolated minute punctate spots neither hinder a formation of a sharply-outlined retinal image, nor do they absorb sufficient light to make a diffuse cloudiness. A saturated cloudiness may reach a considerable degree, and if in the axis of the lens (the various forms of axial cataract) will have no effect other than to dim the retinal image.

The attempt has been made to find the cause of congenital nystagmus in the presence of this axial cataract, but, aside from the fact that axial cataract is not always accompanied by nystagmus, we also find that not infrequently nystagmus occurs without the presence of axial cataract. It was demonstrated by Ammon and Reuff long ago that it is not necessary to turn the eye sideways in order to get a sharply-defined image of the macula. This can be experimentally proven to be correct.

Under certain conditions, a central cloudiness may lead to a spontaneous appearance of the "Purkinje-Arterial" pictures. Reute (l. cl., p. 277) relates the case of a lady, who had posterior synechia after an iritis; also, cataracta centralis (spuria (?). If light entered the eye, she experienced a sensation, as though a dark, purple-colored pane of glass were placed directly in front of her eye, on which there seemed to be a large number of tree-like figures, which she compared to twigs of myrtle, waving in a soft breeze. The illuminated capsular cataract (?), acting as an original source of light, reflected the shadows of the retinal vessels on the posterior layers of the retina. The picture was produced by conditions similar to those, where by means of a lens, the light of a candle is thrown on the outer surface of the sclerotic.

Where the cloudiness of the lens remains stationary, vision remains the same during life, or is subject to only those changes, which are due to advancing age. Here one can estimate the refraction, width of accommodation and the amount vision, by the usual methods.

The same must be done in cases of advancing cataract, with this difference, however, that the examination must be repeated at intervals of several months. These repeated examinations give us an estimate as to the rapidity with which the cataract is developing. Even before all the cortical substances has become cloudy, vision for smaller objects is destroyed, (even for the largest test type). (Yaeger, No. 24; Snellen, 60). One must then let the patient begin to count figures, and it may be taken as a sign that the lens is totally opaque, when the patient, with his back toward the light, can no longer count the number of outstretched fingers.

It will always remain characteristic of the disturbances of vision due to grey cataract that the perception of light is never abolished. A cataract patient should always be able to recognize both qualitative and quantitative (color) differences of incident rays of light.

The lowest degree of illumination which can still be recognized from absolute darkness, is but partially dependent on the character and formation of the cataract, but in reality is largely dependent on the condition of the retina and the degree of its sensitiveness to light. Taking this factor into consideration, we are enabled previous to an operation to form an estimate as to the degree of vision we can expect after the operation. Whereas the total absence of sensation to light, indicates total amaurosis, one is enabled to determine by the degree of quantitative perception of light, the presence or absence of more or less important complications. To determine this, it is necessary to estimate the degree of light perception. In former times, one was satisfied to simply estimate the sensitiveness of the retina by watching the reaction of the pupil when an eye was exposed to various strengths of light. Another method was, to have the patient rapidly open and close his eyelids and thus watch the pupillary reaction, thereby gaining an estimate as to the sensitiveness of the retina. This method may be advised today where the pupil is not bound down. Even in a case where the pupil is bound down, if the pupil of the other eye is free, the consensual reaction will decide the question, whether or not there is any light perception. Aside from the fact that in old people the action of the pupils is sluggish, one can not by this method gain an idea as to the degree of light perception. Hence the suggestion of Von Graefe, which appeared in the first volume of his Archives, (p. 328), must be looked upon as a great step toward advancement. His method was to examine the patient in a darkened room, and let him decide at what distance he could distinguish the light of a small lamp or candle; also, when it is alternately covered and uncovered. The distance at which he can distinguish the light, depends on the intensity of the light used, on the construction of the cataract, and the sensitiveness of the retina. In order to obtain results, which should be estimated on a basis universally employed, it became necessary to construct a source of light which should always and in all places have a given strength. The same result could be obtained, if the distance remaining the same, the intensity of light could be changed according to a measureable scale. This course of reasoning lead Von Graefe to construct the photometer.

As source of light, a wax candle of known thickness is used. This illuminates a ground-glass quadrant over which two metal right angles, with the angles opposite each other, glide toward each other, so that a quadrangular figure of known size is always illuminated. Notwithstanding the ingenuity of the construction of this apparatus, owing to its cost and because it is an inconvenient instrument to handle it has not come into general use. For practical purposes it suffices to examine the light sense of all cataract patients with a light which has a known degree of intensity. A lamp has the advantage, that one may increase or diminish the intensity of the source of light by turning it on full or turning it down. By practice, one finally gets in a position to be able to make a useful estimate. This, however, can not be expressed in figures. At the present day the argand burner light, as used in making opthalmoscopic examinations, is used, and gradually turned lower and lower until light perception no longer exists.

The lowest degree of light still discernible is registered as smallest lamp-light, medium, or bright light. As indicated above, the whole examination is only then of value when vision has diminished to such a degree that the patient can no longer count fingers. In certain forms of total cataract, this in fact never occurs. The greater a nucleus in a senile cataract, the thinner consequently must be the amount of cortical substance, and the farther will the light of a candle flame be recognized. The character of the cloudiness of the cortical substance likewise has its influence. If this has developed slowly so that the general cloudiness and radial striations are very fine, they will permit more light to penetrate, than the rapidly developing, cloudy, mother-of-pearl or silky, glistening bluish-white, widely-striated cortical substance. In such forms of cataract the distance at which a light is recognized varies from 20 to 30 feet. In fully-developed soft cataracts, in which, owing to youth, a real nucleus is not present, as a rule the light sense is not so distinct. In this form, one should not at once judge a complication on the part of the retina to be present, even if the light be only recognized at 16 to 18 feet. In the forms of fluid or emulsion cataracts, as well as in the cataracta Morgagni of the aged, as in the cataracta lactea of youth, it may happen, that the light disappears at 8 to 10 feet, whereas the retina is found intact after an operation. If in over-ripe cataracts, after a time the swollen cortical substance thickens again and becomes more homogenous, the distance at which the candle can be seen, may again increase. Under certain circumstances this becomes a symptom of an over-ripe cataract. In exceptional cases it may even reach the point where fingers can again be counted.

Naturally, calcareous lenses do not permit the passage of any light. All light which reaches the retina must pass to the side of the cataract, consequently must penetrate through the sclerotic. Even though the retina were still capable of performing its function, its perception to light would necessarily be of a very low degree. But *cataracta gypsea* and *calcarea* are almost exclusively found in amaurotic eyes. Von Graefe drew attention to the fact, that occasionally the refraction of the eye exerts an influence on the results of these tests. High grades of myopia, when equipped with concave glasses, not infrequently give the differences between light and darkness at a much greater distance than without them; likewise, the hyperopic with convex glasses. The more inexact the focus of the various rays of light, the weaker will be the illumination of any particular part of the retina.

Eyes which are affected with non-complicated cataracts, can decide the color of the light, even when there is a total cataract. The perception of color, however, is influenced by the color of the nucleus. If the nucleus is yellow or brown, the perception of color will be the same as in a healthy eye looking through yellow or brown glass. The more intense the color of the nucleus the more blue light will be absorbed. Therefore, if a cataract patient looks through a cobalt-blue glass, a candle flame will appear as violet, or even red. The same will follow to a lesser degree if the patients look through a blue glass at a white cloud. But by using glasses of other colors, the influence of the yellow nucleus becomes manifest. A bluish-green glass appears yellowish-green to him, a red glass assumes great brilliancy. If one shows to a cataract patient sheets of variously colored paper, (each of a single color), every answer will go to prove, that he sees it as though looking through a yellow glass.

Therefore, a cataractous eye, as one is wont to express it, has not only quantitative light sense, but is also, as we have seen, not without perception for quality of incident rays of light. The commonly used expression, *qualitative perception of light*; that is, the recognition of objects by their contour, in contra-distinction to quantitative perception of light used to designate the proper exercise of judgment depending on the amount of light which penetrate the eye, should be dropped, since it not only gives rise to a misapprehension, but aside from this is incorrect.

If one will move his hand from above downward before a cataractous eye, which no longer can recognize an object, if no complication is present, in nearly every case the patient will be able to perceive the direction of the motion. This will at once be evidenced by the eye following the hand. If, instead of the hand, a lighted candle is used, the direction will always be correctly given. The examination becomes more accurate, if, in moving the light from one position to another, one covers it with the hand, because where the perception is incomplete, the gradual transition from one place to another leads to conclusions, whereas the perception is more independent (for each portion of the field) where the light appears first in one direction, then in another. For the same reason, the most accurate results are obtained when the light is reflected from the various directions by means of the opthalmoscopic mirror. It then becomes impossible for the patient to follow the light from one position to another.

From this experiment it becomes evident, that the power of projection of light of the eye and the retina is not impaired by the cataract. This is explained by the fact that the cataractous lens does not become non-transparent, but remains translucent, for notwithstanding the fact that to our eye there appears to be a complete cloudiness, "molecular paths" of lens substance still remain, through which the refracted light can regularly pass. Hence the cataractous lens still acts as a collecting lens, does not light up the interior of the eye uniformly, but concentrates the incident rays of light, (depending on the position of the source of light), on a particular part of the retina. Attention was drawn above to the fact, that this occurred with greater accuracy the more the distance of the source of light coincided with the refractive conditions of the eye.

If now, on making such an examination with the candle, one finds that the patient fails to locate the position of the light in some particular portion of the field, or if he fails to locate it properly in any portion of the field, one concludes, that the particular portion, or the entire retina no longer perceive the light. On can, therefore, notwithstanding the presence of a cataract, diagnosticate contractions or defects in the field of vision. On making a very careful examination, it becomes possible, and with a considerable degree of accuracy, to map out the form of the defect or contraction, so that it further becomes possible to determine whether we are dealing with a case of glaucoma or a detachment of the retina.

As a rule, one is satisfied to determine whether the periphery of the retina has suffered, since this complication is the most frequent. However, if one fails to examine for the presence of central defects, this may lead to unpleasant disappointment, when, after a successful operation, one finally comes to test the vision.

In the year 1871, I (Becker) operated the prioress of a convent. Her eye had the myopic build, and she said that she had always been myopic. On the left eye I found a diffuse posterior cortical cataract, on the right a *cataracta accreta*. The examination of the light sense and projection left nothing to be desired. After a preliminary iridectomie, I made a successful extraction. Nevertheless, the patient could not read. Opthalmoscopic examination d'sclosed a large defect of the retina and choroid, which undoubtedly was due to a previous hemorrhage. A special examination in regard to this condition would undoubtedly have led to its detection before the operation.

In order to obtain some idea as to the size of the smallest defect which it would be possible to detect, notwithstanding the presence of a cataract, Becker attempted to see if cataract patients could be made aware of the presence of Mariottes' spot. This was shown to be an impossibility—hence a demonstratable defect must be larger than the entrance of the optic nerve. The experiment can also be successfully practiced, by testing the distance at which the flames of two candles will become fused into one. If these examinations are always carried out with the candles at a certain distance from the eye, one can obtain quite accurate results regarding the extreme delicacy of the perception of the retina.

"When, after the above methods, there is still a doubt remaining as to the light sense, one can determine, by the occasional appearance of phosphenes around the entrance of the optic nerve, (more definitely, however. by the presence of phosphenes as suggested by Serres de Uzeo), if there is any sensitiveness of the retina remaining or not. This matter, however, can never gain any particular or practical value." [36]

AETIOLOGY OF CATARACT. In the previous chapters, taking senile cataract as the prototype, we have cited all those factors which lead to the formation of cataract. We have seen (page 59) that the initial opacities are due to chemical changes in the stagnant fluid which occupies the interspaces, the fibres secondarily becoming cloudy, due to their chemical decomposition and mechanical disintegration. The formation of these interspaces being due (page 76) to interference with the regular sclerosis of the lens and to mechanical causes.

Where both lenses become cloudy, one after the other, we may conclude that this is the result of constitutional disease. Generally speaking, one may assume that the formation of cataract is influenced by a constitutional disease or diathesis, especially since we know that these diseases may lead to other diseases of the eye, which in their turn lead to cataract, as occurs in diabetes, albuminuria and syphilis. However, I do not wish to be misunderstood as stating that every disease of the eye due to constitutional disease will eventually lead to cataract. In his "Pathologie and Therapie," page 224, Becker states, that, strictly speaking, there is no such thing as a primary cataract, the expression "primary" simply hiding our ignorance. If at this time he tried to locate the cause in the eye, at the present day, though we still seek it in the eye, we do so, in an altered chemical constitution of the vitreous, which influences the nutrition of the lens.

It is especially worthy of note to observe whether the cataract occurs in both eyes or not. Where the disease occurs only on one eye, the assumption is a perfectly natural one, that this is due to a local cause. But in those cases where the cataract occurs in both eyes we must seek for some causative factor in the general system, even for the cases in which the eye disease influences the nutrition of the lens. A very pregnant example is the cataract which develops in retinitis pigmentosa. The occurrence of this disease in several members of the same family, seems decidedly to favor this hypothesis.

Under these conditions, it does not seem to be going too far, to assume a like cause for all cases of cataract which occur in both eyes, or in one shortly after the other, and in which age, together with other peculiarities of the entire organism, play a prominent part.

"This idea, whether consciously or unconsciously, has been prevalent

---

[36] Vgl. v. Graefe, Klinische Monatsblatter, 1865, S. 140.

for the past thirty years. Whereas Sichel, Verneuil [37] and Tesnier [38] confine their remarks to attributing their poor results after extraction to constitutional peculiarities; others, following Mooren,[39] have attempted to find the cause in a previous or general disease existing at the time of its development. Rominee [40] records 44 cases of cataract on both eyes in youthful individuals, their average age being thirty years, 31 women and 13 men); these were preceded by typhus 17 times, variola 3, chlorosis and loss of blood 7; purulent discharges, rickets and heart disease 10. These few cases do not give these causes any particular weight. In most of these cases the history fails to state whether or not the cataract had, or had not been preceded by another eye disease, which in its turn might have led to the cataractous formation. Rominee designated these cataracts as "cat pointilee"; in several cases as "demi molle." In that he makes the following statement, "gu'une maladie dibilitant l'organisme pent produire la cataracte," he goes a step further than Foerster, who states,[41] "If a cloudiness of the lens is just beginning, very severe bodily ailment may hasten the development of the cloudiness. Dor [42] declares that all cataracts of youthful individuals (occurring in both eyes) are due to a diathesis. In eight cases he found phosphaturia seven times. I am aware that the opinions on this subject are very conflicting, and it is quoted here, simply to show the existing desire to prove that cataract formation is dependent on constitutional causes. Lately, Deutschman has attempted to demonstrate an actiological connection between chronic nephritis and senile cataract."

The constitutional disease manifests itself in its action on the lens in such a manner, that it either first causes disease of other portions of the eye, thereby leading to a pathological changed vitreous, which, in its turn leads to a disease of the lens and cataract formation, or the lymph of the entire organism becomes changed, thus leading to cataract formation without any other disease of the eye having previously existed.

"The term complicated cataract," in its more restricted sense, is used

---

[37] Note sur l'Operation de la Cataracte chez les Diabetiques. Revue de Med. et Chir., 1877. No. 7.

[38] De la Phosphaturie a Forme Diabetique el de son Influence sur le Resultat de quel ques Operations de Cataracte. These de Lyon.

[39] Opthalmiatr. Beobachtungen. Berlin, 1867.

[40] Cataractes Consecutives a la fievre Typhoide el a la Variole. Recueil d'Opthal., 1879. p. 586.

[41] Beziehungen der Allgemein-Leiden und Organ-Erkrankungen zu Veränderungen und Krankheiten der Sehorgans. Graefe-Sam'sch Bd. VII. Kap. XIII, p. 231.

[42] De la Cataracte chez les Diathesique. Revue Mensuelle de Med. el de Chir. 1878. p. 322.

to designate all those cases of cataract which develop in eyes which have had a previous local disease, such as a detachment of the retina, absolute glaucoma, intraocular tumor or cysticercus. Here also belong those cases in which the iris has become attached to the capsule of the lens, or where, following an irido-cyclitis, a new-formed mebrane becomes attached to the posterior surface of the lens. In all these cases abnormal circulatory conditions are developed. The processes of secretion and assimilation take place under changed conditions. The local cause is attested by the fact of the cataract remaining limited to the one eye.

Of all the forms of cataract, those easiest to understand are those due to trauma. This seldom occurs where there has been a simple concussion of the eye without rupture of the capsule and consequent pathological entrance of the fluids of the eye. Perhaps these exceptional cases can be explained in this way, that the epithelial lining becomes separated from the capsule and fails to become adherent again. If the suspensory ligament tears, the lens becomes luxated and comes into different relations to surrounding parts. The capsule coming in contact with solid parts, the nutritive processes are interrupted. A perfectly analogous result follows where spontaneous luxation of perfectly transparent lenses occurs. This last condition, however, is the result of some previous disease.

If the capsule is ruptured, the dissolving action of the aqueous and vitreous is made manifest at once by the cloudiness, the swelling and the processes of absorption of lens substance.

CHAPTER II.

A SYSTEMATIC CONSIDERATION OF THE VARIETIES OF CATARACT.

THE MALFORMATIONS OF THE LENS.

If, as formerly, we were to state that all anomalies of the lens which are present at birth are congenital, and all those which develop after birth are acquired, we would simply be ignoring the underlying causes of these conditions. A portion of the abnormalities can be traced to anomalies in the development of the lens and the eye; another portion arises after the lens has been fully developed; that is, during the foetal period of growth in a manner similar to analogous diseased conditions which occur in extra-uterine life, in consequence of pathological conditions of the entire organism, or especially in the eye. There is simply this difference, that in the former we must conclude from the residue and consequences, whereas in the latter case we are in a position to make direct observation and to follow their course. Though they are congenital, they do not belong to the malformations. All malformations are congenital, but all congenital diseases of the lens are not malformations. Hence the congenital diseases will be considered along with the analogous diseases which occur in extra-uterine life.

MALFORMATIONS OF THE LENS SYSTEM WHICH ARE ASSOCIATED WITH ANOMALIES OF THE HYALOID ARTERY OR THE VASCULAR CAPSULE OF THE LENS.

Owing to the important role which the lens takes in the formation of the entire eyeball, the mutual action which lens and globe exert one on the other cannot be surprising. In a whole series of anomalies it is very difficult to decide whether the abnormal process in the development of the lens influenced the formation of the eye, or whether the interference with the development of the eye influenced the formations of the lens.

Anatomical examinations of congenital cataracts have for some time past caused attention to be directed to the fact that certain forms are combined with an interrupted retrograde change of the vascular capsule of the lens. The colombata of the eye, in which most peculiar anomalies in the formation of the lens have been observed, are likewise attributed to abnormal conditions, those of the arteria hyaloidae and vitreous playing an important role. We are indebted to Manz[1] for a very thorough and complete investigation of the conditions which lead to these anomalies. From these investigations we learn that the invagination of the epithelial plate into the hollow space of the secondary vesicle may give rise to interference with the proper closure of the fissure of the eye. With the closure of this fissure follows a complete severance of the communication between vitreous and the surrounding "head plate." a process which may be but illy accomplished, owing to the advanced stage of development of the pedicle. Above all, Manz reminds us of the blood vessels which gain entrance along this foetal fissure and which are found so abundantly developed in the foetal eye. This is attested by the conditions found in the few cases of *coloboma bulbi* so far accurately examined, and in which the vascular system of the vitreous still contained the branches of the arteria hyaloidea extending from the walls of the globe to the capsule of the lens.

Whereas, as we see, Manz seeks the primary cause in an excessive vas-

[1] "Die Missbildungen des Menschlichen Auges." Graefe Samisch, Bd. II, 2, Leipsig, 1876.

cular development of vessels which enter from the mesoderm, Hess [2] attributes this to an excessive development of connective tissue in this vascular structure. Others, again, as Deutschman,[3] Holtzke,[4] and Falchi,[5] attempt to prove that these conditions are due to intrauterine inflammation. In his second contribution on the subject, Hess says, "The change of the foetal connective tissue to vitreous does not take place, so that the vascular foetal covering of the lens, which is intimately connected with the former, since the development of this tissue is retarded, the latter, likewise does not keep pace with the changes in other parts of the eye, remains behind and the secondary vesicle can not close properly; sclera and choroid are not properly developed at this point." Everything points to an abnormal development in the secondary ocular vesicle. It may be difficult to determine just what it is that causes the secondary ocular vesicle to fail to close, but it certainly is not of inflammatory origin.

In a later paper by Hess,[6] and in a recent publication by Ludwig Bach,[7] the position is taken and upheld by a series of very interesting anatomical and histological examinations, that all the varieties of colobomata of the eye are due to an abnormal development of the foetal lens, which, owing to its abnormal size, interferes with the proper invagination of the mesodermic tissue, destined to become changed into vitreous, thus leading to cases of so-called anopthalmus, orbitalcysts or micropthalmos. The delayed retrogression of the vascular capsule of the enlarged lens may act as a mechanical obstacle to the entrance of mesodermic tissue at any point along the equator, thus causing the many typical cases of colomba of ciliary body, iris and the lens itself. The cases of various colobomata along the lines of the ocular fissure are explained as the result of failure of the fissure to close at the proper time, either as the result of an abnormal-sized lens, a failure of vitreous to differentiate at the proper time, or of blood vessels too actively developed, and which fail to retrogress. Though inflammatory causes are not denied, they are not looked upon as the usual cause.

---

[2] Zur Pathogenese des Micropthalmus. Arch. fur Opth., Vol. XXXIV, Bd. 3, 1888, and "Weitere untersuchungen uber angeborene Missbildungen des Auges. Graefe Arch., Vol. XXXVI, B. 1, 1890.

[3] Zur Pathologische Anatomie Iris und Aderhaut Coloboma; also Grundlage eines Erklarungsversuchs der sogenante Hemmungsbildung uberhaupt. Klinische Monatsblatter. XIX, p. 101.

[4] "Mickropthalmus und Colobomain Kaninchen." Arch. fur Augenheilkunde. XII.

[5] "Microfthalmo Congenito." Annal di Ottamologia, XIII, 1888.

[6] "Pathologische Anatomische Studien uber einige seltene angeborene Missbildungen des Auges, etc." Graefe Arch., Vol. XLII, part III, 1896.

[7] "Path. Anat. Studien uber verschiedene Missbildungen des Auges." Graefe Arch., Vol. XLV, part I, 1898.

THE CONDITION OF THE LENS IN CASES OF ANOPTHALMUS AND MICROPTHALMUS.

It would scarcely seem necessary to state that, where the eye is absent, the lens must also be absent, if it were not for the fact, that the word 'anopthalmus,' originated by Adam Schmidt,[8] is used to designate a malformation of the eye where an abnormally small and poorly developed eye is present, which does not push the conjunctival sac forward in the usual manner, but rather lies behind and below the conjunctiva. It is in just such eyes, which belong to the *micropthalmus* and *coloboma totali oculi* (Arlt) class, that we find the lens or its analogue in places where we least expect to find it.

In his Anatomie and Pathologie, page 126, Becker states: "The frequently described cases of cysts behind the lower eyelid are always found in cases where there is a rudimentary eye. The gradually developing sac-like process springs from the sclerotic, owing to inadequate closure of the ocular fissure in cases of highly developed choroidal or optic nerve coloboma. To how great a degree the vitreous and the vessels of the optic nerve are implicated in the formation of this anomaly, can not be decided in the individual case. It is, however, a fact that in many cases of *micropthalmus* and so-called *anopthalmus, the coloboma oculi totale* of Arlt, the lens or its rudiment, is still in contact with the retina; or is posteriorly held fast by the arteria corpus vitrei, and anteriorly in contact with the iris by means of the vascular membrane of the pupil. The inverted pupillary edge of the iris is always abnormally removed from its proper position. It is the rule, to find a portion of the hyaloid artery, and at least a portion of the vascular capsule of the lens persisting."

"Examination of an eye in which the lens was adherent to the optic nerve showed that the lens was a round body made up of variously-formed large cells surrounded by vascular villi. The lens was in a condition analogous to that of the Second Period of Development. This period corresponds to the time when, under normal conditions, the vessels and the vitreous begin to extend into the eye along the fissure in the optic nerve, getting in between retina and lens. Where the lens is found in the centre of the vitreous in a case of micropthalmus, it is found to be smaller than under normal conditions. However, it does happen, that notwithstanding the persistence of the connection between the hyaloid artery and the branches of the vessels of the membrane-pupillaris, its development is equal to that of the lens, at the end of the foetal period of growth.

In the above-quoted paper of Bach, he states:

"Owing to the prolonged period of time during which the lens fills

---

[8] Himly and Schmidt Opth. Bibl., III, 1. S. 190.

out the interior of the globe, the vitreous does not develop at the proper time, adhesion between mesodermic tissue along the ocular fissure and the foetal vascular capsule of the lens are not separated, and as the immediate result, the retinal fissure does not close properly—as a natural result, the other coverings of the globe along its under side are influenced and retarded in their growth. One can well see how, as the result of the size, altered and swollen structure of the lens, and further as the result of the hindrance to the separation of the vascular capsule of the lens, from the surrounding mesoblast; this can lead to an increase of intra-ocular tension, in consequence of which; the defective lower wall of the eye in its entirety, or only at one point, gives and becomes excavated." If this condition is long continued, it may lead to a total colomba oculi, and an orbital or subconjunctival cyst. At times, the action ceases after a time and the very small micropthalmic eye is connected by a pedicle with a very fine lumen, with the cyst proper.

In his Therapie and Pathologie, Section 52, Becker states: "Up to the present time, a malformation of the eye consisting of a total absence of the lens has not been observed, and considering the part the lens plays in the formation of the embryonic eye, it surely will be a difficult matter to explain." Dr. Carl Hess, (Beschreibung des Auges von Talpa Europaca und von Proteus Auginens Graef Arch, Vol. XXXV., B. 3, 1889), as the result of his studies of rudimentary eyes, states that "the indenting of the primary vesicle is not caused, as is so universally taught,[9] by the indipping of the lens," and it is especially interesting to note this fact, since H. Becker [10] came to the same conclusion by an entirely different route, since he had the opportunity of examining a micropthalmus (with a total indipping of the ocular vesicle), in which there was a total absence of a development of the lens." Kolliker likewise believes that it is possible for the primary vesicle to be indented, without the presence of the ectoderm. In a later paper, Hess once more draws attention to this fact.[11]

He describes a chick 120 hours old, which had been developed in an incubator. The left eye was perfectly developed, whereas on the right side perfect anopthalmus existed. Examination showed that there was not even an outgrowth of the primary optic stalk from the brain; excluding a theory of development with subsequent loss as the result of disease. The microscopical examina-

9 Schwalbe Lehrbuch der Anatomie des Auges.

10 Ein Fall von Micropthalmus congenita uniliteralis, nebst einigen Bemerkungen uber die vermutleiche Aetiologie und Entwickelungs geschichte desselben. Graefe Arch., XXXIV. B. 3, 1888.

11 Beitrage zur Kenntniss der Pathologischen Anatomie der Angeborenen Missbildungen des Auges, Graefe Arch., Vol. XXXVIII. B. 3, 92.

tion proved all of this; also, the absence of a sign of the lens on the right side. This is undoubtedly a phenomenon of the greatest interest, and should be remembered when we try to study the relations between the development of the eye and lens.

In this same paper he reports a case of *cyclops,* (in a pig), *the single eye containing two perfectly-formed lenses.* So far as I have been able to discover, this is the only case of the kind reported in literature. Hence I will quote it in full:

"The specimen was sent to me (Carl Hess) by Dr. Ruge, of Amsterdam. The single eye was placed just above the very prominent snout. The eye was almost globular in shape, and had a diameter of 22 mm. The almond-shaped lid fissure was about 27 mm. wide. It was impossible to detect a line along which there had taken place a fusion of the lids. Puncta lachrymalis wanting.

The cornea was transversely oval, and disclosed a slight depression in the center, likewise above and below the edges. These indrawn places were connected by a very fine vertical line, so as to give the impression that along this line the two cornea had joined. Both halves were of equal size; their total diameter equal to 17 mm. Otherwise, one finds no signs suggestive of two eyes being joined together. On dissecting the eye, find but a single optic nerve, and transverse serial sections appear normal. The retina is detached, but shows no evidence of separation into two halves. In the anterior half of the eye the conditions are somewhat more complicated, owing to the presence of *two lenses.* One finds two perfectly developed lenses, situated about 4 mm. from each other. Laterally, from each is a normal ciliary body, and a normally developed iris. Corresponding to the vertical fine line on the external surface of the cornea there appears on its posterior surface a T formed prominence, looking upward and downward. This prominence is smallest at the center; thus forming for each lens a pupil of about normal size. These prominences consist partly of vascular connective tissue, partly of nonstriated vascular fibres, like those found in the ciliary body. The prominence which extends backward is covered with a thick pigment layer of epithelial cells, as seen on the pars ciliaris retinae.

The anatomical conditions of the brain were especially interesting. On removing the calvarium, the cerebellum and corpora quadrigemina were found to be normal. At the anterior end of the brain the cerebrum appeared as an undivided mass, filling up the anterior fossa completely, but only about one cm. in thickness. As a result, the corpora quadrigemima were completely uncovered. The upper surface showed a number of shallow depressions, but no real sulci or convolutions. The mass lying anterior to the corpora quadrigenima was only connected with the latter by a very thin lamella of nervous tissue. The posterior margin of this single sphered cerebrum was covered by the pia mater, from which, on both sides of the median line, a small choroidal plexis had developed. On making a frontal section through the center of this cerebrum, a very fine horizontal fissure, which appeared to communicate with the third ventricle was discovered. The following conditions were found at the base: The middle and posterior portions of the brain were apparently normally developed. The position of the optic tracts and chiasm was occupied by a single medianly placed nerve, which anteriorly passed through the single optic foramen. Posterior to the optic nerve, at the base of the brain, a single corpus mamillarae was found; oculomotorius, trochlearis and abducens were all arranged double. A very delicate furrow running along the under surface of the brain, was the only indication of a division of the cerebrum into two hemispheres. The exact condition of the olfactory nerve could not be definitely determined.

Accordingly, the posterior and middle portions of the brain were normally developed; whereas, the cerebrum and all the parts which develop from it, the olfactory and optic nerves and retina were developed as a single one, whereas, *the parts of the eye developed from the ectoderm were again double.* It is indeed astonishing that no signs of fusion can be noted on the eyelids.

The attempt has been made to explain the formation of cyclopie. Hushke assumed that it was due to an abnormal or incomplete division of the general ocular germ. According to this view, cyclopie would be a true interference in development. Opposed to this view is that of Merkel, Geoffrey. Saint Hillaire and others, who assume that the cyclopic eye is the result of a fusion.

Lately, Dareste has conceived a view which leans toward that of Huschke. According to his view, the cyclopie is due to an interference in the development of the anterior cerebral vesicle, which is due to an abnormally early closure of the vesicle. Hess states that he can hardly join the one view or the other, but emphasizes the fact, that this case is more easily explained as the result of an interference in development, rather than on the hypothesis that this is due to a fusion of two originally separate organs.

CATARACTA MEMBRANACEA CONGENITA ACCRETA.

In 1861, Wilde [12] drew attention to the fact that some of the forms of congenital cataract are associated with anomalies in the retrogressive changes of the hyaloid artery, respectively, the vascular capsule of the lens. Becker described the examination of such a cataract as follows: "I examined such a cataract and found a wavy, folded capsule of normal thickness and transparency; also a well-preserved single layer of epithelial cells: aside from these, very regularly arranged fibre-like cells extending from behind forward, showing beautiful nuclei. In the aequatorial region in the situation of the lens whorl were found disintegrated masses. On the ex-

[12] Congenital diseases and malformations of the dioptr. media. Dublin's Quarterly Journal, No. 61, 1861.

ternal surface of the posterior capsule were found numerous patent blood vessels. These conditions are exceedingly interesting, because they indicate that the cause of the disease could not have exerted its influence long after the beginning of the third period of foetal development. This must coincide with about the second month of foetal life." (See Manz, page 82). The persistence of the hyaloid artery places this malformation, which may be designated as a failure of the lens to undergo further development after having reached a certain stage of development, in the category of the above-described sequelae of coloboma formations. W. von Grollman [13] describes a case in which the posterior capsule was wanting, the hyaloid artery had grown into the lens, which was filled with connective tissue, blood vessels and a few lens fibres.

The fact, that branches of the hyaloid artery still containing blood are found on the posterior surface of a certain class of congenital membranous cataracts, indicates, since the hyaloid artery has no accompanying vein, that a number of venous branches of the vascular capsule also remain. And, as a fact, in this form of cataract one does frequently find that a connection between the capsule and the iris still exists. Hence this form is also designated as *cataracta membranacea conjenita accreta*, in that this connection is looked upon as a posterior synechia, the result of a foetal iritis. Further anatomical examinations of entire eyes containing cataracta membranacea accreta are necessary in order to show whether there are other remains of a foetal iritis. This touches on the question of the cause of the *membrana pupillaris perseverans* and the deposits on the outer surface of the anterior capsule which thus leads to the *cataracta capsularis anterior spuria*. It is possible that a disturbance in the retrogressive change in the vascular capsule is to be sought in an inflammatory process in this capsule. This would also explain the genesis of the *cataracta polaris posterior spuria*. All the cases so far described are deposits on the outer surface of the posterior capsule and usually are found in the region of the posterior pole of the lens. They are characterized by the white shining color which this form of cataract reflects. It is seldom very small, often the size of a hemp or poppy seed, and frequently by focal illumination one can see that anteriorly it is concave and smooth as a mirror. On using the opthalmoscope it can be seen to taper toward the vitreous. Generally its contour is round, though in the individual case it may show a few pointed striations.

It might possibly be mistaken for a posterior cortical cataract such as occurs in choroidal disease and disease of the vitreous, more particularly

---

13 "Uber Mickropthalmus und Cataracta Congenita Vasculosa." Graef Arch., Vol. XXXV, B. 314. 1889.

the form occurring in retinitis pigmentosa. It is, however, not difficult to differentiate, since in posterior cortical cataract the glistening white color and mirror-like smoothness are wanting, and the latter form generally goes over into the general cortical cataract while under observation. The presence of radiating striae favors the diagnosis of posterior cortical cataract, on the outer surface of the posterior capsule.

Von Ammon[14] was the first to draw attention to the fact, that abnormalities at the posterior capsule could be traced to disease of the hyaloid. In the eye of a rabbit born blind, he found the obliterated central artery, together with a central opacity of the posterior wall of the capsule. He gives an illustration (Fig. 12, Plate 15) of a case of congenital thickening of the hyaloid artery and a resulting cataracta centralis, showing a portion of the artery attached posteriorly to the conical lens, through the axis of which an opacity exists. Von Ammon diagnosed opacities in the posterior portion of the lenses of living men, which he ascribed to early obliteration of the central artery.[15] H. Muller (l. c., p. 86) described such a posterior polar cataracta in both eyes of a goat. Both lenses showed a two-fold cloudiness. He also observed a case in which there was a greyish opacity in the centre of the lens, (cataracta centralis), together with a flattened cone at the posterior surface, yellowish in its centre, yellowish white at the periphery and protruding backward through the vitreous to the papilla; from the centre of this cone the hyaloid artery could be seen. The eyes, though of normal shape, showed the evidences of a previous inflammatory infiltration. The central artery was surrounded by inflammatory products and could be distinctly seen to pass between the nodule and the lens substance. Therefore, the opaque mass had its seat at and in the remains of the embryonal capsule of blood vessels, and it can scarcely be doubted that this peculiar formation is due to an interference with the embryonal development of the organ. Finally, we are indebted to Berthold[16] for the exact examination of such a cataract, obtained from a congenital buphthalmus, and the origin of which he likewise traced to a persistent arteria capsularis. He found beautiful epithelial cells along the posterior capsule, the lens otherwise being perfectly normal. He adds, "It is remarkable, that this epithelium which is found along the posterior capsule during foetal life should not have entirely disappeared," but, according to our understanding of the subject today, this epithelium must have been

---

14 Klin. Darstellung, III, p. 67.

15 See also Bech, "De Cataracta Centrali." Inaug. Dissert. Lips. 1830.

16 "Beitrag zur Pathologische Anatomie des Auge." Graefe Arch., Bd. XVII, p. 174, 1871.

newly formed. This would then be the first and only case in which such a newly formed epithelium was found in a transparent, non-cataractous lens. Berthold's observations become still more interesting since Becker (Anatomie, p. 70) observed a like condition in both lenses of a dog, but he is unable to give a satisfactory explanation. A later observation and examination by Oeller,[17] in the case of a boy, also one in the eye of a pig, here noted, are certainly worthy of being read.

Since attention has been directed to this subject, the opthalmoscopic examination has disclosed very fine foetal remains of the hyaloid and its branches, such as cause no interference with sight and which ordinarily would have been overlooked.

Case Report. Miss R. S., aged 18, came to have her eyes tested in November. 1895. Opthalmoscopic examination of fundus disclosed a somewhat irregular heart shaped choroidal atrophic area to the upper and slightly to the nasal side of the papilla. This area is snow white, surrounded by a deeply pigmented margin, and about the size of the papilla. During the examination a peculiar striation seemed to veil the distinct view of the fundus, but on gradually adding plus glasses, until the posterior surface of the lens was accurately focused (plus 10 D), these striations gradually became distinctly visible as black lines. They take their origin from a knob-like protuberance, which curves backward into the vitreous. It passes on to the lens and gradually spreads out fan-shaped. taking in a section of about 30 degrees. Directly below this, leaving an intervening space of about 2 mm., another similar figure begins, but soon disappears. These undoubtedly are the remains of the hyaloid, which during foetal life were present on the posterior surface of the lens.

In a monograph by Dr. David DeBeck,[18] all the literature on this subject was compiled, and in his classification he speaks of (I) strands attached to the lens alone; (J) posterior capsular cataracts; (K) striae on the posterior lens capsule.

CHAPTER III.

MALFORMATIONS OF THE LENS IN CONSEQUENCE OF UN-SYMMETRICAL DEVELOPMENT OF THE ZONULA ZINII.

COLOBOMA LENTIS. (Arlt). One of the causes of this malformation of the lens, which is due to an unsymmetrical ligament. is sought in the late closure of the ocular fissure, as is at times seen in cases of coloboma iridis. This is nearly always combined with a slight malformation of the orbicularis ciliaris, in that at the point where the ocular fissure closed one or more ciliary processes are wanting and the ciliary body is simply indicated. In consequence, the zonula, if present at all, is less tense, though in

---

17 Zur Aetiologie der Cataracta Polaris Posterior. Dissert Munchen. 1878.
18 "Persistent remains of the Foetal Hyaloid Artery." Cincinnati. 1890.

all probability it is wanting at this point. As a result of this reduction of tension, on opthalmoscopic examination the line of this defect is marked by a black line, the lens appears notched at its edge, and there is an indenting of the contour as a result of increased reflexion.

Heyl[1] developed the ingenious theory, that this malformation is due to a lack of nutrition, due to a defect in the anterior branches of the hyaloid. This surely can not have much in its favor.

Treacher Collins gives quite a different explanation for the occurrence of this malformation, as has already been fully explained on pages 29 and 74.

According to the latest work on this subject by Dr. E. Bock,[2] congenital malformations of the lens belong to the rarest of ocular findings. The author reports six cases of his own and forty-six other cases occurring in thirty-eight persons reported in literature.

At the meeting of the American Opthalmological Society, 1894, Dr. C. F. Clark, Columbus, Ohio, reported a case of binocular coloboma lentis in which the accommodative power was retained.

THE GENESIS OF COLOBOMA LENTIS. Bach seeks the cause in a delayed closure of the ocular fissure. The process of mesodermal tissue which extends as a process against the edge of the lens, acts as a *mechanical* obstruction at the respective point. As a result of this pressure along the foetal fissure, the lens substance deteriorates, is altered in its constitution, and may simply assume a cloudy aspect; or the more actively affected portion may disintegrate and be absorbed, and along this line one will observe a vacant space or fissure.

Bach accepts this explanation, but goes still further, stating that the fundamental cause is to be sought in an abnormally-developed lens, which in early foetal life opposes the advancing mesoblast, which in its turn presses against the gradually enlarging lens, or vice versa. Further, if the adhesions between the vascular capsule of the lens and the mesoblast do not dissolve along the entire equatorial region, this must lead to a transient tension at the respective point where this attachment persists, which in its turn leads to a disintegration, eventually to a destruction of lens substance. The capsule may even be pushed aside from the region of such a lenticular defect, or the defect may be covered by this membrane. Since the formation of the capsule of the lens is now proven to be the product of the capsular cells, and since nucleated lens fibres must still be present in the neigh-

---

[1] Coloboma Lentis. Report of Fifth International Opth. Congress, 1877. p. 16. Annal d'Oculist, 1877. p. 206.

[2] Die Angeborenen Colobome des Augapfels Wien, 1893.

borhood of the same, hence one may readily understand how the capsule may subsequently form again. Bach concludes, "I assume purely mechanical causes for the production of coloboma of the lens, and am of the belief that primarily we are not dealing with a defect. Coloboma of the lens is not the result of a formative error in the lens proper, but due to an *altered, deteriorated lenticular mass,* which subsequently gradually disappears."

ECTOPIA LENTIS. Closely allied to the two above-described abnormalities is the well-known *anomalie in the formation of the eye,* known as *ectopia lentis.* It can not be looked upon as an anomalie of the lens, unless there is present at the same time a change in the form of the lens, which is seldom the case. The only known difference seems to be that the lens is smaller or thicker than normal. Nothing, however, goes to prove that the architecture or the arrangement of the fibres deviates from the normal. It must therefore be assumed, notwithstanding the unequal length of the zonula fibres, that the pressure exerted on the lens is everywhere equal. And the fact, that the lenses which have been ectopionated, do not especially often become cataractous, seems to indicate, that the nutrition of the lens during life is normal. Nothing special is known concerning the cause of the unequal length of the zonular fibres. Here, once more, attention is drawn to Treacher Collins' explanation, page 74. Since the displacement in both eyes is almost invariably symmetrically upward; either directly upward, or upward and to one side, it does not seem difficult to assume, that here likewise, closure of the ocular fissure plays an important role.

Attention is first directed to this condition from the fact, that the patient sees very poorly, and that vision can not be improved with glasses. Vision can only be improved by the use of strong concave glasses. A practiced eye at once perceives that the anterior chamber is of unequal depth, in that one portion of the iris is situated more anteriorly than the other. The more deeply seated portion trembles on moving the eye. On opthalmoscopic examination, one will see at once, or possibly only after dilating the pupil, the edge of the lens passing through the pupil, as the segment of a black ring along the line where the iris lies deepest. If the attempt is now made to get a view of the fundus, this can be accomplished in a two-fold manner. If one looks through the lens, using the correction for a myopic eye, one obtains a view of the papilla, and on looking to the side of the lens, using the aphakic correction, one gets another view of the papilla. If we now make tests for vision, the presence of this condition can be proven for distance, by concave glasses, where the patient looks through the crystalline lens; the same result, however, may be obtained by using cataract glasses, the patient looking to the side of the lens. If by the one method or the other the anomalie of refraction is neutralized, the second possibility will interfere but little. However, without a correction a true monocular diplopia will occur. This condition can not always be made apparent to the patient at once. It depends upon the distance at which the light is removed from the patient, whether both images will become apparent or whether one will be suppressed. If one had previously determined both conditions of refraction, one can easily find the distance at which both images must become apparent. At this point, as a rule, the patient will see both images at once. The image which is formed without the aid of the crystalline lens is projected correctly, whereas the crystalline lens acts as a prism. Hence the image which passes through the crystalline lens is projected falsely and in exactly the opposite direction to that in which the lens is luxated. This knowledge can be used in assisting the patient to find the second image.

On moving the eye or changing the position of the head, the lens may also change its position. The degree of mobility varies greatly. In extreme cases the lens not only changes its position in the vitreous, but it may also enter the anterior chamber. This latter condition Heyman has described under the title of "spontaneous mobility of the lens." (Spontane freie beweglichkeit). Such a condition must necessarily be preceded by an extraordinary lengthening of the zonula fibres. Such a condition has been anatomically described by D. E. Muller, and thus placed beyond the reach of hypothesis. Horner had already drawn attention to the fact, that the unequal development of the zonula, as well as a tendency to dissolution of the same, may be inherited. This seems to be attested by its occurrence in both eyes. Eduard Meyer has reported an undoubted case of congenital ectopia, in which, in course of years, the displacement increased on the one eye; whereas, in the other eye, the lens, without having lost its mobility, when the head was held erect, returned to its normal position.

(Becker.) I am acquainted with a family, in which a brother and sister show in both eyes a symmetrical ectopia lentis. Ten years ago both could overcome the interference with vision by cylindrical glasses. At present this is no longer possible. The children of the sister, a boy and a girl, both are astygmatic, and were corrected four years ago by cylinders. At that time, I measured the cornea with the opthalmometer, and could not discover any asymetry. On dilating the pupils of both children one could see downward and inward a dark spot at the edge of the lens, which I pronounced a congenital partial cataract. Now the cylindrical glasses are no longer of use, and the trouble is continually becoming more pronounced, as a luxation of the lens. Undoubtedly the zonula first began to give downward and inward, and is gradually becoming elongated.

Von Graefe[3] was the first to accurately describe a case of congenital

---

[3] Arch. fur Opth., I, S. 343.

luxation of the lens. The peculiarities of vision in these cases are here found accurately described; he,' however, failed to state whether this is a congenital condition or not. He seemed to believe that the cause is a fluidity of the vitreous, and a defect in the natural partition wall, though, on using the opthalmoscope, he could not discover the slightest trace of a flaky or membranous cloudiness in the vitreous, and the fundus appeared perfectly normal. In the same year (1854) E. Yaeger described a case, which bore a close resemblance to the one mentioned above, and he described it as a case of congenital displacement of the lens system. Stellwag [4] was the first to describe an abnormally small lens as a congenital anomaly, and to use the word "ectopie" in the sense we use it today. From now on, the reports of cases of luxation of the lens began to increase; also explanations as to its cause. Dixon, the Englishman, as the result of a report of a large number of cases, added much to the methods of diagnosing congenital luxation of the lens. Hippel [5] finally took the last step, when he said that "*spontaneous luxation*" and "*ectopia lentis*" are two entirely different conditions, in that the former is due to diseased conditions in the eye, whereas the latter is a malformation.

CHAPTER IV.

ACQUIRED ANOMALIES IN THE POSITION OF THE LENS, NOT DUE TO MALFORMATIONS.

LUXATIO LENTIS—LUXATION OF THE LENS.

Anatomically considered, the acquired anomalies of position of the lens, can not in any sense be considered as malformations. Nevertheless, owing to the great similarity of the symptoms, both subjective and objective, they will be considered at this point.

The term "*luxatio lentis*" embraces not only the cases of spontaneous displacement of the lens, originally in their normal position, but those cases which occur in consequence of violence which causes the lens to partially or totally leave the fossa patellaris. Blodigo suggested that we use the term "*dislocatio,*" instead of "luxatio lentis," and this name might with great propriety be used in cases of secondary luxation.

SPONTANEOUS LUXATION OF THE LENS. LUXATIO LENTIS SPONTANE. DEPLACEMENT SPONTANE. We are indebted to

4 Wiener Med. Wochenblatt, 1856.

5 "Die spontane luxation der linse und ihre angeborene ectopie." Marburg. 1859.

Sichel[1] for the first accurate descriptions of spontaneous displacement of the lens. This can only occur when the *zonula zinii* has been partially or totally destroyed. If such a defect in the zonula takes place to the side of, or below the lens, a change in the position of the lens does not necessarily follow at once. True, owing to the specific weight of the lens, on moving the eyes, even after they have again come to rest, the lens will continue to make movements. In consequence of these oscilating movements, the lens may become turned on its axis, so that its one edge may come nearer to the cornea than the other: but a real displacement to the one side or downward will not occur as long as the portion of the zonula zinii above, remains intact. As soon as this becomes affected the weight of the lens will begin to exert its influence, and as a result, the lens will begin to sink downward. No matter where the zonula has been affected, owing to the oscillation of the lens, in course of time the zonula will give above, and the lens will become displaced downward. It will then depend upon the conditions of the lateral portions of the zonula whether this sinking will take place exactly downward, or downward and inward, or downward and outward. This is a very important fact, since a lens can never be *spontaneously* luxated exactly upward.

The cause of this spontaneous displacement lies either in the condition of the vitreous and the zonula, or in the lens system itself.

The disease which is considered to be most frequently followed by a spontaneous luxation is a general fluidity of the vitreous. (*Synchysis corporis vitrei*. Aside from the fact that the clinical picture of this disease is by no means a definite one, it is impossible for the lens to sink down without the zonula zinii suffering in its continuity. Although up to the present time it has never been quite clear in what manner a fluidity of the vitreous could affect the zonula, especially since there is no reduction in volume of the vitreous when it is in a fluid state, we are entitled to make the assumption; since, as we have seen, the zonula is of mesodermic origin, as is also the vitreous; hence the same causes which lead to fluidity of the vitreous, may at the same time dissolve the zonula fibres. Hence, in cases of spontaneous luxation, we are not dealing with a tearing, but with a *dissolution of the zonula*. However, when we say this, we are only saying that the same cause, of which we are as yet ignorant, causes a like change in both vitreous and zonula.

A spontaneous luxation may as well take place when the lens is perfectly transparent, as when it is cataractous. Further along, a different factor will be shown to be at work in influencing the spontaneous luxation

---

[1] Oppenheim's Zeitschrift, XXX, 3 Heft.

of a cataractous lens, which factor has nothing to do with the above-mentioned manner of occurrence, since in these latter cases there is no fluidity of the vitreous.

The symptoms of spontaneous luxation necessarily vary, depending on the fact, whether the lens is transparent or not.

In cases of transparent lenses, the symptoms are very much like those of ectopia lentis; they differ, however, from these, in that the symptoms develop in a proportionately shorter time. True, as a rule, this sinking down takes place slowly, though always more rapidly than in the cases described under congenital ectopia lentis.

In order to make a differential diagnosis, it is of great importance to be able to determine, if for a certain period of life, vision has been normal. In just such cases, where formerly vision was perfectly normal, the patient will become aware of the change, vision is not so sharp, and in trying to see accurately, objects seem to oscillate. The lens begins to move about behind the iris, and in consequence the iris begins to tremble. Examination of the refraction discloses the fact that the far point has come nearer to the eye. If the lens has sunk down so far that a part of the pupil is free, a double refractive condition will result, together with true monocular diplopia, as in ectopia lentis. A further striking symptom is now added, since vision changes with each change in the position of the head, for on bending the head forward the lens comes up close to the iris, whereas on bending the head backward, the lens falls back into the vitreous. In the first case the already unequally deep chamber becomes shallower, whereas in the latter it becomes much deeper. Where there is a great mobility, symptoms of irritation on the part of the iris and choroid may develop. This is preceded by a variety of ectopic phenomena. The patient becomes aware of the presence of the lens as a grey disc, or as a similarly colored segment of a circle, and at the same time he begins to see flashes of light and flame like figures; likewise, irritability to light, tearing, and pain may be added.

If the zonula zinii has been entirely dissolved, the slightest jar may cause the lens to fall into the anterior chamber.

In course of time, lenticular and capsular cataracts always follow in cases where there has taken place a luxation of the lens system.

The spontaneous luxation of the *cataractous* lens is produced in an entirely different manner. This is not true of all cataracts which spontaneously leave the pupillary area, for it is possible for the vitreous to become fluid in cases of cataract: without taking into consideration those cases, in which the displacement is of such a slight degree that it has been overlooked, but nevertheless, in consequence of which the lens has become cataractous.

It has long been known, as an established fact, that after a fully-developed senile cataract has existed for a long time, the cataract may spontaneously leave the pupillary area. Before this can occur, it is necessary that a loosening take place, between the zonula zinii and the lens on the one hand, and between the posterior and the concave vitreous depression on the other. Wenzel, Beer, and others have reported that not infrequently, on making a flap incision, the lens, together with its capsule, would pop out of the eye with considerable force. This can only be explained, by assuming that the tension on the zonula zinii, and perhaps also the sudden change in the position and form which takes place in the lens, the moment the aqueous is evacuated; and also due to the pressure the vitreous exerts anteriorly, is sufficient to tear the lens from its connections. It must have been these observations which led to the development of those methods which had as their object the removal of the lens together with its capsule.

The anatomical cause of such a loosening of the lens from its attachments is not to be sought in a fluid vitreous. Not only are we in possession of reports of cases in which the removal of the lens in its capsule was not followed by an evacuation of vitreous, operators know only too well, that a fluid vitreous has a tendency to get in front of the lens and cause the lens to fall backward into the vitreous. However, one must not lose sight of those senile changes in the zonula fibres already described, which makes them stiffer and more brittle, so that they are less able to resist a sudden force acting on them. However, the greatest stress must be laid on the condition of the anterior capsule. If our conception regarding the formation of capsular cataract is correct, the formative stage is followed by the stage of shrinkage, just as we see it in cicatrical tissue. Since we know that the capsular cataract does reach its limit, in that it does not grow in the periphery, as it does in thickness ad libitum, it must necessarily finally become reduced in volume after it has reached its maximum growth. Further, since it is formed on the concave side of the anterior capsule on shrinking, it has the tendency of becoming tense like the string on a bow, and hence exerts a certain amount of tension on the capsule. As a result of this tension, capsular cataracts of long standing appear folded. H. Muller, l. c., pp. 281 and 284). This has been looked upon as one of the causes of pyramidal cataract. Such shrinkage likewise becomes a very important factor in the production of the various forms which secondary cataracts assume. The greater the amount of lens substance absorbed, the greater will be the effect on the shape of the entire lens, in cases in which the capsule has not been injured. The development of *cataracta tremula, natalis* and *elastica* will now be more easily understood, since these are principally capsular cataracts.

The spontaneous luxation of senile cataract is undoubtedly favored by changes in the zonula fibres, and could with difficulty occur without the intervention of some form of accidental traumatic cause, such as vomiting, convulsions or concussion of the entire body and the eye; this is, however, always preceded by the formation of a capsular cataract. The tension which is exerted on the anterior capsule during the process of shrinkage must all the more assist in severing this connection between the anterior capsule and the fibres of the zonula zinii, because this shrinking capsular cataract extends just to the peripheric endings where the zonula fibres are inserted into the anterior capsule.

This view is strengthened by the fact, that in cases of spontaneous luxation of senile cataract, as a rule, one finds extensive capsular cataract; further, that not only in spontaneously luxated lenses, but also in cases where at the extraction, the lens in its capsule escapes by itself, one can never discover any remains of zonular fibres on the capsule. This also shows that the connection is severed at the capsule and not along the length of the zonular fibres.

a. LUXATIO LENTIS TRAUMATICA—TRAUMATIC LUXATION.

Traumas, which may cause the lens to leave its normal position, are either contusions of the eyeball in which the coats of the eyeball may or may not be opened, or the zonula is ruptured by the direct action of a foreign body which has penetrated the eyeball. In the latter case the foreign body may either remain within or again leave the eyeball. If a foreign body penetrates the eyeball in such a manner as to sever the zonula zinii in only a circumscribed area, it goes without saying that besides the zonula, cornea, iris, and also the vitreous are always involved. If the injury is caused by a pointed instrument, (such as a needle, the shoemaker's awl, a steel pen, or a pointed knife-blade), this will again leave the eye and the injury may heal in a few days without any special reaction. Frequently the case comes under observation only after the wound has healed. The statements of the patient then lead us to make a very careful examination. Here we find a cicatrix in the cornea, a hole in the iris, through which, when properly examined, light can be reflected from the fundus. If the hole in the iris is larger and extends perpendicularly to the radiating striations of the iris, the pupil at this point will not be so wide, and consequently not perfectly circular. Possibly one can detect a number of flakes in the vitreous. Aside from disturbances of vision due to opacities in the vitreous, inaccuracy of vision may develop as the result of astygmatism. At the point where the Zonula has been severed, it will exert less pressure on the lens. At this point the lens becomes thicker, and in this meridian, the eye will become myopic. Attempts at cylindrical correction are as a rule attended with but slight success, since the entire meridian does not alter its refraction, the opposition end of the respective meridian remaining fastened in its normal condition. The result of such an injury, therefore, is a permanent reduction of vision. As to whether or not an iris prolapse follows the injury depends entirely on the size of the corneal wound. If this occurs, under certain conditions this must be exercised. It may necessitate an iridectomie.

If, aside from the above-mentioned tissues, the lens and *corpus ciliars* are injured, the process of healing becomes proportionately more complicated, and the sequelae for sight—in fact, for the whole eye; indeed, the second eye, since this may be sympathetically affected—may be of the very worst kind. Hence injuries of these parts are of the very greatest importance, and mention is made of this here so that it need not be referred to again.

Though it clearly is not within the province of this work to enter into the subject of SYMPATHETIC OPTHALMIA, still it seems but proper to state that most authorities today acknowledge that this disease is clearly an infection. Where a foreign body, as indicated above, penetrates the eyeball and is retained, be this a minute spicule of iron, steel, lead, copper, glass or stone, it may remain free in the vitreous or stick fast in the posterior wall of the eye; and, if aseptic, it may become encapsulated and remain latent for years. However, it may be her stated that even these capsules lead to tension on the vitreous and eventually to loss of the eye, notwithstanding the isolated cases reported in literature in which this result did not follow. Leber,[2] as the result of eleven years of experimental investigation with every conceivable substance, studying its action on the interior of the eye, states, that all the metals, even gold and silver, glass, etc., are gradually acted on by the fluid media of the eye, minute quantities gradually dissolved off, and thus act as an irritant causing a purulent inflammation which may be *aseptic* in its nature. The recognition of aseptic pus chemically produced, he regards as of the greatest therapeutic value. But where micro-organisms are carried into the eye with the foreign body the conditions are different and the occurrence of sympathetic opthalmia becomes a

---

[2] Die Enstehung der Entzundung und die wirkung der Entzundungs eregende Schadlichkeiten. Leipsig, 1891.

possibility, if not a probability. Becker considered this subject of such great importance that he devoted an entire chapter to its discussion.[3] He critically analyzed some twenty-two cases, and finally concluded that the tension of cicatrical bands on the ciliary body led to chronic irritation and sympathetic opthalmia. Many of these earlier experiences, read in the light of our present understanding of the subject, are clearly an infection.

"On New Year eve, 1870, a piece of a percussion cap flew into the eye of a twelve-year-old boy in the neighboring county of K. I (Becker) found, downward and inward from the edge of the cornea, two millimeters distant from its transparent edge, a wound about three millimeters long, into which the iris had prolapsed. After excising the prolapse, a coloboma was found extending to the periphery. After the wound was healed, on looking through this coloboma, one could see a distinct indentation of the edge of the lens, *Coloboma Lentis Artificiale*, and this also caused astygmatism. This piece of percussion cap became encapsulated without injury to the eye, and after a lapse of five years the eye still performs its function."

If, aside from cornea, iris, zonula and vitreous, *the lens* and *ciliary body* are involved, the prognosis and the duration of the trouble will materially depend on the extent of the injury to the parts. It then would certainly be advisable to cut short a long and painful stage of healing and forestall a possible sympathetic affection of the other eye by an immediate enucleation.

A contusion of the eyeball is frequently followed, without the coats of the eyeball being ruptured at any point, by a stretching and final separation of the fibres of the zonula zinii, and as a consequence, exerting a temporary or permanent influence, on the form and position of the lens.

It is questionable, and has not as yet been proven, whether or not the individual fibres of the zonula possess the property of elongation or distension. It is stated that where the anterior chamber is evacuated, the anterior capsule of the lens comes in contact with the cornea, and that this could not possibly occur without the elongation of the zonula fibres. It is only certain that the zonula fibres do not tear, otherwise the lens could not retain its normal position with a complete retention of its normal functions. Instead of an elongation of the zonula fibres, such a considerable moving forward of the lens (about 23 mm.) could be caused by an anterior movement of the ciliary body, together with the iris, and the increased convexity of the anterior surface of the lens.

"It would not have been necessary to mention this elongation of the zonular fibres, if it were not for a case reported by Aub,[4] which he tried to explain by

[3] Pathologie and Therapie des Linsensystems, p. 408.

[4] Arch. f. A. und O., II, I, p. 259.

using this hypothesis: A man, 35 years of age, while out hunting was struck on the eyeball by a shot from a shotgun. A single shot was removed from the outer portion of the conjunctiva the next day. On the fourth day after the operation a pronounced circum-corneal injection was present. The cornea was clear, the anterior chamber about one-half filled with bloody serum, pupil narrow, and iris changed in color. At the upper and outer half, the iris, equal to about one-sixth of its circumference, was prominent. After the use of atropine, the lens was disclosed uninjured, but pushed forward in its upper and outer portion. On the seventh day the inflammatory condition seemed to subside. The pupil was dilated ad maximum, but above and outward the lens still continued to press the iris forward. A stick held diagonally before the eye appeared thicker at its upper and outer end than at its lower and inner. Turned 90 degrees the stick appeared everywhere of equal thickness. By the use of a concave cylinder 1-20, placed in the corresponding axis, vision was improved to 20-100. On the thirteenth day the prominence of the iris and the metamorphosie had disappeared. Owing to a slight degree of myopia, V. equal to 20-30, and the cylinder no longer improved vision. Aub declares that this condition of the lens was caused by a partial relaxation of the zonula; but he fails to state in what manner he imagines this to have occurred. Arlt [5] translates 'relaxation' by the word distension (or elasticity), and without the slightest hesitancy accepts this as a condition. But returning to Aub's case I wish to draw attention to the fact that he has not proven that the zonula is elastic, and further, that a partial paralysis of the ciliary muscle, at the point where the shot struck the eye, would explain all the phenomena which he reports."

TRAUMATIC LUXATION is always the result of a tearing of the zonula zinii without an injury of the lens capsule. Since it can not be assumed that tears in the zonula can heal, we are justified in making a diagnosis of a partial tear of the zonula, in all cases in which, in consequence of a contusion, the phenomena of a dislocation of the lens system appear and do not retrogress. In the beginning, these phenomena are the development of a myopia and the gradual shortening of the distance of the far point of the eye. If the tension which the zonula exerts on the crystalline lens is abolished, owing to an extensive or possible total tear, the equatorial diameter will be diminished and the axial diameter will be increased. Owing to this change in the form of the lens, the far point will approach closer to the eye. But where there is a total, or even a very extensive tearing of the zonula, accommodation becomes impossible, and there will be but one point, which will neither coincide with the former far or near point, at which it will be possible to see distinctly. The former symptom will, however, only then become valuable for differential diagnosis, where

5 Uber die Verletzungen des Auges in Gerichtsarztlicher Zeziehung. Wiener Med.-Wochenschrift, 1874, No. 15, S. 296.

we know, what the refraction of the eye was previous to the accident. In many cases, however, by comparing the eye with the uninjured one, we can, with a considerable degree of certainty, form an estimate. (It must, however, not be forgotten that not infrequently the refractive conditions of the two eyes are not alike; hence it can never give more than an approximate result.)

If the lens is not held equally tense in all directions by the zonula fibres and held fast in its connection with the ciliary processes, on moving the eye, the lens will begin to make independent movements, in which the iris will participate. (Trembling of the iris—*iridodonesis*). However, this symptom alone does not decide anything as long as the lens is transparent. For the iris may independently make such movements if the pupillary margin is free and an abnormal amount of aqueous is behind it. In exceptional cases, this can be observed; as, per example, where there is a large cornea and a relatively small lens, in cases of myopia with relatively deep anterior chamber, in cases of buphthalmus, and in cases of *synchisis corporis vitrei*, where the lens lies deeper than the normal.

b. SUBLUXATION OF THE LENS.

In cases in which there is a partial tearing of the zonula, the lens may retain its position unchanged in the concave hollow of the vitreous for an indefinite length of time. In most cases, however, after a time the lens in a two-fold manner changes its position, in that it not only turns on its equatorial diameter, but also moves toward the side where the zonula is still intact. Due to this oblique position or turning of the lens, the iris is pressed forward at one point, and consequently the anterior chamber at that point is shallower. The opposite edge of the lens approaches the axis, and on using the opthalmoscope it may be seen when the pupil is small, and must appear when the pupil is dilated as a black segment of a circle. However small this segment of a circle may be, by means of this, we can definitely determine the position of the lens and the kind of transposition we have before us. The edge may even become visible to the patient, as a black ring. If the edge of the lens passes through a pupil of normal size, naturally, everything will be seen double.

The importance of a subluxation rests on the fact, that under all circumstances there will be permanent interference with vision. Aside from this, experience has taught us, that in nearly all cases, if the patient lives long enough, a total luxation will finally result. Further, in course of time the lens will always become cataractous. This frequently happens before the zonula is completely torn. The latter must naturally follow, since the constant oscillating of the lens, on moving the head and the eyes, necessarily must lead to an abnormal tension on the remaining zonula fibres. The same cause may finally lead to cyclitis, choroiditis and symptoms of glaucoma.

As has already been stated, a restitution of the zonula fibres as the result of healing is not to be expected. Hence one can not speak of a therapie for subluxation. In some special cases the attempt may be made to give aid, by the use of glasses, either by looking through the dislocated lens, or to the side of it. If the lens has become cataractous, the attempt may be made to give assistance by an iridectomie or by an extraction.

The mechanism by means of which a tearing of the zonula is brought about, is as little understood, as is the mechanism of all other internal injuries of the eye, which result from a *contusio bulbi*. It appears most probable, that the globe, owing to its peculiar situation in the orbit, can only be struck in its anterior position, by a blunt force, and most frequently is flattened in a direction from in front, below and outward, backward, upward and inward. Such a flattening, owing to the incompressibility of the media of the eye and the relatively slight elasticity of its coats, can not occur unless the globe is distended in the eqautorial region. If the cornea is the part compressed the distension will take place at the sclero-corneal ring. By this means we can most easily explain, why it is that choroidal ruptures occur most frequently in the equatorial region and very nearly concentric and opposite the place to which the force was applied. This also explains the relatively frequent occurrence of *iridodialysis* and tears of the zonula. Relative to the latter, we must also consider that in every case of concussion of the eyeball, the lens, owing to its greater specific weight, tries to make more extensive movements and hence pulls on the zonula, which tears when a certain degree of tension is brought to bear on it.[6]

The lens may retain its position in the fossa patellaris in cases in which there is a partial, as well as when there is a total tearing of the zonula. In most cases instantly, in other cases after a certain length of time, the lens changes its position, remaining in contact with the patellar fossa or leaving it altogether. The first condition occurs most frequently and will continue longer where the zonula is but partially torn. This may be designated as a *sub-luxation*, (Arlt), in contradistinction to a *luxation*, in which the crystalline body has entirely left the hollow grove of the vitreous, and is found either in the anterior chamber or wedged in the pupii

6 Vergl. Arlt. Wiener Med. Wochenschrift, 1874, No. 12, p. 231.

or in the vitreous, or, finally, that it has been dragged entirely out of the eyeball.

The force which causes a *contusio bulbi*, as a rule strikes the eye in a direct manner. The body coming in contact with the eye may be relatively large as compared with the size of the eye, and have considerable thickness, or have a blunted end on a rounded prominence; and this, aside from causing a general flattening of the globe, may cause a locally deeper impression without penetrating the coats of the eyeball. But it is not necessary that the force strike the eye in a direct manner. Thrusts, blows, gunshot wounds which strike the neighboring bones, may likewise cause a concussion of the eyeball. Finally, it may be mentioned that projectiles flying past, close to the eye, may cause a *commotio bulbi*. During the war of '70-71, I (Becker) saw two cases of injury of the eye which were caused in this manner. True, both cases were ruptures of the choroid, not tears of the zonula, but since the former did occur, it can not be doubted that the latter is a possibility.

c. TOTAL LUXATION OF THE LENS.

Everything which has been said regarding the manner in which subluxation may be caused, is also true in this instance. A trauma of greater intensity, instead of causing a subluxation, causes a luxation. As a rule, a total luxation is preceded by the entire tearing of the zonula zinii; however, one can understand, that a few fibres may remain intact, though the lens be entirely removed from the fossa patellaris.

On which factor, the direction of the luxation of the lens depends, is not known: the symptoms naturally vary and depend entirely on the position of the lens. *When the luxated lens is found in the anterior chamber*, as the direct result of a trauma, we see a round body, with an almost golden colored ring which lies concentric to the base of the cornea, and it has a very deceptive similarity to a drop of oil. This body does not entirely fill the anterior chamber, but the iris is not visible, since it has been inverted. Aside from this phenomenon of total reflection of the edge of the lens, one can see, on focal illumination, in the transparent body, radiating striations and splits, which can be traced to the lens. If such an eye is examined shortly after the injury, one sees the results of the action of the direct trauma, in the neighborhood of the eye, whereas the eye itself is free from any irritation. Later, however, (in most cases, after a few days), ciliary injection and even swelling of the conjunctiva bulbi sets in, and the globe becomes glaucomatose and exceedingly painful. Then the cornea becomes cloudy at the point where the lens is in contact with it, and finally, as the subjective symptom and infiltration go on increasing, perforation takes place. The final result is, escape of the lens and purulent phthisis of the globe.

The lens does not always completely enter the anterior chamber, owing to the spastic contraction of the sphincter iridis, for just as the lens is passing through the pupil, it may become fixed. Here the picture is highly characteristic and can not be mistaken. Nearly always do we see a more or less transparent, round and flattened body extending obliquely into the anterior chamber, and at its edge can be seen the well-known shining, reflected ring. In most cases, such a condition is transitory. If the spasm continues, pain will be added to the interference with vision. The patient seeks relief, which can be given him by the energetic use of atropine. If this is not done, glaucoma will follow, and finally, as the result of ulceration, the eye will become phthisical. It appears, that exceptionally this condition may be tolerated for a considerable length of time. Bader [7] describes an eye, which is in the museum at Moorfield's Hospital, London, showing a lens in its capsule, fixed in the pupil, and which had taken on permanently a biscuit form. He fails, however, to state whether the lens attained this position as the direct result of a trauma, or whether this was simply the result of a change of position of a freely movable lens, which had become wedged in the pupillary area.

The lens is most frequently luxated into the vitreous. Since it has a heavier specific weight, hence after a time, if not at once, we may seek it in the lower portion of the vitreous space. It will now depend largely on the condition—that is, the consistence—of the vitreous, and most probably also, whether or not a portion of the zonula fibres have remained uninjured, if the lens, on moving the eyes, will remain quiet, relatively speaking, or if it make very wide excursions. We must also remember, that, owing to these active movements of the lens, the vitreous must gradually become diseased; that is, fluid. The lens, enclosed in its capsule, may remain transparent for a long time; it will, however, finally become cataractous. Though the capsule prevents the lens from being absorbed, it will nevertheless, gradually become smaller. It is not known whether the intracapsular cells will undergo a hyperplasia where a normal lens sinks into the vitreous, as the result of a trauma. Luxated lenses examined showed incipient capsular cataracts. However, it could not be determined whether this was the result of, or had existed previous to, the luxation. This is mentioned simply to draw the attention of my colleagues to this question, owing to its great importance.

---

[7] The natural and morbid changes of the human eye, etc. London, 1868, p. 266.

d. FREELY MOVEABLE LENSES.

Under this name, a condition has been described and illustrated by innumerable case reports, which may result just as well from congenital ectopia lentis, as in consequence of spontaneous or traumatic luxation. This name was introduced by Heyman. The cases belonging to this category date back a very long time. The common symptom of all these cases is, that the lens, no matter what the position of the head or eye, always takes a position relative to its weight. This does not only refer to a change of position in the vitreous, but the lens may also become wedged in the pupillary area, or even get into the anterior chamber.

In cases of congenital ectopia we must assume that the zonula fibres have an abnormal length. As a result, the lens may slip into the anterior chamber or fall back again into the vitreous. "Such a case, I (Becker) saw at Arlt's clinic, where a boy, eight years of age, could easily accomplish this change. Since, when this small lens was in the anterior chamber, fine indentations were observed all around the periphery of the lens, which undoubtedly were due to the tightened, tense zonula fibres; hence this case served to remove any doubts in my mind, that there are cases of freely movable lenses in which the zonula is not torn."

The symptoms which such a freely movable lens cause, are in part purely optical in their nature; in part pathological, since they cause pain, and other subjective symptoms which give rise to the necessity for operative interference if we desire to prevent total destruction of the eye.

Arlt reported a case.[8] illustrating the first mentioned symptom. A carpenter, 48 years of age, who had always been in perfect health, and who during his school days had had good vision, gradually later on became nearsighted. In his 45th year he suddenly developed monocular diplopia in both eyes. At the end of one year the double sight disappeared again. If he lay on his back he imagined that he saw in front of each eye a round disc, almost like a drop of oil, having a dark edge. For a time, for distance he used convex glasses; he, however, had to discontinue their use. Generally, however, he could read ordinary printed reading matter without spectacles; only, however, when he held it close to his breast. In directing the eyes downward he caused the lenses to apply themselves closely behind the iris, in the pupillary area, and thus he was enabled to read.

The following case is reported by Noyes.[9] A man 45 years of age was struck in the left eye by the fist of another. Three weeks later the diagnosis of luxation downward into the vitreous was made. His refraction was that of aphakia. A week later the patient reported that he saw good again. The crystal-

---

8 Die Krankheiten des Auges, III, p. 5, 1856.

9 Auch. fur Augen und Ohren. Heilkunde, I. 1, p. 134.

line lens, as could easily be determined by the condition of the iris, which was pressed backward, and by the light edge of the lens, had slipped into the anterior chamber. It was still in its capsule, and had a faint amber color, but absolutely transparent, corresponding to the age of the patient. The change of position was brought about by the patient sneezing violently after taking a pinch of snuff on leaving the clinic, where his pupil had been widely dilated by atropine. Immediately thereafter he noticed that vision was improved. Examination of his refraction disclosed Hm. equal to 1-18; V. equal to 20-40 on his right eye; his left injured eye M. equal to 1-9, As. m. .24, V. 20-50. The myopia is explained by the advance of the nodal point, also as a result of the increase convexity of the lens, which had been loosened from the zonula attachment. Noyes states that the astygmatism is due to the fact that since the lens does not completely fill out the anterior chamber, it sinks down; hence, its axis and that of the cornea do not coincide, but that of the lens lies somewhat deeper. There are, however, most certainly other factors at work which cause the lens to suffer in its symmetrical form.

The presence of the lens in the anterior chamber may be born for a long time without destroying the eye; in fact, for years. It is hardly possible for the condition to exist without disturbing the functions of the eye. The pathological changes which follow affect the cornea, which becomes cloudy when the lens comes in contact with it; the iris becomes hyperaemic and loses its color, and cyclitis is developed. Without the development of an exudate—that is, the development of true iritis, a severe ciliary injection develops, and to this chemosis may be added. At the same time, the globe becomes tense and hard, and the other symptoms of secondary glaucoma develop. In some cases, in a proportionately short space of time, the globe changes its form, the area of the sclerosis close to the cornea becomes bluish in color, and a staphyloma intercalare develops. The globe becomes pear-shaped and the axis of the globe may become enormously elongated. The inflammatory symptoms increase and finally either lead to ulceration of the cornea, with loss of the lens, so that *phthisis bulbi* results, or the inflammatory symptoms gradually subside, leaving an amaurotic ectatic globe, which gives rise to no further trouble. In such a case one will find the lens considerably diminished in size, adherent to the cornea.

It appears, that in cases in which the zonula is intact, the permanent presence of the lens in the anterior chamber (free mobility of the lens, owing to congenital lengthening of the zonula) will much sooner lead to intense symptoms of reaction, than in cases in which the lens is perfectly free from its suspensory ligaments. It is most probable, that the great danger of a partial luxation, is due to the constant tension which the remaining portion of the zonula exerts on the ciliary body (Von Graefe).

Hence the lens, which is luxated into the anterior chamber, may involve the cornea and iris, owing to direct contact, and the ciliary body as the result of tension of the zonular fibres.

As long ago as 1856 Arlt [10] described such cases of persistent luxation of the lens into the anterior chamber. The occurrence of growing together of lens and cornea was noted by von Graefe (Arch. fur Opthal., XV, 3, 158), and he states that such cases are the result of dislocation of the lens in the early years of life. Such lenses can be successfully extracted. As regards vision, we can only expect good results before staphyloma intercalare has developed. I (Becker) have been given the accurate history of a case and the operative result, through the kindness of Prof. Mauthner. The nine-year-old N. N. is said to have seen well up to her eighth year. From this time on her vision began to diminish, said to have resulted from a fever. In the left eye the iris, in its upper half, is more anteriorly situated than in its lower half. The pupil is black, and somewhat displaced upwards, irido-donesis. The refractive media are clear. The eye is highly myopic, irregularly astygmatic, but shows no staphyloma. With—$\frac{1}{5}$ vision can be improved to $\frac{18}{8}$. On use of atropine, full dilation of the pupil is obtained, but the lower margin of the lens can not be seen. The right eye shows a normal conjunctiva and cornea; no ciliary injection. Near the highest point of the anterior chamber is located the greyish white and cloudy lens. It is closely adherent to the posterior surface of the cornea, and is immovable. It is smaller in all its diameters, and is shrunken to about two-thirds its normal size. The iris, as far as can be judged, shows no abnormality. The pupil, which can not be dilated by use of atropine, is completely covered by the lens. On May 23, 1870, Mauthner extracted the lens of the right eye by means of a peripheric linear incision. The Graefe knife passed through the *Aequator Lentis*, and the part of the iris which was pressed forward was excised. The lens, which on pressure did not come out, was finally removed with a Yaeger's circular spoon. Nevertheless, a portion of the lens remained adherent to the posterior wall of the cornea. A portion of this was removed with a Daviel's spoon, without, however, causing the cornea to give up its non-transparent and cloudy appearance. No special reaction followed the operation. At the end of five days a severe episcleral injection developed; on the seventh new vessels became visible, extending from the line of the corneal incision up to the part where the cloudiness existed in the posterior portion of the cornea. The lower half of the pupillary margin is adherent to the cloudy corneal tissue. In about one week the episcleral injection and new formed vessels disappeared. By means of a broad iridectomie downward, made on the 22d of June, vision was increased to $\frac{18}{8}$ by use of -|-1-4, equal to -|-10 D.

The pathological and anatomical conditions of the case may be explained by the examination of an eye, which, I am sorry to say, was sent to me (Becker) without a history by Dr. Schmidt, of Odessa. It is exceedingly pear-shaped,

[10] Die Krankheiten des Auges, II. 274.

has a deep excavation of the optic nerve, and shows a detachment of the vitreous, ciliary staphyloma, and in its anterior chamber, almost at the anterior pole, is a lens 3½ mm. in thickness, and 4½ mm. in width. The lens is enclosed in its capsule, which is shrunken at some points; it is cataractous, and adherent to the posterior surface of the cornea. Examined with the naked eye, the lens appears held adherent to the cornea by a mass of exudate. The microscopical examination of the half of the eye placed at my disposal was made by my assistant, Dr. Raab. This showed that at the point of attachment, the corneal cloudiness extended almost to Bowman's membrane, and that this was permeated by blood vessels. At which point these vessels stand in connection with the vessels of the cornea, can not be decided from this half of the eye. The descemetis had been severed over a wide extent of surface, had drawn back and was folded upon itself upward, and downward it had rolled itself up spirally in a most characteristic manner. A new formation has pushed its way in between the descemetis and the original corneal tissue, which also extends in various directions and to a varying extent over the outer surface of the shrunken capsule. The lens has no connection with the iris, which passes transversely across the anterior chamber from its place of origin at the corneal edge (5½ mm. behind the pole of the cornea). The cornea is thicker in the center than at its periphery. *The Corpus Ciliare* is exceedingly atrophic, the ciliary processes appearing as thin ridges. A most exact description of the case, together with the illustrations, can be found in the second edition of Becker's Atlas (Die Pathologische Topographie des Auges), Plate XVIII. This case differs from Mauthner's, in that in the former a ciliary staplyoma had not as yet developed, and consequently one could expect an improvement in vision.

The phenomena which were observed during and after the operation at the line of attachment, especially the persistence of the cloudiness at the point and the development of vessels and their disappearance again, are fully explained by the foregoing examination. Where violent symptoms of reaction begin to develop, both in cases of spontaneous luxation, as well as traumatic luxations in the anterior chamber, a threatened ulceration of the cornea, ending in phthisis, and a total loss of vision, due to secondary glaucoma, can only be averted by an early extraction. Hence, Arlt advised the use of a small Beer's knife, and in each case he decides according to the special features of the case, whether or not the capsule should be opened at the same time. If we desire to excise the iris after the lens has been extracted, this can be grasped by a hook. It will scarcely be possible to avoid escape of vitreous. In order to avoid a possible choroidal hemorrhage, it is advisable to first induce deep narcosis. If the operation is made before the development of glaucoma, the result will be better. The peculiar features which may develop during the process of healing, where glaucoma has already set in, are illustrated by the following case:

The seventy-three-year-old wife of a gardener, while chopping wood, struck herself in the right eye. In the beginning the pain was not severe; she could see, "only different," as she expressed it. On the third day the pain became very violent, and vision was almost totally abolished. On being called, I found the lens in the anterior chamber, the iris pushed back and the entire eyeball red and hard. She could still count fingers. On the eleventh day I made the extraction upward by means of a flap incision. The lens escaped easily without loss of vitreous, and the iris was not excised. Pain ceased at once, the wound healed very quickly, and the patient was ready to be discharged on the tenth day. Since she could not receive proper attention at home she remained at the clinic. I made a trip, and to my astonishment on my return, after an absence of three weeks, found her still at the clinic. Owing to increased intraocular tension, the wound which had healed so quickly commenced to give, and without a perforation having ever taken place, or the iris cicatrized in the wound, I found an ectatic condition of the cicatrix. Notwithstanding the most intense pain the patient would not permit me to enucleate. Therefore, I made an incision through the cicatrix, and permitted sufficient vitreous to escape, so that phthisis bulbi followed.

If, at the time of the trauma the luxated lens is already cataractous, the diagnosis is easy. Owing to its cloudiness, no matter where located, the lens can be found. The subjective symptoms are subject to change, insomuch, that the lost vision may be restored. Respecting the aetiology, one must only be reminded of cases of long standing cataract, where, owing to the shrinkage of new formations on the inner surface of the anterior capsule, the connection between the capsule and the zonula are loosened, and in these cases a contusion of the eyeball, or a concussion of the entire body may be the exciting cause to bring about the condition. Here the luxation is really not spontaneous, but one must assume that if the accidental cause had not taken place, the same result would nevertheless have occurred in course of time. The operative procedure of reclination must also be looked upon as a cause of luxation. The occurrence of luxation into the anterior chamber during the operation of reclination became a matter of great importance in the history of opthalmology. Even in extraction, luxation of the cataract plays a prominent part.

A freely movable cataractous lens is also described, especially the calcareous cataract. As vision, as a rule, is totally lost in cases of calcareous lenses, it is simply a question of removing a calcareous lens which has fallen into the anterior chamber, or become wedged in the pupil, either for cosmetic purpose, since the white or yellow amber-colored, wrinkled body disfigures the eye very much; or one operated on account of the pain or inter-current inflammation. In such operations one must be prepared, not only for the escape of vitreous, but for large choroidal hemorrhages. For this reason, the prognosis as the result of an operation is exceedingly dubious.

If, at the time of the contusion of the globe, the sclera is ruptured, in nearly every case the lens will be removed from its normal position. It may remain in the eye, and thus become a new source of danger, for in nearly every case the capsule is opened. The prognosis, however, does not entirely depend on the lens; hence we need not consider these cases any further. It is, however, not an infrequent occurrence for the lens to be forced out of the eye at the time of the accident. The sclerotic is nearly always ruptured in a direction which is concentric to the base of the cornea, at about 2 (at most, 4) mm. distance from the base of the cornea, most frequently upward, and upward and inward; only isolated cases have been reported where such a rupture has taken place downward. Whether the conjunctiva ruptures at the time or not, depends on the force of the blow. In the first case, the lens will be found in the conjunctival sac, or it is never found. Iris and corpus ciliare, as well as a good portion of the vitreous, prolapse from the wound, and the entire globe collapses. Blood is found in the anterior chamber and, as can be seen in cases which heal, the vitreous is permeated with large clots of blood. Treatment consists in excising the prolapsed uvea and vitreous and applying an asceptic dressing to the eye. The application of cold, especially ice compresses seem to be of great benefit. If the conjunctiva has not been ruptured we will find under a vesicle-like elevation of the conjunctiva, the lens in its capsule, appearing like a round, transparent body, which on focal illumination gives the well-known shining circle. In this location, the lens may retain its transparency for weeks, so that the rupture of the sclerotic, through which the lens escaped, may become entirely healed. It is a striking fact, that in these cases of luxation under the conjunctiva, neither iris nor vitreous prolapse from the wound. The iris, however, is frequently inverted at this point, and simulates a coloboma. Where the sclerotic closes again before the lens is removed, the process of healing is a much simpler one, the conjunctiva acting as a barrier against infection.

SECONDARY LUXATION OF THE LENS.

DISLOCATIO LENTIS.

Among those pathological conditions of a complicated character, which lead secondarily to a luxation of the lens, those which lead to staphylomatous formations occupy the first position.

If, owing to the perforation of a corneal ulcer, the aqueous escapes, or if as the result of a trauma, the anterior chamber is opened, the iris and lens will apply themselves to the posterior surface of the cornea. If the opening closes again, so that no more aqueous escapes, under certain conditions both iris and lens will return to their normal position. But just as the iris, owing to an anterior synechia, may be held in the wound, the lens may likewise, with or without a previous opening of the capsule, be held fast by new-formed cicatrical tissue and thus be prevented from fully returning to its normal position.

It is well known that cases of large perforating wounds of the cornea lead to partial or total corneal staplyloma. The influence which this exerts on the position of the lens depends entirely on the fact whether the entire lens escaped at the corneal perforation or whether the capsule was simply opened, and a portion of the lens was evacuated, or whether the lens, either intact or opened, has become cicatrized to the bulging cornea; and, finally, where all these conditions are not present, whether the corneal staplyloma does not secondarily lead to a dilation of the *annulus ciliaris*, and thus cause a partial or total tearing of the zonula zinii. Accordingly, we may find in the staphyloma either no lens at all, or a *cataracta secundaria*, or the lens is adherent in front, or it may be perfectly unchanged in its normal position, or it may finally be found floating in the vitreous, still attached to the remains of the zonula. In cases of buphthalmus, just as in cases of staphyloma intercalare, the zonula finally tears, and the lens is luxated.

If the pus, in case of panopthalmitis, or purulent hyalitis and choroiditis, forces its way out of the eye, in the majority of cases it will do so, so close to the periphery of the cornea as to partially distroy the zonula. The lens will be displaced and imbedded in a purulent mass, which is partially derived from the vitreous and ciliary body, partially from the iris. In these cases, the lens assumes the most peculiar shapes, which no doubt result (being preceded by softening) from an unequal pressure exerted in a purely mechanical way. Finally, new formations which originate in the retina and choroid, as soon as they come in contact with the lens, force the lens from its normal position, and can cause it to assume the most wonderful shapes. A *hydrops camerae anterious* will press the lens backward; a *choroiditis serosa* or *glaucoma* will force it forward. In a case of spontaneous abscess of the vitreous which followed years after an operation for glaucoma, I observed how the lens was pressed forward until it touched the posterior surface of the cornea, even before a change in the shape of the eye occurred.

CHAPTER V.

**MALFORMATIONS OF THE LENS WITHOUT DEMONSTRATA-
BLE PATHOLOGICAL CHANGES IN THE OTHER
PORTIONS OF THE EYE.**

INDENTED OR NOTCHED LENS. Owing to their great rarity, anomalies in form of the lens in otherwise healthy eyes are exceedingly interesting. The case which Becker describes in both his works is evidently one and the same. In his Anatomy, he states that it occurred in a syphilitic child a few weeks old, whereas in his "Pathology and Therapy," where the case is fully described, he says that it occurred in a boy eight years of age. Both cases are referred to in the same illustrations. (See Becker's Tafl., XII., Fig. 3, 4, 5).

"I (Becker) am in possession of both eyes of a boy 8 years of age, who had congenital syphilis, and who died in the hospital of Vienna in 1866. The eyes were sent to me because, during life, the boy had seen very poorly, without any outward cause being discernible. The lenses in both eyes were found to be of normal size, the anterior capsule of normal thickness and curvature. On the posterior surface, however, 1.25 mm. from the edge, there existed a horse-shoe like indentation open toward the bottom. As preparations of Dr. Goldzieher disclosed, the course of the fibres in the interior of the lens was an anomalous one, and thus accounted for the external appearance."

Knies [1] believed that he had seen a similar case, because he observed peculiar shadows on making an opthalmoscopic examination.

The anatomical connection between this anomalie and central cataract, spindle cataract and zonular cataract will be referred to further along, when these various forms come under consideration. A particularly instructive case (page 186) has been anatomically considered by Schirmer. which illustrates the possibility of its production in a manner analogous to that of a spindle cataract. This has likewise been referred to by Knies (quoted above).

LENTICONUS. CRYSTALLOKONUS. ANTERIOR ET POSTERIOR.

The entire literature on this subject comprises but sixteen cases, hence it will be seen how extremely rare is its occurrence.

The first case was described by Webster [2] as one of *lenticonus*, and the

---

[1] Uber den Spindelstaar und die Accommodation bei demselben. Arch. f. Opth., Bd. XXIII, 1, p. 219.

[2] Ein Fall von Lenticonus aus der Prexis der Dr. C. R. Agnew, Arch. fur Augen und Ohren. Knapp, Moos B. IV, 1874, p. 262.

second by Van der Laan and Placido[3] as *crystallokonus*. Both of these cases were *anterior lenticonus*, and from their descriptions it does not appear that this was a congenital anomalie, though in Webster's case, he describes a small posterior polar cataract and a punctate cloudiness of the posterior capsule. Both cases were observed in men between 23 and 24 years of age. In Webster's case, the history permits of the belief that it was congenital, whereas in Van der Laan's case the statement is made that the disease began to develop some eight years before the patient came under observation. Both authorities state that the lens extended outward, into the pupillary area as a regularly formed cone. Its appearance was like that of a keratoconus, and seemed to indicate a genetic similarity.

Becker states: "We would have no idea concerning the arrangement of the lens fibres in such a lens, had the opportunity not been given of studying the lens of a rabbit, sent to me by Scholer and Uthoff, and later of studying the second eye, which was sent to me, in which likewise there was no persistent hyaloid present, and in which the lens covered with its normal capsule extended conically *into the vitreous*. Unfortunately, the lens sent to me was very friable, and notwithstanding the utmost care, not a single perfect section extending through this process could be obtained. Hence the description is confined to Uthoff's sections, which were thick and unstained. By repeated examinations I convinced myself that the course of the lens fibres in the anterior portion of the eye was normal. Whereas, at the posterior pole there is a cone 1.5 mm. in height, and somewhat constricted at its base, into which the central sagittal fibres of the second period of foetal development extend. In the region of the posterior pole the concentrically arranged fibres are not in apposition with those of the opposite side, but appear to clasp this cone. It gives one the impression as though the lens as an entirety had suddenly been impeded in its further development (the sagittal fibres of the second period having been pressed backward). In the specimens examined, the conical process was almost completely covered by the capsule, though it is presumed that in a more perfect specimen the capsule would have been shown in its entirety. It need hardly be mentioned that the reference as to its origin is purely hypothetical."

This is the first report of a case of *posterior lenticonus*, and, so far, is the only case which has been anatomically examined. In January, 1888, Becker examined the first case observed in man. Owing to the very careful examination made, and the accurate description of the clinical features, this case is quoted in extenso.

Case of Posterior Lenticonus. Dr. F. Meyer, Assistant der Universitats Augenklinik zu Heidelberg.[4]

[3] Una nuova anomalie, etc. Period de Opth. Pract., No. 3. Lisbon, 1880. Nach Nagel's Yahresbericht, 1880, Bd. XI, p. 360.

[4] Arch. fur Augenheilkunde. February, 1888.

Carl E., 10 years of age, consulted Geh-Rath Becker January 7, 1888, who kindly permitted me to publish this case. His father states that for the past three or four years he has observed that his son's right eye deviates outward, but he is not positive whether the eye was perfectly straight previous to that time. Some six or nine months ago, while playing at ten-pins, the son had played so poorly that his (the father's) attention was drawn to his poor vision, and at the same time he discovered that he saw double. The son told him that he always saw double, and was surprised to learn that every one did not see as he did. The parents, brothers and sisters of the boy, all have good vision.

Status Praesens. The boy, a healthy blonde, shows no signs of ricketts, and has never been ill. The right eye shows a moderate degree of strabismus divergens. Externally there is nothing particularly noteworthy as to size or shape of the eye. Left eye Em. V. equal to 6-6. Right—counts fingers at 3.5 mm. The patient states he sees better with 12 D, but this is not really true. With the left eye he reads Y. No. 1 at 36 up to 37 cm., whereas on the right, No. 9 at 5 cm. with difficulty. Hence, he has full accommodative power on the left eye. As a rule he does not see double; but by placing a colored glass before the one eye, crossed double images can be produced, which can be fused by prism of 30 degrees for distance and 37 degrees for near.

Left Eye. Media are clear. Fundus slightly pigmented, the choroidal vessels being visible everywhere. Emmetropia.

Right Eye. Aside from its faulty position nothing pathological is to be observed. As compared with the cornea of the other eye there is no difference, and the keratoscope gives perfectly round rings. On casting the light into the eye with the opthalmoscope, a most interesting picture is disclosed, which becomes more distinct on atropizing the eye. In the center of the red reflected disc one sees a second, smaller circular figure, surrounded by a changeable dark ring. Its diameter is equal to about one-half the diameter of the surrounding lighter ring. It would not be quite correct to compare this inner circle to a drop of oil, since we get a picture more like that of a keratoconus (Webster). The dark encircling shadowy ring is really never seen as a perfect circle, it is rather a semi-circle; which, however, on the slightest movement, either on the part of the patient's eye, or of the observers, changes its position around the central disc. The central disc is not only distinct, as a result of this encircling dark ring, but also from the fact that with every movement of the eye, restless movements are made which are difficult to describe. Thus a series of light and dark circles are produced, which in one sense may be said to be making continuous movements, in that new ones are always appearing while others disappear.

Almost in the center of this inner disc one sees, slightly upward and outward, a sharply defined black speck, which is about 0.5 mm. in length and about one-half as wide, the long diameter extending from above and outward, downward and inward. This is surrounded above and inward by a dark line, almost as far removed from it as its diameter. Inward from this dark line is another dark spot, about as far distant as its length and about one-half as large. This latter, however, is not sharply defined, and aside from this are numerous fine punctate opacities.

On moving the eye the opacities undergo such a high degree of parallactic transposition in the opposite direction that one must secure very slight movements to prevent entire loss of these opacities out of the pupillary area. These movements are decidedly more marked than we are accustomed to note them, when there are opacities at the posterior pole of the lens, and hence permit of our drawing conclusions as to the probable seat of these opacities. One can safely say these opacities are further back than is the usual position of the posterior surface of the lens.

The Purkinje-Sanson pictures are present. The one belonging to the posterior surface of the lens makes very rapid movements on changing the position of the lamp.

On focal illumination we at once see the cause of the peculiar pictures noted above. One sees a funnel-shaped body deep in the sagittal axis of the eye, which reflects the light. The base of the body, as far as on can judge, is at the posterior surface of the lens, and from here it projects backward into the vitreous. This funnel-shaped body is perfectly transparent, and is continuous with the otherwise totally transparent substance of the lens, and its limiting surfaces show the same spots observed with the mirror, only where they were dark they now appear white, strongly reflecting the light, the one first described above appearing almost exactly at the tip of the funnel. Hence there can be no doubt as to the diagnosis of *lenticonus posterior.*

Opthalmoscopic examination in the direct method, to the side of the funnel, permits a good examination of the fundus, which shows nothing abnormal. In the direct method only the periphery of the fundus can be examined, and shows Em. It is impossible to gain a sharp image of the papilla; the best can be obtained by a 12 D or 13 D. The large opacity at the tip of the funnel is best seen with a $+$ 28 D.

That lenticonus posterior is neither a formative nor a developmental anomalie, but rather a pathological process, seems to be attested by the fact that opacities were present on the posterior capsule. One could then compare this condition to that of keratoconus, where, as a result of softening and thinning of the capsule, less resistance is offered to the presence of the growing lens.

Prof. Knapp[5] reported a case in 1891. He considers the conus congenital and stationary, and suggested the term *"ectasie"* or *"excavation of the posterior pole of the lens.* Since then, but three cases have been reported, one by J. Mitvalsky,[6] one by Eisach,[7] and one by Dr. Gullstrand.[8]

[5] Knapp's Arch., Vol. XXII, p. 28, 1891.

[6] Ein Neuer Fall von Lenticonus Posterior mit theilweiser persistence der Arteria Hyaloidea. Centralblatt fur prak Augenheilkunde. Mars, 1892.

[7] Ein Fall von Lenticonus Posterior. Zehender's Klin. Monatsblatt, March, 1892.

[8] Ein Fall von Lenticonus Posterior. Nordisk Opth. Tidskrift, V. 1, Centralblatt, p. 177, 1892.

In a recent paper by L. Bach,[9] the entire subject of lenticonus posterior is reviewed.

He states: "Up to the present time, but sixteen observations of lenticonus posterior have been made, and recently but three anatomical examinations." [10]

Clinical observations disclosed the fact, that this malformation occurred in twelve cases; eight times on one eye, four times on both. In the eight cases, the other eye was pronounced normal seven times. In the four cases, the statement is made that one case is, positively, and the other three cases, in all probability, congenital.

In eight cases a cataracta polaris posterior is said to have been present, together with the lenticonus posterior. In two cases, other opacities of the lens were present. In two cases, remains of the hyaloid artery were found, and in one, a rudimentary persistent pupillary membrane on the other eye.

Bach examined two cases occurring on two rabbits, and, as a result of his anatomical examinations, draws the following conclusions:—

"A disturbance in the development of the eye is the cause of lenticonus posterior. Sufficient facts are at hand to justify us in asserting that during the development of such eyes, there is an anomalous formation of the lens, possibly a slight disintegration at the posterior pole, together with a persistence of the vascular capsule of the lens, which latter remains in contact with a foetal vitreous strand. Then, as the eye increases in size, this strand exerts tension on the posterior capsule, drawing it out, and finally rupturing the same: at the same time the posterior cortical substance, following the direction of least resistance, diffuses itself posteriorly, and forms the lenticonus. Further, the lens substance may swell up, and thus lead to rupture of the capsule. There seems to be no doubt that lenticonus posterior is due to tension exerted on the posterior capsule by the connective tissue strand, which runs through the center of the vitreous. Disturbance in the retrogressive changes in the hyaloid artery, is certainly an aetiological factor in the genesis of lenticonus posterior."

9 Path. Anatomische Studien uber Verschiedene Missbildungen des Auges. Graefe Arch., Vol. XLV, Part I, 1898.

10 Pergeus Ed. Buphthalmus mit Lenticonus Posterior. Arch. f. Augenheilk. XXXV, 1 Heft, S. 1; Hess C. Path. Anat. Studien, etc. Graefe Arch., Vol. XLII, Part III, p. 214.

CHAPTER VI.

PARTIAL CATARACTS.

A.

AXIAL CATARACT. CATARACTA AXIALIS.

Only such cataracts should be considered as *partial*, which have remained as such for many years or during the whole of life; hence they are also stationary. All partial or stationary cataracts which are not the result of a trauma, are congenital or develop during the years the lens is growing (zonular cataract). The forms of partial cataract which occur most frequently are found on a line connecting the two poles of the lens. Hence they are called *axial cataracts*. Formerly they were called *cataracta centralis*, without regard to the fact, whether they were in the centre of the lens, or at its anterior or posterior pole; the centre of the pupil and the centre of the lens being looked upon as identical points. But as long ago as 1814, Benedict[1] drew attention to the uselessness of such a nomenclature, and he proposed that *centralis* should be applied, only to those rare cases in which an opacity of foetal origin, and confined to the nucleus of the lens remained. Those opacities due to inflammation of the capsule of the lens and located at the anterior pole are designated as *cataracta capsularis punctata*.

The axial cataracts are situated either in the centre of the lens, or at its anterior or posterior pole.

1. CATARACTA CENTRALIS (LENTIS).

CONGENITAL, CENTRAL LENS CATARACT.

During life the central cataract appears as a small, white, globular opacity in the nucleus of the lens, exactly in that place, where genetically one would expect to find the oldest fibres. The glaring white light which the central cataract reflects gives evidence of the intensity of the opacity at that point.

Such central cataracts have repeatedly been observed at birth, hence they are most certainly congenital. There are, however, cases (as will be shown further along) in which the opacity of a zonular cataract is so intense as to simulate a central cataract.

The remainder of the lens may be perfectly transparent, and vision excellent. From this we may also conclude, that the curvature of the anterior and posterior capsule is normal. In such cases the central cataract

---

[1] Monographie des Grauen Staar's. Breslau.

is often discovered by the merest chance: often not until very advanced life. More frequently, however, this form of cataract is complicated by other forms, together with *nystagmus*. Reute [2] believes that the nystagmus is not due to the cataract alone, but to some disease of the muscles or nerve inervation.

The seat of this form of cataract must be situated where, according to the development of the lens, one would expect to find the oldest lens fibres; those which had grown in a saggital direction; hence, we must come to the conclusion, that it was the fate of the lens fibres which belong to the second period of foetal development to form this variety of cataract. In very thin meridional sections of human lenses taken from the end of foetal life and the beginning of extra-uterine life, one can recognize these fibres enclosed in the concentric lamellae. It is especially worthy of note that in the sheep during the second period of development there is at times an entirely perverse position and unequal growth of the proximal cells. Though we can not conclude from this, that the cloudiness is the result of the abnormal position, nevertheless, the observation has shown, that at times the abnormal changes do take place. If, however, one is not inclined to believe that subsequently there is cloudiness of this conglomeration of cells; one can conceive of a condition here, as it occurs in lamellar cataract, where, over a mass of lens cells which have become cloudy, new lamellae of lens fibres are deposited, which have abnormal shape, position and transparency. This always presupposes that the productive viability of the epithelium of the anterior capsule and along the whorl has not been disturbed by the formation of the central cataract. The time of development of this form of cataract is placed during the second period of development of the lens; hence, about the sixth or seventh week of foetal life of the human embryo.

Arnold's idea, [3] that the lens is originally cloudy and later clears up from the periphery, must be dropped. For, as has been shown on page 51, this central cloudiness which Fr. Arnold found in the central portion of the lenses of young animals is due to the presence of a fatty substance which melts at a low degree of temperature, and this substance is only found in the centre of young lenses where the temperature is reduced; this coagulates, and the centre of the lens becomes cloudy: whereas, on heating to the temperature of the body, the lens clears up again, the substance returning to the fluid state.

---

[2] Walter von Ammon's Journal, f. d. Chir. and Augenheilkunde. XXXII, p. 524.

[3] Untersuchungen uber des Auge des Menschen. 1832, p. 154.

H. Muller [4] described a case occurring in a young goat, with cataracta polaris posterior and persistent hyaloid. But he was so taken up with the description of the posterior polar cataract, that he simply mentioned the presence of the cataracta centralis lentis.

Carl Hess reports an exceedingly interesting congenital anomaly in a chick 150 hours old.[5] The essential features of this malformation consisted in a delayed and incomplete closure of the lens vesicle, as it is derived from the epithelial plate. In consequence of this incomplete closure, the lens fibres were not held in by the enclosing capsule, and, undergoing hyperplasia, found an exit through the opening in the ampulla; as a result, the normal nutritive conditions were markedly disturbed, and a diffuse disintegration of the elongated fibre followed.

This description is exceedingly interesting, since it offers us an explanation as to the cause of certain forms of congenital cataracts, which up to this time has been purely speculative. It is possible, if the development of the chick had not been interfered with, that later on this lens vesicle might have become constricted and closed, after those fibres which had grown out of the ampulla had totally disintegrated, and a hindrance to a closure which they offered had been totally removed. The fibres within the ampulla (those which later on would have formed the nucleus), would also have disintegrated. If now, later on, new fibres had developed in a perfectly normal manner, a normal cortex would have formed around a diseased nucleus, thus giving us the picture of a true congenital central (nuclear) cataract. Hess further suggests the intimate connection between this form of cataract and zonular cataract, and he further states that anterior polar cataract could easily be explained as the result of a delayed closure of the lens vesicle. Spindle cataracts could be explained in a like manner.

2. CATARACTA POLARIS ANTERIOR. CATARACTA CENTRALIS CAPSULARIS ANTERIOR. CATARACTA CAPSULARIS PUNCTATA. ANTERIOR CENTRAL CATARACT. CATARACTA PYRAMIDALIS. CATA-RACTA PYRAMIDATA.

Frequently we find a small, glistening, white, and (as a rule) round opacity at the anterior pole, which reflects the light. This opacity varies in size from that which is just perceptible, up to one having a diameter

---

[4] Gesammelte und Hinterlassene Schriften Herausgegeben von O. Becker, 1872, Bd. 1.

[5] "Zur Pathology und Pathologischen Anatomie Verschiedener Staaar Formen." Graefe Arch., XXXIX, 1893, B. 1, p. 183.

of from 2 to 2¼ mm. At times this white spot is smooth on the surface; again, it may extend out into the anterior chamber the distance of a milometre. When the pupil is contracted, it touches this on all sides, whereas when the pupil is enlarged it always remains situated in the centre of the same. In the "flat varieties," if they are not too small, we can at times demonstrate by focal illumination a slight folding of the adjacent parts of the capsule. Those which extend into the anterior chamber are known as *cataracta pyramidalis* or *pyramidata*. Very often the cataracta pyramidalis is the only anomaly of the eye. In such cases the amount of vision depends largely on the size of the cataract, and the conditions of its adjacent parts of the capsule. Cases have been repeatedly observed in which vision was perfectly normal. More frequently, however, it is associated with the opacities of the lens, such as cataracta centralis. In all such cases, attention should be directed to the transparency of the cornea; also, careful investigation for remains of a pupillary membrane should be made.

In his "Anatomie," Becker divides anterior polar cataracts into three groups—the congenital, the acquired, and those due to adhesions between capsule and iris.

a. CATARACTA POLARIS ANTERIOR (PYRAMIDALIS) CONGENITA.

All the varieties of cataract noted at this point are *capsular cataracts*. In all cases of *congenital anterior polar cataract*, the lens is otherwise normally constructed. Hence the cataract must have developed after the concentric formation of the lens had begun; hence in the third period of foetal development, possibly at the close of the second. In the foregoing division, attention is drawn to a case observed by Hess, and the possibility of a late closure of the lens vesicle being the cause of an anterior polar cataract. It appears that neither these congenital anterior polar cataracts, nor the acquired forms seem to interfere with the further growth of the lens, and, finally, since the growth of the lens follows as a result of indirect cell division of the anterior epithelium, a partial loss of this epithelium can not interfere with the further growth of the lens. The histological structure of these capsular cataracts differ in no way from capsular cataract as already described.

The capsule itself is not drawn out as a regular one, but seems rather to be folded, and on section shows very pretty pictures. Frequently the base of the pyramidal cataract is round, and extends for some distance into the lens substance; in fact, the central portion seems to extend a little deeper, so that its edge appears curved and distinct against the surrounding transparent lens substance. Where there is a constriction near the

anterior capsule, this curvature becomes especially marked, and it appears
as though this constriction were the cause for the curvature of the deeper
layers of fibres. At times one observes that the pyramidal cataract, as well
as the flat ones, are continuous with a sharp process, which extends backward into the lens substance. Such forms are the transitional step to the
formation of the spindle cataracts.

b. CATARACTA POLARIS ANTERIOR. (ACQUISITA). ACQUIRED ANTERIOR CENTRAL CAPSULAR CATARACT.

The aetiology of the acquired form of central capsular cataract has
been the subject of a great deal of study and investigation. According to
Arlt, it develops in children, seldom in adults, as a result of a perforating
central corneal ulcer. He was of the opinion that a portion of the exudate
remained adherent to the capsule. It is not to be denied that this can
occur. The cases of cataracta pyramidalis in which a shred of scar tissue
extends from the cornea to the capsule, and thus, by this means, draws the
lens and iris forward and holds them in this position, demonstrates that
scar tissue which is formed by cornea and iris can take part in the formation
of the pyramidal cataract. This, however, is not necessary. Schweigger
convinced himself, that corneal ulcers which are not situated in the centre of
the cornea and perforate may give rise to central capsular cataract. Hulke
(O. H. R., p. 189) does not consider it necessary that a perforation should
occur in order to give rise to a central capsular cataract. Owing to the
extreme shallowness of the anterior chamber in the child's eye, especially
in the new-born, a simple swelling of the corneal tissue during an inflammatory process (as, per example, in bl. neonatorum), is sufficient to bring
the lens and cornea in contact (Mackenzie, Ed. IV., p. 469). In both cases
—either where the aqueous is drained off, or where the inflammatory irritation causes a contraction of the pupil—only the centre of the anterior
capsule is permitted to come in contact with the inner surface of the cornea, and it appears, if this takes place for a sufficient length of time, it
will induce a hyperplasia of the capsular epithelium. According to Knies,[6]
but a few days of actual contact of the pupillary portion of the capsule of
the lens with the surface of a corneal ulcer are sufficient to cause a hyperplasia of the epithelium on its inner surface. Knies succeeded in examining
this hyperplasia at such an early stage that the cloudiness only set in during the hardening process. Deutschman's statements are of equal importance. He observed that in acute purulent processes of the anterior

6 C. P. Anterior und C. Morgagni. Zehender's Klin. Monatsblatter. 1880, Bd. XVIII, p. 181.

segment of the globe, only the portion of the globe corresponding to the free pupillary area was affected by the pus, the posterior surface of the iris protecting the remaining portion of the capsule for a long time, undoubtedly because, as a result of iritis, the posterior surface of the iris became adherent to the capsule. Deutschman further observed that the production of a chronic inflammation of the vitreous likewise caused a hyperplasia of the anterior capsular epithelium, leading to the formation of a true capsular cataract.

The local and circumscribed area of development of the capsular cataract, all favor the local and the temporary action of the cause, and this is to be found in the contact of the anterior capsule with the pathological products of the corneal ulcer. As a result of direct contact of the capsule with the vascular pupillary margin of the inflamed iris, and with the inflamed and vascularized cornea, a portion of the lens receives its nourishment as it did in foetal life; namely, by means of the vascular capsule. Here, again, the epithelial cells receive their nutriment directly through the capsule, and as a result there will be an increased production of cells; which, since it will be in excess of the regular development of fibres at the whorl and the gradual movement of the entire epithelium, will naturally lead to a local hyperplasia, which becomes changed into a capsular cataract; which, as a result of its own products, limits its own growth. The various forms of punctate, flat, pyramidal, congenital and acquired central capsular cataracts, are but differently developed products, of the same process.

Sight must not be lost of Hulke's observations, that during foetal life, in which a true anterior chamber does not exist, every affection of the cornea leading to swelling, would be sufficient cause, to excite that portion of the lenticular epithelium lying in the pupillary area to undergo a hyperplasia. Hence Becker states that he "inclines more and more to the belief, that both the congenital and the acquired capsular cataracts are due to the same cause."

Though it is the rule that congenital central capsular cataract is present on both eyes, this is not necessarily always the case.

c. CATARACTA CAPSULARIS ANTERIOR. (ACCRETA.)

There is a variety of circumscribed capsular cataract, which occasionally comes under observation, which results from permanent adhesions between capsule and iris. True simple synechia seldom lead to the formation of capsular cataracts, which are occasionally observed at the point where the remains of a persistent pupillary membrane is still adherent to the capsule, the lens being perfectly transparent.

3. CATARACTA POLARIS POSTERIOR-VERA.

The differential diagnosis between this form and the spuria, was given on page 144. In reality, the diagnosis was made between the latter and posterior cortical cataracts, as observed in retinitis pigmentosa and choroidal disease. The posterior cortical cataracts will be considered further along.

Becker states, (Anatomy, p. 122), "that, based on his examination of preparations of posterior cortical cataract, he considers that he has shown that a true posterior polar cataract may result from a stagnation, (possibly a coagulation), of the tissue fluids, even at the temperature of the blood. (Page 206.) He also reports the case of a dog, where the diagnosis of posterior polar cataract was made. In both eyes, on examination, the foetal fissures were found filled with Morgagni's globules. These, he states, one would not assume were albuminous globules originating from partially destroyed lens fibres, since these ended in the well-known manner, with broadened ends. To his surprise, as far as the fissures touched the capsule, this was covered with a beautiful epithelium, which he suggests might be an anomaly or a malformation."

Knies describes a true posterior polar cataract in connection with a spindle cataract. Becker states that "the formation of a true posterior polar cataract in man would undoubtedly originate during the third period of foetal development. Where due to some unknown cause, the saggital fibres of the second period remain in contact with the capsule and posteriorly prevent the new fibres of the third period from coming together from opposite directions, and pressing these saggital fibres toward the centre, we have the ideal example of a cataracta polaris posterior *vera*. Such a case has been anatomically examined by Schirmer, and will be fully described along with the lamellar cataracts. (Page 186.)

CATARACTA FUSIFORMIS. SPINDLE CATARACT.

Associated with one or more forms of axial cataract, a form of cloudiness occurs, which extends through the entire length of the axis of the lens. Ammon mentioned this form. Pilz [7] was the first to give it a more accurate description and name. In the eye of a boy who had suffered from a scrofulous conjunctival disease, he found an anterior polar cataract about the size of a pin-head, and going out from this a cloudiness which extended backward exactly in the axis of the lens, simulating very much a thread having a smoky or topaz color.

Whereas the case of Pilz was most probably an acquired form, Becker

[7] Pathology des Krystallinsen System. Prag. Viertelyahrschr., 1850, 1 S., 33.

observed a case, in both eyes of a young man, in which a complicated congenital spindle cataract existed.[8] This extended from the posterior surface of the anterior capsule, exactly in the pole of the lens, as a solid, and by focal illumination, as a bluish white, non-transparent process, which gradually widened into a bluish white, very delicate and veil-like transparent bubble, enclosing the innermost portion of the nucleus, and this, continuing again beyond the bubble in the axis of the lens, again becomes a solid strand, which finally attached itself to the posterior capsule. Within this transparent bubble, separated from it by transparent lens substance, was a characteristic *cataracta centralis.*

Previously, E. Mueller had illustrated and described cases in which both *spindle cataract* and *zonular cataract* were present at the same time. He observed a case where three sisters, the mother of whom likewise had a very high degree of reduced vision, had *zonular cataract*, and in three eyes there was also a *spindle cataract* present. The second eye of the youngest also had a posterior polar cataract which he attributed to an obliterated central artery.

It is characteristic to find a central cataract fused with an anterior and posterior polar cataract, as in the case described above. At times, in connection with the globular cloudiness, there may be a number of cloudy lamellae situated more peripherically. Knies has described the spindle cataracts with especial care, and it is interesting to note that in the mother of the children who had this affection he found incomplete *zonular cataract* on both eyes, whereas the father had become blind as the result of *consecutire cataract.* (Right eye, cataracta tremula; left, cataracta accreta). Since the eyes which have been examined show no signs of foetal disease, the anomaly can only be ascribed to an anomaly in the development of the lens. Above all, heredity seems to favor this view. Cases in which the spindle-formed cloudiness gradually goes over into a *central cataract* are explainable on the theory, that at the time when the concentric arrangement of the lamellae begins (third period of development) the product of the second period (which does not clear up, or which possibly only later on becomes cloudy) remains adherent to both poles of the lens capsule, so that it becomes impossible for the new lens fibres to come in apposition at the anterior and posterior pole, but remain separated by this cloudy strand.

Leber has described a *spindle cataract*, which he produced experimentally by injuring the capsule of the lens.[9] His investigations corroborate to a certain degree Knies' views in reference to its formation.

[8] Berichte der Wiener Augenklinik. S. 990.

[9] Kernstaarartige Trubung der Linse nach Verletzung ihre Kapsel nebst Bemerkungen uber die Entstehung des Stationaren Kern und Schihtstaar's Uberhaupt. Arch. f. Opth., Bd. XXVI, 1, p. 286-289.

B.

LAMELLAR CATARACT. CATARACTA PERI NUCLEARIS.
CATARACTA ZONULARIS.

Ed. von Yager [10] presented to us the topographical relations of a variety of forms of stationary cataract, which, though known before his time, were explained by him in a different manner. He observed a uniform cloudiness of several isolated lamellae of the lens, which at a certain distance therefrom surrounded the centre of the lens; and these lamellae were surrounded, both without and within, by transparent lens substance. "It had the appearance of a bright grey, almost transparent, accurately bounded cloudiness of the lens, of exactly uniform size, and rounded off at the edges, having a thickness of from $1\frac{1}{2}$ to 2" in the midst of an otherwise normal lens system, and appeared according to its form and character like a very faintly saturated, uniformly clouded cortical cataract, of a lens system of about $1\frac{1}{2}$ to 2" in size." The examination of extracted cataracts bore out his observations.

The following year, Von Graefe [11] wrote a more exact, and, at the same time, an almost exhaustive treatise. He pointed out the fact that *lamellar cataract*, as it is now known, is, of all the varieties of cataract, the one which develops most frequently in childhood. Since that time, the number of observers of lamellar cataract has greatly increased, so that we are now in a position to divide them into three classes. [12]

After the use of atropine, one observes behind the pupil, a faintly saturated cloudiness, which has a sharply defined line of demarcation from the adjacent transparent peripheral lens substance, and has a diameter varying from 5 to 8 mm. The degree of saturation of this cloudiness gradually diminishes as it proceeds toward the centre of the lens. By this means the *zonular cataract* is most markedly differentiated from a nuclear cataract. In the latter, the cloudiness becomes more saturated as it proceeds toward the centre. On opthalmoscopic examination, the entire cloudiness gives a dark reflex and is sharply defined; whereas, on focal illumination, it appears grey, and the centre of the lens gives a brownish red reflex. The cloudiness is not equally diffuse in all cases, and made up of scarcely recognizable punctate opacities; but there may be two lamellae, one in front of, the other behind the nucleus, made up of a variable number of radially placed cloudy striations. Under such conditions, the lamellar cataract bears

---

10 Staar und Staaroperationen, 1854. S. 17.

11 Arch. Opth., I. 2, 234.

12 Vergl Liebreich, l. c., p. 480.

a very close resemblance to some forms of incipient senile cataract, only in the latter these radially placed striations are more peripheric. But since transparent lens substance is found between these striations, they permit of a clear insight into the formation of this variety of cataract. One is enabled to see through the anterior convex cloudiness into the concave side of the cataract behind the nucleus.

The number of lamellae involved and the density of the opacity may vary, so that one may meet with all gradations, from the scarcely recognizable smoky cloudiness to the complete opacity.

This latter form was first illustrated by Von Ammon,[13] and also described by Wernek.[13a] Arlt described this as a form of stationary nuclear cataracts of youth.[14] Von Graefe was the first to apply V. Yager's anatomical data to Arlt's stationary nuclear cataract, and since then the existence of a stationary solid nuclear cloudiness has been described. So that even Tetzer's compendium of Arlt's Aegide, places these two forms together. Only Hasner still contended that an independent stationary nuclear form could occur. Becker draws attention to the fact that the density of the cloudiness may be so great as to make it impossible to decide whether or not transparent lens substance is enclosed in the center of the lens. This has since been shown to be true, as the result of the anatomical pathological investigations of Schirmer, presently to be quoted.

Von Graefe, Sichel and Ed. Muller were the first to describe a *double lamellar cataract*, the last named even a triple one. It is seldom observed fully formed. It can only be diagnosticated, when the outer cloudy lamella is still transparent. Frequently, however, we observe how around a well developed lamellar cataract, a second one is beginning to develop. The latter is evidenced by the fact that between the lamellar cataract and the equator of the lens, we find isolated, delicate, fork-like, cloudy striations beginning to penetrate the anterior and posterior cortical substance. On focal illumination, one observes that these fork-like striations seem to ride on the lamellar cataract; hence they have also received the name of "*Riders.*" Such partially cloudy, more peripherically situated, lamellae may likewise remain stationary in this condition.

Liebreich has illustrated such a case. These riders, however, only appear later on, and are significant, in that they foretell that the stationary cataract is about to become a total one.

Finally, Liebreich drew attention to the fact, that the lens is less developed in volume in cases of lamellar cataract.

Lamellar cataract nearly always occurs simultaneously in both eyes. Where trauma leads to the development of lamellar cataract on one eye, this is not the case. Becker states that a case of monolateral lamellar cat-

13a Ammon Zeitschrift, III, p. 480.

13 Yager's Atlas, III, Taf. XIV, Fig. 114.

14 Die Krankheiten des Auge, II, S. 250.

aract, the other eye remaining perfectly normal, has never been observed. Schirmer [15] reports a case which is especially interesting, since the cataract was only present on *one* eye; further, while under observation, the cloudiness of the inner zone increased, the originally transparent zonular cataract being changed to an opaque one, (*"nuclear cataract"*), and because there could be no doubt as to the late development of the outer cataractous zone, this having developed after the seventh year, and while under observation. The originally healthy eye remained so.

Schirmer's Case No. V.—Case Report. Heinrich Ernst, aged 14 years, was first seen in this clinic in his seventh year, October 14, 1884. At that time the diagnosis of zonular cataract on his right eye was made. This was of moderate size, sharply defined, and permitted the transmission of light through the center. V—fingers at 1 mm. The left eye was *not* cataractous. In early life the patient had suffered from *rachitis*, and at the time changes could be observed in the cartilaginous portions of the ribs; also the characteristic anamolies of the teeth. An iridectomy was made downward and inward. Vision was not improved.

The boy was seen again June 7, 1891. There is still present on the one eye a double zonular cataract, the inner of which is totally opaque, and according to the usual nomenclature this would be designated as a *nuclear cataract*. The lens is moderately shrunken. The outer not very opaque zonular cataract has a diameter of about 7½ mm.; the inner at 4½ mm. Both are sharply defined, but their contours are not perfectly circular, but more or less wavy or protruding. July 8, 1891. Extraction was made through the old coloboma, after a piece of the capsule had been extracted. On exerting but slight pressure almost the entire lens was successfully extracted without the loss of vitreous.

The cataract, which was extremely soft, was carefully cut in halves, and the one half at once placed in a 60 per cent. alcohol solution; the other half was examined in the fresh state. On transverse section one at once recognized the cloudy rings, and that which is still more important, is that one sees at a glance the center of the lens is perfectly clear and transparent. Hence, this is not a nuclear cataract, notwithstanding the opaque condition of the inner zone. In the fresh sections one finds the droplets between the fibres, the number and size varying, according to the location from which the section is made. They are very numerous in particles taken from the cloudy zone, very few in the transparent zone between the two cloudy zones, and still less so in the nucleus.

The fibres are everywhere smooth, and in places where there are many droplets they are wavy and swollen, but nowhere are they serrated.

The hardened portion was cut in sections. Thick sections show the two cloudy zones very distinctly, with the transparent interspace between them, also the clear nucleus. Under the microscope one finds both made up of numer-

---

[15] Zur Pathologische Anatomie und Pathogenese des Centralstaars, Graefe Arch., XXXVIII, B. 4, 1891.

ous minute drops lying between the fibres, and these are markedly more numerous and smaller in the inner zone, 0.0015 to 0.003 mm., whereas in the outer zone, they range from 0.006 to 0.003 mm. Externally the rings are sharply defined, whereas inward the number of drops is markedly decreased. The characteristic changes are noted to a less degree in the nucleus in the zone between the two zonular cataracts, they are somewhat more numerous.

Schirmer reports a similar case, which, owing to the rarity of this condition, likewise deserves mention.

Case No. VI. Anna Durch, aged 17 years, presented herself at the clinic with a double zonular cataract in the right eye. The outer zone was extremely delicate and transparent, but showed no defect at any point. This surrounds very closely a large disc 6 mm. in diameter, which is totally opaque. The patient had had convulsions in childhood, and her teeth showed the anamolies described by Horner. The clinic records show that this patient had been examined twelve years previously, and the diagnosis reads: *"Simple zonular cataract."* At that time a discission was done on the left eye, and at present a delicate secondary cataract exists.

In this same paper, Schirmer reports another case equally important, because it throws light on the aetiology, not only of central cataract, but also of true posterior polar cataract; the conditions present coinciding entirely with those described by Arlt[16] and Tetzer[17] as the usual ones for the formation of a central cataract; namely, associated with congenital anomalies—in this case, a micropthalmus.

The anatomical basis for the nuclear cloudiness consisted of fine drops which so completely filled the centre of the lens, that the cloudiness of the fibres could be made out with difficulty. "They are equally dispersed throughout the cloudy area; external to this, they suddenly cease to appear. The fibres are greatly changed and transformed in the most peculiar manner. The physiological changes which one would expect to find in a patient 51 years of age did not appear. The minute droplets are arranged as described in previous cases, only in this case, owing to the pushing aside of the central cloudiness, they follow a somewhat irregular course. The interspace between this zone and the central cloudiness shows but slight changes. Hence here we find enclosed in a *zonular cataract* a *nuclear cataract*, an intense equally diffuse cloudiness of the centre of the lens, the anatomical construction of which is analogous to the changes noted in the cataractous zone of a zonular cataract.

Notwithstanding the peculiar position of the cloudiness, this is a central cataract. Anatomical examination showed that the oldest lamellae of

---

[16] Arlt-Krankheiten des Auge, Bd. II, p. 250. Prag., 1854.
[17] Compendium der Augenheilkunde, 4 Aufl., S. 282. Wien, 1887.

the lens were affected by the cataractous process, and its adherence to the posterior capsule explains its dislocation posteriorly. This process is analogous to the one found in spindle cataracts, and this latter form is found associated with zonular cataract. In this case the abnormal adhesions did not lead to a drawing out of this to a thread, since this adhesion only existed at the posterior capsule; hence, as the leaves of the capsule continued to separate farther and farther from each other, there was not sufficient tension exerted, and the posterior ends of the fibres, which should have pushed themselves in between the posterior and the central cataract, were apparently not strong enough to stretch this adhesion, which seems to be a possibility where the adhesion is narrower, as shown by Knies.[18]

Schirmer's Case No. IV. George Naujoks, 50 years of age, born of healthy parents; all of his brothers and sisters, except a stepsister, died in early childhood of diseases unknown to him. This sister, since early childhood, can only see objects which are in close proximity. Whether this is due to myopia or interference in the refracting media, am unable to learn.

Patient states that he never had convulsions. Since early childhood he has only seen sufficiently to grope his way about. In his twentieth year iridectomy was done on both his eyes, and vision was thus somewhat improved. The left eye remained in this condition for many years, and only lately has vision diminished. Several years after the operation the right eye became totally blind.

March 10, 1891. Active horizontal nystagmus on both eyes; pronounced micropthalmus. Right eye, artificial coloboma, downward and inward, in the middle of which one can see the edge of the shrunken lens. Left eye, the cortical substance is totally transparent, with the exception of a delicate cloudiness downward and inward. One can easily discern a *central cloudiness of the lens*, which appears to be markedly posterior to the plane of the iris. This can be separated into a central yellowish white small portion, surrounded by a 3 mm. in size whitish lamella, which everywhere surrounds the edge of the internal cloudy portion. Both are sharply defined; their contours are not entirely circular, but here and there show slight projections. No distinct pictures of the fundus can be obtained, though a red reflex of the fundus can be obtained through the periphery of the lens. There is also a very delicate diffuse cloudiness of the cornea. V.—fingers at 2½ meters.

Right eye. Conditions about the same, with absolute amaurosis, subsequent to a very active chorio-retinitis.

May 22, 1891. Left Eye. A discision was done. Very slight tumescenes and slow cloudiness of the cortical layers followed. Since in the course of a few weeks this did not progress, but began rather to clear up again, an extraction was made through the old coloboma, June 30, 1891. After extracting a large

---

18 Uber Spindelstaar und die Accommodation bei Denselben. Arch. fur Opth., XXIII, 1, S. 217.

piece of the capsule, the spoon was introduced, and the cloudy nucleus, together with the cortex, removed; and the remains largely removed by massage. By June 18, 1891, the cortical remains were totally resorbed, so that the pupillary area was perfectly free back to the posterior capsule. On this could be seen distinctly, centrally located and intensely white, a small posterior capsular cataract, which had been observed shortly subsequent to the extraction; likewise, the two flaps which lie closely to the coloboma appear greyish white. Vision with $+ 12$ D, fingers at three meters. This thickening of the capsule was extracted with but slight loss of vitreous.

July 15, 1891. Course of healing normal. Large, clear space in the pupillary area. The capsule was examined in its fresh state under the microscope, and disclosed a wide-reaching, capsular cataract, in which was found a large quantity of pigment granules. At one circular, circumscript spot, on top of this, is found a conglomeration of most peculiar, short cylindrical structures, which are irregularly placed one over the other. They remind one of greatly thickened lens fibres, which contain large numbers of small and large albuminous drops, and then attain most irregular contours. This circumscript condition and microscopical appearance corresponds posteriorly to the one noted in vivo as a white central cloudiness. Hence the belief that this peculiar formation is the remains of the center of the lens, which, as the examination will show, was adherent to the posterior capsule of the lens, and remained adherent to it at the time of the extraction, and assumed this peculiar change as a result of its contact with the aqueous. The capsule was stained, imbedded, and cut into sections. Sagittal sections showed that between the above spoken of remains and the capsule, true non-pigmented capsular cataract tissue existed. The two flaps likewise contained capsular cataracts, and the pigment undoubtedly was derived from the iris. From this it follows that the pigment only entered subsequent to the extraction.

The extracted lens was cut in half in the fresh state; on section it disclosed an almost globular, intense cloudiness, $1\frac{1}{2}$ mm. wide and 1 mm. thick, which borders posteriorly at the posterior pole, at the point where the piece of capsule was extracted. It gives one the impression as though the nucleus had been forcibly pressed backward. This cloudiness is further surrounded by a second cloudy zone, which anteriorly is separated from the former by a transparent zone, whereas laterally it is directly in contact with, and posteriorly entirely wanting.

The other portion was imbedded and cut into sections. The microscopical examination offers the same explanation for the striking position of the central cataract. In fact, the entire nucleus has been dislocated posteriorly. The anterior cortical layers are especially thick, whereas posteriorly they are very thin, and cease at a certain distance from the posterior pole, so that at that point the nucleus lies entirely free. The study of the equatorial region, where the fibres turn, is especially instructive and conclusive for this condition. The fibres do not lie as in the normal lens, in a plane which is slightly bent backward, but they only follow their normal position in the periphery; the older the fibres the more centrally they lie, and the farther back their point of bending is placed, and finally they border on the equator of the nucleus. A plane drawn through all the points of curvature would assume posteriorly a very decided funnel-shape, facing posteriorly, as though the nucleus had been exerting traction backward. As has already been stated, the posterior surface of the nucleus is centrally perfectly free, simply covered by an albuminous film, and here the fibres have not the concentric arrangement, but are arranged vertically or almost so, and are torn in a jagged line, along which are numerous sharp points. This in connection with the posterior polar cataract, gives us the explanation for the position of the nucleus. *There was an adhesion between the oldest fibres and the posterior capsule of the lens, which at this point held the nucleus fast, and offered an insurmountable obstacle to new forming lamellae, so that these could develop normally only in the anterior half of the lens.*

Otherwise, the examination disclosed nothing other than has already been observed in teased sections. The zonular cataract shows the same small droplets coalescing to form larger ones in the interspaces. The apparently clear zone between the cloudy zone and the central cloudiness, likewise shows similar formations. The outer cortical lamellae are normal in appearance, the inner show signs of advancing age. Where the discission had been done the fibres show signs of disintegration.

The amount of vision depends on the density of the cloudiness, and the equatorial diameter of the cloudy lamellae. It may occur that children with double lamellar cataract may go through school without suffering any material interference during their entire school life. Becker operated a married woman, in whom a lamellar cataract had become progressive, and a man 24 years of age was taken up in the clinic for the same reason. The rule, however, is that the defect becomes noticeable when the studies begin to make greater demands on the eye. Hence most cataracts come under observation between the tenth and twelfth year. If the cloudy lamellae are very centrally located, hence especially small, the eye, where there is a moderately wide pupil, can see past the cataract, and the degree of vision may be relatively high. Becker very carefully examined a series of such cases, three at Vienna, and in all of them, found a slight degree of myopia. Owing to the reduced vision, such an examination offers great difficulties. Nevertheless, eliminating all source of error as much as is possible, it is still possible to estimate the refraction. On using atropine, a case which at first was myopic was found to be hyperopic.

Nearly always, the condition of refraction is found to be a slight myopia, and the width of accommodation is exceedingly narrow.

"With the exception of the three Vienna cases which I examined, being assisted by Dr. Schulek, the utmost care was used to eliminate every source of error. All the estimates of refraction were made with the opthalmoscope. As a rule, no staphyloma was found at the entrance of the optic nerve, but slight evidences of choroidal atrophy were observed. Aside from this nothing abnormal was found in the fundus. The overwhelming occurrence of slight myopia without the opthalmoscopic evidences of a myopic eye, can be explained by the spherical aberration of the lens, since all the rays of light which pass near the center of the lens are deflected."

"Nevertheless, the myopia may be acquired in the usual way, since, owing to the poor vision, objects are brought closer to the eye. In the cases examined vision varied from $\frac{18}{18}$ to $\frac{10}{100}$, and was lowest in hypermetropic eyes. Without exception, the width of accommodation is reduced in eyes having lamellar cataract. This is not surprising, since one does not have to go far to understand that in cataractous lenses, even where the cataract is partial, that but few eyes are suitable for the observation of processes of accommodation, especially where the iridectomy is made for lamellar cataract; hence, the results of the investigations of Coccius [19] are to be critically examined, since they were made on just such eyes."

Lamellar cataract occurs almost exclusively on both eyes. This of itself seems to indicate that the causative element is present in the general condition of the patient. This belief is strengthened by the fact, that frequently there seems to be an hereditary influence. Hence until lately it remained an undecided question as to whether *lamellar cataract* is congenital. Just during the time Becker was occupied in studying this subject, a child fifteen weeks old was brought to him, which had, in both eyes, a small, but not to be mistaken, lamellar cataract, which the parents observed the day the child was born. According to the general opinion, however, lamellar cataract does not develop until after birth.

Von Graefe considered it a fact, that during the first years of life this cloudiness continued to increase in saturation, only later on to remain stationary. Hence so many lamellar cataracts are overlooked during the early years of life.

Great credit should be given to Arlt, who was the first to formulate our ideas as to the aetiology of lamellar cataracts, and he was the first to direct our attention to the frequent occurrence of lamellar cataract in individuals who had suffered from convulsions in infancy. Horner also noted this fact, but added, that many also suffered from deformities of the teeth, of the cranial bones, and were mentally weak. In the 65 cases recorded by Arlt and Horner, in 48 cases the coincidence of lamellar cataract and convulsions were noted. Horner's 36 cases showed deformities of the teeth in 25 cases, in 16 cases anomalies of the cranial bones, and 4 were mentally

[19] Der Mechanis mus der Accommodation des Menschlichen Auges. Leipsig, 1868.

deficient. In 1883 Max von Aix [20] reported 189 cases of zonular cataract, observed between 1865 and 1883, in the private clinic of Prof. Horner. Of these, 107 (56.61 per cent.) had had convulsions in earliest youth; 111, (66.07 per cent.) which in 1865 were designated as having *rachitic teeth*, 60 (31.76 per cent.) showed malformations of the bones of the skull, consisting of more or less assymetry; 40 (21.16 per cent.) showed marked signs of rachitic deformities of the extremities. In 152 cases (80.42 per cent.) the patients showed at least one, usually two or more, symptoms of constitutional disease, whereas but 37 showed absolutely no signs of rachitis. In the entire statistical table, there is not a single case recorded in which the characteristic uveal disease, or interstitial keratitis diffusa, was noted; hence in all probability zonular cataract is the result of rachitis, and not syphilis."

The cases of multiple lamellar cataract are not less important aetiologically than the above, since they show, owing to the presence of the cloudiness in more than one lamella, that the cause of the disease must be of a remittant and recurring nature.

Arlt did not consider lamellar cataract as congenital, but imagined that the shock which the eye received during a convulsion was sufficient to cause a sliding past each other, as it were, of the elements of the lens, just at the point where the most compact and heavy nucleus came in contact with the softer and more delicate cortical substance. This change in position he considered sufficient to cause a cloudiness of the lamellae which lay next to the nucleus. Becker likewise, basing his conclusions on Von Graefe's three cases, where, following an injury to the eye, the lens was dislocated and gradually a lamellar cataract developed, and one of his own in which a lamellar cataract developed after a trauma, came to the conclusion that this form of cataract may be due to trauma, as well as convulsions, the lamellae nearest the capsule being disturbed in their nutrition, and in consequence of this, becoming cloudy. Then, again, the occurrence of a number of lamellar cataracts could be brought in connection with the intermittent character of the convulsions. The inner lamellae being the oldest, depending on the size of the cloudy zone, one could to a certain extent, determine at what time of life the convulsions occurred.

Horner laid great weight on the fact that, aside from the convulsions, other signs of rachitis could be found. It was mainly the result of his observation that attention was first drawn to the rachitic form of teeth found in these cases. Owing to the great importance which attaches to the simultaneous presence of this form of teeth and this form of cataract, I quote his description.

---

[20] "Zur Pathologie des Schicht Staars." Inaug. Dissert, unter Horner.

"On close examination of an inciser tooth one will observe, in a perfect specimen, that the enamel gradually thins off toward the neck. The enamel is shining and smooth, and on focal illumination has a satiny gloss. This satiny appearance is due to a system of transverse furrows, which encircle the crown of the tooth. The less completely a tooth is formed, the less this tooth will show this wavy finish, and by close observation one can see that this is due to the greater distance at which these furrows are one from another. These furrows may be exceedingly delicate, and so closely packed together as to require a magnifying glass to see them; and again, they may become gradually more distinct and coarser, so as to become visible to an observing eye. Now, in rachitis an anomaly presents itself which is easily recognizable. The teeth are plump and thicker. Instead of the elegant chisel-shaped teeth we find them cubical or ill-shapen. Nevertheless, the form as a whole may resemble the ideal. The most interesting feature, however, is the departure from the normal of the surface of the tooth; the enamel instead of gradually disappearing toward the neck, nearly always ends suddenly in a thickening. The above mentioned furrows are heaped up to an enormous height; sometimes we find, especially toward the cutting edge, instead of a furrow, in the same place, a row of round holes, as though they had been gouged out with an awl. Toward the cutting edge the body of the tooth terminates with a convex edge. The union of the lingual and the labial plates of enamel are joined over the body of the tooth in irregular or jagged lamellae. In extreme cases, at some points, the enamel may be entirely wanting, and mostly in such a manner that the base of the denuded spot coincides with a very large transverse furrow; while in other places it is heaped up wave-like; whereas again, at the cutting edge, it seems to be washed away. The denuded bone of the tooth then, as the result of the action of the damp warm air in the mouth, turns brown, in striking contrast to the white enamel. Only individual teeth seem to suffer in a characteristic manner from this anamoly, and these seem to be affected only to a certain degree.

"In contradistinction to this anamoly stands the one due to hereditary syphilis, and which occurs almost exclusively on the upper incisors, and appears even in the permanent teeth.

"The upper teeth are short, narrow, their angles rounded off, and their edges exhibiting a broad, shallow notch. Usually one or two teeth converge toward each other; in other cases they stand apart with an interspace, or they diverge. The simple broad notch of greater or less degree of depth, is hardly ever wanting. The teeth are almost always of bad color. They may, however, in some instances, be of very fair whiteness. On looking carefully at the surface of the notch, there is almost always the evidence of wearing; that is, the enamel is not perfect in the scooped out border of the tooth." [21] Hence, these teeth seem to be wanting in just the most characteristic point in differential

21 Hutchinson-Trans. of Pathological Society of London. Vol. X. p. 294.

diagnosis, for in rachitic teeth we find the heaping up and ridge-like formation, and in places the total absence of the enamel. *This enamel, like the lens, is of epithelial origin, and it must certainly appear as an astonishing fact that both should show a zonular abnormality.*

Previous to this time, H. Schmidt had drawn attention to the fact, that in youthful individuals, in affections of the teeth in which there was irritation of the alveolar branches of the trigeminus, not infrequently the near point became further removed and the width of accommodation narrowed. He looked upon this as due to a reflex increase of intraocular tension. Lately, he has attempted to explain lamellar cataract by referring to an interference with the nutrition of the lens system, due to teething, and he also pointed out the fact, that during the progress of glaucoma, opacities invariably develop in the lens. He considered himself justified in drawing the following conclusions; namely, that the branches of the alveolar nerves reflexly interfere with the processes of nutrition in the eye during the time of teething, and in some individuals this interference may lead to the formation of cloudiness of some of the lamellae. Thus Schmidt attempts to connect the formation of lamellar cataract with the development of the teeth.

In reference to this matter, the investigations of Arnold have led to a most surprising discovery, and supported in a most unexpected manner the views held by Horner; proving that the simultaneous occurrence of lamellar cataract and rachitic tooth formation is something more than a coincidence. Both abnormalities have a common cause—ricketts; and it can be no longer a matter of surprise that other sequelae of this disease, such as abnormalities in the formation of cranial bones, convulsions, etc., occur in the cases in which we find lamellar cataract. Further, we will no longer consider convulsions as a necessary step between ricketts and lamellar cataract. It is also worth noting, that the time of the development of the enamel of the second, or permanent, teeth is coincident with the formation of those layers of the lens which become cloudy where lamellar cataract forms. The permanent teeth alread exist, fully formed at birth, and gain continuously during the next few years their later shape. Therefore, during the time of their greatest development, they are exposed to the action of the same noxious influence.

Up to 1888, Horner's theory, which was coincided in by Leber,[22] was in vogue. At that time, Beselin [23] published the results of his microscop-

22 "Kernstar-artige Trubung der Linse nach Verletzung ihre Kapsel," etc. Graefe Arch., XXVI. B. 1. p. 283, 1880.

23 "Ein Fall von extrahirtern und microscopisch untersuchtern Schichstaar einer Erwachsenen." Arch. fur Augenh., Bd. XVIII, p. 71, 1888.

ical-anatomical-pathological examination of a case of lamellar cataract, in which he claimed that it was formed just as in the senile cataract. He states that he not only found fine continuous splits between nucleus and cortex, which he considered the anatomical substratum of lamellar cataract, but also changes in the nucleus, which was filled with a great number of minute splits and interspaces, all of which were filled with granular matter. Though he considered the changes in the nucleus of post mortem origin—whereas he looked upon the large concentric splits as having occurred during life—*from this he believes that he can positively conclude that they are due to the chemical change of the nucleus which leads to its more active shrinkage.* The new-formed outer lamellae can not follow the contracting nucleus, but separate from this, hence the development of the interspaces between the two—and these interspaces are the expression of what is known as *zonular cataract.*

The essentially new part of Beselin's theory is the assumption, that the detrimental cause, at the time it is exerting its influence, affects a fully formed lens; and, secondly, that the cloudy zone is not the immediate result of the detrimental cause nor produced at the time of its action, but only follows later on, as the result of the shrinkage of the nucleus. This is not in keeping with Deutschman's statements,[24] who found the nucleus unchanged, and who likewise coincided with Horner's theory. Lawford,[25] who examined three cases, likewise states that he found the nucleus changed and found splits and interspaces. He does not state that he agrees with Beselin's theory, but states that he looks upon the formation of fine splits running concentrically to the surface of the lens, and between the nucleus and cortex, as the cause of lamellar cataract.

As the result of his examinations, Schirmer[26] states that in four cases which he examined he found three constant conditions: First, a totally, or almost totally, normal cortical substance; second, beneath this, what microscopically appeared as a cloudy ring running parallel to the surface of the lens, a layer of compactly arranged minute interspaces, and, finally, similar, but larger and less frequently distributed interspaces throughout the nucleus. Microscopically, a sharp line of demarcation did not exist, but the transition from the large to the minute interspaces is quite rapid.

In this work of Schirmer's and the one quoted above, and from which

---

[24] "Pathologische Anatomische Untersuchungen eines Menschlichen Schichtstaars." V. Graefe's Arch., XXXII, B. 2, p. 295, 1886.

[25] On the Pathological Anatomy of Lamellar Cataract or Zonula. Royal London Hospital Reports, Vol. XII, Part II, p. 184. 1888.

[26] "Zur Pathologischen Anatomie und Pathogenese des Schichtstaars." Graefe Arch., Vol. XXXV, B. 3, 1889.

.the case reports are taken, the most modern views concerning the aetiology and pathogenesis of this form of cataract and its relation to central cataract are expressed. A number of later investigators, Bernhard Dub,[27] Carl Hess,[28] and Albert Peters,[29] though differing with him in some minute details, essentially agree with him—hence Schirmer's views expressed in his later work,[30] are quoted in full.

"In accord with Horner's theory, I conceive that a zonular cataract is due to the action of a passing noxious principle which manifests itself by the formation of little droplets in the lens as it exists at that particular time. The droplets appear in greatest numbers in the youngest lens fibres and lamellae, so that clinically we find a demonstrable cloudiness; whereas the oldest fibres, in which less interchange of products is going on, are but slightly affected, and microscopically these latter show no change. The fibres which form later do not suffer in their normal transparency. This explains in a perfectly rationally manner, why it is that the cloudy zone in lamellar cataract has the form of the lens, that the intense cloudiness is confined to one sheath (as it were), and show but slight changes in the nucleus. In very early foetal life the lens is not only smaller, but much more globular than at birth. Hence a zonular cataract which forms very early in life will not only be smaller, but must be more globular, than where formed in extra-uterine life. At such an early period of development the fibres throughout the entire lens possess an equal amount of life, and all demand an equal amount of nutrition; at this time, they do not as yet exist as fibres, which are changed, shrunken and removed from the action of the nutritive processes. This same noxious principle, which later on simply affects the youngest lamellae, causing these to become cloudy and only slightly affects the central portion of the lens, which is removed from the influence of the nutritive processes, here affects the entire lens, leads to a foetal total cataract, over which gradually new transparent lamellae are deposited, and thus in time a central lens cataract is formed."

Hence the theory of the pathogenesis of zonular cataract can, without further discussion, be adopted for central cataract, and the following statements apply to both forms:

"Any noxious principle, the exact nature of which is as yet unknown,

27 Beltrage zur Kentniss der Cataract Zonularis. Graefe Arch., XXXVII. Vol. IV. 1891.

28 Zur Pathologie und Pathologische Anatomie Verschieden Staarformen. Graefe Arch., Vol. XXXIX. B. 1, p. 183. 1893.

29 Uber die Entstehung des Schichtstaars und Verwandte Staarformen. Graefe Arch., Vol. XXXIX. B. 2, p. 221. 1893.

30 "Zur Pathologische Anatomie und Pathogenese des Centralstaars. Graefe Arch., Vol. XXXVIII. B. 4, p. 1. 1891.

will, in all probability, interfere with the proper nutrition of the lens and in the lamellae already formed at the time of its action, as well as in those just forming. These changes lead to the formation of minute drops, which in the beginning are probably in the fibres, but which later on, as these shrink, are pressed out; it is, however, possible that they were outside the fibres from the beginning. Only those fibres, which are fully alive and still in the midst of the nutritive processes, at the time this noxious principle is acting, contain such numbers of minute drops as to lead to a clinical cloudiness, the older fibres depending on, to how great an extent they participate in the nutritive processes are proportionately affected. The cause for the formation of this form of cataract seems to abate quite suddenly, as attested by the sharp line of demarcation which exists between the opaque and transparent zone.

"Depending on the time and intensity of the action of the noxious principle, an entire series of varieties of cataract may develop. At one end of the series is the small white globular central cataract; at the other, restricted to but a few lamellae is the very delicate, large, almost transparent zonular cataract. The former are due to a very decided and very early interference with nutrition—(as is universally conceded, central cataracts are congenital)—the latter are due to a very low grade, and relatively late, disturbance. Zonular cataract appears to be developed at birth, but probably developes more frequently in extra-uterine life, and as to how late in life this may develop, the above cases of zonular cataract demonstrate. Between these two forms are ranged the large cataracts, which show the configuration of a zonular cataract and are totally opaque."

"It is true that a similar pathogenesis for both forms of cataract, is no proof of a similar causation, for there does not appear to be such a great difference as Schnabel contends.[31] Schnabel contends that nuclear cataracts, as well as punctate and congenital total cataracts, are due to an abnormal condition of the original epithelial germ, whereas zonular cataract is due to disturbances occurring in intra or extra-uterine life." As proof of this, he states that one frequently finds nuclear cataracts in different members of the same family, or in various generations of the same family, but zonular cataract, never! Hirschberg adds a note to this reference, stating that he has operated grandmother, mother and child for zonular cataract and that he has also seen similar forms in mother and son; and other opthalmologists likewise have had the same experience. Opposed to this latter view, one must mention Knies' spindle staar family. Three brothers

31 "Vortrag Gehalten in der Sitzung des Vereins der Aerzte Steiermarks," November 24, 1890. Referat in Centralblatt fur Augenheilkunde, April, 1891.

had central cataract, together with a simple or double zonular cataract. Since anomalies of the lens existed in the three sisters of these brothers, in their mother, and the mother's grandfather, this case does seem to indicate some abnormal condition of the original epithelial germ. But to me, notwithstanding the larger number of members of one family so affected, it does not prove an abnormal condition of the lens germ, but leads rather to the assumption, which I believe is justifiable, that this is due to a general dyscrasia (rachitic disposition?) in the original germ, which is inherited, and that the anomaly of the lens is secondarily induced by the former. It is undoubtedly true that central cataracts are especially frequently found associated with other congenital anomalies of the eye, but it is undoubtedly likewise true, that at times its formation has the same underlying basis as a zonular cataract. Therefore, I do not believe that, generally speaking, we can accept Schnabel's axiom. As he expresses it, it can not be sustained, but rather, zonular cataract, as well as central cataract, may be due to various causes. Both may be due to abnormal conditions of the original lens germ, but also to intra- or extra-uterine disturbances."

It is impossible to draw a sharp line of demarcation between zonular and central cataract.

C.

A VARIETY OF FORMS OF CONGENITAL PARTIAL CATARACTS.

There is probably no portion of the lens in which, at some time, a circumscribed opacity has not been observed, and which does not change its relative position and size. A whole series of such have been observed.

a. DOTTED CATARACT. CATARACTA PUNCTATA. CATARACTA COERULA. CATARACTA SENILIS PRAEMATURA PUNCTATA.

This form of cataract is seldom seen, because it is usually overlooked. Liebreich was the first to accurately describe it.[32] In his "Anatomy of the Lens," page 174, Becker considers this form of cataract along with the constitutional cataracts, and designates it as cataracta senilis praematura punctata. He says, "Constitutional diseases, especially albuminuria or diabetes, may be excluded. I have not examined for phosphaturia. Syphilitic infection as a rule was not denied. The peculiarity lies in the presence of circumscribed punctate cloudy areas in the anterior, rarely in the posterior cortical substance, and their excessively slow increase in size.

"I had a typical case under observation for fully thirteen years. It begins

---

[32] Nouveau Dictionaire de Medicine et de Chirurgie Prat., par J. B. Barlliere et Fils, VI, p. 480.

with minute punctate opacities near the anterior capsule. In the course of the following four or five years other opacities were added, until the entire anterior and posterior cortical substance was permeated with them. In the tenth year cloudy streaks first began to develop, until finally, owing to the cloudiness of the entire anterior cortex, the cataract looked like a senile cataract, with a yellowish white nucleus and blueish white cortex. The patient was operated on in her forty-eighth year, and although healthy was prematurely old; 6-6 vision was obtained. I make this statement because it goes to show that the posterior segment of the eye was healthy."

Dr. Waldhauer, Sr.,[33] states that in 900 cases operated for cataract, he found two of this variety and neither had constitutional disease. He also reports the case of a colleague suffering from Bright's disease, operated by Von Graefe in 1860.

Dr. Carl Hess [34] examined eleven cases clinically and six anatomically. He gives the following description: "All showed small circular, sharply defined cloudy areas, the largest of which did not appear to have a greater diameter than 1 mm. and are found in the perinuclear lamellae, and decrease rapidly in numbers as they approach the poles. They seem to be more numerous in the anterior cortical substance than in the posterior. As a rule, they are differentiated from the usual grey spiculae of grey cataract by their greyish green color. In all cases the equatorial region is as good as free from these, or completely clear and transparent. In some cases the spiculae of grey cataract may be added. The age of the patients varied from 34 to 64 years, and all the cases were characterized by this exceedingly slow development. General diseases, such as albuminuria and diabetes, could not be discovered. In all cases, vision was such as to permit of concluding that the condition of the retina was normal."

"In all cases the lens was easily extracted, though the usual clinical signs of a ripe cataract were wanting, the peripheral cortical layers still being totally transparent. From this we may conclude that there existed an unusual consistence of the cortical lamellae in a relatively young individual. In all his cases which he examined anatomically, he found these to be elliptical spaces filled with homogenous or very finely granular masses."

Hess divides this form of cataract into two varieties—the *congenital* and the *acquired*.

He made the first anatomical examination of the congenital variety, the clinical history showing that both mother and daughter had, besides

---

[33] "Zwei Falle von C. Punctata." Graefe Arch., Vol. XXXI, Bd. 1, p. 249.
[34] "Zur Pathologie und Pathologischen Anatomie Verschiedenen Staar Formen." Graefe Arch., Vol. XXXIX, Bd. 1, p. 183. 1893.

this condition, a central cataract. He states, "Close to the nucleus irregularly distributed spaces, filled with granular masses, were found, which did not take up the haematoxylin stain satisfactorily. The fibres surrounding these spaces were more or less "gnawed at." From this, he states that he feels justified in assuming that the congenital form is anatomically essentially different in its character from the acquired.

For the *acquired form* he assumes that the lentiform spaces were preformed, but did not lead to any disturbance, being filled with clear, transparent fluid. The punctate cloudiness followed, where this fluid underwent a chemical change, possibly a coagulation. He further suggests that these eliptical spaces might result from an irregular shrinkage of the nucleus, but it must be remembered that they are arranged in a special portion of the lens, "abnormal structural conditions of the perinuclear lamellae."

b. CATARACTA STELLATA.

According to Liebreich, this is a special variety of cataracta punctata. Hasner described two such cases, and illustrated one.[35] His description coincides with that of Liebreich. It was observed to be nearer the anterior pole, and had a much more complicated figure; whereas, in cataracta punctata, the opacities, as they approach the poles, form a three-pointed star-figure, forming angles of 120 degrees. At the anterior pole this figure forms a Y, and at the posterior pole this is turned at about 60 degrees. In the cataracta stellata the figure is a more complicated one; the radii are but 60 degrees apart, and from these a second series extend. Becker states, that he observed a very pronounced case at Arlt's clinic.

CHAPTER VII.

CATARACTA ACCRETA. CATARACTA COMPLICATA.

In consequence of direct, permanent contact with diseased, firm, vascular, normal or pathologically changed portions of the eye, the lens becomes cataractous—cataracta complicata.

All forms of cataract belong here which occur in consequence of disease of the retina, or the formation of extensive cyclitic, irido-cyclitic or iritic bands of new-formed connective tissue. Hence the causative diseases are detachment of the retina, intra-ocular tumors, glaucoma absolutum, cysticercus, cyclitis, iridocyclitis, and the unknown changes which lead to buphthalmus and other ectatic processes in the eye.

Iwanoff was the first to make anatomical examinations of this form.

---

35 Klinische Vertrage, p. 270. 1866.

In all these cases the cellular hyperplasia is incited by the abnormally constituted nutritive fluid which, though entering along the normal channels, is derived from a pathological vitreous. Further, the continued contact of the lens with vascular, normal or pathological structures, even in a circumscribed area, will once more incite the embryonal mode of nourishment.

A number of cases will serve to illustrate these points:

INCIPIENT TOTAL CLOUDINESS OF THE LENS, THE RESULT OF ADHESIONS OF THE LENS WITH A GRANULOM OF THE IRIS.

In consequence of a granulom of the iris, adhesions formed between the pathologically changed iris and the capsule of the lens. As far as this adhesion extended a capsular cataract and folding of the capsule had followed, and along the equatorial line large vesicular cells had developed, whereas the remainder of the lens remained transparent. No doubt, with the growth of the new formation, the extent of the lenticular cloudiness would have increased.

CATARACTA COMPLICATA (BUPHTHALMUS).

H. Z., a boy 8 years of age, was taken up at the clinic June 13, 1878. The right eye was emetropic, V equal to 6-6. Regarding the left, the parents state that when the boy was one year old they began to notice that this eye was larger than the right. At the age of seven years Dr. Pauli, of Landau, saw the child, and found buphthalmus, trembling of the iris, floating opacities in the vitreous, amaurosis. Owing to the opacities in the vitreous the fundus could not be studied. The eye was free from all signs of irritation. Four months later (October, 1878) inflammatory symptoms suddenly developed in the left eye. At the time of his entry (June 13, 1878), the lids were swollen, chemotic and anterior chamber filled with blood. Pain in ciliary region T.—2. June 17, 1878, enucleation; sagittal diameter, 30 mm.; equatorial, 29 mm.; base of cornea, 15 mm. The horizontally dissected eye disclosed a large anterior chamber filled with blood, anteriorly bounded by a very thin, vascularized cornea, posteriorly by a transversely stretched membrane, which takes its origin from the iris and Fontana's spaces, and consists of a thickened, inflammatory, vascularized formation on the iris. This new formed layer of inflammatory tissue fills the pupil, and in this area is firmly adherent to the lens. The posterior surface of the iris, its pigment layer, for a short distance is likewise adherent to the lens. More peripherally the posterior surface of the iris apparently is unchanged, and a posterior chamber exists. With the exception of its anterior chamber, which is somewhat flattened, the lens has retained its shape. Its equatorial diameter is 8.4 mm.; its polar, 4.3 mm. The fibres of the zonula are well preserved, and can be distinctly seen in the stained sections. The ciliary processes are pressed anteriorly, and are long and thin. Petit's Canal is 2.7 mm. wide.

Aside from an intense cellular infiltration, the ciliary body shows no changes. In the posterior segment of the eye the choroid is adherent to the sclera. Equally infiltrated; nevertheless, at several points nodular like thickenings exist. Anteriorly, posterior to the orra serrata, to the temporal side, osseous tissue is developing. The entire atrophic retina is detached, and near the papilla shows numerous folds. These partly cover a deep excavation of the papilla, which is distinctly visible in the sections. Both the flat space between the choroid and retina, as well as the entire vitreous space, Petit's Canal included, and the posterior chamber, is filled with a fluid which has coagulated in the Muller's fluid. This undoubtedly chemically changed fluid in the eye lead to such a complete imbedding of the lens, that after the lens had been cut in four parts and imbedded in stearin, it was possible to make fine sections (Kuhnt Ludwig). The other half of the lens was put up in calabar substance, and then cut (Dr. Pinto). From the description it follows that the lens was held fast in the pupillary area and its immediate nighborhood, and that it was connected with vascularized tissue, and was further imbedded on all sides by pathological humor aqueous and vitreous. The changes in the lens are highly interesting, and fit in exactly with those already above mentioned in the case of the granulom of the iris.

A capsular cataract, 8 mm. long and 0.4 mm. thick, occupies the pupillary area. This shows all the attributes of a conglomeration of cells without the presence of intercellular substance; hence, this in the first stage of development. In the equatorial region are vesicular cells. The inner surface of the posterior capsule is clothed with epithelium, which is undergoing hyperphasia. The lens whorl is but partially recognizable. The changes in the fibrous portion of the lens are likewise characteristic; separated lamellae, between which are highly light-reflecting globules of coagulated albuminous fluid, and the presence of innumerable vacuoles in the peripheric fibres all indicate that this cloudiness of the lens has developed rapidly. This agrees with Dr. Pauli's statement. In June, 1877, the iris trembled, the pupil was free, and the lens transparent. In October the first signs of changes in the eye were noted, which lead to the formation of the cataract. As the immediate cause of the same, one must designate the local adhesions which the vascular pseudo membrane in the pupil and the pathological nutritive supply on the part of the vitreous.

CATARACTA CAPSULO-LENTICULARIS COMPLICATA (DETACHMENT OF THE RETINA).

Mrs. K., about 40 years of age, was treated by Steffan, to whom I am indebted for this eye. I take the following from his notes:

October, 1873, staplyoma posticum progress. Choroiditis disseminata. Cataract polaris posterior. Inner half of field of vision wanting. Externally she still counts fingers at 1.5. Right eye. Irido-choroiditis, cataracta capsularis accreta. Ciliary irritation. Amaurosis. This eye was enucleated October 7, 1873. Two years later, October 7, 1805, the eye was opened horizontally. The retina was totally detached, the entire space between this and the choroid was filled with cholestearin crystals. The retina, together with cyclitic bands, encloses completely the posterior section of the eye. Anteriorly it is covered by the irido-cyclitic new formations, which also cover the pupil. As the result of these bands the iris in its periphery is drawn posteriorly; as a result, the anterior chamber is unusually deep. It is especially worthy of note that the pupillary edge of the iris, together with the sphincter, is drawn backward by the cyclitic bands. Hence, I observe here for the first time a condition directly the opposite of that so frequently observed in glaucoma. Microscopically one can see that the lens consists of two distinct parts. The entire anterior and posterior capsule is covered with a capsular cataract. On fine sections one can see that it is formed like all other capsular cataracts. At some points, however, small and large particles of amorphous, chalky microscopical granules are deposited. This always occurs first in the spaces between the tissue, and surround and gradually displace the nuclei. The farther inward we proceed the larger and more compact do these concretions, which gradually assume the shape of Drusen, become. Almost the entire space within the capsule sac not occupied by the capsular cataract is filled with the chalky deposit.

In this case entire calcification of the lens ensued, without a rupture of the capsule having taken place.

CALCIFICATION OF THE LENS. Since deposits of lime salts within the capsular sac most frequently occur under the above considered conditions—that is, where the cataract occurs consecutive to some previous disease of the eye, which has led to permanent firm adhesions between the lens and pathological vascular tissues—this condition will be considered here. It has also been described as a *petrification* of the lens.

Under these conditions, the deposits of lime salts always occur first in the new-formed tissue, which is derived from the hyperplasia of the intracapsular cells. Nevertheless, a deposit of lime salts not infrequently does occur, but where the lens is simply fixed in its position by a simple synechia, or in cases where a youthful individual has suffered destruction of the deep-seated structures of the eye; hence, under conditions to be considered presently. Under such conditions, the deposit of lime salts is not preceded by an extensive capsular cataract. The deposit of the amorphous granules of lime takes place first on the inner surface of the epithelium of the anterior and of the pseudo epithelium of the posterior capsule, and extends gradually from the periphery to the centre of the lens. This is demonstrated by the fact that at times, the innermost nucleus is not calcareous, but consists of an amorphous, smeary, at times waxy, mass. This is certainly worthy of note, since one must assume, that though this gradual petrification is steadily going on, from without inward; that though finally there must be a very considerable crust of lime salts, this must still be permeable to the inorganic constituents of the nutritive fluid. Minute calcareous deposits are at times noted in over-ripe, senile, non-complicated cataracts. They always appear as thin lamellae of highly refracting granules close to the capsule, and at times they look like crystals. Nevertheless, I have never been able to distinguish crystals with certainty. A total calcification always requires a long time—months, and even years. This is due to the slight amount of organic constituents of the vitreous, and the always sluggish interchange of nutritive fluid in a diseased eye.

The petrification of the lens is either local, or the entire lens is involved. The former condition is observed in the over-ripe senile cataract, the latter in the consecutive and complicated cataracts of youth. In children, the contents of the capsule may remain fluid and gradually become inspisated, (*cataracta lactea*), or the formation may be a solid, strong one from the beginning, (*cataracta calcarea*) (*gypsea*).

Beer noticed that when the eye is kept perfectly quiet for a time, a color difference develops in these milky cataracts, in such a manner that the lower half gets chalky white, whereas the upper half, has a more yellowish color. If one waits long enough, this line of separation will become an almost straight line. This phenomenon is due to the precipitation to the floor of the capsular sac of the heavier calcareous granules. Naturally, this difference can only become distinct where the fluid portion is relatively great. Hence, the milky cataract does not always appear to have sediment, and it is not always an easy matter to differentiate between a *cataracta lactea* and a *cataracta calcarea*. One must judge by the uneven tuberous surface of the latter, as compared with the perfectly even surface of the former. Also, the more exact light sense in cases of cataracta lactea may aid us in making a correct diagnosis.

OSSIFICATION OF THE LENS. The question of the possibility of an ossification of the lens, naturally follows upon the consideration of *cataracta calcarea*. Technically speaking, the question is not, whether at the place where the lens normally is found, a deposition of true bony substance is found, but whether bone can be found inside of a lens capsule which has never been ruptured. The latter proposition is denied by me (Becker), the former is not contradicted. Where this bony body simulates the form of the lens, it will always be found that the space which the latter originally occupied is entirely surrounded by pathological tissue, forming a perfect mold of the lens. The following case will demonstrate in how remarkable and rapid a manner this can occur: Ward Holden,[1] in a pathological report, confirms these statements:

[1] A case of Ossification of the Lens. Clinical History by Dr. John Dunn. Pathological Report by Ward Holden. Archives of Opthalmology, Vol. XXVII, No. 5. 1898.

Case. September 28, 1882, a father accidentally struck his son in the right eye with a pitch-fork. On September 29, 1882, the conjunctiva bulbi was found oedematous, and downward and inward in the cornea was found a right-angled flap wound. Blood in the anterior chamber. Globe soft. Perception of light present. Projection wrong. September 30, 1882, at 12 o'clock; hence, forty-three hours after the injury, the eye was enucleated and placed in chromic acid. December 14, 1883, the eye was cut and imbedded. Macroscopically we believed that the lens was applied to the posterior surface of the cornea. Under the microscope it was shown that simply the capsule was present, but that the lens had been extruded at the time of the accident. The capsule had filled with blood, and thus had simulated the presence of the lens. The vitreous was very much infiltrated, and the pars ciliaris retinae was being changed into a cyclitic band. It can scarcely be doubted but that this space which the lens had occupied, and which was now filled with blood, in course of time would have been occupied by new-formed tissue. If this later had become changed to bone, we would have found a bony formation occupying the position, and having the exact form of the lens; but this certainly would not have indicated that the lens had been changed into bone.[1a]

PERFORATION OF THE LENS BY A GLIOMA OF THE RETINA.

"Iwanhoff [1b] speaks of this condition, and makes the fine distinction, that contact of a tumor could be looked upon as a trauma. First, it arouses the intra-capsular cells to a hyperplasia; after a length of time the new formation destroys the capsule by usur; after this nothing impedes the entrance of the cellular elements of the new formation as well as lymphoid cells, and finally the new formation and its stroma and vessels within the capsular sac, until finally the entire lens, like any other tissue, is entirely destroyed.

"My former assistant, Dr. Bettmann, examined such an eye, in which the usur of the capsule undoubtedly occurred only a short time before the enucleation. The epithelium has given rise to the already so often spoken of hyperphasia of pseudo-epithelium and vesicular cells. At the point of perforation somewhat anterior to the equator, a broad strip of round cells is working its way toward the center, whereas another is pushing its way along the inner surface of the anterior epithelium."

PERFORATION OF THE CAPSULE OF THE LENS, AS THE RESULT OF THE TRACTION OF CYCLITIC BANDS.

In this connection, Becker discusses a case described by Haab.[2] He concludes that the cyclitic bands, together with the vessels they contain, are the result of a foetal irido-choroiditis. As a result of the traction of

---

[1a] See reference in Yahresbericht fur Opthal., 1880, p. 367.

[1b] Beitrag zur Pathologischen Anatomie des Hornhaut und Linse Epithelels Pagenstecher Klinische Beobachtungen, Bd. III, p. 126.

[2] Uber Angeborene Fehler des Auges. Arch. f. Opth., Bd. XXIV, 2, p. 274.

these bands on the posterior capsule in an eye which had become ectatic, the posterior capsule burst.

In his "Pathology and Therapy," page 284, Becker gives the following hints regarding the operative interference in these various forms of *cataracta accreta*: "It is not without good reason, that every one expresses fear in operating cataracts which have formed adhesions. However, only those offer a bad prognosis which have as a basis an extensive traumatic cyclitis. Whereas the presence of a single capsular synechia can easily be overcome by the cystitome, at the time of the capsular incision, it certainly is very easily understood, that the more extensive the adhesions, the greater will be the difficulties encountered in loosening them. In cases of a broad adhesion, it will be advisable to make a preliminary iridectomie before the cataract operation. Arlt drew attention to the fact, that by this means, not only were a large number of adhesions broken up, but also the predisposition to an iritis was lessened. The danger in the operations undoubtedly is due to the fact, that an inflammatory process which has just about subsided or is even yet present in the latent form, is lighted up again. Whereas the presence of cyclitis most emphatically contra-indicates operative interference, this is allowable in simple iritis; hence this gives us the measure, as to the course to be pursued in cases of *cataracta accreta.* Hence, where there is the slightest doubt as to a cyclitis, the operation can not be delayed too long; the longer one waits, the more certain can one be that the cyclitis has really ceased, and the less is its recurrence to be feared."

CHAPTER VIII.

CATARACT DUE TO DISEASE OF ONE EYE, WITHOUT THE PRESENCE OF ABNORMAL ADHESIONS.

In these cases the cause of the cataractous formation is to be sought in the vascular system of the eye.

CATARACTA MOLLIS EXCHORIOIDITIDE.

In 1880 I (Becker) operated on a man 62 years of age for cataract, V—¼. During his convalescence he was called on by his daughter, 24 years of age, who had on her left eye a posterior cortical cataract, which also extended into the equatorial region, but was not ripe. I kept her under observation till close of 1881, and repeatedly had her general condition examined into; also her urine (for albumen and sugar), but this was always negative. The cataract was extracted as soon as vision sank to the recognition of the movements of the hand. I wish to state positively that before the operation projection was perfect, the field of vision free, and the smallest candle flame was visible in the entire room. The operation and time of healing were without mishaps; but after complete restoration the patient could only count fingers, and then only when they were held to the temporal side. A subsequent discissio cataractae secundariae did not improve her vision. The cause was found in a great number of vitreous opacities, and it was impossible to tell whether a detachment of the retina had occurred.

There can scarcely be a doubt but that during the operation, a choroidal hemorrhage had set in, and that this was due to a disease of the choroid. Cataract formation on the one eye undoubtedly was due to the presence of choroidal disease; the other eye, the right, was, and is at the present time, perfectly healthy.

Becker reports a second case, in which vision was better and the intensity of the disease less. He concludes, "The presence of cloudiness of the lens does not depend alone on the intensity of the disease, but probably on the length of time a less severe disease or some special unknown constituent of the vitreous is acting.

Knapp[1] states that he believes that the formation of senile cataract is more frequently associated with opacities of the vitreous than one would imagine. In many cases of incipient cataract he was able to diagnose opacities of the vitreous.

CHAPTER IX.

CONSTITUTIONAL CATARACT.

Constitutional disease, the nature of which is still unknown, may lead to disease of the choroid and retina, and this, in turn, to cataract.

A.

CATARACTA POLARIS POSTERIOR IN RETINITIS PIGMENTOSA.

For a long time past, oculists have recognized a form of cataract, which seems to depend on choroidal disease, which develops spontaneously in individuals who have not reached advanced age, and which characterizes itself by the fact that it develops in the posterior cortical substance, remaining stationary for a long time, or relatively early, going on to the completion of a total cataract. As the result of the studies relating to the mode of nutrition of the lens, this assumption has been verified.

The clinician has based his reasons for this belief on the occurrence of a choroiditis before the formation of this form of cataract, or the finding

---

[1] Bericht uber das Siebentes Hundert Staar Extractionen. Arch. f. Opth., Bd. XI, 1, p. 49.

of its results after a successful extraction. One often finds disease of the vitreous, and since we have grounds for believing that the disease of the vitreous is dependent on disease of the choroid, these facts strengthen the above argument. Scarcely a clinical fact seems to attest this more, than the occurence of a posterior cortical cataract in a case where retinitis pigmentosa has existed for a long time.

At first there appears at the posterior pole a round, almost button-like, opacity. To this is added, at first, one; later, a number of opacities radiating and running to a point. These striations gradually elongate, until finally a total cataract is developed. This cloudiness never reaches the greatest degree of saturation, but always remains more or less transparent.

As long as this opacity is present only at the posterior pole, a doubt might arise as to whether we are dealing with a deposit from the vitreous or with an opacity in the lens. But the appearance of the radiating striations at once tells us, that the cloudiness is in the cortical substance of the lens.

Landolt has afforded us the anatomical demonstration. Transverse sections of the lens, taken from an eye which had retinitis pigmentosa, show in both the posterior and anterior cortical substance, a separation of the various lamellae without any true molecular cloudiness of the lens fibres. In the spaces between the lamellae of the lens he found coagulated Morgagni's globules. Both posteriorly and anteriorly, he found a thin section of clear lens substance adherent to the capsule.

Other forms of cataract are seldom added to the post polar cataracts of retinitis pigmentosa. Mooren[1] once observed a case which developed into a total cataract. Becker examined a case of capsular cataract, showing great folds in the capsule, the posterior segment of which had been examined twenty years before by Czerny on account of the pigmentation of the retina. Unfortunately the lens was so small that one could not discern positively whether there was not also a posterior polar cataract.

B.

CATARACTA CHOROIDEALIS. CHOROIDAL CATARACT.

This form of cataract is differentiated from the above form of choroidal cataract as seen in retinitis pigmentosa, by its more rapid progress. In this form, the cloudiness which is at first confined to the posterior cortical substance, relatively speaking, rapidly becomes changed to a total cataract. In this form we find that the nucleus, even in individuals advanced in life, becomes cloudy and has even been observed to become soft.

[1] Opthalmiatr. Beobachtungen. Berlin, 1867.

207

(Becker.) In the fall of 1881 a lady, 29 years of age, came to me for treatment. Vision had been good, but after having lived through times of great fright, sorrow and trouble during the war, she noticed that vision was failing in both eyes. This was found to be due to opacities in the. vitreous and posterior cortical cataract. I made a preparatory iridectomy on both eyes, and subsequently practiced discission. To my astonishment, after complete resorption, I found the vitreous clear. I imagine that aside from hastening the ripening of the cataract, the iridectomy had a favorable influence on the choroidal disease, which was the cause of the opacities in the vitreous.

· Those who have experimentally studied the nutritive processes in the lens, have also turned their attention to the relation existing between posterior polar cataract and the diseases of the choroid and retina. (Choroiditis disseminata, chorio- retinitis, retinitis pigmentosa, etc.) Thus Kneis[2] and Ulrich[3]. The latter says, "At best, even under normal condiditions, the posterior pole, as far as its nourishment is concerned, is unfavorably situated, and if we stop to consider, that in cases of so-called choroidal cataract those conditions are found in which the function of the choroid, as the source of nutrition, has suffered, (chorio-retinitis and retinitis pigmentosa), to use a short expression, we might designate this form of cataract as *inanition-cataract*.

C.

TOTAL CONGENITAL CATARACT.

CATARACTA CONGENITA TOTALIS OCULI UTRIUSQUE.

The total congenital cataracts are always present on both eyes. They may be soft, even fluid; of firm consistence, or shrunken, and are often adherent to the iris.

Up to the time of the publication of Becker's work on the anatomy of the lens, no cases of congenital total cataract had been studied anatomically. He was given the opportunity of examining five eyes obtained from three children, in whom cataract existed at birth, and who had died from intercurrent diseases. It will be of great practical value to cite these cases in full, since they will give us the key to the proper understanding of a number of congenital cataracts, which were examined after they were extracted.

CASE 1.--CATARACTA CAPSULO LENTICULARIS CONGENITA.

Peter Buttmann, of Opan, twenty weeks old, was brought to the clinic July 29, 1877. He was a pale anaemic child, and was being raised by artificial

[2] Die Ernahrung des Auges und die Abflusswege der Intra-ocularen Flussigkeiten. Arch. f. Aug., Bd. VII, p. 340.

[3] Uber die Ernahrung des Auge Graefe Arch., Bd. XXVI, Bd. 3, p. 43.

feeding. According to the statements of the parents, at birth his pupils were black. At the end of two months they observed that the pupils appeared cloudy. From the fact that the child no longer followed a bright object with its eyes, they concluded that either the child did not see well, or possibly was blind. On examination both cornea, iridis and anterior chambers were found normal. Both pupils were equally grey, and reacted promptly to light. Before an operation could be done the child died of marasmus on July 2d. Shortly after death both eyes were enucleated and preserved in Muller's fluid. In January, 1882, the right eye was cut in half horizontally. The retina was in position, the vitreous slightly detached. The lens and capsule had retained their normal shape. The lens showed a diffuse grey cloudiness close to the anterior capsule, and this was surrounded by a darker homogenous mass. Both portions appeared equally hard. Examination of the vitreous in the fresh state disclosed innumerable round and proliferating cells.

Both halves were first imbedded in glycerine mass, then cut in the equatorial region, and the anterior half reimbedded, and on January 30th cut with the microtome. Whole series of sections 0.01 mm. in thickness were easily obtained.

The equatorial diameter of the entire lens equals 7.77 mm., whereas the equatorial diameter of the microscopically cloudy portion equals 6.3 mm. The length of the axis of the entire lens equals 4.5 mm., whereas the cloudy portion equals 4.13 mm. The microscopical examination shows that the form of the lens is due to the uninjured capsule. The thickness of the latter varies. At the anterior pole it is 0.01 mm. in thickness; posterior to the equator this increases to 0.017 mm., and at the posterior pole scarcely reaches 0.0023 mm. The cloudy portion is really the part of the lens which is made up of lens fibres; the darker mass which surrounds this consists of coagulated amorphous fluid, in which, here and there, a loosened lens fibre is imbedded. Anteriorly the lens is adherent over an area of 5.6 mm., to a developing capsular cataract of more than 0.2 mm. thickness. The epithelium is wanting in the area of the capsular cataract. In the interspace of the fibrous capsular cataract, innumerable nuclei are found, which are beautifully shown by double stains of haemotoxylin and oesin, or with alum carmin. Close to the capsular cataract the capsular cells are well preserved. They are still cubical, and whereas the capsule shows thickness of 0.01 mm., they are equally thick and high. The nuclei show a diameter of 0.005 mm., and occupy the center of the cells. Soon the height of the cells increases, and reach a height of 0.002 mm. At the same time the nucleus does not increase in size. but approaches closer to the upper end. At the same time the capsule grows thinner, and measures 0.007 to 0.008 mm. In the equatorial region the capsular cells attain a height of 0.038 to 0.04 mm., whereas the capsule diminishes in thickness to 0.004 mm. It is to be noted that the line along which the cells begin to apply themselves slanting lies far posterior to the equator.

Inward from the capsular lamellae lies a much more extended second layer of quite regularly arranged epithelial cells of much larger size. These cells attain a height of 0.05 mm., and a width of from 0.02 to 0.04 mm. The nucleus has the same diameter, 0.05 mm., as the epithelial cells. These are situated along a line of the capsule which only possesses a thickness of 0.009 mm., and the epithelium a height of 0.025 mm.

At some points groups of these epithelial cells lie on the true epithelium. That these cells are derived from the true epithelium appears from the fact that some of the latter can be observed undergoing vesicular-like changes (goblet cells). The formation noted in all the sections in the equatorial region in all probability are produced in like manner. They consist of a tissue which reminds one of a capsular cataract (containing more cellular elements and lens fibrous tissue), and are rich in coagulated Morgagni's fluid, which fills the interspaces. As far as these structures extend the epithelium is wanting. Since the configuration in all sections is the same, hence a thick process extends posteriorly within the capsule toward the center of the lens into the coagulated fluid. The centrally located solid body, on very fine meridional sections, discloses beautifully the structure of the embryonal lens. Lamella after lamella can be traced; anteriorly they meet in a narrow fissure, posteriorly ending in an open triangular fissure. The fibres on both sides of the fissures appear to be attempting to approach each other, but are prevented by a 1 mm. wide solid nucleus, which consists of sagittal curved fibres. In this nucleus one can easily recognize the lens fibres of the second period of foetal development, whereas the fibres on either side of the fissur belong to the third period. Nuclei in the final stage of retrogressive metamorphosis are only recognizable in the outer lamellae. On transverse and vertical sections the fibres disclose a peculiar condition, which becomes especially distinct by the double stain. The entire tissue is permeated by numberless minute drops, which at first give us the impression of being nuclei which have taken the stain more deeply. This inequality of size, lack of structure, and their position between the fibres, precludes the possibility of their being nuclei. They remind one of globules of fat, a condition which was lately referred to again by Henle and Michel as occurring in the embryos, and the new born chickens, cats, goats, calves and rabbits. Loosened lens fibres extend out into the fluid which surrounds the body of the lens, and these plainly indicate the progressive disintegration and solution. They do not show the well known fibre endings, but the edge appears as though they had been "gnawed at."

If we would now attempt to formulate an opinion as to how this condition was brought about, the first thing to be done is to fix the time when this disease process began. The concentric structure of the lens, the presence of the tri-star figure, are positive indications, that the formation of the lens had gone on uninterruptedly with the third period of foetal development. The size of the lens is but slightly less than that of a new-born infant, hence the date of the beginning of this disease could not have been far from the date of birth. In fact, there is no reason why we should doubt the assertion of the parents, that the disease began in the first days or weeks after birth. I look upon this cataract as congenital, and designate it as such; and I feel justified in so doing, since Knies[1] has observed that a capsular cataract may remain perfectly transparent for a long time. Though one must acknowledge the possibility, that even in this case, which we have had the opportunity of examining, that this disease only set in subsequent to birth, there is no reason—since, as has been observed, there was neither any other external or internal disease of the eye nor general disease—why it could not be possible for a perfectly analogous disease condition to develop during the last month of intra-uterine life. Undoubted cases of congenital cataract can be explained by this method of development.

Since the examination of the entire eye did not disclose a very florid disease, which could be looked upon as the cause of the cataract formation, this would, on the other hand, indicate that the cataract formation dated back to foetal life and was due to a constitutional disease, the traces of which could no longer be discovered.

CASE 2.—CATARACTA MORGAGNIANA CONGENITAL O UTRI.

Max Merz, aged seven weeks, died January 10, 1883, of cholera infantum, at 3:30 a. m., and the post-mortem was held in the afternoon at 2:30. Both eyes were enucleated, and at once placed in Muller's fluid, where they remained for six weeks. They were imbedded in celloidin and cut. At birth the observation was made that the pupils were not black but grey. A few days before death atropine was instilled into the eyes. The pupils dilated but slightly. The cataract had a milky color, evenly diffused, and showed no striations. The lens had the same appearance after enucleation. After the one eye had been prepared so as to permit of imbedding, the entire lens was examined by focal illumination and by transmitted light, using a Hartnack objective 2 and Oc IV. The periphery of the lens, which was not much reduced in volume, was transparent, and along the equator one could recognize cellular elements. Eccentrically situated and apparently fixed, one could observe in the transparent capsular sac, the reduced in size and transparent nucleus. Owing to the manipulation preparatory to imbedding and placing in absolute alcohol, the entire lens appeared somewhat shrunken, so that on section the natural form of the lens had suffered somewhat. The microscopical conditions can be briefly given. They are essentially those of the previous case; only that the capsular cataract in the pupillary area is not so well developed, and restricted to a few nodules. As a result, the nucleus is not adherent anteriorly, lies obliquely in the capsular sac, and is completely surrounded by a coagulated homogenous fluid. The nucleus discloses the same beautiful structure. A layer of large,

---

[1] Cataracta Polaris Anterior und Cataracta Morgagniana. Zehender's Klin. Monatsblatt, 1880, Bd. XVIII, p. 181.

tumescent cells lie on the epithelium, and posterior to the equator form similar pictures. With these, however, the formation of cells does not cease, but clothe the greater part of the posterior capsule with epithelial and vesicular cells. Aside from this a number of hyaline excrescences (Drusen) are just beginning to develop in the anterior capsule, so that it may be noted that these also occur in young individuals.

CASE 3.—CATARACTA FLUIDA CONGENITA O UTR.

Lena Schaul, four years of age, was brought to the clinic November 1, 1882, from the Mossbach Institute for mentally deficient children. She was so inanimate that she had to be fed artificially, since she would not swallow. On November 7, 1882, the left eye was operated for cataract. The second eye was not operated, since the patient died May, 1882, of diarrhoea, fatty liver and "Schluck pneumonie." The right eye after hardening was imbedded and cut. It was then examined with a Hartnack obj. 2, Oc. IV, and was found but slightly reduced in volume. During life the diagnosis of a shrunken, membranous cataract, with anterior capsular cataract, had been diagnosed. On dilating the pupil the observation had been made, that in the middle of the anterior capsule, equal to about a medium-sized pupil, a white light was reflected, whereas in the periphery it was transparent. We believed we were dealing with a form of cataract presently to be described, notwithstanding the fact that while operating the left eye it was only possible to extract the anterior capsule with the cellular hyperphasia adherent thereto. This capsule, hardened in alcohol and stained, showed a moderate cellular hyperphasia without formation of fibres.

Sections of the lens show very considerable shrinkage, as the result of manipulation previous to and subsequent to imbedding. This shrinking has assumed a higher degree than in the previous case, since it was shown that the nucleus of this cataract, which at other times bears the greatest resemblance to the previous cases, was entirely resorbed. It is to be noted that aside from the cellular hyperplasia, here also "Drusen" are present; the whorl along the equator can still be recognized to a certain extent, and as a rule, there is no epithelium along the posterior capsule. The capsular sac is partly filled with coagulated, homogenous fluid, partly with vesicular cells.

CASE 4.—CATARACTA MEMBRANACEA CONGENITA.

Louise Flesch, aged twelve months (Fischbach), was taken up in the clinic in March, 1880, with total cataract on both eyes. There was slight nystagmus on both eyes, cornea clear, no synechia; both pupils reacted rapidly to light. Both lenses were moderately cloudy, and reflected a grey light. The eyes followed the light. After a previous iridectomy discission was done. Apparently the capsule was incised, but no cataractous masses escape. The child was sent home again, and subsequently, first on the right and then on the left eye, an incision was made with the lance, and the thickened capsule extracted with the forceps. In both eyes portions of the capsule and tumescent substance remained behind. The extracted portions were preserved in alcohol, and were not imbedded until the spring of 1882. The thickness of the capsule equaled 0.008 mm., the height of the epithelial cells a little more than 0.01 mm. In the center of the anterior capsule lies a thick capsular cataract, whereas the latter portions are free of the same. At the border of the capsular cataract one can observe how a very thin lamella of the capsule separates from the remainder, and covers the cataract on its inner surface. (N. B.—See the pathology of capsular cataract for the later and more correct ideas on this subject.)

These four cases undoubtedly illustrate various stages of the same process. The general conditions found present in all these cases consist in the taking up of an abnormal quantity of fluid inside of the capsule of a fully developed lens (foetal period of growth). This fluid accumulated between the lens and its capsule, which separates the former posteriorly from the capsule; anteriorly and in the equatorial region, from the epithelium. In all these cases this condition leads to a hyperplasia of the intracapsular cells. In the case, *Buttmann*, this process was so active in the pupillary area, as to lead to the fixation of the lens proper by means of the forming capsular cataract; in the case, *Merz*, a like condition is noted, but it appears after the body of the lens had been separated completely from the epithelium, more active changes had followed. The lens proper sank to the bottom of the capsular sac, hence lies eccentric and is much reduced in size. In the case, *Lena Schaub*, the nucleus was completely resorbed. At the same time, one must bear in mind that this patient was four years of age, hence the cataract was much older than the others. In the fourth case we may assume that the body of the lens was likewise absorbed. The capsular cataract was highly developed, and on its inner surface one can still observe vesicular cells. Though only the anterior capsule was extracted, one finds recorded in the history of the case, on the date of her discharge from the hospital, the remark, that the pupil of the left eye is totally black and that it is impossible to detect any cataractous remains and that the right eye shows but slight remains posterior to the iris.

In the first three cases in which the lenses were observed during the life of the patients, they appeared as vesicles having the normal form of the lens. Though the lenses appeared somewhat smaller than one would expect to find them at that time of life, they nevertheless did not present the appearance of a *cataracta membranacea*, a condition which, from their appearance during life, one would have expected to find.

As to the aetiology, the occurrence on both eyes favors a cause present in the general organism. The nature of this, since the cause appears to have been active during foetal life, can not be stated. But that nutritive conditions seem to play an important role, appears to be attested by the fact, that in all three cases in which we examined the cataract in the eye, the vitreous showed marked changes. In both the cases, *Buttmann* and *Merz*, the vitreous was permeated by proliferating cells, which frequently showed long, swollen processes. In the case of *Lena Schaub*, the cells were more sparsely distributed, but all showed numerous and dilated processes.

Besides this, the fact is especially worthy of note, that in all these cases so far examined, the eyes showed no other signs of an inflammatory process. In order to be perfectly certain in this matter, I examined the vitreous of a large number of eyes taken from the new-born and very young children, and though I always found in this fluid an increased number of cellular elements, as compared with the vitreous of the adult, in not a single case did I find those forms which justify us in stating that there is an inflammatory irritation of the vitreous. From this, one may conclude that where the vitreous shows the evidence of an active cellular proliferation, by the presence of large numbers of cells, the vitreous fluid is chemically altered, and hence supplies to the lens an abnormally constituted nutritive material.

Had the second and third cases coincided entirely with the first, one might form an idea as to the point where the first pathological changes begin in such a case. The absence of epithelial cells along the posterior capsule and the presence of the peculiar hyperplasias of cells along the whorl—hence there, where, under normal conditions, the nutritive stream gains entrance to the lens—indicate very strongly that it is just at those places where the initial changes begin, making it impossible for new fibres to form, and prevent the further surface advance of the dividing epithelial cells, so that the new-formed cells are piled up on top of each other, and finally lead to the formation of a capsular cataract. The difference in the case, *Merz*, may be explained as due to a less intense action along the whorl, so that, though the formation of new lens fibres was prevented, it was not so with the further advancement and formation of new epithelial cells. In the case, *Lena Schaub*, since no perceptible changes were found along the whorl, this explanation could not be accepted without further explanation.

It appears that in the above-described cases, in which neither remains of the hyaloid artery, nor the vascular capsule of the lens, nor a foetal iritis are present, the genesis of all those cases of congenital or total cataract occurring on both eyes during the first years of life is given. This is true as well of those in which a portion of the lens is still present as in those which simply consist of capsule, hyperplasia of capsular cells and fluid, which latter we have been in the habit of designating as shrunken cataracts. It is possible, in course of time, according to the mode of development, for *shrunken cataracts* to form. Nor can it be denied that where such a cataract is not operated and remains in situ to very advanced age, the fluid in the capsule may be absorbed, and then appears as a membranous cataract (*cataracta membranacea*). Only differing from *cataracta membranacea*, are those forms which, on account of their similarity to fruits dried in the pod, have been given the name, *cataracta arida siliquata*, by Adam Schmidt. Such a cataract, including its capsule, seems to have a thickness of 2 to 3 mm., is a perfectly opaque, yellowish white, caky mass, and appears to be composed principally of dried-up lens substance. Frequently one observes, associated with such a cataract, a more or less extensive tearing of the zonula zinii, and then it trembles with every movement of the eye; and it is then called a trembling or floating cataract. (*Cataracta tremula vel natatilis*). Arlt drew attention to the fact that such "dried-pod" cataracts, as well as the membranous, seem to adhere to one or more places in the periphery, and hence, where repeated attempts are made to depress them into the vitreous, they always seem to rise up again. (*Cataracta elastica*). This, however, can be partially explained by the fact, that both of the forms, owing to their being so dry, are specifically lighter than the vitreous. Here at least the suggestion of Pauli may be adopted, to perform reclination upward. Where the contents of the *cataracta tremula or natatilis* is fluid, this cataract will assume the shape of an almost globular relaxed bladder (*cataracta cystica*). This capsule filled with fluid appears always to seek its equilibrium. In his "Pathology and Therapie," page 249, Becker describes the following interesting case:

In 1874 I extracted from the eyes of a woman, 36 years of age, two congenital, shrunken, membranous cataracts, which were not adherent to the iris. Her statement that these cataracts had existed since birth was worthy of belief, since she also had nystagmus. The question as to whether both these cataracts were shrunken, or whether they were soft cataracts which had subsequently during extra-uterine life become membranous, may be set aside. Both cataracts answered the above anatomical description exquisitely. Especially well shown were the cellular elements in the fibrous tissue. I do not doubt but that the entire cataract took its origin from the capsule cells. Dr. Raab made the examinatio. (N. B.—This same case is cited in Becker's Anatomie, p. 40, Figure 22, as "Cataracta Capsularis Congenita."

The operation was done as follows: First an iridectomy was made; the cataracta membranacea was then grasped by forcing one branch of the forceps through the zonula, so that it passed behind the cataract and into the vitreous, and then by slow and steady traction the cataract was gradually extracted. After an interval of several months, when the patient again presented herself, a most peculiar condition was present. After dilating the pupil the *zonula of zinii* came into view. This had remained in position, had a faint grey color, and presented the appearance of a striated fill for the neck. This had a perfectly circular central hole about the size of a moderately dilated pupil, and on moving the eye no motion of its own could be detected. Consequently the zonula had not retracted. That this was so plainly visible is no doubt due to a pathological thickening which took place at the time the shrinking process of the cataract was going on.

Finally, the cases *Buttmann* and *Merz* offer an explanation for a large number of clinical observations, which formerly were designated as *Cataracta Morgagniana in Children*. Both Janin and Arlt have reported cases in which they have operated for cataract, where on opening the capsule a cloudy, milky or blueish fluid escaped, a transparent nucleus remaining behind, which later on became cloudy. A cataract, as observed in the case *Merz*, might take such a course, if one will assume that the nucleus, as far as this still exists, permits to a degree the transmission of light.

CONGENITAL HARD NUCLEAR CATARACT. Graefe's Cases, 1 to 3, have awakened another train of thought which I would fain express here. In the year 1879, Alfred Graefe drew attention to a form of congenital cataract which up to this time had seldom been recognized,[4] but which previously had been recognized by Mooren.[5] This form was characterized by its excessively hard, wax-like consistency. This form always occurs on both eyes as a total cataract, and the volume is always equal to that of the physiological lens. The cloudiness is more homogenous, or possibly increases, toward the centre. It is a greyish white, or perfectly grey in color. It has no tendency to shrink or to complications. Capsular cataracts do not occur. Since discissions are of no avail, extraction must be done. Just[6] corroborates these statements, and reports seven extractions done on four children, all between the seventh and the fifteenth month. In all these cases, according to the statements of the parents, the cloudiness in the lens did not develop until after birth. In two of the cases the thickened capsule was subsequently removed with the forceps. Just's cases differ from Von Graefe's insomuch that the former reports the presence of capsular cataract.

Just was kind enough to send me four of the cataracts and the two capsules for microscopical investigation. The latter showed capsular cataracts, without the presence of much intercellular substance. Unfortunately the nuclei were too friable to permit of making of fine sections. In teased specimens no abnormal formation of the lens could be detected. Hence, the examinations gave but a negative result.

These Graefe-Just congenital nuclear cataracts can scarcely be looked

---

[4] Uber Congenitalen harten Kernstaar Sitzungs Bericht der Heidelberger Congress, 1879, p. 25.

[5] Opthalmiatr. Beobachtungen, Berlin, p. 209. 1867.

[6] Kernstaare im Kindesalter. Centralblatt fur Aug., January, 1880.

upon as anything other than cataracts agreeing with the type, *Buttmann.* If one will assume that a lens which has become adherent to the anterior capsule by means of a capsular cataract, is not reabsorbed, but persists and becomes saturated with a fluid which coagulates easily, one can easily understand how this will become changed in a more homogenous waxy mass, and then we have before us the *congenital hard nuclear cataract.* If, on the other hand, the nucleus is not fixed, one can further assume, as in cases, *Merz, Schaub* and *Flesch,* that this will gradually be dissolved and resorbed. Thus, in congenital total cataract, we would have a two-fold final stage, one corresponding to the *cataracta hypermatura reducta,* and the other to the *cataracta Morgagniana.*

CATARACTS OF SUDDEN DEVELOPMENT.

In one of Just's cases, the mother saw the cataract develop during the time the child had a convulsion. He cites another case, according to which the mother likewise saw the cataract develop in the course of a few minutes. The child (her sixth) was eight weeks old; two other children in the same family had congenital cataract. Just, who had previously examined the child, and found the eyes healthy, saw the case two hours after the occurrence, and found a ripe cataract on the left. Such occurrence may likewise be explained by our anatomical examinations, if one will imagine that just at the moment the mother observed the cloudiness, the nucleus of the lens changed its position in the capsule.

TOTAL ACQUIRED CATARACT (ON BOTH EYES).

D.

CATARACTA MOLLII JUVENUM. (CATARACTA DIABETICA.)

As the result of direct observation, we know as yet but little of the changes which the elements of the human lens undergo during the formation of a soft total cataract. Those authors who have attempted to experimentally produce cloudiness of the lens, either as the result of the withdrawal of water, or of the action of intense cold, report the formation of vacuoles in the epithelium and in the lens fibres. In both of the spontaneously developed soft human cataracts which I have been enabled to examine in their normal position in the eye, I was enabled to find these vacuoles in and between the fibres, but not in the epithelial cells.

Besides the case of rapidly developing soft cataract subsequent to a detachment of the retina, in a woman forty years of age, (reported on page 200), I (Becker) have had the opportunity of examining one other soft, tumescent cataract, in a nineteen year old diabetic patient. Since, aside from this, the diabetic cataract is the very paradigma, par excellence, of a constitutional cataract, it will be eminently proper to describe this form more fully. And an unrestricted elucidation of the various controversies existing concerning the genesis of diabetic cataract will aid us in formulating an opinion as to the manner in which constitutional cataract develops.

Case. R. W., 19 years of age, from H., a blonde, poorly nourished girl, with a dry skin, suffered from diabetes. Two days after an extraction had been done on the left eye, and a preliminary iridectomy on the right, she died of diabetic coma. The eye, which was removed twenty-three hours after death, remained in Muller's fluid seven years before it was examined. (Figures 24, 25, 26 and Plates V and VI were made from the sections.) The corneal epithelium was plainly preserved, notwithstanding the long time the specimen had been in Muller's fluid, and showed perfectly distinctly the nuclei undergoing division. The epithelium had begun to grow down into the iridectomy. wound. The stump of the iris, as well as the posterior surface of the same, show an enormous tumescence of the pigment cells. These are so large that one can easily see the nuclei, a thing which under normal conditions is very difficult. Likewise the portion of the iris on which the pigment rests is oedematously swollen. Around the periphery of the iris there is a pigment ring, which is raised to an almost veritable swelling, as the result of an infiltration with an amorphous fluid. There must have been pathological changes in the posterior segment of the eye previous to the operation, for immediately behind the lens traces of blood can be found in the vitreous. I have not been able to decide from which vessels this has come.

We are, however, interested more especially in the conditions of the lens. This has an equatorial diameter of 8-2 mm. and a sagittal of 4-8 mm. This almost globular form is due to the excessive taking up of water inside the capsule, which is partly situated between the lamellae and lens fibres, and partly in larger quantity between the lens proper and its anterior and posterior capsule. Anteriorly this layer equals 0.53 mm. in thickness, posteriorly, 0.65 mm. Only along the equator do we find the nuclear zone and whorl still in contact with the capsule. This fluid, which has been taken up in the capsule, is firmly coagulated; hence, has not fallen out of the finer sections. At the anterior pole the capsule has a thickness of 0.019 mm., at the posterior, 0.008 mm. If one examine carefully with a high power the epithelium of the anterior capsule, one will find it undergoing a hyperplasia at the anterior pole. As yet, neither pearls nor large accumulations of cells have formed, but at numerous points several layers of cells can be found. Internal to the layer of cells is a regular layer of albuminous globules. Toward the equator the epithelium is beautifully and regularly arranged, and the whorl is of extraordinary beauty. A number of sections show, immediately posterior to the whorl, an extensive formation of large vesicular cells. Toward the center of the lens the fibres and lamellae of the lens are separated from each other, and as a result large spaces have formed, which are filled with coagulated fluid. This has a tendency to form globules similar to the tissue fluid of the lens. Whereas the normal width of the lens fibres equaled 0.010 mm., the smallest diameter found equaled 0.019 mm. Only in the peripheric fibres did I find any signs of deterioration, disintegration of the lens fibres, formation of vacuoles, or punctate cloudy spots.

The reaction of the various stains on the lens was especially interesting. Alum carmin, which otherwise is exceedingly good for staining nuclei, stains the entire specimen equally, but does not show the nuclei with any prominence. Likewise haematoxylin. But beautiful and useful specimens are derived by the use of double stain haemotoxylin eosin. But even in these the nuclei at times hardly take up sufficient stain to make useful specimens. This is very remarkable, since only here and there over the entire capsule, certain nuclei take the stain more intensely and appear larger. The number of these darkly stained nuclei increase toward the equator. At the whorl, however, all are pale, showing the various stages of degeneration to veritable death of the nuclei. As a result of this double stain, we discern delicate chemical differences, which would not otherwise have been discovered. Thus we find in all peripheral sections, which have not been extensively fissured, dark blue dots and spots, which have a great resemblance to the fat drops observed in youthful lenses. Likewise, the spindle-shaped bodies or interspaces appear blue. But it must as yet remain undecided whether or not this is the result of sugar contained in the tissues, or whether this is simply the result of the action of the hardening material.

But in applying the results of the anatomical examination to the clinical observations made on the living eye, one must not forget that this was a cadaverous eye. which had been preserved seven years in Muller's fluid. The girl died January 11, 1874, at 1:45 p. m., and t he post-mortem examination was made the following day at 12 o'clock. Notwithstanding the low temperature during the month of January, sufficient time has elapsed to allow the formation of Morgagni's globules on the inner surface of the epithelium; nevertheless, the time was certainly too short to permit of so large an amount of water being taken up in the capsule. Nevertheless, hundreds of specimens which have been preserved in like manner do not show such a condition. Hence, we may assume that the hydropsia occurred during life.

Ossowidzki [7] collected all the historical notes relating to the occurrence of grey cataract in patients suffering with diabetes mellitus. From the more recent literature, I will only quote that which seems to be most important.

1. Reports vary greatly concerning the frequency of cataract in dia-

---

[7] Uber die bei der Zuckerruhr Vorkommenden Augenkrankheiten. Berlin. 1869.

betic patients.   Fauconneau-Dufresne [8] found them in 0.6 per cent., J. Mayer [9] in 3 per cent., Seegen [10] in 4 per cent.; whereas, Von Graefe estimated its occurrence in as high as 25 per cent. of cases.[11]   In $14\frac{1}{2}$ years, I (Becker) have treated 60,000 eye patients, and among these I found twelve cataracts in six diabetic patients; on five of these patients I made seven extractions during this time.   Hirschberg [12] claims to operate six to eight diabetic cataracts yearly, and among the last 150 cataract patients consulting him in private practice, six had diabetes.

2. The diabetic grey cataract may occur at any period of life; it is stated, however, to occur most frequently in youth.   The youngest patient with cataract reported is a girl twelve years of age.   (Seegen, No. 23).   My (Becker's) patients were, respectively, 19, 27, 38, 40, 62, and 63 years of age, whereas I recollect that formerly I operated a number between the ages of 18 and 35, and some of these were blood relations.   Seegen's six diabetic cataract patients were, respectively, 12, 39, 47, 53, 56, and 64 years of age.

3. More women seem affected than men.   Among Seegen's cases, four were women, two men.   In my cases, the number was equal.

4. In diabetes more frequently than in other conditions, the cataract develops simultaneously in both eyes, or only a very short interval intervenes before its development on the second eye.   Seegen's twelve year old girl is said to have had cataract only on her left eye, but it appears that she remained under observation but a short time.

5. Usually one finds large quantities of sugar in the urine, and the general condition of the body very much reduced.   The cases in which this is not found to hold true, is in older people; Seegen, 53; Foerster, 52; my own cases, 62 and 63 years.

6. The form of cataract which develops in a diabetic patient, as a rule, depends on the age of the patient at the time of its development.

In his "Pathology and Therapie," page 270, Becker states, "Since the causative disease is not limited to any particular period of life, hence the cataract may develop in different varieties; in young individuals as a total soft cataract, in the aged as a mixed cataract.   Hence, from its general

[8] Leber.   Uber die Erkrankungen des Auges bei Diabetes Mellitus.   Arch. f. Opth., Bd. XXI, 3.

[9] Uber die Wirksamkeit von Karlsbad, Diabetes Mellitus.   Berlin Klin. Wochen., 1879.

[10] Der Diabetes Mellitus.   Leipsig, 1870.

[11] Foerster-Beziehungen der Algemein-Leiden und Organ Erkrankungen zu Veranderungen unf Krankheiten des Sehorgans Graefe Saemisch, Bd. VII, Cap. XIII, p. 219.

[12] Uber Staar Operationen und Diabetisch C.   Deutsch. Med. Wochenschrift, No. 37, 1889.

appearance, one is not enabled to make the diagnosis of diabetic cataract. One does, however, frequently observe tendency to a rapid retrogressive metamorphosis." Foerster states, "that in the great majority of cases in old people, the cataract develops just as it would in the senile form. There are, however, cases in which the cataract develops in an entirely different manner. This form of diabetic cataract may be recognized, and has something peculiar in its formation. First, the cortical lamellae immediately beneath the capsule become cloudy; a thin, bluish grey film permeates the entire anterior surface of the lens, and its position immediately behind the edge of the pupil demonstrates that the most external layers of the cortex are involved. Its color, so far as it is confined to the sections of the superficial lamellae, is homogenous. Whereas in other cases this facetting of the sectors of the superficial layers of the lens is one of the last acts in the formation of cataract, it is here noted as one of the first. The nucleus and the deep lamellae are not entirely transparent, as can be seen by focal illumination. In the course of a few weeks, the deep layers are involved, and finally a bluish, soft, non-nuclear cataract results, which can not be differentiated from the cataracts of youthful individuals. This always occurs simultaneously on both eyes. I have only observed this form in young individuals up to the twentieth year, and at the very beginning the appearance of the lens is so characteristic, that from this alone on several occasions I have predicted sugar in the urine.

As my (Becker's) observations do not agree with the above description, and as we shall see that other authors likewise lay great stress on the appearance of the cataract, I will give the description of all my cases.

Case No. 1. R. W., of H., aged 9 years, was the youngest individual. The cataract on the left eye was extracted January 8, 1874, and had the appearance of a lens which had become cloudy very rapidly, was a tumescent, bluish white soft cataract. The iris shadow was very pronounced. Examination for sugar was not made. On December 4, 1873, the right eye was noted as cataracta corticalis posterior. At the time of the extraction of the first the second had materially increased; nevertheless, she still counted fingers at 5-6 feet.

Case No. 2. A. S., a farmer from W., aged 27 years, has had diabetes for a long time. At times 8½ per cent. sugar in the urine. In 1882 he noticed that the sight of the right eye was failing, and on December 16th he could only recognize the movements of the hand. Projection good. The cataract had a mother of pearl appearance, tumescent, and the lens star is darker and seems to stand out from the cloudy fibres. The iris shadow is well marked. The left eye has a. M. 3. V. equals $\frac{6}{4}$ Lens is clear. March 19th, three months later, the patient was examined again. On the right eye the cataract was somewhat shrunken. Anterior chamber deep. Iris shadow marked. The dark grey lens could only be detected by oblique illumination. The substance of the lens shows fine radiating striations. Between these striations are white punctate dots. Vision is not materially altered. Left eye, the anterior chamber is of normal depth. In the pupillary plane on focal illumination one notes a veil-like bluish-grey cloudiness, as though the lens had been breathed on. The lens star shows a somewhat more saturated greyish white color. The nucleus is transparent. On dilating the pupil with atropine, find that the equatorial zone of the lens is cloudy in a broad zone. Vision reduced to $\frac{6}{14}$.

Case No. 3. A. E., a farmer, 38 years of age, came under observation March 6, 1873. The left lens showed signs of an immature soft cataract. The anterior corticalis was still soft. Counts fingers at 4-5 feet. Right lens. Cataracta incipiens H 2 V$=\frac{1}{15}$; urine, S. G., 1042. November 27, 1873, could only recognize movements of the hand. S. G., 1033. The lens was extracted November 28th. Owing to a slight iritis during the process of healing, a preliminary iridectomie was made on the left eye January 5, 1874, and February 27, 1874, the extraction followed. Discharged with O. D. V.$=\frac{2}{3}$, O. S. V.$=\frac{1}{15}$. Kuhne, who examined both lenses for the presence of sugar, found the same present. (Pathologie und Therapie des Linsen System, p. 271.)

Case No. 4. J. S., a day laborer, 40 years of age. Sight began to fail in 1880. Since December can only count fingers. Was taken up at the clinic March 7, 1881, at which time he could only recognize movements of the hand. Lens is completely cloudy; exceedingly tumescent. Anterior chamber shallow. Urine acid. S. G. 1030. Quantity passed in twenty-four hours equaled 6720 cm.; contains 6.7 per cent. sugar, equal to about 450.2 grms. Extraction was made on the right eye March 9th; left eye March 29th. Healing perfectly. Vision equalled to $\frac{1}{2}$ The daily amount of sugar varied. On the day of his arrival, owing to the journey and poor nourishment, the quantity of sugar was 450.2 grms., whereas the usual quantity was from 200 to 300 grms. On the day before the first operation, failed to estimate the amount of sugar. The amount of urine passed was 2780 and 1080 ccm. In the next few days the quantity of sugar fell to 80.98 and 86 grms., but rose again during the following ninety days to 161.3 grms.; sank once more, but rose again during the last few days before the second operation to 173.3 grms. After this there was again a decrease. These results are interesting because they indicate the influence of diet during his trip and the first few days after the operation, and in the days previous to the second extraction, during which time the patient was given a mixed diet, in order to strengthen him. In both cataracts sugar was found. (See page 67 of text.)

Case No. 5. Mrs. B., of W., aged 62 years, for the past three years has suffered from a very intense degree of diabetes, with never more than 0.9 per cent. sugar in the urine. She has repeatdly been to Carlsbad. For a year past has noted the decrease of vision in both eyes. Was seen for the first time November, 1882. O. D. cataracta incipiens; O. S. cataracta nondum matura. In both eyes found the posterior cortical substance and the equatorial zone very cloudy, and the nucleus highly refracting the light. Right eye counts fingers at 2.3 m.; left eye at 1 m. In 1883 the cataract on the left eye had advanced so far that the radii could be seen when the pupil was dilated. Extraction was done under narcosis March 7th. Process of healing uneventful. During the operation the aqueous was aspirated with a pipette from the conjunctival sac, and together with the lens was examined by Kuhne and found to be free from sugar.

The amount of urine passed, the specific weight and the amount of sugar, especially the latter, during these days, though slight was at no time very great. March 7th, amount of urine=1110; S. G.=1020; sugar=0.22 per cent. March 8th, 1860, 1018. and 0.3 per cent. March 9th, 1250, 1013, 0.1. From this time on the urine was free from sugar (March 15th), only on March 17th, 22 per cent., did the urine show signs of sugar.

Case No. 6. Mrs. J. D., of Z., a wealthy woman 63 years of age, was operated on by me November 16, 1871. According to appearances this was a cataract senilis simplex. Left eye shows a cataract incipiens. This lady has had diabetes for a number of years. Quantity of sugar not estimated. $V. = \frac{1}{16}$. Opthalmoscope revealed a retinitis diabetica. Kuhne, who examined the lens, found no sugar. (P. and Th., p. 271.)

Jany [13] gives us a very accurate description, in which he especially emphasises the fissuring of the cortical substance, which gives it the appearance as though discission had been practiced. In both his cases the anterior cortical substance was but slightly cloudy, whereas posteriorly there existed exquisite choroideal cataract. "The entire posterior corticalis simulates "the pod of a fruit," in which the peculiar asbestos gloss was particularly noteworthy. Owing to the scarcity of personal observations, I have called on my colleagues. Horner writes, "I find cataracta punctata, especially posterior cortical cataract, equatorial cataract and anterior cortical cataract. The age of the patient appears to influence varieties. In young diabetic individuals there appears to be a more rapid disintegration of the anterior corticalis, whereas in older people (and in fact, in very severe cases) the posterior corticalis may first be affected. According to my observations, there is no particular rule."

Leber lays stress on the same picture which is observed in youthful diabetic patients and in other rapidly developing cataracts occurring in youthful individuals. "The cloudiness is close to the capsule and there is always a tumescence and shallowness of the anterior chamber, but I do not find that the anterior corticalis is always first involved." Concerning the cataract of a young woman at present under observation (about 4,000 cm. urine, with 10 per cent. sugar) and suffering with a high degree of diabetes, Leber writes, "In the right eye the cloudiness exists just as Horner has described it, consisting of broad, bluish, wavy sectors; which, if not immediately beneath, are at least close to the capsule. Through this cloudiness one can plainly see the cloudy striations in the posterior corticalis.

13 Zwei Falle von Beider Seitige Cataracta Diabetica. Arch. f. Augen, Bd. VIII.

On the left eye the anterior corticalis is as good as totally transparent; whereas the posterior shows the shell-like cloudiness, disclosing the delicate, moderately broad striations of which it is made up."

Dr. Max Perles [14] reports the following remarkable case. In a patient sixty-two years of age, he discovered a very peculiar change in the lens. By daylight the pupils give back a peculiar greenish-black reflex. On focal illumination and examination with the corneal loup, the anterior corticalis and the nucleus are found to be clear. In both eyes, however, the temporal portion of the posterior substance discloses an almost completely symmetrical deposit of rust-brown coloring matter, which is arranged like a closely woven network of mycelium. This deposit is located immediately beneath the capsule, is most dense along the temporal edge, becomes thinner toward the middle, and finally is lost in the finest threads. In this network these dark brown granules are deposited. Neither vesicles nor droplets, as is usual in beginning cataract, can be seen. The vitreous is free from cloudiness; both eyes are emmetropic. View of the fundus is difficult, but shows no visible change. There is no albumen in the urine, but about 7 per cent. of sugar; no abnormal pigmentation of the skin. Microscopical examination of the blood shows the haemoglobin normal. This pigmentation of the lens positively only set in after the diabetes had existed in this severe form for several years. Perles concludes: "These changes, in all probability, are due to the diabetes, since a like pigmentation of the skin in this form of disease is not unusual. However, an expression of opinion as to the nature and source of this pigmentation can not be made until anatomical examinations have thrown some light on the subject."

Regarding the presence of sugar in non-cataractous lenses of diabetic patients, we possess but a single observation made by Deutschman. [15] In the lens of a ten year old girl who had died of diabetes, he could not discover any sugar in the lens, whereas the urine contained 0.5 per cent. From the following it will be seen how important it would be to make a large number of analyses in analogous cases.

In the following table, arranged according to their age, will be found a report of all the accessible cases of diabetic cataract in which the lens was examined for sugar after the extraction. Assuming that the table represents all the reported cases of diabetic cataract extracted and examined for sugar, one finds that in the great majority of cases sugar was found present. In both of the senile cataracts extracted by me November 30 and 31, no sugar was found. Since negative results are reported for all ages, one is justified in assuming, that the presence of sugar in cataract has nothing to do with the age of the patient, and since at times in the soft, rapidly

14 Pigmentstaar bei Diabetes. Hirschberg's Centralblatt, p. 171. 1892.
15 Untersuchung zur Pathogenese der Kataract. Arch. f. Opth., XXIII, 3, 1, p. 143.

clouding and tumescent cataract, sugar was not found at other times; hence the variety of the cataract can not be looked upon as indicating the presence of sugar in the lens.

In all the positive results, there has been a high percentage of sugar in the urine, and in the negative a low percentage. If one will stop to consider the large quantity of sugar voided the day of, or the last few days previous to the operation, as an indication of the quantity present in the blood and tissue fluids; also, as has been observed time and again, that the cataract formation only occurs where there is a large excretion of sugar, hence one will understand that in these cases, sugar will be found in the lens. From this it would also follow that sugar will not be constantly present in the lens, but will vary, depending on the general condition. This fact is particularly demonstrated in Case 4, No. 25 and 26 of the table, in which special attention was given to this fact:

No.	Name of Operator.	Name of Examiner.	Age.	Sex.	Kind of Cataract.	Urin. S. G.	Urin. Percentage of Sugar.	Result.	Sugar was present in the vitreous.
1	Schmidt.	Zincke.	15	F.	Cataract hypermatura reducta.	Much Urine	Large quantity of sugar.		
2	"	"	15	F.	Cataract hypermatura reducta.	Much Urine	Large quantity of sugar.	1?	
3	Viol.		16	F.	Cataract hypermatura reducta.	1040	Large quantity of sugar.	1?	
4	"		16	F.	Cataract hypermatura reducta.	1041	Large quantity of sugar.	1	
5	Jany.	Buchwald.	17	M.	Ant cortical delicate, post cortical dense cloudiness, nuclear clear.		0.7-5.61 in the days of the oper 2.0.		1
6	"	Muller.	17	M.	Lens densely tumescent, thick cloudiness of cortex.			1	1
7	Viol.		18			1042		1	
8	"		20			1045			
9	Stober.	Hepp.	21	F.	White, cloudy, soft, tumescent cataract.	1041	4,807	1	
10	Jany.	Muller.	22	F.	Tumescent milky.	1040	0.15-8.6		
11	"	"	22	F.	Anterior corticalis delicately clouded, posterior corticalis shell-like cloudiness, nuclear clear.	1034	0.15-8.6 3%	1	
—		Hepp.	23	F.				1	1
12	Stober.		23	F.	Soft, milky.	1052	8.8-9.7	1	
13	Teillais.		23	F.	" "	1052	8.8-9.7		
14		Carins.	25	M.	Greyish white opalesence to yellow. o.5.	1052	8.9	1	
15	Knapp.	..	25	M.	Cataract hypermatura reducta.	1052	8.9	1	
16	"		28			1052		1	
17	Viol.	Klinger.	31	M.	Catar. nondum matura o. w.	1052	7.8	1	
18	Berlin.	"	31	M.	Catar. nondum matura o. w.	1052	7.8	1	
19	"	O. Liebreich.	34	F.	Catar. mollis matura o. w.	1040	8.6	1	
20	Schmidt.	"	34	F.	Catar. mollis matura o. w.	1040	8 6		
21	"		35	M.		1040	8.6		1
22	Nagel.	Kuhne.	38	M.	Both eyes, soft tumescent cataract.			1	
23	Becker.	"	38	M.	Cataract.	1040	8.6	1	
24	"	"	40	M.	Both eyes, soft tumescent cataract.	1040	8.6		1
25	"	"	40	M.	Both eyes, soft tumescent cataract.	1040	6.7	1	
26	"		40		Moderately soft cataract, with clear nucleus.	1040	6.7		
27	Berlin.	Fehling.				1040	6.7		1
28	Leber.		53	F.	Rapidly developed, double, soft cat., not entirely ripe.	1040	4-7		1
29	"		53	F.	Broad mother of pearl striations.	1040	4-7		1
30	Becker.	Kuhne.	62	F.	Cataract senilis matura.	1040	4-7		1
31	"	"	63	F.	Cat. senilis non dum matura.	1040	0.1-0.9		1

Therefore, to summarize all that has been said as the result of personal observation and the observation of others, one would say that in youthful individuals the diabetic cataract develops about as follows. First there is a cloudiness in the equatorial zone, in most cases followed by a cloudiness in the posterior cortical substance, and after this had developed the anterior corticalis is attacked. This rapidly progresses to form a soft cataract, at first attacking the lamellae immediately beneath the capsule. At this time there is neither a tumescence nor a shrinkage of the lens system, but it is true that very soon the star figure is developed. This latter symptom, as in all other soft cataracts, I look upon as the first indication of the taking up of water. The tumescence goes on rapidly and steadily, as the result of the taking up of water in the capsule, and at the same time the lens is fissured and split into sectors. The tumescent lens always shows a very marked iris shadow, because there is a very perceptible layer of fluid between capsule and lens. This condition may last one or two months. At the end of this time the volume is reduced, but the iris reflex may remain. The silky gloss is lost and a new picture, (that of the cataracta hypermatura reducta of senile cataract), is developed. The entire lens system is reduced. Schmidt-Rimpler extracted and measured such lenses. Both lenses, Nos. 1 and 2 of the above table had an equatorial diameter of 8.5 mm.; the right a saggital diameter of 2.5 mm., the left of 2.0 mm. (See Becker, Case No. 2). From personal observation, I can not state, nor have I been able to find any statements in literature, as to whether the diabetic soft cataracts of youth can become entirely fluid; whether capsular cataracts may be added to these, or whether calcareous deposits can take place. Berlin writes to me that he operated a diabetic patient for a cataracta Morgagniana; who, however, during the days of the operation had albumen, but no sugar, in his urine.

In the entire sequence of changes which take place in diabetic cataracts, I can discern nothing which differs from the ordinary soft cataracts of youth which occur in both eyes. Therefore, it seems most probable that the cataract results from the entrance of a pathologically changed nutritive fluid, resulting from the addition of sugar, along the normal point of entrance in the equatorial region. The only difference from other constitutional cataracts consists in the fact that we believe that this form is due to the presence of sugar in the vitreous; whereas in the others we have not as yet been enabled to separate the anomalous substance in the nutritive supply.

THE AETIOLOGY OF THE SO-CALLED DIABETIC CATARACT.

Owing to the fact that sugar has been found in all the tissue fluids of the body, and since the now famed experiments of Kunde for the experimental production of cloudiness of the lens, entire series of methods have been devised to explain the cloudiness of the lens which develops in diabetes.

After Leber [16] had expressed the hope, that our knowledge concerning the development of diabetic cataract would be furthered, by experimental investigation, Deutschmann [17] and Heubel [18] entered on this task most fully.

Notwithstanding the difference and the relative values of the methods employed in making these experiments, and aside from the animated discussions which arose between Deutschman and Heubel, it becomes a matter of general interest to note, that both experimenters are in accord in stating that the so-called salt, or sugar, cataracts are produced by the process of diffusion, between the salt or sugar containing aqueous (or vitreous) on the one hand, and the lens on the other; in consequence of which water and albumen diffuse in the aqueous, and the nacl, respectively the sugar, into the capsule of the lens.

According to my (Becker's) judgment, Deutschman's conclusions prove nothing. He placed a human eye, taken from a corpse, in a 5 per cent. sugar solution and after fourteen hours the lens became cloudy, whereas in a highly diabetic girl in whom there was no cataract, sugar was formed in the fluid media of the eye not in excess of 0.5 per cent.; hence he denies that the cataract can result from the extraction of water by means of a large quantity of sugar present in the fluid media of the eye. Though no weight is placed on Heubel's objection that experiments made on enucleated lenses can not be applied to the living eye, he nevertheless is correct, beyond a doubt, when he draws attention to the fact, that smaller quantities of sugar solution acting for a relatively longer time, may cause even more

---

16 Uber die Erkrankungen der Augen bei Diabetes Mellitus. Arch. f. Opth., Bd. XXI, 3.

17 (1) Untersuchungen zur Pathogenese der Cataract. Arch. f. O., 3, 1. (2) Zur Wirkung wasser entziehender Stoffe auf die Krystallinse. Arch. f. d ges Phys., Bd. XX. (3) Entsteh die Diab Kataract beim Menschen in Folge von wasserentziehung der Linse seitens zucker haltiger Augenflussigkeit? Eine Entgegnung an Prof. Heubel in Kiew. Arch. f. d ges Phys., Bd. XXII.

18 (1) Uber die Wirkung Wasserentziehender Stoffe insbesondere auf die Krystallinse. Arch. f. d ges Physiol., Bd. XX, p. 114-118. II Bemerkungen zu Deutschmann's Aufsatz. (2) Arch. f. des Physiol., Bd. XXI, p. 153-176. (3) Antwort auf Dr. Deutschmann's Entgegnung. Arch. f. d. ges Physiol., Bd. XXII, p. 580-590.

extensive changes, than large quantities acting for a short time. The lesser quantity of the active substance is compensated for by the longer time it is active.

"With all due respect to Heubel's talent, both as an experimental investigator and critic, I feel called upon to raise a few objections from a clinical standpoint, to the application of his experimental results to cataract as observed in diabetic patients."

"In his first critical essay, in reply to Deutschmann, (2, above p. 175), he sums up his views, stating that, "in the formation of the *true* diabetic cataract, the sugar contained in the aqueous and vitreous (be it as such or in Combination with Na. Cl.), is of the very greatest importance, and the first and most important change which the lens undergoes is the withdrawal of water as the result of the action of the sugar." "The *genuine* diabetic cataract develops in an unusual and in a peculiar, entirely different manner, and in this mode of development the aqueous positively exerts an influence in producing this cloudiness." "There is a complete analogy between the mode of development of the diabetic cataract and those cataracts which are experimentally produced by the dehydrating action of sugar and salt solutions. This cloudiness always involves, first, the external cortical layers; at the beginning the nucleus remains clear and the surface of the lens shows the sector-like facetts." "Competent observers have stated that with proper diathetic and therapeutic treatment, by which the amount of sugar can be considerably reduced, the lens may be made to almost completely clear up again, a condition which has hardly ever been observed in other forms of cataract. There, also, do we find another remarkable coincidence between diabetic cataract and those experimentally produced by the dehydrating action of the sugar and salt solutions."

"One must here note that Heubel lays particular stress on the expression, 'genuine *dialetic cataract*.' By this he can only have reference to the diabetic cataract of youth as described by Foerster. Heubel possibly unconsciously has given up complete agreement with Foerster, for he states that sugar in the vitreous may also lead to cataract formation. (Cited above, p. 187.) He describes an experiment in which, if the aqueous is permitted to escape, the cloudiness only appears at the posterior pole. But, aside from this, I believe that I have shown above that "*genuine* diabetic cataract," as a special variety, does not exist, but coincides in form with the majority of cataracts developing in youthful individuals, as rapidly developing soft cataracts, also as to their course and final end. Heubel's arguments, based on the experimentally produced cataracts and their subsequent clearing up, is even on a weaker basis. The cases on which Heubel bases his arguments (cited above No. 1, p. 176, II, 176), Becker reported years ago.[19] Seegen's case [19a] occurred in a man 39 years of age; Gerhardt's in a woman 56 years; and, according to Foerster's statement, these could not have been cases of genuine diabetes, since they do not occur past the middle of the twenties. Heubel himself states that "hardly ever" has a non-diabetic cataract been known to clear up. "Will anyone think hard of it, if oculists refuse to accept this fact as proven? I hardly doubt that both Gerhardt and Seegen will acknowledge the possibility of their having made a mistake. At the same time, one must not doubt but that vision was improved by Carlsbad salts. It has simply not been proven that a disappearance of cloudiness of the lens bettered vision. It is far more probable that this was due to a clearing up of the vitreous and the improvement of a case of retinitis; causes which ought not to be set aside."

In his reply Heubel drew attention to two other possibilities. Zehender's remarks did not escape him, namely, that the soft, tumescent condition of most diabetic cataracts seemed to refute the idea that there is a withdrawal of water from the lens. This thought, later taken up by Jany and myself, was answered by Heubel (one cited above), by his drawing attention to the fact "that in beginning cloudiness and in new cases the dehyration is but partial, is restricted to a small portion of the lens; whereas, the remainder of the lens substance retains its normal or possibly a reduced consistency." Heubel considers it as more than probable, that as the result of the withdrawal of water the changed, cloudy (or shrunken) "lensrads," after the lapse of a certain length of time, even where there is abundant addition of water, can not be cleared up again; and after diabetic cataract has existed for a certain length of time, such manifold changes do not set in as can easily lead to a soft and watery consistence of the cloudy lens substance." As a fact, one must acknowledge that in soft diabetic cataract, as in any other spontaneously developing cataract, the tumescence is the first stage of cataract formation.

In his first essay on this subject Deutschman pointed out the fact that the microscopical conditions noted in the experimentally produced salt and sugar cataracts does not coincide with those of the true diabetic cataract. True, at that time he only had for comparison the short communication of Knapp [20] concerning the condition of extracted diabetic cataract. Here I must again agree with Heubel (two above). "We can scarcely form an idea as to the manner in which diabetic cataract develops by examining a diabetic cataract in its latter stages." There is always this difference, the experimentally produced diabetic cataract develops acutely, whereas the diabetic cataract develops in

[19] Pathologie and Therapie, p. 272.

[19a] Der Diabetes Mellitus. Leipsig, 1870, p. 212.

[20] Bericht uber ein siebentes hundert Staar extractionen. Arch. f. Opthal., Bd. XII, p. 49.

a chronic manner; hence, it seems questionable to me, though it would be possible to examine microscopically a developing diabetic cataract in its capsule, whether one would even be able to formulate a theory which could not be attacked. Our science is certainly deeply indebted to Heubel for the thorough and objective criticism, and the manner in which he refuted Claude Bernard's hypothesis, that *cataracta diabetica* is solely and alone due to the increased amount of sugar in the blood.

In 1887, Deutschman again took up this subject,[21] and formulated the following hypothesis as to the genesis of this form of cataract. He states, "Owing to the dyscrasia, the lens, which is an epithelial structure, is subject to the same disintegration as other epithelium. The lens fibres undergo the same local death as does the epithelium of the kidney, and with this death of the cells begins the anomalous process of diffusion; but the moment the lens fibres begin to die, just as in the cadaverous lens, changes follow in consequence of the processes of diffusion, and cloudiness and tumescence of the lens follows. Hence I assume a primary death of the lens, which is an epithelial structure, in diabetic cataract. This must not necessarily be a total death; a partial death is sufficient to permit of a change in the process of diffusion. I am opposed to the theory of "the withdrawal of water from the lens."

Likewise, Leber, by demonstrating that the fluid media in diabetes have an alkaline reaction, has refuted Lohmeyer's hypothesis,[22] that sugar in the aqueous and vitreous becomes changed into lactic acid, and the action of this leads to the cloudiness of the lens, hence we are as far today as ever from finding the intermediate link between the pathological condition in which sugar is found in the nutritive fluid and the cloudiness of the lens. In the case of the diabetic cataract, we are no farther than in other forms of constitutional cataract.

There is an entire series of constitutional diseases, in which the constitution of the blood and lymph is altered, hence in which the lens receives an abnormally constituted nutritive material, which in some cases leads to cataract formation. Diabetes mellitus belongs to this class of diseases.

PROGNOSIS OF CATARACT OPERATIONS IN DIABETES. "Even at the present day some operators look upon operations for cataract in diabetic patients as offering a poor prognosis. This is evident from the oft-

[21] Pathologisch-Anatomische Untersuchungen Augen von Diabetikern, nebst Bemerkungen uber die Pathogenese der Diabetischen Cataract. Graef Arch., XXXIII, Bd. 2. 1887.

[22] Beitrag zur Histologie und Aetiologie der Erworbenen Linsenstaare. Zeitschrift fur Rationale Medicin., N. F., Bd. V, p. 99. 1854.

repeated printed statement, "Luckily operated." As is well known, Von Graefe was very guarded in his statements, and though others, as well as myself, have pointed out the fact that the incision even in very emaciated diabetic patients, heals very kindly, nevertheless, Jany advises, after a peripheral incision, the extraction be made by suction subsequent to a preliminary discission. But if any one will read Jany's description of his four cases operated in this manner, he can only conclude that eyes which can undergo such manipulations are really less vulnerable than healthy eyes in which an ordinary senile cataract has developed. From a large number of experienced operators, I have been privately informed that, just in diabetes, an unusually good process of healing follows. It is possible that the presence of sugar in the lymph causes the edges of the wound to become rapidly agglutinated. The only possible complication (where the operation is correctly done) is an iritis. This has occurred once to me; also to Horner, and likewise to Leber. Snellen writes to me, "I often find the pigment at the edge of the pupil very loose, as in macerated eyes." I (Becker, "Pathologie and Therapie," p. 272) before this time had drawn attention to this fact, namely, that in cases of tumescent diabetic cataract, the pigment around the edge of the pupil is very broad, and that even after an iridectomie the same condition is noted along the edges of the coloboma. This peculiar condition of the iris, and the hemorrhages into the vitreous, even though extremely slight, indicate that a diabetic cataractous eye is not only a diseased eye, but possibly also explains the occasional occurrence of iritis after an extraction."

There is another circumstance to which I desire to call attention. In the literature on this subject I find four cases reported, in which a few days after a cataract extraction, the patient died of diabetic coma. One ought to tell the relatives, as well as the patient, of the possibility of such a termination, in consequence of the excitement incident to an operation and the dietary restrictions which become necessary.

E.

CATARACTA SENILIS PRAEMATURA.

Between the soft cataracts of youth and the senile cataract, a form of cataract develops which occupies a mediam place between the two forms, both as to the time of its development and its seat in the middle of the lens. The aetiology seems to be closely linked with a general reduction of the nutrition of the body. Foerster considers the cause of the cataract formation to be a premature marasmus of the body. He also draws attention to Hogg's statement of the frequent coincidence of urethral stricture and hypertrophy of the prostrate with the marasmus praematuris, (among 56 patients, he found 17 cataract cases). However, this does not prove an exact relationship between the two. There is, likewise, a total absence of symptoms by means of which one may with certainty recognize the premature marasmus or premature senility. Up to this time, it has not been possible to do more than make some general statements. Nevertheless, Becker states, he has attempted to make a diagnosis of such a cataract from the manner of its development.

CATARACTA (SENILIS PRAEMATURA) NUCLEARIS.

This form of cataract characterizes itself by developing in the nucleus of the lens, between the fortieth and fiftieth year, a time of life when the sclerosis of the nucleus of the lens is already far advanced; and this cloudiness gradually extends into the transparent cortical substance. It has a peculiar white, almost milky, color. This cataract, at an exceedingly slow rate, finally becomes a total cataract. The individuals show in their general appearance that their health has been disturbed for a long time. They are people who have been reduced by general marasmus, disease, excessive bodily exertion, many and difficult labors, material want, grief, and care; and frequently the clinical history shows that the patients (women) have suffered from hysterical convulsions.

Becker states that he has only been enabled to examine teased specimens of extracted cataracts of this form, but has not been able to discover any distinctive peculiarity. A positive judgment must be withheld until a complete eye containing such a cataract can be examined. In his "Pathology and Therapie," [23] he suggested, that possibly a chemical examination might throw some light on the subject.

He further suggests [24] the possibility that, in contradistinction to all other conditions, there has never been a true formation of a nucleus in a lens which becomes diseased in this manner. It would, then, not be a difficult matter to understand how, owing to this exceptional condition of the lens, there should follow a peculiar cataract formation.

Without in such cases being able to demonstrate a diseased condition of the nutritive fluids of the entire body, (since we find neither albumen nor sugar in the urine), we might look upon the general marasmus of the entire body as the cause of a failure to form the nucleus. The subjective symptoms are those of so-called nuclear cataract. The prognosis is not as good as in simple senile cataract. It is not dependent, even partially, on the general condition of the individual, nor on the general tendency of

---

[23] S. 73, p. 270.
[24] S. 73, p. 270.

the healing of wounds; but on the fact that the outer non-cloudy lamellae of cortical substance necessarily remain behind in the eye, or are removed with difficulty. In no other form would Von Mutter's proposal—to puncture the capsule, so as to hasten ripening of the cataract—be as applicable as in this form. In such cases it would be worth the attempt, in advanced cases, to practice discission. At the present day, no doubt, artificial maturation would be practiced.

F.

SENILE CATARACT. CATARACTA SENILIS.

As the name indicates, this form of cataract occurs in the aged, and as a rule one should hesitate to designate a cataract as senile if the patient has not passed the fiftieth year. It is not correct to state that an earlier ageing of the entire body would predispose to senile cataract. There are no observations reported where in so-called "youthful aged ones" an earlier sclerosis of the lens occurred or developed more rapidly than under normal conditions.

Just as far as the sclerosis of the lens extended at the time the cataract formation began, just so far will the lens remain as good as unchanged during the entire time those processes take place which are associated with and take place during cataract formation. In consequence, after extraction we find, even in the most varied forms of senile cataract, that the nucleus is bi-convex, more or less intensely yellow, or even red; always transparent, but *not* cataractous. Both Malgaigne and Foerster pointed out the fact that in senile cataract the cloudiness develops first in the cortical substance, but this did not receive the deserved recognition.

In the second part of this work, the pathology and the most important forms of senile cataract were so exhaustively considered that a short resume of the clinical data at this point will suffice.

The very first recognizable signs during life, of a beginning senile cataract, are the very delicate fissures in the deeper portions of the cortical substance, which totally reflect the light. These are followed by the "riders," which develop in the equatorial region. These cloudy striations are due to the presence of a chemically changed fluid which accumulates in the interspaces as the result of processes of diffusion going on between this fluid and the lens fibres. This fluid had an index of refraction differing from that of the neighboring lamellae. The cause of this formation of interspaces is to be found in the pathological shrinkage of the nucleus, which seems to be a preparatory condition to the formation of cataract. As a rule these interspaces make their first appearance in the cortical substance, in the equatorial region, because in the region of the poles both capsule and cortex can more easily follow the shrinking nucleus than along the equatorial zone, where the zonula of zinii exerts traction in an opposite direction. As a result of diffusion between these spaces and the contents of the fibres, the latter suffer changes which lead to molecular disintegration.

During the time these processes are going on, possibly even preceding them, without exception, hyperplasia of the capsular epithelium is progressing, which is looked upon as an atrophic hyperplasia.

The general picture which these striated opacities in the cortical substance present at this time, whether observed by the direct illumination with the mirror or by focal illumination, is always that of the well-known arrangement of the lens fibres. The careful observation of this gradually developing total opacity of the cortical substance which surrounds the sclerosed nucleus, has led oculists to a series of names which designate the condition of the cataract.

As long as the above anatomically described condition persists and but few cloudy striations appear in the periphery, either in front of or behind the nucleus, one speaks of a beginning cataract (*cataracta incipiens*). Where this cloudiness has advanced further, we use the expression, "unripe cataract," (*cataracta nondum matura*). Although there can be no sharp line of demarcation between these two stages, nevertheless they can be kept apart by speaking of *cataracta incipiens* as long as the greater portion of the cortical substance is not cloudy. When the entire cortical substance has become totally cloudy, we speak of *cataracta matura*. At times, a further distinction is made; a stage immediately preceding that of ripeness is described as *cataracta maturescens*. The molecular disintegration of the lens fibres is accompanied by a tumescence or swelling of the lens, due to the taking up of water, and this process may go on more or less rapidly. This may proceed so rapidly and the polar diameter of the lens so increase, as to become evident to the naked eye; and press the iris forward, so as to lessen the depth of the anterior chamber.

This taking up of water is followed by a giving off of the same; the tumescence, by a reduction in volume. If from the depth of the anterior chamber one can judge that the size of the lens is equal to that of a normal lens we call this a *cataracta matura*, when this has fallen below the normal volume we speak of an over-ripe cataract, *cataracta hypermatura*.

The stage of ripeness is recognized, on focal illumination, by the sign, that one can no longer recognize dark sectors; and on using the opthalmoscope, even when the pupil is dilated, we no longer get a red reflex from the fundus. One must, however, direct attention to the most anterior lamellae, since these are of the greatest importance. Owing to the extreme thinness of the capsule of the lens, the pigmented edge of the iris will seem to lie in contact with the lens when the cortical substance is totally opaque. If transparent cortical substance is still present behind the iris, on focal illumination a black interspace will appear between the pupillary edge of the iris, and the most anterior lamellae which reflect the light. This is known as the projected iris shadow, and by this means one can determine how much cortical substance still remains non-cloudy.

The ancient operators observed, that where the lens had become completely cloudy, it would, comparatively speaking, be as easily removed from its capsule as a ripe fruit be shelled out of its pod; hence the expression, "ripe cataract. And this is found in the writings of Baron Wenzel, the father (l. c., p. 14); also of Percival Pott, 1779 (Morgagni, XIII, 18). It appears after the expression "ripe cataract" had for a time fallen into discredit, it again came into general use, and in reality there can be no objection raised to its use, if we associate its use with a well defined condition, such as was described, and for which we are indebted to Arlt (l. c., p. 260).

Our knowledge concerning senile cataract has advanced in more ways than one. We are indebted to Priestly Smith for one important step forward. He succeeded in demonstrating that the cloudiness in the senile lens is preceded by a reduction in its volume. *This shrinkage* of the nucleus, which I had looked upon as proceeding to a like degree in all similar lenses, and which I had utilized to explain the occurrence of the first fissures and splits in the equatorial region as the result of the fixed position of the equatorial region in consequence of the zonula zinii, *is now shown to be developed to a greater degree in those lenses which later on become cataractous, than in those which remain clear.*

On pages 66, 67 it has been shown that the nucleus of a senile cataract has a different chemical constitution, than the senile nucleus of the non-cataractous lens. Hence one might assume that the cause of the increased shrinkage of the nucleus is due to its abnormal chemical constitution. But since this has only been proven in the case of cholesterine and only as exceedingly probable for albumen, (Cahn, Knies); hence it yet remains, to make the same chemical analyses of the nuclei of senile non-cataractous lenses, so as to compare the two.

"According to Jacobson and Cahn, we may assume that both the cholesterine and the modified albuminous substance are not carried into the lens from without by the nutritive stream, but are developed from the albuminous substances which are normally present in the lens. Since the changes which take place begin in the nucleus of the lens (hence in its oldest and inmost lamellae), and no doubt proceed, just as do the normal processes of sclerosis, very slowly; hence we may draw the surprising conclusion that the preparation for the formation of senile cataract has been going on for a long time. That is, *the beginning of the abnormal chemical changes in the nucleus of the lens, which are a departure from the normal sclerosis of the ageing lens, and which lead to the senile cloudiness of the lens, do not coincide in time, to the period when we observe the first cloudiness at the border line between nucleus and cortex, but precede this by many years.* Whether or not a person shall become affected with cataract in his sixtieth year, in all probability is decided at forty. Stress has already been laid on the fact, that senile cataract always occurs on both eyes, though one lens may be affected somewhat later than the other. The cause of this must be sought in an altered constitution of the nutritive fluids of the entire organism. True, we do not as yet know what this something is. This is probably to be explained by the fact, that we have not as yet sought at the proper time or place, when this preparation for the future cataract formation is going on. It is just possible that these departures from the normal, which later on lead to cataract formation, might be found in the lenses of persons just reaching the age in life when presbyopic functional symptoms manifest themselves, and just in those lenses which apparently one would suppose would remain perfectly clear, even in very advanced old age. It is certainly more than a mere coincidence that just those processes, which take place in the nucleus of a *premature senile cataract*, and which differentiates it from the senile cataract, should occur just in these years, when we suppose this preparation for the formation of a senile cataract is taking place."

The question of hereditary predisposition to cataract, might likewise be elucidated, if we would try to discover a common constitutional peculiarity. If one finds a family, as I have, in which the grandmother developed double senile cataract without any known complication, at 57 years, the father at 48 years, and the son at 26 years, one can not help thinking that there must be some hereditary constitution cause.

The subsequent taking up of water is not inconsistent with Priestly Smith's assertion. The taking up, is to be looked upon as a process of diffusion going on between the fluid media of the eye and the already partially cloudy, hence chemically changed, lens. This is looked upon as the second stage of senile cataract formation.

THE AETIOLOGY OF SENILE CATARACT. As we have seen, there is a chemical and a physical difference between the nucleus of a simple senile lens and the nucleus of a senile cataract. As a result of this chemical difference, as Priestly Smith has shown, there is an increased shrinkage of the nucleus of the lens, which later on is to be attacked by cataract, and this, on the other hand, has given additional support to Becker's theory. The anatomical proof of the hyperplasia of the intracapsular cells which invariably accompanies the formation of senile cataract, aside from the above, is in accord with the theory of shrinkage.

ALBUMINURIA AS A CAUSE OF SENILE CATARACT.

"Deutschman, since he found albumen in the urine of a large percentage (33 per cent.) of patients suffering from senile cataract, attempted to set up a special form of cataract—*cataracta nephritica*. After attention was drawn to this fact, the percentage in my clinic also rose; thus, in 1881 it was 2 per cent., whereas in 1882 it was 18.8 per cent. Though chronic nephritis does occur frequently in old people, this does not by any means prove that there is a causative relationship between the two. And if the above explanation, as to the time when the basis is laid for the later developing cataract, is not totally erroneous, the mere fact that both these diseases are present at the same time, does not by any means prove a causative relationship between the two."

"Although chronic nephritis and albuminuria belong to the constitutional diseases, which, as we know, may at times lead to deep-seated and almost always, disease of both eyes, and which may easily affect the constitution of the vitreous, for the present, at least, the causative relation between chronic nephritis and cataract can not be looked upon as proven."

ATHEROMA OF THE CAROTID AS A CAUSE OF CATARACT.

"Michel's statement,[25] "that atheroma of the carotid is a very intimate causative factor in the production of senile cataract, as well as in the production of cataract in one eye," seems to find but slight support, in fact. Based on a collection of the cases reported, and a few experiments of his own and clinical histories, some with, some without, post mortem examination, Michel assumes as proven, that pronounced interference with the circulation in the carotid may cause very great interference in the eye on the same side; and he further believes that where the circulation in both carotids is interfered with for a long time, this will gradually lead to an increase of those pathological processes which characterize themselves by interference with the nutrition of the eye. Michel says atheroma of the carotid is such a disease, and such a nutritive disturbance leads to cataract."

"Michel goes on to state, "owing to the rigid walls of the arteries, the pulse waves are not carried sufficiently far, and in consequence of the loss

---

[25] Das verhalten des Auges bei storungen im Circulationsgebiet der Carotis in Beitrage zur Opthalmologie als Festgabe fur Friedrich Horner. Wiesbaden, 1881.

of elasticity, the column of blood is not propelled onward. *Hence, a certain slowing up of the movement of the blood follows*, and, as a result, changes of nutrition follow.

It is easily seen, that the explanation is based on a false premesis, for *ceteris paribus*, a column of fluid will rise, not slower, but more quickly in a rigid tube; but when the propelling force acts periodically, the column will not ascend continuously, but intermittently. When fluid is forced into a tube periodically it will also flow out periodically, since the same amount of fluid must flow out at the one end of a tube as is forced in at the other end, under a certain degree of pressure.[26] However, in rigid tubes, the changes in the degree of pressure is greater than in elastic tubes. Where the outflow is not a free one, the conditions are not the same. Where the interference is very great, the advancement of the column of blood is slowed, and the blood in the left heart is under heavier pressure. In atheroma, owing to the diminution of the lumen of the smaller arteries and capillaries, this resistance is increased. Whereas an atheromatous degeneration of the vessels of the eye, whether this be combined with an atheroma of the carotid or not, would influence the nutrition of the eye, more especially the lens.

"However, notwithstanding the want of a proper explanation, the connection between atheroma of the carotid and cataract is still pointed out, hence I have had the last fifty-three patients taken up at the clinic for spontaneously developed cataract examined in this regard in order to test Michel's statements. I was all the more induced to do this, owing to an experiment known to me which appeared to have some direct bearing on the connection between one-sided atheroma and cataract on the same side, and which seems entirely to have escaped Michel's notice. Heubel [27] writes: "One can easily bring about a cloudiness of the lens, truly only after the death of the rabbit, if one injects a concentrated sugar solution in the peripheral end of the common carotid. Death nearly always follows immediately after the injection, but simultaneously or a few minutes later one always observes the lens on the same side assume at first a faint, gradually-increasing cloudiness, and hence one may assume that this form of cataract develops just as it does in the rabbit."

"Perhaps I would not have decided to place my negative results opposite the positive results of Michel were it not for the recent publication of a dissertation by Marion von Karwat, written under Michel's direction,[28] and which indicates that even at the present day he holds fast to his conclu-

[26] See Rollet, Physiologie der Blutbewegung in Herman, Handbuch der Physiologie, IV, 1, p. 177.

[27] Quoted above, 1, p. 164.

[28] Beitrage zur Erkrankung des Auges bei Carotis atherom. Wurzburg, 1883.

sions, and if according to an observation of Mooren's he did not look upon this as a proven fact. In his "Funf Lustren Opthalmologischer Wirksamkeit" he says (page 197): "Michel's beautiful experiments have proven to us the connection between the development of cloudiness of the lens and sclerotic (atheromatous) changes in the walls of the carotid." Such a thoughtless assent on the part of Mooren becomes all the more conspicuous, because Mooren[29] states that atheroma of the carotid is the cause of senile cataract. Michel, however (p. 45), purposely avoids stating that the condition of affairs are such, but that there is a direct connection between cloudiness of the lens and atheroma of the carotid, but not that where this condition exists, there is also a like change in the vessels of the choroid. But he distinctly states: "In not a single case where it was possible to make an opthalmoscopic examination after an extraction could changes be found in the arterial vessels of the retina." He further points out the fact that if this were the case, the functions of the eye would suffer more frequently than is the case.

In order that this examination should be conducted in the most perfect and reliable manner, I begged of Prof. Adolf Weil to conduct the same. He was kind enough to do this with the greatest conscientiousness, and has permitted me to publish the results, together with his views on the subject.

"Michel's ideas have awakened a number of priori thoughts. In the first place, it is difficult to understand how, with the existing anastomosis between the two carotids and the vertebral arteries, an atheromatous change in one carotid artery, the vessels of the eye itself being normal—and such he expressly states to be the case—could bring about disturbance in the lens. It is also remarkable that though he continually speaks of a connection between cloudiness of the lens and sclerosis of the carotid, he fails to state whether he has reference to the common carotid, the internal or external. The internal carotid, even in thin people, is not accessible to palpation; hence, we must assume that his remarks refer to the carotis communis, or the external. The relative frequency of atheroma in young people, the isolated, more especially the involvement of the carotid, the occurrence of arterio-sclerosis on one side, the absence of all other symptoms which would point to atheroma of the carotid in which we find true aneurysmal formation. It is, however, as unknown for an aneurism of the carotid to bring on a cataract. Notwithstanding these objections, it nevertheless seemed proper to determine by renewed investigation whether these two conditions really existed at the same time, though no direct connection between the two could be proven. For this purpose the circulatory system of fifty-three cataract patients was examined, without the examiner knowing any-

---

29 Opthalmish Beobachtungen. Berlin, 1867.

thing concerning the special condition of the cataract. (As to which side the cataract was confined, whether it was on one or both sides, etc.) Examination was made of the heart, the brachial and the radial arteries, and the portion of the carotis communis and externa which were accessible to palpitation, to determine whether the carotids were atheromatous or not. This palpitation, however, is much more difficult than in the case of the radial or brachial arteries, which can be more easily encompassed and compressed. Judgment as to whether the carotid is more or less tortuous, or whether the pulsations are more marked, must surely be more uncertain, unless the degree of change is very great or unless comparison between the right and left offers a very great difference. It must, however, not be forgotten that even under normal circumstances the right carotid communis is often thicker than the left. And a moderate dilation of the upper end of the common carotid—a sort of bulb—according to the general opinion of anatomists must not be looked upon as pathological. Every experienced examiner will agree with me when I state that the width and the tension in the arterial tube, as well as the height of the pulse wave, not only in different individuals, but even in the same individual, varies greatly at different times. Hence, one will only be able to diagnose with certainty changes in the walls of the arteries (thickening and rigidity), when the anomalie of width and tension of the arterial tube, as well as the pulse wave, exceed a certain degree."

The following table gives the results of Weil's Examinations:

Age.	Male.	Female.	Total.	Normal Condition.	Atheroma of the Carotid without Heart Disease.		Atheroma of the Carotid with Heart Disease.		With Struma.	Heart Disease without Atheroma of the Carotid.
					On the side of the first diseased lens.	Not on the side of the first diseased lens.	On the side of the first diseased lens.	Not on the side of the first diseased lens.		
1–10	1*	2*	3	3						
11–20	2		2	2						
21–30	1*	1*	2	2						
31–40	1		1	1						
41–50	2	3	5	3		1				1
51–60	6	8	14	11	2	1				
61–70	8	9	17	8	2	4		1		2
71–81	1	7	8	2	2			1	1	2
81–90		1	1			1				
Total...	22	31	53	32	6	7		2	1	5

1. The asterisk marks the four cataracts which occurred only on one eye.

2. Both of the boys' eyes eleven and twenty years, had zonular cataract.

3. The man of thirty-eight had albuminuria.

4. Of the five patients between forty and fifty years, three had nuclear cataract (Becker), one had albumen in the urine. One was a rapidly developing tumescent cortical cataract, without the presence of sugar in albumen.

"Hence, in but sixteen cases was there any disease of the carotid to be found, whereas in thirty-seven cases this was not the case. Of the sixteen, but six had atheroma on the side of the lens which first became cloudy; in ten this was not the case. This, however, only occurred in individuals who had passed the fortieth year. In the four cases with cataract on one eye, the condition of the circulatory apparatus, especially of the carotid, was found to be normal. It would hardly seem necessary to examine into this table any further. This much, however, must be patent to every unbiased reader; namely, that both Michel and Mooren have gone too far, in that the former assures us that there is an aetiological connection between the so-called senile cataract and the one-sided cataract of unknown aetiology, and that atheroma of the carotid offers a satisfactory explanation for this cloudiness of the lens, and the latter in giving assent to the utterance."

"Hence, I find myself placed in the peculiar position of defending my position against Mooren by Mooren's own statements made many years ago, and in which he expressed the correct views concerning the aetiology of cataract (1867)."

"In the above I have given my reasons which prevent me from accepting the views of Deutschman and Michel concerning the genesis of certain forms of cataract. There is possibly some basis of truth in both, for chronic nephritis is frequently accompanied by disease of the smaller blood-vessels and capillaries. According to some authorities this disease of the blood vessels is the cause of the nephritis. Likewise, even though Michel can not convince himself of the fact, we may assume that where there is atheroma of the carotid there is likewise disease of the smaller arteries, especially the smaller branches of the opthalmic. *This pathological condition of the vessels of the uvea would then offer us the intermediate link in the chain between cloudiness of the lens on the one hand, and nephritis and atheroma of the carotid on the other.* As I have already shown, both diseases may then be utilized to explain the occurrence of cataract even on the one eye, if statistics made on a large scale once demonstrate the more frequent occurence of either two. And here it is proper to point out the important fact, that in the microscopical examination of cataractous eyes more attention might be given to the condition of the choroidal vessels."

In his Pathology and Therapy (Sec. 67, p. 261) Becker draws attention to some interesting points concerning the aetiology of senile cataracts. He quotes Walter and Arlt, who claim that eyes with a blue iris are more frequently affected than those with a brown iris, for, says Arlt: "the pigment in the iris prevents the lens from being acted on to so great a degree by the light." Though Yager, Arlt, and Hasner conclude that more men are affected than women, in proportion of 4.3, Becker concludes that though this may apparently be a fact, he goes on to state: "Many of the patients taken up in clinics come a long distance to be operated. The most of these are poor people, so that the expenses of such a journey are met under great difficulties. Hence, since vision to man is of greater value than to woman, since he must carry on his occupation, in order to earn money to supply the necessities of life; hence, this fact alone will explain why it is that more men are operated than women.

It has already been stated that cataract occurs with greatest frequency in the young and in the aged, and it is worthy of note that after the seventieth year there is a very marked decrease in the proportion of frequency. In 882 cataracts occurring between 25 and 85 years, 626 occurred between 45 and 70 years (Arlt). The majority of senile cataracts occurred between the 50th and 70th year.

Station and occupation do not appear to exert much of an influence. Cataract has been observed in the English royal family. It is probable that King Wenzel of Bohemia had a cataract. King Don Juan of Aragon was operated by Rabbi Akiabar, of Lerida, for cataract in 1468[29a] Gladstone, the great English Premier, was successfully operated in 1895 by Nettleship. But if senile cataract occurs but seldom among the rich and notable, this may be explained by the fact that this class forms but a small percentage of the entire population.

Dr. Meyerhoefer [30] draws attention to the fact that cataract develops in glass makers. In an examination of 506 persons he found opacities in the lenses of 59, and 4 had total cataract. This he attributes to the excessive heat of the oven, and the exceedingly profuse perspiration, which withdraws large quantities of fluid from the body.

The subject of heredity had already been touched upon. A long list of observers could be mentioned who have recorded cases proving that heredity plays an important role. Among these we find the names of Beer, Richter, Arlt, Dupuytren, Sanson, Streatfield, Susardi, Dyer, Roux, Maunoir, Sichel, Ullmann, Bartard, Hirschberg, Armaignac, Galezowski and others. Carreas y Argo [31] has given us a complete review of this subject, and concludes, that the hereditary cataracts by preference attack individuals belonging to the same sex, as the one so first affected; further, that the cataracts do not always, as many authorities contend, develop at the same time of life as in the previous generation, but quite the contrary at an earlier date, and may even develop at birth. Galeowski places the hereditary percentage at from four to five per cent. It is also noteworthy that the heredity is not always continuous; it may skip a generation.

Galeowski,[32] in the course of nineteen years among 128,000 patients, noted

[29a] Ullersperger A. F. O., 2, p. 272.

[30] Zur Aetiologie des Grauen Staares Jugendlicher Individuen bei Glass macher. Zehender's Monatsblatt, 1886.

[31] Hirschberg's Centralblatt, August, 1884, p. 466. "Von der Erblichen Cataracten und ihrer Ubertragung auf Individuen des gleichen Geschlectes."

[32] De la marche el du prog des Cataract. Recivell d'Opth, May, 1885.

4,776 cataracts (1,646 senile, 199 traumatic, 1,680 cortical, 231 congenital, 130 capsular, 94 diabetic, 128 choroidal). He ascribes the principal aetiological factors, aside from trauma, to heridity, gout, age and the various diseases of the choroid.

G.

CATARACTA HYPERMATURA.

Subsequent to the stage of ripeness of senile cataract, one of two diametrically opposite changes may take place. Either as a result of the giving off of water the cataractous mass may become smaller and inspisated —*cataracta hypermatura reducta*—or the cloudy substance becomes fluid and the nucleus sinks to the bottom of the sac, during which process cholestearin, and possibly fat, are formed, without great development of drusen, capsular cataract, cataracta Morgagniana.

1. CATARACTA HYPERMATURA REDUCTA.

It appears that in a large number of cataracts which have passed the stage or ripeness, the giving off of water continues, and the inspisated cataractous mass consists of degenerated lens fibres. The cataract has the appearance of a drop of dried carpenter's glue, and though the radiating striations do not entirely disappear, these are now associated with a number of quite regularly arranged transverse striations. When the pupil is dilated the appearance is very similar to that of a spiderweb. About this time the cortical substance, and with it the entire cataract, may again become transparent. We may assume this, since at times patients who are waiting for the second eye to become blind before coming for operation, observe that they are again beginning to see something with the first affected eye (Arlt 1, c. p. 260.) The lens may remain in this condition for years. In course of time, however, a capsular cataracta develops. These are the cases of true *phako scleroma.*

As far as microscopical examination goes this has shown the presence of fatty drops, so-called myelin, cholestearin plaques, calcareous granules and pieces of lens fibres.

2. CATARACTA HYPERMATURA FLUIDA.
CATRACTA MORGAGNIANA.

In another series of cases we find that though the volume of the tumescent cataract is reduced below that of the normal volume of a senile lens, it does not become inspisated, but becomes even more fluid than it was during the stage of tumescence. Under these conditions it becomes exceedingly difficult, and in some cases it is impossible, to get anything like a distinct reflex of the nucleus on focal illumination. The cataract has a greyish-yellow color, and one can no longer detect any striations. A different picture can be produced by having the patient bend his head forward for a time. After a time one will then be enabled to observe a brownish, more or less circular disc, which will disappear if he bends his head backward. These changes are due to the fact that the nucleus is floating in a fluid cataractous mass, and hence can change its position. Being specifically heavier, it sinks to the floor when the head is in the upright position, and changes its position with the relative position of the head. Such nuclei have a very similar likeness to a lentil, are perfectly smooth and transparent.

Pathologie and Therapie, Sec. 68, p. 264. H. Muller (l. c., p. 263) had the opportunity of making an anatomical examination. He says: "On opening the capsule, a thin, yellowish pus-like fluid escaped, which seemed to contain only very delicate pale molecules. A dense cloudiness followed the addition of acetic acid, and in excess this cloudiness again disappeared, a few flakes remaining. Under the microscope this pasty fluid was found to contain myelin, fat and cholestearin.

Page 265. I have not been able to positively determine the name of him, or for which particular variety the name *C. Morgagniana* was first used. Morgagni (l. c., Epis. 63, 6) described a case which may have led to the use of this name. He gives the following description of the eye of a man 40 years of age who in youth had had smallpox, and who acquired a corneal cicatrix, in consequence of which he was nearly blind. "Scleroticam igitur cuma tergo vix incidere coepissem; limpida aqua statim effluxit, it quam pass magna vitrei humoris videri poterat abiisse, cum pass reliqua, naturali quadantenus similis, annexa, ut solet, crystallino humori restitisset qui illam cum retrosum traherem, secutus est. Is parvus erat secundum om nes dimensiones, crassit autem vel paulo minor quam ejusmodi oculo conveniret. Facie anteriore in medio cral albus, siucti per corneam transpexeram, caetera albidus; et cum inter digitos leviter comprimerem, mollis. Cumvero ejus tunican incidere coeppisem; continuo apua erupit, nihil purulenti habens, imo pura, el limpida, eague copia pro parvitate crystallini, ut hic statim ad multo minorem crassitudinem redigeretur. Quidquid de substantia ipsius reliqum fuit, lentis pristinam figuram retinuit; el cum per diametrum disse cuissem; utraque sectio quandam quasi seriem mimarum nigrescentiam particularum ostendit, quae per medium recta ab uno ad alterum sectionio ducebatur, cum ubrique alibi color absolete albidus appareret."

Aside from the fact that this is the first report of a case of detachment of the vitreous, one could call this a case of *cataracta Morgagnia*, as we understand it today. Here we find a capsular cataract, a fluid corticalis, and within a regularly floating nucleus. In one point only does it not tally; the fluid which escaped was clear not cloudy. I could find no reference to this case by authors which would tend to show that they based their writings on the above case. Jamin (l. c., p. 243 and 264) describes two cases, in one of which the nucleus was found floating in a milky cortical substance, the nucleus being a regular brown, the other showed a greyish blue, slimy corticalis, after the evacuation of which a perfectly transparent nucleus remained, by means of which the patient is said to have been able to read and see small objects without the use of glasses. In a foot note, speaking of the first case, Jamin says (l. c., p. 244) that the cloudy fluid was simply altered humor Morgagni, and that in the second case the humor Morgagni was simply cloudy. The statements of Morgagni in reference to this matter are found in his "Adversaria Anatomica Sexta Anima Adversa, LXXI," and reads as follows: "Deinde eadem tunicam in vitulis etiam, bobusque sive recens, sive non ita recens, occisis perforata plures animadverti illico humorem quendam aqueum prodire; quodet et in homine observare visus sum." Himly (l. c., p. 229) bases his statements on the writings of Jamin, and is of the opinion that Morgagni was the first to differentiate between Morgagni's cataract and milk cataract, and also accepts the name for the second condition. Beer (l. c., p. 292) likewise uses the one name for both varieties. Notwithstanding this I would have doubted the existence of such a condition had not Arlt (l. c., II, p. 257) described a case belonging to this variety. Owing to its rarity I will give an abbreviated quotation. A girl 9 years of age had cataract on both eyes, and these had developed six to eight weeks subsequent to birth. The cataracts, which were yellowish grey in color, with here and there greyish opacities, were about 1 mm. removed from the iris, and the patient saw sufficiently to get about. On dilating the pupils a milky fluid was disclosed in both capsules surrounding both nuclei, not unlike a hypopyon. The nuclei changed their position with every movement of the head. For two years the amount of vision remained unchanged. In the eleventh year the discission was made. After incision of the capsule a quantity of cloudy fluid escaped, and the pupils appeared black. The child could now recognize the fingers of the hand, a handkerchief, etc. On the twelfth day a decided reaction set in—hydro meningitis. The lens gradually became cloudier and more voluminous, and after three months was totally resolved. Arlt specifically designated this as a *cataract Morgagni*, though his description is exactly that of a cataract Morgagni, as we have described it in the aged. All the late authorities use the name only for those cases where the cortical substance becomes fluid in advanced life, and the hard nucleus sinks to the bottom of the sac. If we wish to do justice to both varieties, one is compelled to include under the name cataract Morgagni all those cases in which the cortex is fluid and the nucleus hard, aside from the color of the nucleus, which in age is sclerosed, whereas in youth this is soft and transparent.

A later examination is by Knies, (p. 182), who examined a case in which Horner had made the extraction; the case of a woman forty-three years of age. "The entire anterior capsular epithelium was normal; in the equatorial region there was an excessive proliferation and many of the well-known large, round vesicles, partly containing nuclei, other new formations, such as we are accustomed to find in the so-called crystalline pearls. As yet we can not state whether we are to seek the cause of the Morgagni's cataract in a perverted crystalline pearl formation in which the epithelial cells have undergone a mucoid or similar change. "The nucleus shows no change different from that observed in other cataracts; the fluid between it and the capsule was coagulated by the hardening fluid, (alcohol and Muller's fluid) ,and consisted largely of myelin globules and detritus, in which nothing special could be recognized."

If we will designate every cataract in which the cortical substance has become fluid as a *cataracta Morgagniana*, we will meet with it at every period of life, even congenitally. Only, the fluid cataracts of youthful individuals do not possess a nucleus. However, in these cases one frequently finds present in the fluid an unusually large quantity of carcareous, finely granular matter, and crystals. If the eye is kept perfectly quiet for a time the calcareous matter gravitates to the bottom; whereas above, there will be, relatively speaking, a clear fluid. If the eye is moved about, the cataract assumes a milky hue. In the few cases of *cataracta lactea* examined, just as in the firm cataracta calcarea, the epithelium of the anterior capsule was found practically destroyed.

In older individuals one always finds a nucleus in the fluid cortical substance. The volume of the nucleus depends on the age of the individual; the younger the individual, the smaller the nucleus. Nevertheless, the age of the cataract must be taken into consideration as a factor; for at times one does find a very small nucleus in old people; so that one must assume that the decrease in the volume of the nucleus is the result of maceration in the fluid corticalis. The smallest nucleus Becker extracted was obtained from a man fifty-seven years, and it weighed in its fresh state 0.07 grm. The normal weight of a lens of the same age is 0.24 grm., and the weight of a large nucleus of a mature cataract about 0.13 grm., so that the supposed melting away of the nucleus must have equaled about one-half in its weight.

I have frequently examined the cortical mass, and have always found cholesterine and fat.

THE CONDITION OF THE INTRACAPSULAR CELLS IN OVER-RIPE CATARACTS.

Almost without exception, in cases of *cataracta hypermatura reducta*; less frequently in cases of *cataracta Morgagniana* which have existed for any length of time, we find capsular cataracts developing. All the various stages which have been described in the earlier part of this work are met with here.

I desire, however, to draw attention to a point in the genesis of capsular cataract, which was probably not sufficiently dwelt upon. If after the volume of the lens is reduced; during the time of preparation for the cataract formation is going on, and the epithelial cells, which have not lost their formative power, are incited to reproduction; the question might be asked, why it is, that the former method of formation of lens fibres at the whorl does not continue and proceed to the laying down of new lens fibres and lamellae. *Undoubtedly the epithelium must have undergone a change which prevents this.* A normal increase is only possible where the formation of new cells is distributed over the entire epithelial surface and where, as a result of indirect nuclear division, the new cells force themselves in between the old, and thus cause a gradual movement toward the equator. If we will now assume that this power to move along the inner surface of the capsule is lost to the cells, which have fallen a prey to the simple senile atrophy; hence the new-formed cells will likewise be retarded in this power of locomotion, and will form, at the place where they are developed, heaps of cells which in the further course of changes, gradually go over to form a capsular cataract. *This loss of power of locomotion hence becomes an essential factor in the formation of a capsular cataract.* This assumption is supported by the fact, that along the posterior capsule, where the hindrance does not exist, one so frequently finds a complete epithelial covering developing from the cells along the equator.

As Knies and Muller have stated, in Morgagni's cataract one frequently finds the epithelium as well preserved as in other unripe cataracts. In all the cases which I examined, as well as in the cases of Kniess and Muller, the vesicular cells in the equatorial region were excessively developed. It appears that, whereas Knies observed their development exclusively in the equatorial region of the lens, Muller claims to have seen them develop in different ways, as did Wedl, from other epithelial hyperplasias and formations along the posterior capsule.

These vesicular formations are a constant production in all cataract formations. Knies was the first who gave utterance to, or more properly speaking, recorded in literature, this thought, which is worthy of respect. Notwithstanding our total ignorance as to the cause, why it is that in one case the corticalis of over-ripe cataract becomes inspisated; in another, notwithstanding the giving off of fluid, it becomes fluid; I can not refrain from expressing the thought, as to whether it is not possible in cases where we find such excessive formation of vesicular cells, for these later on "to flow together," and thus form the anatomical basis for a *Morgagni's cataract.*

H.

CATARACTA NIGRA.

"The name of this form of cataract, as well as its existence, has been both variously applied and understood. Wenzel (l. c., p. 38) describes the extraction of a lens taken from an eye in which vision was very much reduced, the pupil of which did not appear grey; so the existence of the cataract was doubted. A large dark-brown lens escaped from the wound. The wound healed, and vision was restored. This form of cataract he called *cataracta nigra*. The entire description showed that he was dealing with a lens in which the formation of the nucleus extended up to the capsule without the process ever having come to a standstill. Such exquisite examples, in which no cortex remains,, are but seldom encountered. They might also be called *cataracta brunescens*."

"It would be proper to translate *cataracta nigra* as the 'black grey cataract,' but not as "black cataract," since this latter term, even today, is used to define absolute amaurosis. It is interesting to note that in former times both the English and the French used the expression cataracta nigra synonymously with *gutta serena* and paralysis (?) of the optic nerve. I find it is so used by Percival Pott;[33] also by Morgagni.[34] In a dissertation by Von Warnatz (Cataracta Nigra, 1832) is found a very complete compilation of the literature on this subject. In later times Von Graefe[35] accepts the name of *cataracta nigra* for those cataracts in which pigment is found inside the capsule, which he considers as coming from the haematin which has passed through an uninjured capsule. Cases belonging to this class have also been described by Von Beck. Should it become an established fact that pigment does pass through the capsule, it certainly would be proper to call these *cataracta pigmentaire*, or *cataracta hemorrhagica*, rather than *cataracta nigra*. I can not understand how men can be such blind followers of Von Graefe as to persist in writing about the frequent occurrence of cataracts containing haematin."

Since it has been shown that the nucleus of a senile cataractous lens differs chemically from the simple sclerosis of old age, the cataracta nigra must be looked upon as a senile cataract, which, in consequence of the regularly progressing sclerosis up to the periphery, is not accompanied by the formation of splits and fissures, in the most peripheric cortical lamellae.

The most essential points in the senile sclerosis, as well as in the senescence of the lens are the following; the oldest fibres in the centre of the lens lose the serrations which they had attained during the growth of the entire

33 Remarques sur la Cataracte, Traduit de la Auglaisse par Lemoine, 1779, p. 501.
34 Epist., XIII, 13, 14. 1762.
35 Arch., I, p. 133.

organism, and with the steady increase in the index of refraction and the taking on of a more saturated yellow color, until finally an almost homogenous mass is formed, in which the individual elements are scarcely recognizable, or not at all; and, as age advances, this process slowly, but surely, extends toward the periphery. At the same time, the processes at the whorl and along the nuclear zone become less active and consist of but few elements containing nuclei. The epithelial cells become fat, and in many the chromatic substance and the nuclei are greatly reduced. The capsule becomes thicker and tougher. The farther this process extends, the more light will be absorbed, and the poorer will the vision be, where there is a moderate degree of illumination. This explains one of the causes for the reduction of vision in the aged."

"It may, however, happen that, even in very advanced age, not even an equatorial cloudiness may exist—gerontoxon lentis—and the individuals have good vision. Thus I have had the opportunity of examining the lens of a man ninety-four years of age, and on focal illumination found but a scarcely recognizable yellowish reflex; whereas, on opthalmoscopic examination, the lens was perfectly clear, and with a convex glass of 2 D on both eyes, $V = \frac{4}{13}$ to $\frac{4}{5}$.

"Then, again, there are people who see much more poorly at an earlier age—thus I have examined people who, as early as the fifties, could scarcely count fingers at one or two metres; without any cloudiness of the lens being discernable with the mirror; whereas, on focal illumination, there is a deep brownish-red reflex from the lens. Therefore, this remarkable difference in the conditions of the lens, noted during life, is due to the pathological sclerosis and saturated color of the nucleus in cataracta nigra.

I have examined anatomically two lenses extracted in their capsules, and sent to me by Dr. Mittelstadt and Dr. Marckwort, of Antwerp, the diagnosis being cataractae fere nigrae. Very fine microscopical sections, made with the microtome, show that the entire lens up to the capsule are regularly changed to nucleus. The whirl and nuclear zone consist of but few cells. On transverse sections only the nuclei appear on the inner surface of the capsule, the protoplasm of the cells being so greatly reduced. One finds no pictures of splits or fissures in the sections. It is especially worthy of note that there is not a trace of cortical substance between capsule and nucleus. The only difference between this lens and the senile lenses of the same age would be the sparse and frequently interrupted distribution of vesicular cells in the equatorial region. Teased preparations show nothing differing from that formed in normal lenses. There was no particular avidity to the stain.

About the same conditions were found in another lens received from Sammelsohn. In the equatorial region, however, were large nests of vesicular cells.

Therefore, cataracta nigra is a special variety of senile cataract, but differs from the ordinary senile lens of the same age in the pathological nuclear sclerosis, which, as we have seen in the underlying basis in the development of senile cataract. Hence, the same reasons likewise apply here, which lead us to consider senile cataract as a constitutional cataract.

CHAPTER X.

CATARACTA CAPSULARIS. CAPSULAR CATARACT.

As we have seen, capsular cataract is most frequently a sequelae of the over-ripe cataract. If we only waited long enough, we would find that to every lenticular cataract finally would be added a capsular cataract.

The variety generally observed by the oculist is seated at the anterior pole. In the non-complicated, over-ripe senile cataract, it usually acquires about the size of a medium-sized pupil. It then, as a rule, has sharply defined, jagged edges, and it is generally accepted that these jagged edges mark the line of insertion of the zonular fibres into the capsule. Frequently the capsule is folded in the portions which cover the capsular cataract, and in cases of pyramidal cataract, this frequently reaches the height of a millometre. These folds are a proof that this new-formed tissue has a tendency to shrink, and in this shrinkage is to be found the reason for the loosening of the connection between the capsule and its suspensory ligament, and this may lead to cases of spontaneous luxation of over-ripe cataracts. This also makes possible the operation where the lens is extracted in its capsule.

There are many exceptions to the restriction of the capsular cataract to the pupillary area. This is especially true of the consecutive cataracts, for it may extend over the entire inner surface of the anterior capsule, and may even extend over the posterior capsule. It is especially in these forms of capsular cataract that we so frequently find the calcareous deposits. The capsular cataract may remain unassociated with any other form of cataract for many years. When a capsular cataract develops in advanced age, the lenticular cataract will soon follow. The primary development of a capsular cataract is the purest example of what might be technically designated as an inflammation of the lens, (or hyperplasia of epithelial cells), a true phakitis; but where this occurs, the eye is otherwise diseased, even though its exact nature be indefinite. The mere presence of a primary capsular cataract should arouse our suspicions of other complications. If Leber's theory is correct, that these epithelial cells have the function of giving the nutritive fluids their specific chemical constitution, it certainly must be evident that a diseased epithelium must of necessity finally be followed by a lenticular cataract, and likewise it must not be forgotten that a diseased nutritive material (aqueous or vitreous) can stimulate the capsular cells to proliferation.

True capsular cataract does not only occur congenitally as an anterior polar cataract, but it may be acquired primarily at any age of life.

CHAPTER XI.

TRAUMATIC CATARACT. CATARACTA TRAUMATICA.

Mechanical disturbances may lead to an injury of the lens, and thus secondarily lead to the development of traumatic cataract. This may be due to the action of a blunt force, as a concussion, or as the result of a puncture, accidentally; or of an incision, intentionally produced, as where discission is practiced.

A.

CATARACTA EX CONTUSIONE. Here, as a rule, the capsule of the lens is ruptured, and the lens becomes cloudy, in consequence of coming in contact with the fluid media of the eye. In exceptional cases the lens substance becomes cloudy, even when the capsule has not been ruptured. Thus Arlt[1] states, "though we do not as yet possess any reliable reports of cases in which a concussion of the eyeball, in which neither a rupture of the capsule nor a simple tearing of the capsule has taken place, lead to a cloudiness of the lens; still, as a rule, we must acknowledge the possibility of its occurrence." The truth of this statement seems to be proven by the fact, that Berlin[2] produced a cloudiness of the anterior cortical substance by gently tapping the eyes of rabbits with an elastic rod.

Becker reports the following case, in which, as the result of a concussion of the eyeball, without a tearing of either the zonula or capsule, cloudiness of the lens followed:

During the winter of 1870-72, a policeman, stationed at the railway tunnel running under the Heidelberger Schloss, while engaged in removing large icicles which had formed at the entrance of the tunnel, was struck by one of these in his right eye. The pain was not very severe, but vision at once became cloudy. Several days later he presentd himself at the clinic, and vision was found to equal $\frac{18}{8}$. There was no sign of an external injury, luxation or tear of the capsule, but we found a rupture of the choroid. This latter was quite centrally located, but not very large. From time to time he presented himself at the clinic, so that we had the opportunity of carefully observing the gradual development, from the third week on, of an anterior polar cortical cataract,

---

[1] Uber die Verletzungen des Auges in Gerichtsartzlicher Beziegung, l. c., p. 296.

[2] Zur Sogen Commotio Retinae. Monatsblatt, 1873, p. 47.

which assumed the same form as a posterior cortical cataract, after an injury of the periphery of the lens. After it had developed to about one-half the size of a medium dilated pupil it became stationary. After a year the railway company gave him an easier position, so that he passed from observation.

Whenever a unilateral cataract is met with an indefinite time after a contusion of the eye, one should not forget that the cataract may be the result of an injury to the eye other than a lesion of the capsule or zonula. It is only of too frequent occurrence that months pass before the lens becomes cloudy, and then the cataract is to be looked upon as consecutive. However, there must not always be a rupture of the choroid; hemorrhage into the vitreous, with secondary detachment of the retina; but a consecutive cataract may develop, when the only demonstratable sign is a paralysis of the ciliary body, together with an apparent myopia. Hence, great care should be practiced in making a prognosis, even in apparently slight contusions of the eyeball, and this should be especially remembered as a point in medical jurisprudence.

Ruptures of the capsule, independent of a tear in the coats of the eyeball or of the zonula, have been but rarely reported. Isolated cases of tearing of the posterior capsule have been reported by Knapp and Aub.[3]

John R., aged 20 years, the son of a farmer living at Kuhbergershof, while chopping branches from a tree, was struck in the eye by a twig. Vision at once was impaired, without any visible sign of injury. Two weeks later, since vision did not improve, he was brought to the clinic. It was impossible to detect the slightest trace of an injury, either in the lids, conjunctiva or cornea. The conjunctiva bulbae was pale, and there was absolutely no ciliary injection present. Cloudy lens substance was being extended through the narrow pupil into the anterior chamber. Tension was normal. Field of vision intact, and he could count fingers at one foot. He had no pain; there was no irritability to light, no increased secretion of tears. On use of atropine the pupil dilated and disclosed no synechia. Though the patient was repeatedly examined later on, and notwithstanding every possible effort, no trace of an injury, more especially of the cornea, could be detected. And since on dilating the pupil a change of position of the lens system could be absolutely excluded, hence the diagnosis of a simple rupture of the capsule of the lens as the result of a contusion was justified. The progress of the case was an exceptionally favorable one, and the lens was totally resorbed without the occurrence of any complications.

B.

Frequently a simultaneous luxation takes place—that is, a *tearing of the zonula zinii and a rupture of the capsule*. All these cases, in which one is able to demonstrate a subluxation of the lens, and to which already in

---

3 Arch. fur Augen und Ohren, I, 1, p. 20 and II, 1, p. 256.

the first few days, a cloudiness of the lens is added; belong to this class. In most of these cases the lesion in the capsule is in the equatorial region between the insertion of the zonula and its anterior and posterior attachments. All clinical observations show that the cloudiness begins in the equatorial region.

C.

INJURIES CAUSED BY CUTTING OR POINTED INSTRUMENTS NEVER affect the lens alone. The symptoms, the course and prognosis depend entirely on the size of the capsular wound, the depth to which the instrument penetrates the lens, the kind and extent of the injury, which at the same time affects other parts of the eye, and also as to whether the body which causes the injury remains partially or entirely within the eye. Should the body which causes the injury only penetrate the cornea and the lens, and do no other injury, we will have a condition to deal with similar to a *discissio per corneam.* If the corneal wound is a large one, some of the lens substance may be extruded, and hence the absorption hastened, but just such wounds later on materially interfere with vision.

If, besides cornea and lens, other portions of the eye are involved—the iris, the sclera, and *corpus ciliare,* the vitreous, etc.—the prognosis largely depends on the extent of the injuries. Penetrating wounds which at first appear trivial, owing to infection, may become the most serious.

Where the foreign body penetrates through the periphery of the cornea and the ciliary portion of the iris into the lens, so that the lens is struck near the equator, it very curiously indeed happens that, aside from the cloudiness in the neighborhood of the point of entrance, the posterior cortical substance is clouded earlier than anywhere else. On dilating the pupil, it is possible to follow the entire course of the penetrating instrument through the lens, and the same cloudy lens star develops. If the wound is not large it may close again, and the opacity remain restricted to the posterior cortical substance, or eventually clear up again.[4] If small foreign bodies enter the lens, they may either still stick fast in the cornea by the other end, penetrate the iris or extend into the pupil and anterior chamber, and be recognized by the naked eye; or they may be entirely enclosed in the lens capsule; or, finally, they may pass through the lens and be found sticking fast in the posterior wall of the eye, or be found lying free in the vitreous. As long as the lens remains transparent, one can get a view of these foreign bodies by means of the opthalmoscope.

The diagnosis is easy, where it is possible to see the foreign body in

---

[4] Vergl die Berichte der Wiener Clinic. p. 87 and No. 76.

the cornea or iris alone, or in both, and penetrating the lens. That the lens is involved becomes evident, owing to the more or less diffuse cloudiness which in such cases is never wanting. It is more difficult at times to demonstrate the presence of a foreign body which is entirely enclosed in lens substance, especially when the lens has secondarily become totally cloudy. It then depends entirely on the color of the foreign body whether or not one can still see it. However, it is not necessary, nor does it always occur, that the entire lens becomes cloudy. One then sees, either in the anterior cortical substance a circumscribed white cloudiness, with its corresponding capsular wound; or, if the cloudiness lies deeper, we see between it and the capsule a linear cloudy path which indicates the course of the foreign body. If the reports of some authors are to be believed, we can at times recognize the foreign body.

Many observers attest the fact, that the capsule may close again after the entrance of a small foreign body, and this be retained in the lens. Especially where the wound is in the region of the iris, this may form a primary object of closure. When the wounds are in the centre of the pupil, the iris can be of no assistance, and still it is possible for the wound to heal without any lens substance ever having been extruded—*a true sanatio per primam intentionem*. More frequently, the wound only heals after a flake of greater or less size has been extruded and been absorbed. In the vicinity of the wound the capsule is always folded.

Becker states that, from his own experience, he knows that grains of powder may become encapsulated in the lens without causing a total cloudiness of the lens. This, however, is the exception; the rule being that foreign bodies will lead to a complete cloudiness, even where the cloudiness remained partial for a long time. This condition seems to be analogous to the congenital partial cataracts. Hence one must not be astonished if, after an extraction, one finds that the cataract which we considered as an ordinary senile cataract, should be found to contain a foreign body. Workers in metals, who are so accustomed to have particles of metal fly into their eyes, overlook the entrance of such a foreign body into the lens, since the aqueous is not necessarily evacuated, and the reaction must not necessarily be any greater than when a particle is imbedded in the cornea. If now the lens should cloud up but slightly, and in fact, very slowly, the occurrence of the injury will in all probability be forgotten before the disturbance of vision is noticed.

One most frequently observes the retention of a foreign body where it is very small and not too heavy. In these cases, most probably, the sclerosed nucleus holds the foreign body fast. The case of Parnard, in which he was enabled to see, and later extract, a grain of shot out of the lens,[5] deserves to be classed as a great curiosity.

It occurs much more frequently, that the foreign body which penetrates, passes through the lens. Even in such cases, the openings in both capsules may close again. This occurs most frequently when both point of entrance and of exit are in the periphery of the lens, the healing of the anterior capsule being again aided by the iris. The posterior wound, however, is under more favorable conditions, since the vitreous has less tendency to dissolve the lens fibres.

Where the penetrating body is of considerable size, or where by chance the capsular wound happens to be a large one, the lens becomes cloudy in proportion to the area which comes in contact with the fluid media of the eye; and it depends largely on the amount of general injury which the eye has received whether the lens will be partially or totally resorbed, and whether the eye will be destroyed by iridocyclitis, choroiditis or panopthalmitis.

No case has been observed where, following the entrance of a foreign body into the lens, and its remaining in situ, or after its passage through the lens, the lens either spontaneously cleared up again, or remained entirely transparent from the beginning. Hence the cases reported by Desmarres fils [6] can only be looked upon with doubt, as to their correct observation.

Opening of the capsule, in consequence of a perforating corneal ulcer, is likewise to be looked upon as an injury of the lens. The sequelae, as far as the lens is concerned, depend on how much of its substance is lost, or is later on absorbed by the aqueous. Sometimes the shrunken lens remains adherent to the cornea and iris, owing to new-formed cicatrical tissue; again, it returns, in a greater or less degree, to its normal position. Aside from the fact that the lens, together with its capsule, may entirely leave the eye, at times the only remains is a *cataracta secundaria*.

The appearance of a traumatic cataract is that of a soft cortical cataract. The rapidity with which the lens becomes cloudy depends on the extent of the injury and the age of the individual. Since young people are more exposed to such injuries than older, hence in this we find a further reason why the traumatic cataract as a rule is soft. The chemical constitution of the foreign body will affect the color of the cataract, and whenever the well-known color is wanting the suspicion of a foreign body in the lens ought to be aroused.

---

5 Annal d'Oculistic. 43, 23.

6 Le cons Cliniques sur la Chirurgie Oculaire, p. 96.

It is a well-known fact, that traumatic cataract is a perfectly passive change in the lens substance. Immediately upon injury of its capsule, the lens substance comes in direct contact with the aqueous, and as a result the lens becomes cloudy and swells up. As has already been pointed out, in studying capsular cicatrices, page 90, if the opening is very minute, this is soon plugged up by a thin fibrinous covering, and in the course of a few days a cicatrix covers the wound. But where the injury of the capsule has been more severe, the edges retract, curl up outwardly, and the aqueous comes in direct contact with the lens substance. Those portions of the lens which have exuded are gradually resorbed and disappear, while new flakes continue to well forth from the capsular wound. At the same time, due to the taking up of water, the lens continues to swell up and the cloudiness to increase, until in the course of a few days or weeks, the entire lens may become opaque.

But not alone to the aqueous is due the resorption of the lens fibres. In the disintegrating masses of lens substance and around the zone of resorption of larger pieces of lens fibres, one finds numbers of lymphoid cells which take on the most manifold changes in form. These cells contain two nuclei and a dark, granular protoplasm, which might be looked upon as fat granules. These cells and their relation to the resorption of traumatic cataract, are better understood today, as the result of Boe's experimental investigations; and he looked upon them as derived from lymphoid cells. Boe also drew attention to numerous cells containing myelin drops, which subsequently assumed such size as to restrict the protoplasm of the cell to a narrow zone around the myelin drop and pressed the nucleus against the cell wall. Kostenitisch [7] likewise observed the presence of lymphoid cells in the masses of lens substance, and so illustrated them. In a recent work by Wagenman,[8] the presence of these cells, also of giant cells, and their relation to the absorption of traumatic cataract is made the subject of special study. He states, "repeatedly have I found that giant cells stand in very close relation to the absorption of lens fibres, and more especially in this case, in traumatic cataract." In all the cases which he studied he found giant and lymphoid cells. These cells not only contained albuminous and myelin drops, but pieces of lens fibres and quantities of lens substance undergoing all degrees of metamorphosis. He states, that the change within this cell is undoubtedly due to the digestive power of the protoplasm. "This power of bringing about retrogressive changes in the lens substance

[7] Path. Anat. Untersuchungen uber die Zunthutchen Verletzungen des Menschlichen Auges. Graefe Arch., Vol. XXXVII, 4.

[8] Einiges uber Fremdkorper Riesen Zellen im Auge. Graefe Arch., Vol. XLII, Part 2.

or its derivatives taken up by the cells, is especially marked in the giant cells, in which one can find, side by side, the most varied products of disintegration of lens substance, intact, and myelin globules undergoing granular degeneration, hyaline drops, etc.

He assumes that these giant cells possess the power of exerting a catalytic action on the hard lens substance, dissolving and absorbing it, and he ascribes this same power to the smaller cells.

One of his cases is of exceptional interest, because it throws a good deal of light on a subject which has long been in dispute, namely, whether wandering cells could pass through an uninjured capsule.

Case of spontaneous resorption of a luxuated cataract in an eye suffering from chronic irido choroiditis.

"In the lower segment of the globe posterior to the ciliary body, the lens is in such a position that its former lower edge touches the wall of the globe and the lens is directed obliquely backward, with its former anterior surface looking upward. The lower edge of the lens appears to be fixed by new connective tissue, and in the region of the orra serrata it is partially calcareous. and beneath the folded anterior capsule is an old capsular cataract.

"The capsule of the lens discloses numerous interspaces, and in some places splits, due to the action of the lymphoid cells, even in the region of the capsular cataract, defects are found in the capsule. Within the capsular sac are groups of lymphoid cells, especially between the capsular cataract and the body of the lens; likewise, between the posterior capsule and the lens. Over large areas the body of the lens is clothed with a layer of large tumescent, single or multi-nuclear cells, containing an opaque protoplasm, and besides these all stages of lymphoid cells occur.

"Everywhere the cataract has the appearance as though it had been "gnawed at." Cells have worked their way in between the sclerosed fibres and have separated them. Everywhere the cataract is being absorbed. Giant cells are also found, which are closely applied to the side of the fibres. It appears as though the processes of the cells were forcing their way in between the fibres. These giant cells contain a uniform granular protoplasm, and differ from the other cases in that no pieces of lens fibre or myelin drops could be found."

Here the capsule of the lens disclosed numerous perforations, due to the *histolytic action* of the cells. The giant cells possess this same histolytic power of dissolving substances chemically resistant and difficult of assimilation, such as the hyaline membranes. This action on the capsule is catalytic, ("fernwirkung"), and finds its analogue in the action of the lymphoid cells in inflammatory processes, and in the action of osteoclasts in the resorption of bone."

Leber [9] has experimentally shown that the lens reacts but slightly to

[9] Enstehung der Entzundung, p. 254, etc.

the presence of foreign bodies. Where pieces of sterilized copper wire were passed through the lens in an axial direction, the centre of the lens remained perfectly clear, only at the points of entrance and exit in the cortical substance did any swelling and cloudiness take place.

In course of time, as was to be expected, the cloudiness went on to the formation of striae in the anterior corticalis, but the greater part of the lens remained perfectly clear. After a time the lens took on a dirty yellow color. Forlanini [10] showed that at times splinters of wood remained as long as ten days in the lens without producing more than a circumscript cloudiness at the point of entrance. In considering the action of foreign bodies of iron and steel in the crystalline lens, Leber (cited p. 96) states, "It is a well-known fact, that splinters of iron and steel imbedded in the lens may remain permanently, without doing any damage to the eye. The never-failing cloudiness of the lens, in and of itself, is not to be looked upon as the result of the action of the foreign body. But even in these cases, after a time the metal undergoes a partial dissolution, and later a kind of diffusion for a certain distance beyond the foreign body, and thus gives the cataract a rusty yellow color. Von Graefe, in his clinical lectures, often said that the coloring of the lens is so characteristic, that it is certainly pathognomonic of the presence of an iron splinter, where this can not be directly seen or demonstrated. The color is due to the deposit of the most minute granules of the hydrated oxide of iron, as is shown by the fact, that when they are acted on by nitric acid and ferrocyanide of potassium, they give a blue color. This has been repeatedly demonstrated on freshly extracted lenses which contained splinters of iron. Macroscopically, the lens has a peculiar olive-brown color, since the color is diffused for a certain distance beyond the foreign body, the iron must be diffused in the form of the acid carbonate of iron, and this, by further oxidation, is precipitated as the hydrated oxide of iron.

D.

SECONDARY CATARACT. (Intentional injuries). A necessary condition for the formation of a secondary cataract must always be a partial or total retention of the capsule of the lens within the eye after an extraction. Only where the ideal operation is done and the lens is extracted in its capsule, is this formation avoided. Where the lens substance which remains after an extraction and the capsular epithelium alone are involved, we designate the new formation as a *cataracta secundaria simplex*; but where neighboring tissues—as iris, corpus ciliare, and vitreous—are in-

[10] Annal di Opthal., I, p. 145. 1871.

volved, or abnormal adhesions are found, we speak of a *cataracta secundaria accreta, cataracta complicata.*

This condition may develop after a total resorption of the lens substance subsequent to an injury accidentally or intentionally produced, as the result of operative interference when a discission is made or, as is more frequently the case, after an extraction.

Immediately after incision of the capsule and extraction of the lens, owing to the pressure of the vitreous the curvature of the posterior capsule is reversed, its convexity now facing anteriorly. The triangular flaps in the capsule produced by the cystitome are everted outwardly, so that all around the periphery, the capsule is intact; whereas, in its central position there is a defect, the anterior surface of the posterior capsule coming in contact with the aqueous. After the anterior chamber is again restored, the capsule is pressed backward again, so that the posterior capsule is almost perfectly straight and the edges where the anterior capsule is everted come in contact with the posterior, and thus, if we may so express it, a circular pocket is formed all around the periphery, and, as a rule, this pocket contains lens substance which has remained behind after the operation, and the products of new cellular formation originating from the epithelial cells which line the capsule. This formation has been designated, *Sommering's crystalline pearl* (or wulst). Owing to the changed conditions of pressure, these new-formed cells assume a great variety of forms; in fact, all of those already described, the large vesicular cells, Wedl's cells, irregularly developed cells, with protuberances to the one side, etc. This cellular proliferation does not only take place between the leaves of the capsule, but at the edge of the crystalline pearl one finds a hyperplasia of the capsular epithelium going over onto the anterior surface of the posterior capsule. Here they no longer have the shape of the normal epithelial cells, but are more like flat pavement epithelial cells, which likewise undergo a hyperplasia. These cells, after a certain length of time, secrete a vitreous or hyaline-like substance, which forms a covering for these cells and the posterior capsule. It is the product of this hyperplasia of epithelial cells which gradually causes the interference with vision subsequent to a cataract operation. Just exactly what it is that leads to this regeneration it is difficult to state, but undoubtedly the cells possess a tendency to regeneration which is incited by the operation and the changed relations of tension and pressure.

In all these cases one finds the pupillary area occupied by a very delicate greyish, almost transparent, film, discernible on oblique illumination, and which permits of a red reflex from the fundus. All gradations are met with, from this delicate, scarcely visible, greyish film, up to the dense white membranous cataract.

"It not infrequently occurs that the result of a successful operation is reduced by the retention of cataractous masses within the capsular sac. This is especially apt to occur when an unripe cataract is operated, but does occur, even in the ripe. If the opening in the anterior capsule is sufficiently large, the masses which remain swell up and are resorbed. In this case the pupil finally becomes pure black. But where the leaves of the capsule are rapidly closed and the retained masses are cut off from the aqueous, these are not resorbed, but remain behind, forming a white membranous cloudiness, (*cataracta secundaria*). If a portion of the pupil remains free, sight may be good. But if the entire pupil is involved, vision is reduced, depending on the density of the cloudiness. At times the secondary cataract forms later on, as a result of hyperplasia of the epithelium of the anterior capsule." [11]

11 Fuchs Lehrbuch der Augenheilkunde, 1891, p. 763.

PART IV.

THE THERAPY OF THE DISEASES OF THE LENS SYSTEM.

At the present day the therapy of cloudiness of the lens is confined entirely to operative procedure. True, we might consider proplylactic measures—but even these must remain restricted to certain special varieties, such as traumatic cataracts.

CHAPTER I.

MEDICINAL TREATMENT.

"From the earliest times, have not only the most manifold suggestions been offered to bring about, by medicinal treatment, the disappearance of a beginning cloudiness of the lens in cases of partial, and even total, cataracts, but frequently those have come forward who claim good results from such efforts. But I will spare myself and the reader the trouble of enumerating all those things, which have been tried and reported as worthy of a trial, for this would necessitate my beginning with the 'honey and saffron, cooked in the bile of hyenas,' of Plinius (XXVIII., 8), and mentioning all the remedies down to dilute phosphoric acid, which but a few months ago (1876) was praised in many political, and even scientific, papers, both in France and Germany, as a universal remedy for grey cataract; and could thus fill pages with the recitation of such unproven things." More recently, one reads of the beneficial effects of electricity, the mysterious agent to which so many turn when everything else fails. If it is possible anywhere, it is certainly demonstrated here, that unless we possess a perfect knowledge of the causation, no successful therapy can ever be evolved. Hence, all therapeutic attempts rest on the purest empiricism.

"If any one is interested in this subject, and has a desire to look up all these suggestions in detail, he will find all the old literature on the subject collected and made use of in Rosa's 'Handbuch der Heilkunde, 1830, II, p. 710,' and in Himly's 'Die Krankheiten und Missbildungen, etc., II, p. 247;' The latest literature can be found in the bibliography annexed."

Although up to the present time we have not attained any results, we must not entirely set aside the possibility that the time may come, when it will become possible to arrest further development of a beginning cataract, or even clear up an opacity which has already developed. The experiments of Kunde (828) and Kuhnhorn (843) have demonstrated that the lenses of animals which have been made cloudy by drawing out their water can again be cleared up, by simply laying them in water. At this point, I would once more draw attention to the facts recorded in the earlier parts of this work regarding the chemical constitution of the senile non-cataractous lens and the cataractous lens of the same age of life, and that the nucleus of a senile cataract has a different constitution from the nucleus of a senile non-cataractous lens; also, to the wonderful and surprising conclusions to which these facts have led Becker. (See section on "Senile Cataract, on page 234.)

As is evident from a careful study of all that so far has been said, every variety of cataract which is not a congenital malformation or disease, or which is of traumatic origin, is either secondary to some disease, either local in the eye, or to some general disease of the entire organism. With a more complete knowledge of the causation of these latter forms of cataract, we may hope, by applying the proper treatment at the proper time, to prevent their occurrence, but I do not believe that we will ever succeed in causing a retrogression after the processes of cataract formation have once been started.

Eduard v. Yager, out of a large number of cases in which he made a diagnosis of clearing up of a cloudy lens, reports two in detail (p. 917). Both are cases of cortical cloudiness (one anterior and one posterior). The one occurred in a man 25 years of age, whom he had had under observation for four years; the other in a woman 42 years of age, who was under observation for twelve years; however, never, even where the senile change was of the most minute kind, did he see the cloudiness totally disappear.

If we are to designate every true cloudiness which occurs in the periphery of every senile lens as a *cataract incipiens*, I can not agree to the truth of this general proposition. Becker reports the following case: "For the past five years I have known a gentleman and a lady, in whose eyes as long ago as respectively twelve and fifteen years, the opthalmoscopic examination was made by men of reputation and ability; colleagues whose veracity is not doubted, and I hold their affidavits that at that time cataract was diagnosticated, and that the disease has not progressed since that time. But I also possess the most convincing proof in an observation, in which I myself made the diagnosis of cataract on both eyes of a lady, the wife of one of my colleagues, which have since totally disappeared again."

Stellway (p. 663) likewise seems to have frequently observed similar cases. He, however, does not attempt to explain them as true opacities, but considers them as *gerontoxon lentis* (Ammon). Relative to traumatic cataracts we possess the beautiful observations of V. Rydèl (1107), which have since been corroborated by the observations of others. An early closure of the point of entrance is favorable to such a clearing up. The isolated observations which V. Dietrich made, while making his well known experiments, also belong in the category.

Holscher [1] reports two cases where children at birth had cataract, and after the close of the second year these lenses commenced to clear up, beginning at the periphery. In the beginning in simple sectors, until finally they were entirely free of opacities. In the fifth year they had entirely cleared up inside of the capsule.

Under the title of "Spontaneous Cataract Cure," we find reported in literature a series of cases of spontaneous resorption and luxation. These are nearly all cases in which vision was lost, owing to the cataract, and had again been spontaneously restored; not, however, due to a retrogression of the processes of cataract formation. Here in a certain number of cases, without operative interference or trauma, a result was obtained, such as is purposely sought by operative interference. Some of the cases are worthy of being recorded.

The spontaneous resorption of a cataractous lens without an injury of the capsule. A man, 40 years of age, who subjected himself to a "starvation cure" for rheumatism and gout, became affected with soft cataract on both eyes, without suffering any pain or inflammatory symptoms. Without the intervention of any operative proceedure both cataracts were resorbed in the course of a few years, more quickly on the right than on the left eye, so that he was enabled to read without the use of glasses by holding large print closely. (Warnatz, 435.) (This was undoubtedly a cataracta Morgagni, with total resorption even of the nucleus.)

Cataract developed in both eyes of a woman 45 years of age. Setons were put on both arms and laxatives were administered at the same time, and at intervals cups were also applied. After a duration of five years the yellowish white cataract became more cloudy in both eyes; did not, however, become resorbed from the periphery to the center, but had a fractured and divided appearance, a starlike configuration, almost like the figures seen after a keratonyxis. Resorption progressed so rapidly that at the end of six months both pupils were pure black, and every cataractous discoloration of the lens had disappeared. This patient used spectacles. (Warnatz.) (Likewise a cataracta Morgagniani.)

To these cases, taken from the pre-opthalmoscopic literature, Becker adds the clinical report of a case kindly given to him by his friend, Dr. Brettauer, of Triest, which may serve to put these observations of Warnatz in their proper light, and serve to place the possibility of a lens being spontaneously resorbed within its capsule in its proper light.

March 20, 1862, Mr. Z., aged 35 years, came to me for treatment. On the right eye he had a ripe cataract, a milky white corticalis, presenting no special features. Beneath the capsule were a few white chalky nodules, about one-half the size of the head of a pin; and the nucleus could be differentiated. On the 26th of March the right eye was operated by a flap extraction downward, with-

---

[1] Walter and Ammon Journal, XXXII, p. 219.

out an iridectomie. Immediately after introduction of the cystotome the vitreous prolapsed. At the same moment the cataract disappeared out of the pupillary area. Whether the entire cataract was fluid, or whether the vitreous caused the nucleus to be dragged out of the eye, could not be determined, as the accident required my undivided attention. We hunted for the cataract on the bed and on the floor, but it could not be found. During the healing process blood filled the pupillary area for a long time, and the iris cicatrized in the wound. August 4th, with a $+ \frac{1}{5}$ the patient could read Yager No. 3, and with a $+ \frac{1}{6}$ the numbers of the houses across the street. The result was permanent, since with this one eye he was enabled to follow his occupation, that of a hat maker, and at the end of twelve years (March, 1874), with $+ \frac{1}{6}$ V $= \frac{10}{18}$. When he came again, in 1871, to have his glasses changed, Dr. Brettauer, who had not seen the patient since the operation, noticed a trembling and discoloration of the left iris, which was, however, round and reacted to light. In the center of the pupil was an irregular star-shaped membrane. This disclosed, on dilating the pupil, going out from the central-shaped membrane corresponding with the sectors of the lens; a gelatinous mass, hanging from which are an innumerable number of cholesterine crystals, resembling the golden tinsel on a Christmas tree. Between these various sectors of gelatinous substances, we can get a red reflex from the fundus by means of the opthalmoscope. (Becker saw this case in 1872.) March 2, 1874, this trembling of the iris had increased; the gelatinous mass as a whole had grown less, likewise the number of crystals. Downward and outward a sector of gelatinous substance seemed to lie anterior to the plane of the central membrane. Immediately posterior to the lens one could see a number of easily movable and quite large vitreous membranes, all in the anterior portion of the vitreous. The papilla was slightly hyperaemic, and on the outer side a small conus about one-sixth the diameter of the papilla. With $+ \frac{1}{6}$, vision equaled nearly $\frac{10}{18}$. The slightest change in the position of the glass impaired vision; hence, there is no sign of accommodation. How long vision has been improving on this eye Z. is not able to state. During the past two years this absorption and diminution of the crystals has materially decreased. Z. denies ever having received a trauma, and it is not possible to demonstrate, either on the cornea or iris nor on the capsule, a cicatrix, a tear or anything resembling it. Since the patient required on this eye a glass of the same strength as he did on the operated eye, there can be no doubt but that this is a case of *spontaneous resorption of a cataract where the capsule has not been ruptured.* (Brettauer.)

Gilson (p. 722) has reported a case where a congenital cataracta lactea was resorbed, as the result of a blow on the eye, which ruptured the capsule without causing any other injury to the coats of the eye.

Finally, all these cases belong to this class, in which, following a spontaneous sinking of the cataractous lens, vision is restored. Literature is full of the reports of such cases. The oldest reports are by St. Yves, and Janin reports two cases. One of these had a cataract from early youth. Siebold and

Himly (Opthal. Bibl., I, 187. 1801), in the reports of their cases, seem to have come to similar conclusions, in that pre-supposing that a subluxation had occurred, they gave the patient suffering from a "trembling cataract" the advice to take jumping exercises, in order to bring about a total luxation. Later on it became fashionable to apply electricity or to give large doses of strychnia, so as to bring on a separation of the lens from its connection as a result of muscular contraction.

Sperino attempted to clear up a beginning or even fully developed cataract by operative means, though not by a true cataract operation. After Hoquet, in 1729, and Les Col. de Villars, in 1740, had suggested that the attempt be made by means of repeated punctures of the anterior chamber to influence the development of cataract (the experiments of Dietrich also being here), Sperino took up his experiments in a more extensive manner, in that he did not restrict his experiments to cataract alone. His results were excellent. A woman who could no longer find her way about was so much improved by this method that she could read Yager No. 3 without spectacles, and vision was permanently improved. In forty other cataract cases vision was more or less improved. It is definitely recorded that the clearing up was determined by opthalmoscopic examination. These experiments were repeated, especially by Sperino's countrymen. Borelli,[2] in twenty-one cases, had little or no result. Torresini (ilid) even noticed a rapid increase in the cataractous cloudiness. Rivaud Landran reported a case without any results at the Congress held in Paris in 1863.[3] Since that time nothing further has been heard concerning Sperino's suggestions. I do not know whether this subject has received any further attention. Good results were certainly not attained, otherwise we would have heard of them. The great attention which the experiments of Sperino attracted is explained by the fact that the possibility of the nutrition of the lens being affected by the repeated punctures of the anterior chamber, could not a priori be denied. It can not be doubted but that by the repeated evacuation of the aqueous, the chemical formation of the same is altered. We know that by means of puncture of the anterior chamber in cases of traumatic cataract, and after discission, we can hasten the absorption of the swollen up lens substance. Aside from this, every time the anterior chamber is punctured, the lens changes its position, which does not take place without at the same time the lens changing its shape, and consequently the lamellae are pushed past each other. If it is correct that there are always, or at least often, a splitting up of the lens during cataract formation, hence such an abnormal change in the form of the lens, as occurs when the aqueous is evacuated, can not but influence the formation of a cataract. One should at least incline more to the opinion, as Torresini observed, that the cataract formation is hastened by the repeated punctures. This would be in accord with Snellen's verbal statement to me (Becker), that the making of a preliminary iridectomie will ripen an unripe cataract.

[2] Gionale d Ottalmologia Italiano, 1862.

[3] Comptes Rendus, 155. See the discussions in which Raymond, Desmares, Testelin, Borrell, Dor, Ricardo-Secondi Quaglino took part.

CHAPTER II.

THE OPERATIONS FOR CATARACT.

The true operations start out with an essentially different purpose. By their means the cloudiness of the lens is not expected to be cured, but rather the detrimental influence which such a cloudy lens exerts on vision is to be removed. Only exceptionally do we remove a cataractous lens in order that we may abate the disfigurement.

The object of all operative interference in primary cataract is to make it possible for a large amount of regularly refracted light to reach the retina. This can be attained by various methods. We can leave the cataractous lens in the eye, but remove it from the pupillary area, by pushing it to one side, or downward into the vitreous—*depressio, reclinatio, lentis.* We can remove the lens, by making a wound of sufficient size in the coats of the eye, cornea and sclera, and thus remove it at once from the eye— *extractio, suctio, lentis.* By opening the capsule we can bring the lens in direct contact with aqueous and vitreous, and thus bring about a resorption within the eye—*decissio per keratonyxim, et per scleronyxim.* Finally, we may permit the partially luxated or partially cloudy lens to remain without interfering with it, and by means of an artificial pupil, bring the light unimpeded to the retina—iridectomie in cases of cataract.

A.

DISLOCATIO CATARACTAE, DEPRESSION, RECLINATIO C. PER SCLEROTICONYXIM AUT PER KERATONYXIM ABAISSEMENT DE LA CATARACTE. COUCH-ING—SUBLATIO C., RELEVEMENT DE LA CATARACTE.

DEPRESSION.

Definition—Every operation which has for its object the removal of the lens from the pupillary area, and the sinking of it into the vitreous, by means of an instrument (a needle) ,which is pushed through the sclerotic or cornea, is designated by the words, *"depressio cataracta, reclinatio;"* "turning over of the cataract; *deplacement.* By means of the needle, pressure is either brought to bear on the lens from above, and so depressed exactly downward, (*depressio cataracta*—method of Celsius), or the needle is applied to the anterior surfac of the lens, and by this means the lens is turned over backward, so that its upper edge becomes its posterior, and its anterior surface its upper, (reclination according to Willburg, 1785—turning over of the cataract); or the needle is turned backward, outward and below, at the moment the lens is being turned over, so as to cause the anterior surface of the lens to face the *gabella frontis*. (Reclination according to Scarpa, 1801).

There are cases in which a spontaneous process occurs in cataractous eye, which may be looked upon as the prototype of depression, and which really lead to the artificial application of this procedure. These are the cases of spontaneous sinking of cataractous lenses which have already been considered.

From the most ancient times the point for the puncture has always been in the sclerotic, midway between the outer edge of the cornea and the outer canthus. This seemed to be such a self-evident procedure, that this method of puncture was never given a name (*scleronyxis*) until Buchhorn (1805) began recommending that the puncture for the depression be made through the cornea (keratonyxis from χέρας and νύττω punctio corneae). How the method of discission developed from this suggestion, I will explain more fully when we come to the subject of *keratonyxis cum depressione cataractae.*

THE DEPRESSIO CATARACTAE is the only method of which a complete and lucid description has been handed down to us from ancient times. This is found in Celsius (Lib. VII., c. VIII., 14). Owing to the extreme importance which this bears to the history of opthalmology, I will quote it here in full:

"Igitur vel ex ictu concresit humor sub duabis tunicis (κερατοειδή; et κορωειδής), qua locum vacuum esese proposui; isque paulatim indurescens interiori potentiae se opponit. Vitiique ejus plures sunt species; quaedam sanabiles, quaedam quae curationem non admittunt. Nam si exigua effusio est, si immobilis, colorem vero habet marinae aquae, vel ferri nitentis, et a latere sensum aliquem fulgoris relinquit, spes superest. Si magna est, si nigra pars oculi, amissa naturali figura, in aliam vertitur, si suffusioni color caeruleus est, aut auro similis, si labat, et hac atque illac movetur, vix unquam succurritur. Fere vero pejor est, quo ex graviore morbo majoribusve capitis doloribus, vel ictu vehementiore orta est. Neque idonea curationi senilis aetas est, quae sine novo vitio, tamen aciem hebetem habet: ac ne puerilis quidem; sed inter has media. Oculus quoque curationi neque exiguus, neque concavus, satis opportunus est. At que ipsius suffusionis quaedam maturitas est. Expectandum igitur est, donec jam non fluere, sed duritie quadam concrevisse videatur. Ante curationem autem modico cibo uti, bibere aquam triduo debet; pridie ab omnibus abstinere. Post haec in adverso sedili collocandus est loco lucido, lumine adverso sic, ut contra medicus paulo altius sedeat: a posteriore autem parte caput ejus minister contineat, ut immobile it praestet; nam levi motu eripi acies in perpetuum potest. Quin etiam ipse oculus immobilior faciendus est, super alterum lana imposita et deligata. Curari vero sinister oculus dextra manu, dexter sinister debet. Tum acus admovenda est acuta ut foret, sed non nimium tenuis; eaque demittenda recta est per summas duas tunicas medio loco inter oculi nigrum et augulum tempori propiorem, e regione mediae suffusionis sic, ne qua vena laedatur. Neque tamen timide demittenda est, quia inani loco excipitur. Ad quem quum ventum est, ne mediocriter quidem peritus falli potest; quia prementi nihil renititur. Ubi eo ventum est, inclinanda acus ad ipsam suffusionem est, leniterque ibi verti, et paulatim eam deducere infra regionem pupillae debet; ubi deinde eam transiit, vehementius imprimi, ut inferiori parti insidat. Si haesit, curatio expleta est: si subinde redit, eadem acu concidenda et in plures partes dissipanda est; quae singulae ea facilius conduntur, et minus late officiunt. Postea educenda recta acus est, imponendumque lana molli exceptum ovi album, et supra quod inflammationem coerceat, atque ita devinciendum. Post haec opus est quiete, abstinentia, lenium medicamentorum inunctionibus, cibo, qui postero die satis mature datur, primum liquido, ne maxillae laborent; deinde, inflammatione finita, tali, qualis in vulneribus propositus est. Quibus ut aqua quoque diutius bibatur, necessario accedit."

From the above one sees that even Celsius differentiated between the traumatic cataract and the one due to internal causes, and that he considered all cataracts not the result of trauma as due to some disease. He was even then of the opinion to which we are all now returning; namely, that all cataracts are secondary in their nature. He also recognized the importance which the color of the cataract bears to the prognosis. In that he separated the curable from the incurable. He acknowledged that there is hope of a cure when there is still perception of light. We meet with the expression "ripeness of the cataract," and also learn that a preparatory treatment was practiced, and that at the time of the operation, the patient was placed in a position similar to that customary up to a few years ago. (The patient in a low chair, the physician somewhat higher. Desmarres, 1252, p. 15.) An assistant held the head; the other eye was covered with a bandage, in order that the eye to be operated on might remain quiet. The doctor should be ambidextrous. After the operation the patient received only fluid nourishment, "net maxillae laborent." If we look at the very exact description of the operation, one really can not tell at what one shall be most astonished; that Celsius should have had such a complete understanding of the operation of depression, which up to a few years ago was so frequently made, or that this method should not have materially improved until after the discovery of the extraction, which robbed it of its supremacy and caused it to be almost entirely abandoned.

The only change from the methods of Celsius in ancient times, is confined to the instruments. Instead of the round-pointed needle of Celsius, we gradually came to use the myrtle-leaf-shaped needle of Brisseau. This change was first suggested by Gunz (1750) and was first carried out by Willburg (1785), and was the cause of the introduction of the name *reclination*. The lateral displacement of the lens (*depressio lateralis*, 1801) was first suggested by Bell and was first introduced into practice by Scarpa, and this was greatly facilitated by the use of a cataract needle, which was moderately curved on the flat at its point, and even today this needle bears Scarpa's name. The suggestion of Pauli, 1858, (450) is to be looked upon as an error—*sublatio cataracte, relevement de la cataracte.*

The words of Celsius may be interpreted to mean that the needle should be so introduced from the beginning, that the point, by being simply pushed forward, will reach the upper edge of lens. Later on, we diverged from this, in that the needle was introduced perpendicularly through the coats of the eye, and the attempt was made, by just touching the upper edge of the lens, to reach the posterior chamber. If by this means the certainty of depressing the lens was increased, the amount of damage to the interior of the eye must likewise have increased, owing to the movements of the needle. The methods of Willburg and Scarpa must likewise have led to more extensive destruction of the vitreous, than where the typical operation of Celsius was practiced. If, owing to the lens rising up again, they were compelled to break the lens into a number of pieces ("eadem acu concidende et in plures partes dissipanda, Celsius") the destruction of the vitreous could surely not have been less extensive, even where this method was practiced.

Since the time of Buchhorn's suggestion, *depressio per corneam* has also been practiced, (depressio per corneam, per keratonyxim). It appears however, that this method is of earlier date. For it is said, that among nations which are somewhat removed from our civilization (as, for instance, in Roumania) skilled women who are not physicians, even today, practice this method (*depressio per corneam*) by means of thorns of the Lycium Europaeum which have been hardened by fire. Who will fail calling to mind the fable of the goats?

Tradition tells us that the ancients ascribed the discovery of reclination to observations which were made on goats. It is really worth while stopping and critically examining this story.

Plinius[1] tells: "Oculos subfusos capra iunci puncto sanguine exonerat, caper rubi." It is not difficult to form an idea how the sentence came to be written. No doubt goats were observed which had wounded themselves with a thorn, and they must have had a subconjunctival hemorrhage, and at the same time a *suffusio*; therefore, a cloudiness in the pupil, which might either have been a true cataract, or an occlusion of the pupil, or possibly a hypopyon. The traumatic cataract must consequently have been the result of the injury by means of the thorn, and not an injury of the eye by means of the thorn, purposely

---

[1] Ed. Sittig, VIII, 201, p. 131.

produced in order to remove a cataract. Plinius even goes so far as to imagine that the animal had purposely caused a local bloodletting, in order to relieve itself of the eye disease. Plinius, however, says nothing regarding the cure of cataract.

In the "Introductio seu medicus," which is ascribed to Galen, we find, in Chapter 1, the following interesting statements (Ed. Kuhn tom XIV., p. 675): "Quaedam dicuntur ex casu abservata fuisse, ut suffusos pungere, inde quod capra quaepiam ex suffusione male habens, junco aculeato in oculum impacto, visum receperit." Here a cataract operation is spoken of, and since we do not possess any positive evidence that any operation other than depression was known during the time of Galen, hence we may apply these remarks directly to the operation of reclination. It is perfectly natural that such an operation should have been made, and by this means the reasons on which the operation of discission is based were finally arrived at. It must certainly strike every one as a curious fact, that the ancients who displayed such great talent in making observations, and who had every opportunity of observing the frequently occurring cases of traumatic cataract, should not have come upon the idea of purposely bringing about the process of spontaneous resorption as it occurs in traumatic cataract. However, this is easily explained if we will call to mind, that in most of the cases of cataract in which reclination was practiced, the cataract only became partially resorbed, and in many cases of reclination vision was restored only after the remains of the lens which occupied the pupillary area were gradually resorbed, and that frequently, instead of making a reclination, in reality a discission was made. (See Celsius.)

I can not refrain from again most particularly drawing attention to the fact, that this book is only ascribed to Galen; the period when it was written is not fixed. I also desire to quote a passage from Aelian,[2] which has been translated by Schneider: "Caliginem oculorum, quam suffusionem medici vocant, caprinum pecus probe curare scit; et ab ipsa remedium ejusdem homines quoque mutati dicuntur, idque hujusmodi est. Cum conturbatum oculum sentit, eam ad rubi spinam et admovet, et reserandam permittit; haes ut pupugit, pituita statim evocatur, nullaque pupillae laesione facta, vivendi usum recuperat; neque sane hominnum sapientia adfaciendam sibi medicinam eget." This shows that the fable has been perfected pretty well.

According to Scott,[3] the Brahmids of East India depressed the cataract by means of a small cotton tipped probe, which is inserted through an opening in the sclera, after a considerable amount of the vitreous had been evacuated.

---

[2] De Natura Animalium, Lib. VII, Cap. 14. Ed. Schneider. Leipsig, 1784, p. 230.

[3] Journal of Sciences and Arts. London, 1816. No. 3, pl. II, A. B., and Himly's Krankheiten und Missbildungen, Bd. II, p. 297.

According to Engel [4] the same procedure is successfully practiced in Turkey, the Moldau and Wallachei of Laien (Stellwag, l. c. 1, p. 771). The reports deserve to be recorded here, not only because, as Stellwag has pointed out, they teach us how much an eye can withstand without being totally destroyed, but because they teach us that in every country the autochthon cataract operation was the *depressio cataractae* in some modified form.

B.

EXTRACTIO CATARACTAE.

(PER KERATOTOMIAM AUT PER SCLEROTOTOMIAM).

"Extraction" was the expression used to designate every operative method, by means of which a lens of normal size, shrunken, transparent or opaque, with or without its capsule, was entirely or partially removed from the eye through an incised or thrust wound through the outer coats of the eye, (cornea and sclera) and through the (anterior or posterior) capsule, proportionate to the size and consistence of the crystalline body or portion of the same to be removed. According to the position of the incision, the differentiation was established between a corneal, a scleral, and a corneoscleral extraction, and depending on the form of the incision, as a flap, semicircular (Bogen) and linear extraction.

"As a rule, extraction is only practiced where we desire to remove a cataractous lens from the eye. In more recent times we have extracted perfectly clear lenses where particular indications presented themselves, as where sympathetic opthalmia of the second eye had set in (obsolete), or where we desire to reach a cysticercus in the vitreous, or behind the retina. And finally it has been suggested that we remove a normal lens to overcome a high degree of myopia, (Donders, l. c., p. 351). (Fukula.[4a])

To make an extraction by means of an incision behind the ciliary body, as was suggested and often practiced by Freitag, Bell, Butter, Earlie (263), Quadli, Loebenstein-Loebell and Ritterich, has been entirely abandoned, so that I need pay no further attention to this procedure. However, in the last few years (1876) this scleral incision has again come into vogue, in removing foreign bodies from the vitreous, also subretinal cysticercii; hence, this scleral incision is at least worthy of being mentioned at this place.[5] It is not at all improbable that the operation of extraction was known to the ancients. The passage quoted from Plinius (l. c., XXIX, 1, 8) to sustain this assertion, reads as follows:

"Ne avaritiam quidem arguam, rapacesque nundinas pendentibus fatis, et dolorum indicaturam, ac mortio arrham, aut arcana praecepta. Squamam in oculis emovendam potius quam extrahendam: per quae effectum est, ut nihil

---

[4] Gaz. Med. de Paris, 1840.

[4a] Operative Behandlung hochstgradiger Myopie durch Aphakie. Graefe's Arch., Vol. XXXVI. 2 P., p. 230. 1890.

[5] See O. Becker, in Mauther's Opthalmoskopie, p. 467-468.

magis prodesse videretur, quam multitudo grassantium. Neque enim pudor, sed aemuli pretia summittunt." But there is nothing to show that the word "squama," as used by the ancients, was used to designate a cataract (S. Hirsch., p. 285). Then Galen would be the first in whose works I find the extraction mentioned. In "Methodi Medendi, LXIV, c. 13, Ed. Kuhn. Tom. X, p. 986," is written: "Ἔμπαλιν δ' ὡς ἐπὶ τῶν ὑποχυμάτων ἀποπίπτοντες τοῦ πρώτου σκοποῦ· πρὸς ἕτερον ἄγομεν αὐτὰ τόπον ἀκυρότερον. Ἔνιοι δὲ καὶ ταῦτα κενοῖν ἐπεχείρησαν, ὡς ἐν τοῖς χειρουργουμένοις ἐρῶ."

"The extraction is again mentioned in the Continens of Rhazes, who lived in the ninth century. In the Venetian edition of 1506 (Lib. II, Fol. 3. B. 40), we find in 'Latyrion dixit cum chirurgicus vult extrahere cataractam ferro debemus tenere instrumentum super cataractam per magnam horam in loco ubi ponitur illud,' and at another place far from this one we find: 'Dixit Antilus et aliqui opererunt sub pupilla, et extraxerunt cataractam et potest esse cum cataracta est subtilius: et cum est grossa, non potuet extrahi, qui humor egrederetur cum ea.' Both of these passages, since their discovery by Albrecht von Haller, have been quoted in all text-books, and have given rise to a great many false conceptions, in that they have led us to arbitrarily place the time of Latryion's life in the first century after Christ; whereas, the text simply states that he must have lived before the ninth century, and we have likewise brought Latrylon in personal relationship with Antilus, who lived in the third or the beginning of the fourth century." (Hirsch.)

In the eleventh century, it is Avicenna [6] who again takes up the subject of extraction. "There are various instrumental methods of treating cataract, thus there is one in which we sever the lower portion of the cornea, and then pull out the cataract; but this is dangerous, for with the cataract, if it is thick, (agua quado est grossa), the vitreous also escapes." It is worthy of note, and Hirsch drew attention to it, that there is not a single passage extant, which could prove to us that any one of the well-known ancient physicians ever really made an extraction. All reports, taken from that time forward, and on which any reliance can be placed, simply go to show, that the cases which they report are simply hearsay, and others coming after them, have simply quoted their writings.

Avenzor, who lived in the twelfth century, mentioned the extraction, but declares that it is a simple impossibility. He writes (Lib. I, Tract 8, Cap. 19, Fol. 149): "The cataract must not be pulled out until it is fully ripe; if removed sooner it will return, . And when I say pulled out (extrahere), I desire you to understand that this is not possible, as so many believe, but that I push the cataract down into the depths of the eye by means of a needle, and when I have done this I draw the needle out again."

All other evidence of ancient times and the middle ages is not relevant to the operation of extraction. From the time of Avenzor until the close of the seventeenth century, all writers are so completely silent on this subject that we must come to the conclusion that it had fallen entirely into oblivion. Hence,

---

[6] Ed. Venetio, 1544, Fol. 237, Buch 3, Fen. 3, Tract 4, Cap. 20.

we are placed in a position where we can follow closely, even in its preparatory stages, the discovery of the corneal extraction by Daviel. In his dissertation (De Cataracta Argentorum), which appeared in 1721, Henricus Freitag tells us, that in 1694 his father, John Conrad Freitag, removed through the sclerotic, by means of a hook-shaped needle, two cataracts which had again "risen up" after reclination. According to the statements of Albini, in Goskey's dissertation (15), about this time, in 1695, men traveled from place to place (cataract cutters—staarstecher) who practiced extraction through the cornea. Gosky described an instrument something like a pair of forceps, which was used to extract the grey cataract. He gives an illustration of this instrument in his dissertation.

These facts were unknown to the French, to whom we are really indebted for the method of extraction. At the same time that Brisseau made his discovery as to the seat of cataract, St. Yves (1707), Du Petit (1708) and Duddell (1729), extracted, per corneal incision, cataracts which had fallen into the anterior chamber during reclination.

In 1745 Jacques Daviel found himself called upon to practice this same procedure which Petit had practiced, being compelled to remove, per corneal incision, a cataract which had fallen into the anterior chamber while making a reclination.

Jacques Daviel was born in La Barre, Normandy, August 11, 1696. He studied at Rouen, and served at the Hotel Dieu, in Paris. In 1719 he was sent as "plague physician" to Provence, and for the services there rendered he was appointed Surgeon to the City of Marseilles. There he became Professor of Anatomy and Surgery, but from 1728 he employed his time exclusively in the treatment of eye diseases, and he became so renowned that he was repeatedly called to Portugal and to Italy. In 1746 he settled in Paris, and in 1749 he received the appointment of Surgeon Oculist to the King. In 1750 he was called to attend the Kurfurstin at Mannheim; in 1754 to Ferdinand VI. of Spain, and later he was once more called to see the Princess Clemens of Bavaria. To restore his shattered health he went to Bourbon and to Geneva, to take the baths, at which latter place he died in 1762.

A hermit of Aiguilles, in Provence, was operated on the right eye without result, and came to Marseilles, where Daviel was at that time residing, to be operated on his left eye by him. But Daviel had no greater success. A number of pieces of the lens fell into the anterior chamber, which at the same time became filled with blood. Daviel then punctured the cornea with a bent needle, and enlarged the opening with a pair of curved scissors. The pupil cleared up and the patient saw. Two days later, however, purulent inflammation set in, and the eye was lost. Nevertheless, Daviel advanced a step farther, and made the attempt to reach the lens in its capsule by means of an incision in the cornea, and then to permit the lens to enter the anterior chamber through the pupil, and from here to draw (tirer) it out of the eye. He did this operation the first time on a woman. He tells us: "Jouveris la cornee comme je l'ai explique ensuite en portant la petit spatule dont j'ai deja parle sur la partie superieure de la cataracte je la detachai et je la tirai en morceaux hors de l'oeil avec cet instrument. La prunelle parut nette, la malade n'eut la moindre accident, et fut guerie guinze jours apres." After five successful operations he had one failure, and Daviel decided for the time being to give up this method, and returned to reclination. This he likewise did in a particular manner, in that he first opened the sclerotic at the usual place by using a double edged needle; he then entered with a blunt instrument, with which he dislocated the lens. Two years later, in 1747, while operating a gentleman in Paris, to which city he had in the meantime removed his residence, he was again compelled to incise the cornea, in order to permit the cataract, which it seems would not be dislocated into the vitreous, to escape through the pupil and corneal wound. Although there was a slight loss of vitreous, the operation was followed by a successful result. From now on, during the following three years, he from time to time operated through the cornea, in order to attain greater accuracy in this new method of operating. He writes: "Mais ce n'est determinement que dans le cours du voyage que jai fait a' Mannheim (1750), poury traiter, S. A. S., Madame La Princesse Palatine de Deuxponts, d'une ancienne maladie qu'elle avait a l'oeil gauche, que je pris la resolution de ne plus desormais operer la cataracte que par extraction du cristallin."

Regarding this operation, which he made at Mannheim. Remon de Vermale, Physician to the Kurfstin, made a report in a letter to Mons. Chicoyneau, Private Physician to the King of France, and later, in a copy to Van Swieten, Physician to Her Royal Highness in Vienna. There are, all told, but three pure cataract extractions. They were made respectively on "The Court Officer, Schlemmer, of Mannheim, aged 60 years; on "The Master of the Horse," of the Margrave of Baden Durbach, Baron v. Beck, aged 57, and on the journeyman tailor and drummer of the town of Heidelberg, Franz Kertenayer. These three cases are of historical interest, because Vermale's reports are the first literary evidence we possess of Daviel's operation; indeed, of the flap operation. This letter of Vermale is dated November 25, 1750, and it seems that it appeared in print in Paris as his own pamphlet in 1751. Daviel referred to this, and speaks of it as a dissertation in his "Original Investigations," which he presented before the Academy. "Sur une nouvelle methode de uerir la cataracte par la extraction du cristallin (107), which was written in 1752, but was first published in 1753, in volume II of Memoirs de l'Academie de Chirurgie. (The first volume of this memoir bears the date of 1743). To this fact can be traced the errors which arose regarding the date of the first literary reports of Daviel's extraction.

Hirschberg[7] claims that this was not published until 1757. A German translation of this first publication of Daviel's appears in the work of Magnus (1876, p. 265). Unfortunately this contains an ugly error. "The cornea is cut

---

[7] H. Archive, p. 198. 1890. Zur Geschicte der Star Auziehung.

in the shape of a cross." The original statement is, "in the shape of a half moon." From the time of Richter (Gr. Staar. Goettinger, 1773) up to the present day, all writers state that Daviel cut two-thirds of the corneal circumference. Daviel, however, states "only a little more than half."

The idea of this new method was conceived in 1745; for at that time he extracted a cataract which was still in position behind the iris and still enclosed within its capsule. But since he emphatically states that on his trip to Mannheim he made up his mind in the future to employ exclusively this new method; hence, we must designate the year 1750 as the true year in which this method of extraction was born. During this year the new idea received its introduction into practical existence.

It becomes a matter of special interest, as can be seen by reviewing Vermale's descriptions, that just that condition, in the case of a certain Baron v. Sickingen, Lord Steward of the Elector, Carl Theodore, which lead to the painful inflammation from which he suffered for years, as the result of reclination, and to relieve which the most renowned German oculists had been called from long distances, was only relieved after Daviel had extracted the lens, which had again risen up. This circumstance finally lead Daviel to the determination to adopt this method of extraction, and it is this danger which arises from the retention of a cataract within the eye, which in our day has become the main reason for our almost entirely abandoning this operation of reclination.

The details of the operation have naturally been greatly changed since Daviel's time, but in all methods of extraction the main idea has naturally been retained.

Daviel employed an instrument which corresponds to the bent lance in use today, and with this he incised the lower edge of the cornea, and widened the wound to the right and to the left, either by using two blunt knives (aiguille mousse), or by using a pair of curved scissors, which today bear Daviel's name; so that about the lower two-thirds of the corneal periphery was severed. Daviel says: "Et Achevera la section tant d'un cote que de l'autre afin de la porter de chaque cote un peu en dessus de la prunelle." Aside from this, we can get this information by studying his illustrations. He then lifted up the corneal flap with a golden spatula, and cut the anterior capsule with a sharp pointed needle. Finally, in order that the lens might escape, he pressed on the lower portion of the globe.

The changes and improvements which the method of Daviel underwent refer partially to the instruments used, partly to the size, form and seat of the wound.

Just as we find it true in general surgery, so also will we find that the cleaner cut the incision, the greater will be the tendency to heal. On this principle must have been based the idea, which led Poyet and Dr. La Faye to use an instrument like a knife in cutting the cornea, and which finally led to the construction of Beer's cataract knife, which is to be considered a great step toward advancement. By means of Beer's knife, it is not only possible, but it is customary, to make a complete corneal incision by a single sweep of the knife, and by this means, in the great majority of cases it is possible to get a surface wound which lies everywhere on an equal plane. For the same reason, the use of a Graefe's scleratome must be looked upon as a step backward, since it is only possible in exceptional cases to make the entire incision by a single pass of the knife. As a result, the surface of the wound lies in different planes, and may even be jagged or step-like. If, notwithstanding all this, the scleratome has received greater recognition, this surely must be due to other circumstances; more especially since with it, it is easier to make a conjunctival flap.

A similar view has been promulgated regarding the form of the wound, which during the first hundred years, aside from the reduction of the incision, from two-thirds to one-half of the base of the cornea had been but slightly changed, whereas since 1850, especially as the result of the efforts of Von Graefe and his pupils this has been materially changed. (III., l., p. 291). The peripheral linear incision is to be praised as an advancement, owing to its tendency to heal; the height of the flap is lessened, the wound is made in such a place which is at least partially permeated by blood vessels, and in the conjunctival flap was attained a sort of provisional bandage and protection against infected conjunctival secretion. However, it can not be denied that the necessity of the iridectomie lengthens the time of the operation and can not but be looked upon as detrimental, as must also be the 12-15 mm. in length wound of the iris, such as has heretofore been made.

Though the majority of operators accept the wound of the iris as a part of the operation, this fact does not settle the question as to whether the wound of the iris is of a more trivial nature, than the distension and squeezing to which the iris is subjected when a flap extraction is made without an iridectomie, but it rather points to the fact, that in the old flap extraction it is more difficult to cause the lens to come out of a corneal wound of the proper size, where the capsule of the lens has been opened to a sufficient extent, and where all superfluous pressure is avoided during the delivery of the lens, and at the same time cause but a minimum insult to the iris. The complicated effect of a large iris wound can be overcome by making the iridectomie several weeks before the extraction. (Mooren). Undoubtedly the extraction wound will then lie partially in the corneal cicatrix of the iridectomie incision. Apriori, one would imagine that here would be developed a condition which would not be favorable to the healing process. This, however, is rebuted by the results obtained by numbers of operators, who always make a preliminary iridectomie, and have had uniformly good results. The main advantages to be derived from a preliminary iridectomie previous to the delivery of the lens, is to be found in the ease and certainty with which cataractous remains behind the iris may be completely removed from the eye by shoving, stroking and pushing maneuvers; much more so than is possible with a coloboma of the iris. The form of the crystalline pearls which remain, depends largely on the operative method employed. In all the various methods mentioned, in the most successful cases, all that can take place, is a complete evacuation of the lens substance. On the other hand, the retention of the capsule in the eye makes a total evacuation of cortical remains all the more difficult. Those portions located in the equatorial region lie, as it were, in a pocket, and although they may get in the area of the coloboma and be visible to the naked eye, they can not be removed, notwithstanding every effort. Hence one can comprehend why, since Daviel's time, the quest for an operative procedure, by means of which it would become possible to remove a cataract, together with its capsule, has never ceased.[8] Pagenstecher, following this line of thought, has been quite successful. It becomes self-evident that if a method should ever be discovered, by means of which it would become possible in every case to remove a cataract in its capsule, without at the same time more seriously injuring the eye than is done at the present time, or if it should ever become possible to perfect our powers of diagnosis to such degree as to determine if it would be possible to make an extraction in the capsule, such a method would in all time to come, take first rank as an operative procedure in opthalmology.

In 1886, Prof. Hirschberg, of Berlin,[9] published a paper, in which he describes the essential differences between the various operations and the causes which led up to their use. He draws attention, as does also Jacobson,[10] to the jealousy which has been engendered between the French and the German oculists as to the relative value of the operations introduced respectively by Daviel and Von Graefe.

Jacobson states, "In order that I may add something to the history of the past twenty-five years, I will tell my colleagues what the attitude of Von Graefe toward Daviel's extraction was. Forty years ago, (1846), when but few extractions were made in Berlin, and Junken, as the knight of the needle, dazzled large audiences with his recital of the surprising indications for reclination, depressio, sublatio, etc., the teachings of the, at that time, illustrious artist, did not impress Von Graefe in the least. After he

8 Graefe Saemisch, Vol. III, p. 284.

9 Uber Staaroperationen. Deutsche Med. Wochenschrift, p. 410.

10 Ein Motivirtes Urtheil uber Daviel's Lappen Extraction und Graefe's Linear Extraction. Von Prof. J. Jacobson. In Konigsberg. Graefe Arch, 1886.

had finished his studies in Paris, Prague and Vienna, he began, in 1854, to teach, what to him seemed the only justifiable operation for senile cataract, and that reclination was only to be practiced in exceptional cases, as where the first eye had been lost by purulent inflammation. Jacobson tells us that he first made Von Graefe's acquaintance at a time when he was an enthusiastic follower of the French method, and during which time reclination was still being actively employed in Paris and in the Austrian Universities. He devoted the greatest care to the preparatory treatment, the various forms of dressing, and to the after-treatment, but he tried everything in vain. That, which his teachers experienced, he was not spared, about 10 per cent. of his cases were lost as the result of corneal ulceration. From that time on, *his every endeavor was to prevent suppuration.*"

Hirschberg tells us, that the original Daviel incision, made in the first half of the present century, was a *lower half-circular incision made in the corneal tissue,* close to its margin. (According to Richter, one-half; Beer, one-eighth; Arlt, one-half mm. from the limbus; whereas Young's incision was a good 2 mm. from the corneal margin, hence the opening was often too small, and at times he failed to deliver the lens).

We are indebted to the illustrious men, Beranger, Wenzel, G. A. Richter, and Beer, for the perfection of the flap operation, which today, as the *classical,* is compared with the so-called Von Graefe, or *modern,* operation. As a fact, a perfect flap extraction belongs to the most beautiful surgical procedures. The cicatrix is scarcely visible to the naked eye, scarcely more noticeable than the ordinary senile change. The pupil is round, and reacts; at most, the iris may be somewhat displaced backward, owing to the absence of the lens, and by the use of proper cataract glasses, vision is excellent. But this ideal result was attained in but 50 per cent. of cases, and even in the hands of the best operators, purulent destruction followed in at least 10 per cent. of cases. Still no one dared to make the incision smaller. This had long been looked upon as a great mistake and source of loss. At this time, Graefe appeared upon the scene. After a series of attempts made by himself and his pupils, especially Mooren, in Dusseldorf, Von Graefe introduced the preparatory iridectomie in 1864, and Mooren reduced his percentage of losses from 11 per cent. down to 3½ per cent. In 1863, Jacobson, of Konigsberg, made his incision in the sclerocorneal margin, to which he now added the iridectomie under deep chloroform narcosis, and thus, in 100 cases, reduced his losses from 10 per cent. down to 2 per cent. In 1864, Bowman and Critchett, of London, accepted Graefe's modified linear extraction, (incision with a lance knife, *above*; excision of iris, and delivery of the lens with a spoon), and, finally, in 1866, *Von Graefe* published his *"Peripheral Linear Incision,"* which was looked upon as a great triumph, and won the admiration of the opthalmologists of the entire world. "I shall never forget how, in 1867, opthalmologists from every part of the civilized world flocked to Berlin, to see with their own eyes this new method. The Opthalmological Congress at Paris in 1867, and Heidelberg in 1868, brought endless words of praise from Arlt, Knapp, Rothmund, Horing, Nagel, Horner, Critchett, Soelberg-Wells, Ed. Meyer, Wecker, and, what seems more especially noteworthy, from Mooren, and Jacobson, (Arch. f. Opth., XIV., 1868), who preferred this operation to his own."

Albrecht Von Graefe struck the proper chord, when he attempted to *prevent the unnecessary gaping of the corneal wound.* He asked himself, what, in the eye, is the analogous condition to a linear incision, and he recognized the fact, that on a globe the shortest distance between two points is along a segment of the greater circle of a sphere, and he accomplished this by *the narrow knife devised by himself. This incision just cut the upper corneal margin.* It was a linear incision $4\frac{1}{2}$ mm. long, to cover which he also cut a narrow strip of ocular conjunctiva; he then exercised a sector of the iris, opened the capsule with a small curved cystitome, and he removed the lens by soft massage from without, made by means of a rubber spoon on the lower edge of the cornea. This operation, as a rule, was done without an anaesthetic; the four acts of the operation being done while the eyeball was fixed. At times the English speculum was used.

It can not be denied, that this operation reduced the percentage of losses from 10 per cent. to 5 per cent., and losses by suppuration were reduced to 2-3 per cent.

A. V. Graefe, in 869 extractions had 3.8 per cent. loss.
Mooren, in 102 extractions had 2.9 per cent. loss.
Knapp, in 200 extractions had 2.0 per cent. loss.
Arlt, in 217 extractions had 5.5 per cent loss.
Arlt, 1866-73, in 1075 extractions had 5.6 per cent. loss.
Arlt, 1874-81, in 1547 extractions had 2.06 per cent. loss.
Horner, in 100 extractions had 8.0 per cent. loss.
Rothmund, in 186 extractions had 3.8 per cent. loss.
Rothmund, 1869-83, in 1420 extractions had 4.2 per cent. loss.

Possibly, the only one who did not follow the new operation was Hasner, of Prague. He had an exceedingly large experience—6-7,000 extractions—and he always made the half-circle incision.

(NAGEL'S BERICHTE.)

1868—106 flap extractions, only 4 per cent loss.
1877—138 flap extractions, 121 good results, 12 medium, 8.6 per cent. loss.
1879—181 flap extractions, 85.5 per cent. good results, 10.7 per cent. medium, 8.8 per cent. loss.
1880—110 flap extractions, 85.4 per cent. good results, 9.9 per cent. medium, 6.36 per cent. loss.

"But scarcely was the lion dead, than an opposition developed, which formerly did not possess the courage to assert itself. Ten years after the introduction of the Von Graefe method the statement is made, that *nothine remains but the knife.*"

Graefe's life has borne fruit to the cataract operation, and certainly has led to the development of new ideas. His method reduced the percentage of losses, even in the hands of those who have since changed his technique. His influence may be compared to that of Lister, whose fame will live on, long after his ideas have been set aside by the advancement of science. True, time has shown that the principle of the linear incision is not as essential as Von Graefe originally thought. Where not accurately made, the linear incision is often too small, and places difficulties in the way of the delivery of the lens, and leads to escape of vitreous. In the hands of a novice the linear incision may be too peripheric, and as a consequence leads to cicatrization of the iris in the wound, and this to sympathetic opthalmia—an almost unheard-of complication during the time of the classical flap operation.

The new method had the advantage, that the lens no longer had to be forced through a small—in old people, often rigid—sphincter, which can scarcely be dilated, and which now could easily come forward through the slit in the iris, and, further, that cortical remains could easily be removed by simple massage without going into the eye with a spoon.

And thus a sort of compromise procedure has developed, which bears the name of no operator, which is very like the Graefe procedure; has accepted all its advantages, and tries to avoid all the recognized dangers, and has received the name of *the one-third circumference incision.*[11] The incision should always be of sufficient size to permit the largest lens system, though it be hard, to pass easily. *This can be done where the incision equals one-third of the corneal circumference.* In the centre of the incision a section of the iris is removed, then the cystotomie and delivery of the lens follows by simply applying moderate pressure to the lower part of the cornea.

Jacobson (cited above) sums up the subject with the statement that a great many opthalmologists have gone over from the Graefe operation to the *peripheric flap incision in the corneal margin—but not to the Daviel flap.* So that the incision is the one originall suggested by Jacobson in 1863. He states: "*A large incision in the sclero-corneal margin heals better than a Daviel's flap or the so-called corneal linear incision.*

---

11 (1) De Wecker—Annales d Oculistique. 1884, 92. p. 207. and 1885. p. 29. (2) Hirschberg's Deutsche Zeitschrift fur Prak. Med. 1887. Beitrag zur Augenheilkunde Heft., III, 1878, p. 77.

Jacobson summarizes the value of both Von Graefe's and Daviel's work, as follows:

"It will always remain as the undeniable work of Von Graefe, that he did not, as most of his predecessors, content himself with attempts to stop suppuration of the cornea, but after long and systematic attempts, became the originator of a new method of extraction, in which the dangers of wound infection were reduced to a minimum. Though the theoretical premises may have been ever so wrong, still, as a result of this method of extraction, losses by suppuration were reduced from 10 and 12 per cent. down to 3 and 4 per cent., and poor results from 10 or 15 per cent. to about 6 per cent."

"To Daviel belongs the honor of having devised the bold procedure, by means of which all the forms of later times have been made possible, and which totally set aside reclination, depression, and similar methods, which in their old form will never return. It is not the great practical service of having reduced the 25 per cent. of losses down to 10 or 12 per cent., which will make Daviel's name immortal in the history of our science, but rather his clear insight, which showed him the way to the only safe means of extracting the cataract from the eye, and to a perfect method of healing. His boldness, which permitted him to make such an extended separation of the cornea without fear of injury to the eye, his great surgical genius, which lead him to devise from its very beginning the complicated technique of this operation, all pronounce him the father of this operation, whereas to Von Graefe belongs the credit of having removed its most serious dangers by means of his new operation."

C.

DISCISSIO CATARACTAE. BROIMENT DE LA CATARACTE.

DISCISSIO CATARACTAE PER KERATONYXIM AUT PER SCLER-OTICONYXIM.

Where a discission is made, (*discissio capsulae lentis,* incising of the capsule), the intention is, by means of a needle, which is pushed through the cornea or sclera, to open the anterior, also the posterior capsule, so as to bring the lens substance in direct contact with the aqueous humor, or the vitreous, so that it may be absorbed, and also that the anterior capsule may draw back out of the pupillary area.

"Discission is the latest of the three principal cataract operations. It is also, so to say, a daughter of depression. Among the writings of the ancients (Galenus, de Methodis Medendi, XIV, edition Kuhn, tom. X, p. 1019), we find but a single passage which seems to refer to this operation of discission. The translation of this passage, which Anagnostakis (1239) made, seems to have been made with a purpose. Learned philologists whom I have consulted regarding this passage are not at all satisfied with his translation. The whole matter appears to have reduced itself to this, namely; and this we also know from other sources, that the ancients did puncture the cornea. Since all the more exact points of differential diagnosis were wanting for all those diseases which lead to a cloudiness posterior to the pupil, to adhesions and indistinctness of the same, I am no longer in doubt, after a somewhat thorough investigation of the literature that the great confusion which existed concerning these named processes, was the result of the continual confounding of glaucoma, occlusion of the pupil, and hypopyon, one with another. To say the least, it would be exceedingly strange if discission had been known to Galen, and that the knowledge of this would have been completely lost again for hundreds of years."

It must certainly have occurred frequently during the act of making a depression; and, in fact, it must of necessity have occurred in all cases of cataract, that large portions of the same strayed into the pupillary area and protruded into the anterior chamber, or remained in the patellar fossa or in the vitreous itself. Even in Malgaigne's time, where controversies concerning the existence of capsular cataract were going on, such remains of lens substance were looked upon as pieces of thickened capsule. But from these numerous clinical histories, in which we find such accurate descriptions of how these capsules were gradually absorbed, it follows, that they could only have been remains of lens substance. Henkel (1770) was the first, to whom this common occurrence suggested the founding of a new operative procedure. The statements of Percival Pott (1781) are much more exact. He stuck a needle through the sclerotic; with this he impaled the lens, and tried by repeatedly turning the instrument to destroy, as much as possible, the capsule and the lens, so as to prepare it for resorption. This new method found many followers, especially among Pott's countrymen, Hey, Saunders, Adams; and by the latter was improved. The Englishmen, and not without right, claim the honor of inventing this method of breaking up the lens through the sclerotic. However, if we acknowledge Pott as the founder of this method, this is not exactly correct, since when we use the word *"discission"* today it also carries with it the thought of keratonyxis; and, furthermore, the expression, *"discissio cataractae*, as can be proven, was not used until 1824. Hence, Pott's operation should be designated as a breaking into pieces, (*"dislaceratio"*), if we do not wish to take up Himly's suggestion, which will be referred to again."

"Discission through the cornea (*keratonyxis cum discissio cataractae*) is even of later date. This likewise has its previous history. Wenzel and Gleize, in their writings, state that cataracts after the opening of their capsules have been gradually resorbed in the anterior chamber. Conradi and Beer attempted to cut the anterior capsule in a methodical manner. Their results, possibly due to a lack of method, were not favorable, and they gave it up again. In 1806 Buchhorn published the results of experiments made by him, at the instigation of his teacher Reil, in which he incised the anterior capsule of the lens through to cornea (here originates the word keratonyxis), in the eyes of corpses and animals.

"Langenbeck, to whom he sent a copy of his dissertation, then carried out in operative practice, keratonyxis; that is, incising through the cornea and the capsule of the lens. Of all the innumerable writings with which literature is replete concerning this operation of keratonyxis, it is only necessary to mention here the dissertation of Hulverding (Wien, 1824), because it was through him that the word *discissio* (it is to be written with two ss, not one. It is derived from discindere, to split up, to tear to pieces), was introduced into opthalmology. However, we must not lose sight of the fact, that as far as Buchhorn and Langenbeck were concerned, they did not in the beginning look upon it as a new method by which without injury to the posterior capsule, the contents of the capsule, was by means of the aqueous to be resorbed, but they rather looked upon it as a new method in which, by means of a corneal puncture, the lens could either be depressed, as was done by Celsius, or be broken up, as was done by Pott. Only gradually, without any particular person being deserving of the honor, out of this suggestion of Buchhorn, *the discissio cataractae s. capsulae lentis*, as we know it today, was evolved. It would not be out of place to accept Himly's suggestion, and use synonymously with our discissio, *punctio capsularis*, the word *dislaceratio* with discissio. One can hardly refrain from expressing the greatest astonishment that it should have taken so long to come upon a method which we so frequently see clinically exemplified in cases of injury, following which the lens is absorbed.

One must not fail to supplement the above by the *suction method*, a method which Sichel shows us, was known to the ancients, and states that the Arabs learned it from the Persians. In our time, it has been re-invented by Laugier, and, as literature attests, is practiced today. By means of a trocar, which is pushed through the cornea into the lens, the soft and fluid portions of the lens may be aspirated through a canula, and thus an entire cataract may be removed from the eye, just as where an extraction is made. Taking into consideration the manner of procedure, and the size of the wound, this method approaches that of discission. Since today we are in a position in most cases to diagnosticate a soft cataract, it is to be supposed that this method will remain in use for special cases.

CHAPTER III.

THE PROCEDURES AND CHANGES IN THE EYE DURING AND SUBSEQUENT TO CATARACT OPERATIONS.

In order that we may understand, and become fully acquainted with the injuries which an eye necessarily receives while undergoing a cataract operation, and that we may become familiar with those sequelae which do follow, and others which, under certain conditions, are sure to be added, we may follow a variety of plans. Where one possesses an accurate knowledge of the anatomy of the eye, and of the operative procedures, though he may have no clinical experience, he certainly can attain a very clear theoretical conception of all these procedures. Thus, in 1732, Frances Petit, in his published "Reflexions," exerted an influence on practical opthalmology, in that among other things he showed that the iris is not vaulted, as it appears to be when seen through the cornea.

The physician finds a second method of observation in watching the healing process of the operated eye. For this, we are indebted to Von Jacobson, who did this in a methodical manner, beginning with the first hour after the operation. His writings concerning this matter are truly classical.

Finally, here, just as in General Medicine, the study of the pathological anatomy—that is, the anatomical examination of eyes which had been operated on for cataract—teaches us the reasons for our clinical observations, and assists us in drawing conclusions, by means of which the ill results may in the future be avoided or controlled. Both branches of pathological anatomy are here of equal importance; the experimental, as well as the descriptive pathological anatomy.

Along these three lines, all these processes which occur in eyes which have been operated for cataract shall be studied and enumerated, going over, first, briefly, the methods of healing and the sequelae, as observed in reclination and discission. But, since reclination is but little practiced at the present day; hence our personal observations are but limited. Many of the evil sequelae of discission fall in the same category with those of reclination; in part they lead to the same final results, as have been observed when a large portion of lens substance remains after a cataract extraction. In fact, as we shall see further along, there are certain clinical pictures which develop in almost exactly the same manner, no matter which method is practiced. Owing to their great importance, the attempt will be made to give an exhaustive account of our present position and knowledge of the changes which take place subsequent to a cataract operation.

First of all, the reader is reminded of the far-reaching and beneficial effects which the study of bacteriology has had, not only on general surgery, but also on this particular branch of the same. In no other department is such painstaking care requisite to prevent *infection*. Not only must the eye and its adnexa be absolutely free of infection *before an operation* is undertaken, but the same care and attention must be given to the instruments, the bandage and the eye water used *during* and *after* the operation and during the processes of healing. *Truly, to prevent infection, here, if anywhere, the price of success is eternal vigilance.* This one factor, *"infection,"* is responsible for more poor results than all the others combined, and its occurrence will explain many of the pathological conditions to be enumerated. *He who will read between the lines, will, in the following pages, note the effect of infection.*

A.

RECLINATION.

The operative procedures, by means of which a displacement of the lens is purposely and skillfully brought about, differ from each other, as we have seen, in more ways than one, depending on whether the needle-like instrument which we employ is pushed through the cornea, or the sclera, and also upon the position in the eye, into which the cataract is to be brought. The thrust wound through the cornea which is made in keratonyxis is, as a rule, followed by but slight consequences; but, nevertheless, we meet with cases in which the reaction has been very great, and the operation followed by iritis and cyclitis. If the needle is poorly constructed, so that during the operation the aqueous is evacuated, there will be added to the injury of the eye, which must necessarily take place during the act of tilting the lens over, an entire transposition, equal to the depth of the anterior chamber, of the contents of the eyeball, and this transposition, during discission, not infrequently complicates the surgical procedure in a most detrimental manner; however, during extraction, this can never be avoided.

In making a sclerotonyxis, the needle wounds the conjunctiva, the sheath of the *muscle, rectus, externus,* or the muscle itself; the sclerotic, the choroid, and the ciliary portion of the retina. It then reaches the vitreous, and then the danger arises of puncturing one of the ciliary processes, and finally it passes through the zonula zinii. Thereupon, it either enters the lens behind the aequator and leaves it again in the periphery of the anterior capsule, and finally comes in contact with the iris; or, without touching it, makes its appearance in the pupil, with its surface in contact with the anterior capsule, (Willburg, Scarpa); or it grasps the lens at its upper edge, in order to depress it, in which an injury to the lens before the act, is not always necessary. (Celsius). Hence the injury, on making a sclerotonyxis; the simple puncture with the needle, is a more serious procedure, and differs further from the keratonyxis, in that the channel of the wound through vascular tissues and the possibility of puncturing a choroidal vessel (Celsius), or a ciliary process exists, and of thus causing an internal hemorrhage. Nevertheless, experience has taught, that even this method of puncture is frequently tolerated without evil consequences. Where, after reclination in any particular case, inflammatory symptoms develop, we are not able to exclude the fact, that the peculiar nature of the channel of the puncture is in all probability responsible for the trouble. (*Infection.*) Arlt (operations lehre, p. 255) considers it as the usual occurrence, where we operate after Scarpa, that the needle passes through the edge of the lens and the anterior capsule, and on raising the handle of the instrument, the anterior capsule bursts; and if the cataract is hard enough, it will be forced into the vitreous through the previously torn posterior capsule. Hence, in making a dislocation of the lens, we either cause a rupture of the posterior and anterior capsule; or, at times, a partial, at times, a complete detachment of the lens in its capsule from the zonula zinii; with or without at the same time injuring the capsule. Hence the hyaloidea in the hollow groove of the vitreous must be torn, and the tissue of the vitreous forced asunder, in order to permit of the lens occupying a certain amount of space. In which part of the vitreous the lens will finally come to rest, and the manner in which its surface will lie, depends on the method pursued.

It stands to reason, that it is impossible for the capsule to be torn, or for the lens to become detached from the zonula zinii, or for the hyaloidea to be ruptured without at the time exerting a certain amount of traction on the corpus ciliare and the parse ciliaris retinae. The force and influence which the traction will exert on the future welfare of the case depends partially on the certainty and the delicacy with which the operation is made, and partly also on the intimacy which exists between the lens and its suspensory ligament. As we have already seen, this connection becomes looser as age advances; more particularly so, where a shrinking capsular cataract has developed. The performance of the operation and the nature of the cataract, influence the extent of the injury which the vitreous must receive. There will be but slight resistance to the dislocation of a hard, shrunken lens, whereas the traction on the ciliary body will certainly be greater, where a cataract is but partially cloudy, or where the cataract is soft. When the entire lens system has been reclinated, there is less danger for it to mount up again, whereas in cataracts which have a less tough consistence, the capsule is torn in the greatest variety of ways, and a portion of its shreds will remain in connection with the reclinated lens. On this account, in the latter cases, the reclinated cataract more frequently mounts up again, thus necessitating a repetition of the steps of reclination, and thereby increasing the injury to and destruction of the vitreous. The result of the operation depends greatly on the consistence of the vitreous. If it is normal, it will naturally offer greater resistance to the sinking of the cataract; but, at the same time, if the foreign body has once been taken up, it will be held all the firmer, since both its point of entrance and the channel which it made for itself will close up and heal all the sooner. A fluid vitreous will offer but little resistance to the cataract, as we see it in cases of spontaneous luxation of the lens, but on the other hand it will offer no resistance to the independent movements which the foreign body may make. As we shall see further on, fluidity of the vitreous may be a result of reclination, hence this will explain how it happens, that cataracts which have not been fully resorbed may after many years spontaneously mount up again.

Further, it depends on the nature of the cataract, especially its consistency, whether it will be necessary to go through the movements of reclination a number of times, and it depends largely on the factor whether or not the lens will be depressed in the vitreous as a single mass, or divided into a number of pieces. This certainly must exert an influence on the pathological processes which take place in the eye after an operation. From that which has been said, it must become evident, that in this method of operating more than in any other which we will consider, great differences will be found in the results, even of operations which have been most successfully executed. (Stellwag, l. c., p. 771). In considering the processes of healing, it does not suffice to eliminate the operative procedure; but, owing to the reaction of the lens in the eye, pathological conditions are produced which under certain conditions may require weeks, months and even years to subside. The dislocated lens is to be looked upon as a foreign body which possesses the peculiarity that it may be dissolved and absorbed, and this pathological condition may only be looked upon as ended when the above conditions have been fulfilled. But since in these cases such a complete resorption never takes place, hence just such eyes never become free of this diseased condition.

If, by means of these lever-like movements, the lens is successfully removed from the pupillary area, so that it does not mount up again, and no signs of reaction follow, one might almost say that the immediate result of the operative procedure is wonderful. Truly, one must have been present and witnessed such a procedure—something which is hardly vouchsafed the younger generation of oculists—to form any idea of the impression which the suddenly-attained black pupil makes, and to witness the radiant joy of the patient who has had his sight suddenly restored to him. And, in fact, such cases were not of infrequent occurrence.

A reclination which is made without a mishap is often followed by no reaction whatever. The eye remains perfectly pale, the lens does not mount up again, and in the course of a week the patient is permitted to use his eye. In other cases the conjunctiva becomes reddened, the eye irritable to light and tears a few days; this, however, soon subsides, and the use of the eye is delayed a few days.

If ciliary injection sets in, one must decide if this is partial, or if the entire cornea is encircled. Even in the first condition, the conjunctiva begins to swell up; there is considerable secretion, the iris becomes discolored, vascularization becomes distinct and leads to exudation. After a time this abates, leaving a few synechia. After all these inflammatory symptoms cease, we find the pupil drawn in the direction in which the lens was reclinated, and a secondary cataract of greater or less thickness can be seen. The usefulness of the eye will depend on the thickness of this latter cataract.

If the ciliary injection is not restricted to the neighborhood of the point of puncture, the conjunctiva will become chemotic, iritis develops, and one can discern through the pupil that the capsule is involved in the inflammatory process. This disease lasts longer, and not infrequently leads to total occlusion of the pupil. How much of a result can be obtained by a subsequent operation in such a case, to increase vision, I can not state from personal observation, nor have I been able to find any reports in literature. It appears that the so-called subsequent operations have but lately been adopted (1876). If the pupil is not entirely occluded, a greater or less amount of vision may still be obtained. If these symptoms increase, hypopyon develops, and then the pupil will give a yellowish reflex. These cases may terminate in one of two ways. During the gradual resorption of the hypopyon and total occlusion of the pupil, *phthisis bulbi* gradually develops; this process takes months, and is accompanied from time to time by pain; sensibility to light is totally abolished, or may for a time still be present. Or the pus is not resorbed, but evacuates itself at some point, most frequently in the neighborhood of the point of puncture, finding its way outward through the sclerotic. But seldom has ulceration of the cornea been observed. (Daviel). (*This is the picture of an infection*).

The above-named forms of disease may be complicated by portions of the lens remaining in the pupil, floating about in the vitreous, or getting into the anterior chamber. Before a useful amount of vision can be attained these must first be resorbed and eliminated from their respective positions.

These processes may not develop at once in the manner described, but may develop suddenly in an entirely unexpected manner after the lapse of months or years in cases which had apparently terminated most successfully. There are also cases in which, without any premonitory symptoms, or without any outward signs, a serous choroiditis develops, leading to glaucoma and amaurosis. Finally, cases are reported from the remotest antiquity, in which lenses which had been reclinated for thirty years, suddenly mounted up again in a vitreous which had become fluid, and began moving about freely, and for a time return to occupy their former position in the pupil, or by accident getting into the anterior chamber, thus causing secondary glaucoma.

"The anatomical examination of eyes on which the operation of reclination has been practiced has explained to us the reasons for the various clinical pictures that have been described. The literature which reports the examination of eyes on which reclination had been practiced is considerable. The epoch-making examination of Brisseau was made on an eye, on which this operation had been made after death. Maitre Jean, Heister, Morgagni and others corroborated by their post-mortem examinations on non-operated corpses the anatomical nature of grey cataract; these, however, were soon followed by a number of others, Deider, Henkel, Boerhaven, Hein, Pott, Scarpa, Acrel, Earl and Hesselbach, and these again by Soemmering and Textor, who were almost exclusively interested in the fate of the torn capsule after reclination, and also of the reclinated lens; and only in a passing way paid attention to other changes which they found in the eyes. The first accurate examination of an eye on which reclination had been practiced, and which was obtained for pathological examination during the period of reaction, was made by Rienker, in the year 1834. This was followed by examinations made by Von Graefe, Iwanoff and Pagenstecher, so that today we possess quite accurate anatomical information regarding the more important processes, even those which occur in the most serious cases after reclination. A short time after scleronyxis it is often impossible to find the cicatrix of the puncture. Nevertheless, in one case Soemmering was able to recognize the point of puncture thirteen months after the operation; in another, eight and a half years later. This was recognized as a dark spot, one and a half lines from the cornea, and appeared somewhat more transparent than the rest of the sclera. Within, it was hardly a line from the edge of the retina, but on the folded edge of the cornea it could not be recognized. Puncture wounds of the cornea will be presently considered."

The changes which the capsule undergoes after reclination, vary greatly. If the lens, together with its capsule, has been reclinated, naturally no trace of the latter will be found in the pupillary area. The future condition of the eye then depends on the fact, whether or not any considerable inflammatory symptoms follow the operation. In Sommering's fifth operation he found the capsule free from its ligament and its entire circumference except at the lower edge, where it was still attached to the zonula. Sommering leaves the question an open one, as to whether the capsule was separated and depressed without tearing, or if there was originally a small tear which had closed again.

Opinions differ greatly regarding the frequency with which the lens, together with its capsule, is reclinated. Stellwag (l. c., p. 614) declares as the result of his investigations that cases of primary cataract dislocation in the capsule are an exceedingly rare occurrence. Hence, the statement of Beer (l. c., II, p. 364), who in former years found reclinated lenses in their capsules, as also did Richter (Chir. Biblioth., II, 322) and Szokalski (Prager Viertel Yahresschrift), are all the more important, since both after the lapse of many years extracted cataracts which had mounted up again, and were enabled to determine that they were enclosed in their capsules. Stellway states that it is possible to find the "dry pod cataracts."

If the capsule in its entirety, or even a portion of it, remains in direct continuity with the zonula, it is impossible to perform reclination, unless at least the posterior capsule is torn. Five years after reclination Von Grafe found in an eye which he examined the anterior capsule intact; whereas, in the posterior there was a circular opening 2.5 inches in diameter. Hence, the point of the needle used did not touch the anterior capsule, but remained imbedded in the lens substance. Stellwag (l. c., p. 608) stated that such a thing is possible, and Ritter (915, p. 9) proved it experimentally. The opening in the posterior capsule is not always regular. Stellwag found in post-mortems made on cholera patients, that the capsule was torn in many directions. Sometimes the central portion was missing. But even in these cases the peripheral portions adhere to the anterior capsule. If death had followed shortly after their reclination, they were to be recognized as floating shreds. But if the patient lived many years after operation these shreds were always found drawn back, and forming either a part of the crystalline pearl (Wulst), or as the posterior portion of a tattered secondary cataract, resembling in form a *cataracta siliquata*; or they were even found together with the anterior capsule somewhere in the eye rolled up like a ball.

The anterior capsule either disclosed a simple hole, or a piece had been torn out. These shreds which had been torn loose resembling a cloth which had been rolled up, were found folded together in the vitreous; they were, however, adherent to the nucleus of the lens, and were further, still in connection with the uninjured portion of the zonula, and in this manner with the corresponding ciliary processes. In other cases the anterior capsule was partially loosened from the zonula, and floated in the *aqueous humor* of the posterior chamber, either alone or in connection with the remains of the posterior capsule. Stellwag described a case in which reclination had been performed according to the rules laid down, and the anterior capsule was found adherent to the zonula only below, and was floating in the vitreous as a conglomerated folded mass.

In every case in which it was shown that the anterior capsule had simply been torn, but that its connection with the zonula had not been disturbed, a so-called crystalline pearl or wulst had formed. This was first accurately described and defined by Soemmering, and dependent on conditions found in eyes on which reclination had been practiced. The formation and the anatomy of the co-called crystalline pearl has already been described under secondary cataract.

After the lens has been forced out of its capsule into the vitreous, the latter must take the place of the former. Hence, th vitrous will cause the capsule to bulge out anteriorly. But along with the gradual shrinkage and resorption of the reclinated lens, an increased secretion of aqueous takes place, and together with the formation of the secondary cataract, the two halves of the capsule approach each other so as to lie almost in an even plane. This is found in nearly all post-mortem examinations. Earl alone states that after a lapse of five months he still found the space formerly occupied by the cataract filled with transparent fluid vitreous. Whereas, Soemmering states that at the end of thirteen months he found a perfectly even partition wall, made up of the remains of a torn lens capsule, which separated the aqueous from the vitreous.

According to Soemmering and Textor (l. c., p. 32) the opening in the posterior capsule is at times filled out by a very delicate, transparent membrane, which then forms the partition wall between aqueous and vitreous. This can be nothing more than the hyaloidea, concerning the wounds of which Stellwag has observed that they can heal without leaving a cicatrix. It is to be regretted that just in this fifth observation of Soemmering he makes no mention of the relation which he found existing between aqueous and vitreous. The few statements which report that after the close of the process, the vitreous is found bulging anteriorly, are of earlier date. Even in eyes which had very good vision, an abnormal adhesion was found between the periphery of the posterior capsule and the zonula, without the presence of any synechia. Such thickenings of the zonula coming on after a cyclitis are not of such rare occurrence (v. Graeffe).

Nearly all investigators seem to have interested themselves mostly with the fate of the reclinated lens. The position which a reclinated lens will occupy must necessarily depend on the method which is practiced, if the operation has been done in a perfect manner, and further depends on whether the lens does or does not completely or partially mount up again. Examination has shown that the reclinated lens comes to lie directly over the insertion of the *R. inferior* (Soemmering, l. c., p. 30), at times downward and outward in the vitreous (Soemmering, Plate I, Fig. 1 and 2. 4. Plate II, Fig. 5. Textor, Fig. 2, 3, 4). In cases of incomplete reclination, and following partial resorption, the nucleus of the lens may again become so displaced as to get back into the capsule, sink to the bottom, and simulate a Morgagniani's cataract (Textor, Fig. 1). The opportunity has been but seldom offered to accurately determine, at an early date, the position of the surfaces of the lens. Hence, it may be a matter of great interest to state that I (Becker) have been given a specimen by Dr. Manz (scleronyxis), in which the lens lies somewhat below and inward, almost touching the lower edge of the torn capsule, and with its anterior surface turned upward. In Soemmering's fifth case the lens must have occupied a somewhat similar position, and four and five years after a reclination v. Graeffe could determine the anterior (less convex) surface of the lens turned backward and somewhat upward, the posterior surface somewhat forward and downward.

The illustrations of Soemmering and Textor give us a very good idea of the position in which the lens finally becomes fixed. It is also very noticeable that in Soemmering's illustrations we find the lens lying further back than in Textor's illustrations. This is probably due to the fact that Soemmering reclinated through the sclera, whereas Textor did so through the cornea. One can, however, only then form a correct estimate of the position of the lens lies, if we bear in mind the position of the center of the lens, for since the lens shrinks in the vitreous; hence, in order to judge how far the lens is removed from the anterior or posterior portion of the eye, one must not forget that this depends on the degree of shrinkage. In Textor's cases the center of the lens lies on the folded portion of the *corpus ciliare*, whereas, in Soemmering's they lie on the flat portion, so that before resorption his lenses must have been partially on the retina.

All reports agree in showing that the post mortem examinations showed the volume of the reclinated lenses to be diminished. It is only in the fifth report of Soemmering that he emphatically states that though years had elapsed since reclination, the darkened and hardened lens in its capsule was not reduced in volume. Likewise in Manz's case, no reduction in volume could be found. (I regret that I can not give the exact date of the operation.) In all other cases I find it mentioned how great the reduction in volume was, or if the lens had entirely disappeared without leaving a trace. The number of the latter observations, however, is not very great. Such cases have been described by Deider, Acrel, Hoin, Earl, Soemmering, Arlt and Iwanoff. However, it must be stated that in the eyes operated by Soemmering and Iwanoff vision was destroyed as the result of very severe inflammation, so that it is very likely that the lenses were destroyed by the purulent inflammation. Hence, with the exception of Arlt's cases, all those reports of cases in which good vision existed after reclination with total resorption of the lens are of earlier date. However, both Acrel and Arlt make very positive statements. The former says (l. c., p. 109): "I examined the eye on which the patient had good vision subsequent to the operation, and I find that the depressed lens had been totally dissolved and absorbed." Arlt says (p. 346): "In a specimen taken from an insane patient, who had been operated nine years previously, not a trace of the nucleus of the lens could be found, either in the vitreous or on the retina." The volume of the remains of the lens varies greatly, from the scarcely perceptible pieces to pieces the size of millet seeds—greyish white bodies. (Soemmering, Beob. 1.) Beyond a doubt the result is greatly influenced by the consistence of the cataract, and dependent on the fact whether, during the operation. a great deal of cortical substance is stripped off; also, whether the capsule is also reclinated. Time does not seem to be the only factor requisite to bring about resorption of a cataract. Beer says (l. c., p. 364): "In fact, I have never yet seen a cataract which, being held but partially fast, could be entirely dissolved and resorbed, and before I will believe that this can occur, I must personally see a depressed, solid, hard cataract really dissolved and resorbed, which I am sorry to state I have never as yet been able to see." In a case which Hesselbach examined, a lens which had been depressed for forty-four years was not entirely resorbed. However, in these cases of such long standing, examined by Hesselabch and others, deposits of lime salts were found in the remains of the lenses.

Ritter described the processes of resorption of the lens in the vitreous as similar to those which take place in the aqueous. The fibres lose their close and compact arrangement. so that the reclinated lens may later on separate into a number of pieces. The fibres shrink, and whereas the fibres break up and become tumescent, and finally absorbed, the membrane most probably remains unchanged. Opinions differ greatly as to what becomes of portions of the capsule which get into the vitreous during reclination. Stellwag states (l. c., p. 615) that he frequetnly was not able to find pieces of capsule which had been torn away and fallen into the vitreous. Likewise, he frequently found edges of the posterior capsule which were still connected with the anterior capsule much reduced in size. Where the edge of the posterior capsule was wanting, one could never find any remains of the posterior. The portions of the latter which were found imbedded in the crystalline pearl was never as large as those shreds which were found adherent to the edge of the anterior capsule, when the eyes were examined shortly after the operation. From this we can assume that not only dislocated pieces of the anterior and posterior capsule and those which are torn out may be absorbed, but also those which are still adherent. Stellwag himself seems to acknowledge that the whole capsule or large pieces of the same are not only *not* absorbed, but offer great resistance to the resorption of the enclosed lens substance. This general principle of Stellwag's, which is also met with at other places, I desire to contrast with the fact, that at that time the methods of microscopical investigation were not developed sufficiently to distinguish whether or not very fine and delicate shreds of the capsule were still present in the eye. Even in cases where the entire eye is destroyed by purulent inflammation. the *hyaline lamellae of the choroid* withstand solution, as does also the *membrana limitans of the retinae*, even when nothing else remains of these structures. The same is true of *membrana descemeti* and of the *capsule of the lens*, in cases of traumatic cataract. Dr. Goldzieher found, one year after the completion of a cataract operation, a piece of the capsule entirely unchanged, enclosed in the conjunctival cicatrix. Though I have observed very considerable swelling of the capsule of the lens, and though this might be looked upon as a prodromal stage of resorption, still I do not consider this as proven.

As has already been mentioned, a complete healing of the hyaloidea in the hollow groove of the vitreous (fossa patellaris) after reclination, without having a cicatrix, has been anatomically determined. Even the path which the lens followed during the act of depression could in some cases no longer be found. Every investigator has observed, that the vitreous becomes thickened and filled with cloudy threads and membranes, in the immediate neighborhood of the lens. Even Soemmering states that the extent of these pathological formations is proportionate to the degree of inflammation observed during life. Occasionally he observed a positive nest of new formed tissue in which the lens was imbedded. Even in eyes in which the lens was totally resorbed, he could plainly see the groove in which the lens had been deposited. In this tissue Soemmering even found new formed blood vessels. The remark of Stellwag is very interesting, indeed, in which he states that he never found the cataractous nucleus in direct contact with the retina. He always found a measurable stratum of vitreous substance between the surface of the lens and the retina. Since Stellwag's statements only refer to eyes which had been operated successfully, this coincides perfectly with the results obtained by H. Pagenstecher, in his experimental investigations. According to the latter, a foreign body may be introduced through the sclerotic into the vitreous, and tolerated for a long time without leading to a hyperplasia of cells and incapsulation. If this does take place, it always extends from the point of puncture to the place where the foreign body rests. This hyperplasia takes place more certainly and more quickly when the foreign body is in contact with the retina. The view held by many oculists, namely, that the pressure which the lens exerts on the coats of the eye, especially the retina, causes the severe reaction after reclination, is by this means fully explained, as are also the observations of Stellwag. Leber, in his masterly work already so often quoted (Die Entzundung. Leipsig, 1891), has shown that the inflammatory reaction within the eye is due to the action of micro-organisms and the ptomaines which they produce. In his experiments with sterile particles of metals, and with various chemicals, he has shown that the former are gradually acted on by the vitreous dissolved off, and even in the minutest quantities like chemicals exert an irritating influence, and give rise to inflammation of asceptic or chemically produced pus. This inflammation may be of a very low grade and chronic variety, and gradually lead to destruction of the vitreous.

The comparatively frequent observation, namely, that in successful cases of reclination, the reclinated lens is found still held in connection with the lower portion of the zonula, will explain why this detrimental pressure on the retina and corpus ciliare does not so often overstep the limit of endurance.

The zonula fibres act like an elastic spring, counteracting the pressure which the lens would otherwise exert. The elasticity of this membrane, and with perfect right, has been enumerated as one of the causes for the mounting up again of the lens. This, however, is not the only cause.

Time and again post mortem examinations have shown the vitreous to be fluid (Soemmering, Acrel and others). A synchisis before the operation would necessarily defeat the results of an operation. Just as a fluidity of the vitreous is to be looked upon as a cause of spontaneous luxation, it must likewise favor a reclination of the lens; but it will also prevent a permanent result. If the fluidity is a result of the reclination, it will depend on the kind of adhesion whether or not the lens will become freely movable in the vitreous. Various observers have found the reduced lens floating freely in the vitreous.

Stellwag (l. c., p. 618) describes a peculiar form of fluidity of the vitreous, which seems only to affect the anterior and middle portion; but with this I am neither familiar from personal observation, nor from the statements of others. He says: "Very frequently he finds the vitreous reduced to such a degree that, aside from the portion which is applied to the retina, there is a space anteriorly which is filled with watery fluid." And he adds (with perfect right): "and when the portion of the vitreous in contact with the nucleus of the cataract becomes fluid, the position of the latter in the future will be determined by its specific weight. On moving the eye about we can then see it dancing about inside the globe, and it may possibly get into the anterior chamber.

Such a fluidity of the vitreous, coming on long after an operation, has for a long time been looked upon as the cause of amaurosis without cloudiness of the transparent media, or without detachment of the retina. (Secretion glaucoma of v. Graefe). This was first described by Beck and later again by V. Graefe.

The connective tissue threads, which in cases which take a favorable course totally surround the lens and hold it in its position, can be most easily described as the products of a circumscribed cyclitis, and of that particular variety which by preference originates in the pars ciliaris retinae. The amount of new formed tissue permits us to estimate the intensity of the cyclitis, and Soemmering has described and illustrated stages of development of this process. We possess the reports of more exact examinations made by Rieneker, V. Graefe and Iwanoff, in which vision had been totally destroyed as the result of cyclitis and its various complications subsequent to reclination. Rieneker examined an eye on which keratonyxis had been practiced eleven days previously by means of a Scarpa's needle. Violent inflammation followed, intense chemosis, hypopyon and a yellow reflex from the pupil was noted. The eye became amaurotic on the fourth day; the light sense remained nihl, but the inflammatory symptoms subsided a few days before death. On post mortem examination the point of puncture could only be found existing as a fine cicatrix. At the lower portion of the anterior chamber exudate was still present (hypopyon), which firmly adhered to the cornea and iris. The upper half of the iris had a greenish discoloration, and in the neighborhood of the hypopyon were small echymoses. The moderately dilated pupil was in about two-thirds of its area filled with exudate. The retina was loosened up and of a grey color; the choroid was of a brownish red color. Extravasated blood lay between the retina and the vitreous. The vitreous was very consistent. and of a greenish color. To the temporal side was a mass of pus about the size of a bean. In front of this, to the outer and lower side of the uvea lay the lens, on the ciliary band, between hyaloidea and nervea. Close to the lens was an ecchymosis. The lens was swollen, externally soft and flaky, internally hard. In the neighborhood of the lens the sclerotic seemed to be normal. This is the only case, which I have been able to find in literature, in which the sequelae following reclination and acute purulent irido choroiditis, has been described in a perfectly clear and comprehensive manner, taking into consideration the time when it was written. (No doubt bacteriological investigation would have demonstrated the presence of staplylococci and streptococci). It appears that Iwanoff must have examined a similar case. In the eye which Moren examined (l. c., p. 35) the globe had retained its form and size, retina and choroid were in their normal position, the vitreous, however, was drawn forward, so that its anterior posterior chamber measured but 8 mm. Downward and outward, where in Rieneker's case the lens lay, there was found an abscess in the stage of inspisation. The only remains of the lens was a crystalline pearl. This was everywhere enclosed in a thickened, new formed tissue. which posteriorly gradually disappeared in the vitreous, and anteriorly bound this crystalline pearl tightly to the iris. The pathological conditions were just as intimate with the ciliary body, which had likewise been changed by inflammatory products. Both retina and choiroid showed increase of tissue change, more anteriorly than posteriorly. Anteriorly the former showed many spaces filled with fluid, and many round cells, and the latter a more intimate connection of the various lamellae could be made out, especially between the pigment epithelium and the vitreous lamellae of the choroid. We recognize the description as that of a typical case of irido-cyclitis. Von Graefe examined a blind eye four or five years after reclination had been practiced. During life one could not determine any other diseased condition than a rigidity of a moderate sized pupil. In the center of which one could see a secondary cataract. Post mortem examination showed that the iris was not adherent to the secondary cataract. The latter. however, was held adherent to the zonula by means of an exudate, and by means of this also with the ciliary processes. In the retina could be seen countless small and large whitish granules and nodules, and part of these extended into the choroid. At some places they formed large plaques. On microscopical examination all of these were found to form a continuous sheet between retina and choroid, which at the orrata serrata became continuous with both membranes in their entirety. In the vitreous the direction which the lens had taken could be followed by means of a new formed connective tissue mass, which lead to a membranous pocket in the vitreous, and was located downward and outward. In the neighborhood of this pocket, very fine whitish, cloudy membranes in the otherwise colorless vitreous. A considerable amount of carbonate of lime was found between the choroid and retina, as also on the inner surface of the ciliary body, just as in the above mentioned case. Von Graefe draws attention to this diffuse process, extending from the ciliary processes over the entire choroid. Owing to the fact that the new formed connective tissue was in the vitreous, and the iris was not involved, this should be designated as a chorio-cyclitis. The case of Von Graefe, which was examined by Iwanoff, was an atrophied eye, as a result of reclination. Here it appears the reclinated portion of the lens was resorbed. The entire vitreous had been changed into a new connective tissue mass and was drawn forward. Only here and there could the various layers be distinguished in the detached retina, which seemed to be made up of hypertrophied, radiating fibres. The entire choroid was folded, and between this and the retina anteriorly was a thin lamellae of bone. Even in fine sections small abscesses could be detected in the vitreous. The sheath of connective tissue which surrounded the lens seemed to be very tough, and at some places enclosed deposits of lime salts. This advanced calcification seemed remarkable, considering that the reclination had been practiced but nine months previously. The processes which lead to these changes is to be designated as an irido-choroiditis.

B.

DISCISSION.

As a rule, but slight reaction follows discission through the cornea; there are, however, exceptions to the rule.

The kind of instrument used to puncture the cornea, and to open the capsule, is not without its influence. The English discission needle which is now in general use, only became so gradually. This is straight, anteriorly two-edged, and its neck has everywhere an equal thickness, so that, when during the operation the needle is either pressed forward or drawn backward, it always completely fills out the channel of the wound; and, since the wound made by the double edge is just equal to the diameter of the neck, hence it is impossible for the aqueous to escape, during the operation. The older instruments, especially those which, even until recently, were recommended by some English physicians, are conical and increase in thickness. This instrument not only interferes with the free movement in the channel of the wound, but its use certainly favors the bruising of the edges of the wound. · Such a wound will leave a cicatrix, which will be visible for a much longer time. In exceptional cases, the edges of the wound have been observed to swell up and assume a bubble-like prominence. If we will only stop to consider, how kindly frequently repeated punctures of the anterior chamber are borne, (Sperino), we can not assume that the occasional unfortunate mishaps, are entirely the result of the corneal wound. Here again, the effect of an infection, either direct, by use of a non-sterile instrument, or the subsequent infection of the wound from conjunctival secretion, is to be borne in mind.

If, during or after the operation, the aqueous is partially or completely evacuated, the entire lens system must move forward. All the sequelae of this occurrence, the release of the blood vessels from the intraocular pressure, and the consequent hyperaemia, in all the vascular portions of the eye, as well as the tension which is exerted on the ciliary body in consequence of this moving forward of the lens, must be looked upon under certain circumstances as replete with injurious effects. It is well known, that puncture of the anterior chamber during the course of inflammatory affections of the eye, is accompanied by great pain. The moving forward of the entire lens system depends on the extent of the wound in the capsule, the depth to which the needle penetrates the lens substance, the consistence and, more especially, the compactness of the cataract. If one may so express it, the normal process of absorption of the lens, after opening the capsule, has already been fully described in the general consideration of traumatic cataract. But discission does not always follow the normal course there depicted, for symptoms of a violent reaction may develop. The pupil contracts, and, in spite of the free use of atropine, will not dilate. The iris becomes discolored, and, owing to the rapid swelling up of the entire lens, is pushed forward, or a large amount of lens substance enters the anterior chamber and also presses the iris forward. The peri-corneal infection which develops at once, gradually leads to an oedema of the conjunctiva bulbi; the eyes become hard, and the field of vision contracted to the nasal side. At the same time, the patient complains of irritability to light, and intense pain radiating along the branches of the trigeminus. The picture of secondary glaucoma is complete.

It has been supposed that these phenomena are the result of opening the capsule too widely, and of permitting the needle to sink too deeply into the lens substance; nevertheless, they have occurred after the most careful opening of the capsule. Hence, either the eye must be too sensitive or the cataract peculiarly constituted chemically, so as to exert such a detrimental influence. But the increased tension is always brought on by the rapid swelling up of the lens; this leads to the circulatory disturbances, the contraction of the field of vision, the irritability to light and the ciliary pain.

"All these changes are almost exclusively observed in the eyes of youthful individuals, except in cases in which we are dealing with extensive injury. In older persons the opening of the anterior capsule likewise leads to a swelling up of the cortical substance, but if this does not exceed reasonable bounds, it will not lead to a pressing forward of the entire lenticular mass, which does not seem to take place unless the nucleus likewise swells up."

These words of Von Graefe [1] explain why injuries of the lens in older individuals have a better prognosis than in younger individuals; and also why in the latter days of his activity he became more careful in the selection of cases, in which he practiced discission. If we are to look upon the great swelling of the cataract as the cause of the increased intra-ocular tension and its evil consequences, it must become evident, that if the swollen lens, even in its entirety or partially, is extracted at the proper time, the pain, as a rule, will cease at once, the chemosis will gradually subside, and the resorption of any portion left behind will take a regularly normal course. It must, however, become evident, that under just such circumstances a thick secondary cataract will develop, and that this can hardly take place without the formation of synechia.

The spastic contraction of the pupil following discission is caused by a swelling up of the lens, which condition likewise leads to increased tension, owing to the interference with the evacuation of the swollen lens substance into the anterior chamber. The increase of tension is also due to increased secretion within the eye, due to the injury to the lens. Hence the healing influence which an iridectomie, made either at the time of discission or previous to it, exerts on the course of the discission, can be explained in two ways. Owing to the incision in the *sphincter pupillae,* the iris loses its power of contraction, and, aside from this, the excision of the pieces of the iris, acts just as it does in true glaucoma. Hence it is most advisable to make the extraction of a swollen lens through a linear incision, at the same time making an iridectomie. In his last publication on cataract, Von Graefe spoke in the highest terms of praise of this method of treatment, and I (Becker) have repeatedly drawn attention to the same fact.

If the operation made during the stadium glaucomatosum is not made according to this method, advised above, in most cases a very painful, "sneaking" iridocyclitis will follow, leading to occlusion of the pupil and *phthisis bulbi.* In such cases the detachment of the retina usually comes on at a later date. For a long time, a part of the sensitiveness to light remains, even in eyes in which intra-ocular tension is reduced.

There may also develop primarily, as well as following a *status glau-*

---

[1] A. f. O., I, 2, p. 238.

comatosus, a suppurative irido-choroiditis, panopthalmitis, with purulent destruction of the eye.

Where a discissio per scleroticam is made, the amount of vision attained should equal that attained where a soft lens is reclinated. Hence it will be unnecessary to again consider those processes which have already been described, and which make the results of such an operation questionable.

The pathological processes which follow a discission have been practically considered under the head of traumatic cataract. Here we must again refer to the experimental investigations of Dietrich and Ritter. However, to give a synopsis of their work, would be but to repeat many facts which have already been quoted.

Swanzy (Diseases of the Eye. London, 1892, p. 360) states, "This method is applicable to all complete cataracts up to the twenty-fifth year, and to those lamellar cataracts in which the opacity approaches so close to the periphery of the lens, that nothing can be gained by an iridectomie. After the above age, the increasing hardness of the nucleus, and the increasing irritability of the iris render the method unsuitable."

"Discission is a safe procedure when used with the above indications and precautions. The danger chiefly to be feared is iritis, from pressure of the swelling lens, masses on the iris. When this occurs, or is threatened, removal of the cataract by linear incision in the cornea should be at once performed. Another danger consists in the glaucomatous increase of tension (secondary glaucoma); here, likewise, removal by a linear incision is at once indicated."

C.

EXTRACTION.

As we have seen, the original Daviel extraction consisted of a *corneal flap* (*downward*), taking in *two-thirds of the corneal circumference*, and without an iridectomie. The only change up to the time of Von Graefe consisted in the position of the wound (Yaeger, *upward*; Wenzel, *outward*). But the principal objection to this operation always had been, the relatively large percentage of losses as the result of suppuration. Von Graefe early recognized that this was due to the, at times, unnecessary gaping of the wound, to overcome which he introduced what is known as the *linear incision*. Such an incision can only be done, when the incision is made in the "largest circle" of the spherical surface of the eye, because the shortest distance between points upon the surface of the sphere, *i. e.*, the line which is most nearly straight falls in the largest circle. The largest circle which passes through two points on the surface of a sphere, is situated in a plane passing through these points and the centre of the sphere. In order to make this incision, a much narrower knife was necessary, and this Graefe likewise invented, and this today bears his name. This incision was likewise made in the *cornea*, but in order to allow the lens to escape easily the *preparatory iridectomie* was made. Jacobson made his incision in the *sclero-corneal margin*, and this suggestion was adopted by Von Graefe adding to this an ocular conjunctival flap which acted as a provisional bandage. This is known as his *peripheral linear incision*, and was in vogue during his lifetime. After his death, however, operators gradually departed from this operation, going back to the flap extraction, one set of operators making what is known as the *scleral flap extraction*. In this operation, the puncture and counter-puncture are made in the sclera one-half mm. from the corneal margin, and in such a manner that a straight line connecting these two points would separate the upper fourth from the lower three-fourths of the corneal circumference. After the counter-puncture is made, the incision lies close behind the limbus. As soon as the sclera is severed, the edge of the blade is turned slightly backward, so as to form a conjunctival flap, about 2 mm. in width. The iridectomie, capsulotomy, and extraction of the lens follows. The great advantage of this operation lies in the fact, that the incision lies under the conjunctiva, which latter also forms a flap, which soon closes over the wound again, and thus *prevents subsequent infection.*

A second form of operation is the *corneal flap extraction,* (Wecker, Stellwag). Here the entire incision is made in the corneal limbus and in such a manner that one-third of the cornea is separated from the sclera. In this operation no conjunctival flap is obtained; or, if any, but a very slight one. *The iridectomie may or need not be made,* depending on the desire of the operator. Fuchs says, (Lehrbuch, 1891, p. 759), "Since this incision is less peripheric. prolapse of the iris is less apt to occur, than where a scleral incision is made. Whereas, when no iridectomie is made, the patient has the advantage of a round and movable pupil, it also brings with it its disadvantages: First, the delivery of the lens without an iridectomie is more difficult, since it must be forced through a narrow pupil, which procedure requires considerable pressure. Hence, this method is not indicated in cases which depend on a very delicate delivery of the lens, as, per example, where the lens trembles and every increase of pressure is apt to lead to tearing of the zonula and the hyaloidea, and at the same time lead to a prolapse of the vitreous. Second, extraction without iridectomie is not advisable in complicated cataracts, in which synechia exist between lens and iris. Third, notwithstanding the use of eserine, prolapse of the iris may occur in the first few days after an operation. Under such circumstances the prolapsed iris must be excised. Hence, extraction without iridectomie is not indicated in cases which show a tendency to prolapse of the iris, or where the patient is restless. Hence, one may conclude that the corneal flap extraction, where the conditions are favorable, gives the most satisfactory results; it is, however, not adapted to all cases, nor does it insure those almost positive results, as does the scleral extraction with iridectomie." Swanzy (Handbook. Fourth Edition, 1892, p. 355) states, "As a set-off against the circular pupil, the extraction without iridectomie exposes the eye to the serious danger of prolapse of the iris into the wound. These operators make it a rule to perform an iridectomie in all cases where they can not satisfactorily repose the iris after delivery of the lens; but even where they can repose it well, they are not, they state, secure against the occurrence of a prolapse within the first two or three days after the operation; nor do they find that eserine, or any other means, provides the desired safeguard. It is admitted that prolapse of the iris takes place after a number of these operations, and that there is no foretelling in what eyes it will occur. The prolapsed portion of the iris heals in the wound, which then, in a few weeks, becomes more or less cystoid and bulging, causing displacement of the pupil, and irregular curvature of the cornea, with resulting deterioration of vision. Nor is this all; for such eyes are liable, weeks, months, or even years after the operation, to take on severe iridocyclitis, ending in total loss of sight. Another disadvantage of this operation is, that removal of cortical remains can not be so effectually performed, as where a coloboma has been made."

"Therefore, while admitting the charm of a circular pupil, I am of opinion, that the question is not, whether the appearance of some eyes operated on is pleasing to us, and to others who inspect them; but rather, what advantage the greatest number of persons operated on derive from the operations. With sentimental talk about "mutilation" of the iris, I can not sympathize. If the advocates of the method under discussion should find a means of insuring the eye against prolapse of the iris, the operation will be placed upon a different footing; but, until then, the procedure can not, I think, be recommended."

"It is easy to understand why, in the simple extraction prolapse of the iris, with subsequent incarceration, is so liable to occur, even some days after the operation, and why it is so difficult to devise a sure means for preventing the accident; as, also, how it is that even a very narrow coloboma is sufficient to protect the eye from the disaster. And yet I am inclined to think, that among the oculists who have reverted to the simple method, there are some who do not realize the *modus operandi* in either case. Within a few hours after the operation, the wound in the corneal margin most commonly closes, the aqueous humor collects, and the anterior chamber is restored. But it takes many hours more for the delicate union of the lips of the wound to become quite consolidated, and during that time it requires but little—a cough, a sneeze, a motion of the head, the necessary efforts in the use of a urinal or bed-pan, no matter how careful the nursing—to rupture the newly formed union; and, as a matter of fact, this often does take place. The aqueous then flows away through the wound with a sudden gush, and, where the simple extraction has been employed, carries with it the iris. Doubtless, in this event, it is that portion of the aqueous humor which is situated behind the iris, which is chiefly concerned in the iris prolapse; the aqueous humor in the anterior part of the anterior chamber probably flows off without influencing the position of the iris. The advocates of the simple operation endeavor to prevent secondary iris-prolapse, by a spastic contraction of the pupil, produced by eserine, which is instilled at the conclusion of the operation, and again, by some operators, a few hours afterward. In most instances, the desired end is by this means effected."

"But there is a considerable percentage of cases in which the contraction of the sphincter iridis is overcome by the pressure of the aqueous humour from behind, and iris prolapse takes place."

"How, then, does the formation of a coloboma prevent prolapse of the iris when the wound bursts, as I have described? Not because the portion of the iris which is liable to prolapse has been taken away. That would mean nothing less than the whole of the part of the iris which corresponds to the length of the opening in the corneal margin. But the coloboma averts secondary iris-prolapse, because it provides a gateway, a sluice, for the aqueous humor contained in the posterior part of the anterior chamber, to escape directly through the wound, without carrying with it the iris in its rush; and it is evident, that the narrowest coloboma which can be formed will be amply sufficient for the purpose. To my mind, a narrow iridectomie here is no "mutilation of the iris," but rather a measure which rests upon a sound scientific basis, and which is calculated to insure the safety of the eye in an important particular."

"As a disfigurement of the eye, there is practically none, when the coloboma is so narrow, and is situated in the upper part of the iris. The pupil, too, is movable; almost, if not quite, as much so, I venture to say, as in most cases of simple extraction. For it is entirely a mistake to suppose that a narrow coloboma renders the pupil immovable. Where there are no adhesions between the pupillary margin and the capsule, as frequently happens, the reaction to light is active; a drop of atropine will dilate the pupil widely, and a drop of eserine will contract it."

Naturally, every incision must be of sufficient size to permit the cataractous lens, whose horizontal section is an ellipse, to emerge conveniently. Schmidt-Rimpler states,[2] "In the flap incision, extraction is performed by bending the flap of the cornea away from the sclera. The length of the incision must here approximate the diameter of the cataract from right to left; for example, 8 to 9 mm., while the height of the flap must at least equal the antero-posterior diameter of the cataract; for example, 3 to 4 mm. If we assume the horizontal transverse diameter of the transparent cornea —excluding the sclera limbus, which can be moved over about 0.5 mm. on each side—at 11 mm., height of the flap above, 5 mm.; a flap incision made here would even exceed the dimensions of the largest cataract. But it must be remembered that the size of the wound in the membrana descemeti (inner corneal wound) is somewhat smaller than that in the outer corneal layer (external corneal wound). If the cataract is to pass through a linear incision, the latter must be made to gape. This is done by bringing the ends somewhat closer together, so that an ellipsoidal opening is formed. The length of the incision must therefore be greater than the diameter of the lens from right to left. Its size is determined when we know the circumference (u) of the ellipse necessary for the passage of the lens. It equals $\frac{(a+b)\pi}{2}$; where "a" is the smallest diameter, "b" the largest diameter of the ellipse. If the cataract is 4 mm. in thickness, and 9 mm. in diameter, $U=\frac{(4+9)\pi}{2}=6.5+3.14=2.041$. The linear incision, which is to be converted into an ellipse by the approximation of its ends, must therefore, be half as long, or about 10 mm. (In this calculation, we disregard the fact that we have to deal with ellipses or incisions, not upon a plane, but upon a spherical surface). A linear incision of such length can only be made by passing through the transparent corneal tissue. If the incision is made in great part in the edge of the cornea, as is usually done, we must abandon an absolutely linear character; the majority of so-called linear incisions are really flap incisions, although of small flap height. It is to be regarded as a special advantage of linear incisions, that they have a less tendency to gape, than flap incisions; strong intra-ocular pressure is capable of lifting up the flaps."

"The length of the incision must depend on the size and consistence of the cataract. Thus, a soft cortical cataract, which is displaced during extraction and changes its shape according to the wound, requires a smaller opening than a hard cataract. The size of the nucleus is also important."

Ph. Steffan [3] has given us a very interesting table of measurements of

[2] Handbook, 1889. English edition, p. 326.

[3] Weitere Erfahrungen und Studien uber die Kataract Extraction, 1882-1889. Graefe Arch., Vol. XXXV, B. 2. 1889.

500 extracted cataracts. But 13 per cent. of these had a maximal diameter of 8.5-9.0 mm. and a thickness of 4 mm.; further, whereas, after the forty-fifth year, we must be prepared to find the maximal size, up to the forty-fourth year the diameter equals 8 mm. and a thickness of 3 mm.

Diam. of Cataract in mm.	Under 30 Years.	30-34 Yrs.	35-39 Yrs.	40-44 Yrs.	45-49 Yrs.	50-54 Yrs.	55-59 Yrs.	60-64 Yrs.	65-69 Yrs.	70-74 Yrs.	75-79 Yrs.	80-84 Yrs.	85-89 Yrs.	Total.	Mean thickness of the Cataract.
5.5-6.0		1	1			1		2		1				6=2%	
6.5-7		5	4	7	10	13	23	21	14	11	2			110=22%	
7.5-8		3	2	4	16	38	47	71	76	35	21	5	5	320=64%	3 mm.
8.5-9					3	2		6	15	12	5				
In the capsule						3	2	1	3	3	5	2	2	64 12.8%	4 mm.

· Hirschberg (quoted above) states, "In order to attain good results in cataract extraction, three things are necessary; care before the operation, care during the operation, care after the operation. The two greatest attainments of modern surgery, namely, anaesthesia and antisepsis (new, asepsis), have not failed to bear fruit in opthalmology."

The patient should never be operated on the day of his admission to the hospital. One day of preparation is sufficient; to wait longer, causes the patient to become impatient, and this is detrimental.

The day previous to operation the patient receives a dose of oleum ricini (or some other luxative) and in the evening a light repast. The day of the operation, three hours previous to the same, a cup of coffee (or milk) without bread; and, subsequent to the operation, during the first few days, a bland diet which does not require much mastication and produces but little faecal matter; hence, during the first four or five days during which the patient is confined to bed, there is seldom a desire to empty the rectum. Finally, the evening previous to the operation, the patient receives a luke-warm bath, especial attention being given to a thorough washing of the head.

The operation is to be done in a well-lighted room, the best light being the north light.

The operator's hands are to be thoroughly washed with soap and water, washed in sublimate 1:1000 and alcohol, and the finger nails cleaned with nail brush and file.

The instruments are to be tested by the operator himself. All instruments which enter the eye must be made thoroughly aseptic. *Boiling water destroys the pus-formers*, so that instruments which are kept clean may be considered sterile, after being placed in boiling water for one-half to one minute. All glass or porcelain utensils are to be previously cleansed in a 1:1000 sublimate sol. All glasses, dishes and droppers are previously placed in a 1:1000 sublimate sol., and prepared fresh for each patient, and just previous to the operation are washed out in a warm 1:5000 sublimate sol. The three fluids (absolute alcohol, 96½ per cent.; sublimate water, 1:1000, and sublimate water, 1:5000) are kept in well-stopped bottles. A small bottle of a 5 per cent. cocaine sol. is prepared fresh, just prior to the operation.

The operations are always done early in the morning, for to do such delicate operating the operator should feel fresh. Knapp,[3a] however, believes it better for the patient to be operated in the afternoon, because the usual five or six hours of smarting will then be followed by an undisturbed sleep, during which the union of the wound has the best chance to take place and become permanent.

With a sterilized dropper, at intervals of five minutes cocaine is dropped into the eye three or four times. (When the iridectomie is made, four times is sufficient; the touching of the iris with the forceps will scarcely be felt).

During the intervals in which the cocaine is being dropped into the eye, the lids should remain closed. Immediately after the last drop has been dropped into the eye, the lids and conjunctiva are to be carefully washed with absorbent cotton and fresh sublimate water, and then dried. The patient is then placed horizontally on the operating table, with the head slightly raised. An assistant holds the head, his one hand on the temple on the side opposite the operator, and the other on the forehead. (A nurse usually holds the patient's hands.)

The eye which is to be operated, is placed toward the window. The operator, who always operates with his right hand, sits behind the patient when operating the right eye, and in front of the patient when operating his left.

A short speculum, one which separates the lids widely and keeps them at a good distance from the eye, but which opens and closes easily, is then introduced; the screw, however, should never be closed, so that it may be removed quickly by a single movement at any time; and which, as a rule, is done immediately after cystotomie, and in exceptional cases where the patient presses very hard, even before the iridectomie.

With the left hand, the operator now takes a short pair of fixation forceps with a spring to close them, and with these grasps a fold of the ocular conjunctiva just below the horizontal meridian. In his right hand he takes his cataract knife, which is 1½ mm. in width; this is delicately held, like a pen, the cutting edge naturally upward, toward the upper corneal margin.

[3a] Norris and Oliver System of Diseases of Eye. Vol. III, p. 797.

In this manner, the anterior chamber is punctured, s) that the back of the knife separates one-third of the corneal circumference. (The pulling downward of the eyeball by means of the fixation forceps, as well as the pointing of the knife toward the centre of the pupil, as advised by Von Graefe, are unnecessary, and, if anything, detrimental.) The cocainized eye is completely tolerant to the fixation forceps, so that one may at once make puncture with the cataract knife. The practiced eye will at once see at a glance whether the width of the pupil is equal to one-fourth or one-third of the height of the cornea, (3 or 4 mm.); hence, whether the edge of the knife should be tangent to the upper edge of the pupil or a mm. below this; and along this line the knife reaches the symmetrical point opposite to that of its entrance into the anterior chamber, in order to gain the correct point of contra-puncture; the handle of the knife is depressed slightly toward the temple, and then the point of the knife is pushed forward a few milometres. The handle of the knife is then made to make a quarter turn on its axis, so that the cutting edge comes against the posterior surface of the cornea, and then, by means of a slight sawing motion, the corneal incision is completed, the line of the incision falling close to the limbus.

The assistant, who sits or stands on the opposite side of the operator, takes the fixation forceps out of the operator's hand from beneath the operator's hand, and holds them. The operator lays his cataract knife on the porcelain plate at his side, and takes up the curved iris forceps with his left hand, the scissors with his right. (The instruments are often handed to the operator by an assistant). The iris almost never prolapses, but in the exceptional cases it is first carefully replaced, after waiting a few moments to see if it does not do so itself. The curved iris forceps is then introduced, *closed*, at the centre of the incision in a radial direction, and opened a few milometres from the edge of the sphincter; and iris fold is grasped, withdrawn, and cut off by a single clip of the scissors. Since the introduction of cocaine, bleeding from the iris almost never occurs; the incision in the globe likewise never bleeds, since it is made entirely in the cornea, and the conjunctival flap given up. As a rule, the coloboma is small, with converging or parallel edges; its definite form, however, is dependent on the exit of the lens.

The assistant now carefully opens the spring on the fixation forceps; at the same time, the speculum is gently closed, and while the patient is being told to slowly look downward, these are also removed. The assistant now gently holds the lids apart, far enough to expose the entire cornea. Thereupon, the operator again clasps the ocular conjunctiva exactly the vertical meridian, with a pair of forceps held in the left hand, while in his right hand he takes the cystitome (the hook of which is longer and sharper than in the original Graefe model, whereas the straight portion is shorter). With this, a T-shaped incision is made in the capsule; the horizontal portion first, and this is made to lie in the coloboma. Finally, the operator reverses the instrument, and with the convex surface of the rubber spoon (or metal), makes gentle pressure on the external lower portion of the cornea, whereupon the lens rises up, during which time the spoon slowly follows, until the lens is totally delivered. The patient is told to close his eyes, and the operation is practically completed.

Where the operation is made without the iridectomy, Knapp lays particular stress on the manner in which the capsule is to be opened. He says: "The cystotome so advances that the tip goes underneath the upper part of the iris, turns it, and with the tooth makes the incision into the upper part of the capsule, parallel with with the corneal section, about 6.7 mm. in extent. As soon as the capsule is opened, the lens makes a visible forward motion. Then the cystotome is withdrawn again with the knee forward, so that the point does not injure the iris." [a]

Today the operation requires scarcely as much time as it does to read its description; less than one minute, when the preparatory iridectomie has been made; less than two minutes for the complete operation.

The operator holds a small pledget of cotton, which has been dipped in sublimate water, for a few moments over the patient's eyelids, and then the patient looking downward, by slight pressure on the lower lid, which pressure is transmitted to the cornea, the cortical remains are removed. This gentle massage also aids in replacing the iris in its proper position. After the cystotomie, the entrance of any instrument into the eye should be avoided. True, one should always have the blunt spatula and the Weber's Loop close at hand on the porcelain dish, but they seldom are called into use. A small pair of scissors should also be at hand to enlarge the wound, if the contra-puncture should happen to be too far in the cornea; and if, on gentle pressure with the spoon, the lens does not present itself. After the operation, the wound which should coapt well, be smooth and free from coagula, is irrigated with a sublimate sol. 1:5000; likewise, the entire conjunctival sac. The eye is then covered with an aseptic dressing, and, together with the non-operated eye, is bound up.[b]

The after treatment is very simple. The after pains are very slight since the use of cocaine, and especially where mild antiseptics are used. The first dressing is removed at the end of twenty-four hours. During the

---

[a] System of Diseases of Eye. Norris & Oliver. Vol. 3. p. 798.

[b] Modern operators apply a simple broad dressing, held in place by strips of court-plaster.

first and second days, a dose of chloral hydrate is given, and the nurse is especially watchful. The bandage is renewed each day until the twelfth day, but the patient is not permitted to touch the eye.

At each removal of the dressing, the lids are first gently washed with pledgets of cotton dipped in sublimate water. Atropine is not used before the first day, and, in fact, only then when there are cortical remains or irritability of the iris."

"Reaction seldom follows. The two principal forms are iritis, due to swelling up of cortical remains, and septic infection, which nearly always leads to destruction of the operated eye, and can but seldom be stayed."

"THE LINEAR EXTRACTION is only adapted to soft and fluid cataracts in young persons. Here the incision is made with a broad lance-shaped iridectomie knife; either in the outer horizontal or the lower outer quadrant. The knife penetrates about 4 mm. from the corneal margin, and is pressed forward in the plane of the iris, until the corneal incision has attained a width of 6 or 7 mm. The point of the knife being now laid close to the posterior surface of the cornea—in order that no injury may be done to the iris or lens, when the aqueous humour commences to flow off—the instrument is very slowly withdrawn, so that the aqueous humour may come away gradually without causing prolapse of the iris. In withdrawing the knife, it is well to enlarge the inner aspect of one or the other end of the wound, by suitable motion of the instrument in that direction.

The knife being now put aside, the cystitome is passed into the anterior chamber as far as the opposite pupillary margin, care being taken, by keeping the sharp point of the instrument directed either up or down, not to entangle it in the wound or in the iris. The point is now turned directly on the anterior capsule, and by withdrawing the cystotome toward the corneal incision, an opening in the capsule of the width of the pupil is produced. The cystotome is then removed from the anterior chamber with the same precaution as on its entrance.

The edge of the spoon is then placed on the outer lip of the corneal incision, and the latter is made to gape somewhat, gentle pressure being at the same time applied to the inner aspect of the eye by the fixation forceps and in this way the lens is evacuated. When the pupil has become quite black, the operation is concluded. If pressure does not at first clear the pupil completely, the speculum should be removed, the eyelids closed, a compress applied, and a few minutes allowed to elapse, in order that some aqueous be secreted. A renewal of the effort to clear the pupil will probably now be successful; if not, another pause may be made, and then fresh attempts employed, until the pupil is quite clear. It is unwise to insert the spoon into the eye to withdraw the fragments; and, if some of these should be left behind,. no ill results need necessarily follow, although iritis is more apt to supervene than if the lens be thoroughly evacuated. Fragments left behind become absorbed. If there be a prolapse of the iris which can not be reposed, it must be abscised." (Swanzy, p. 336.)

This same operation is applicable to *membranous cataracts*, with a sharp-pointed hook or forceps, which is passed through the wound; the membrane is grasped and withdrawn. The advantages of this incision consist in its relatively small size, and the readiness with which it closes. No iridectomie is necessary. But, owing to the size of the corneal incision, this operation is only applicable to the membranous and soft cataracts; that is, in those which do not possess a nucleus.

By increasing the size of this original linear incision, moving it back farther, and making it above and combining it with an iridectomie, Von Graefe originated his *peripheral linear incision*. But this incision was often too small, so that Jacobson moved it still further back into the sclera. He, however, abandoned the linear incision, and made a flap incision and the iridectomie.

Graefe made his opening in the capsule with the cystitome, others with a discission needle or a small, sharp hook. A decided improvement has been the introduction of the *capsular forceps*. By means of this instrument, not only is the capsule opened, but a piece of the anterior capsule is withdrawn from the eye. This prevents a rapid closure of the capsule and permits of a greater resorption of retained lens substance. This procedure has lessened the number of secondary cataracts. It has, however, one objectionable feature; namely, it is possible, in tearing the capsule, that the rent will be too extensive, extend too far into the equatorial region, even into the posterior capsule, and thus produce conditions favorable to prolapse of the vitreous.

During the sitting of the Seventh International Opthalmological Congress, held at Heidelberg, in 1888, Schweigger wrote the following sentence on the blackboard: "The bad results are not dependent on the position or the size of the incision." Since the application of antiseptic and *aseptic* methods to eye surgery, most of the complications occurring subsequent to a cataract extraction have ceased to exist; namely, the whole train of diseases due to septic infection. It seems rather a sad commentary that all the efforts of Von Graefe and his school should have passed away and have been set aside. Still, to him remains the credit of having greatly reduced the percentage of losses in the pre-antiseptic days.

In considering the changes which the lens undergoes during an extraction, we must differentiate between those of the capsule, of the intracapsular cells, and of the true lens substance. The size of the wound in the capsule has but an indirect influence on the process of healing. This membrane, aside from rolling and folding itself up, remains perfectly indifferent to the changes in its vicinity. The intracapsular cells, the so-called single layers of epithelial cells which line the inner surface of the anterior capsule, as also the cellular structures along the equator, on opening of the capsule and extrusion of the lens, are disturbed in their regular continuity and brought in contact with a heretofore foreign fluid. The manner in which they react has already been considered under "Secondary Cataract" and the "Crystalline Pearl."

Only exceptionally is the lens removed in its entirety. As to what will remain in the capsule depends largely on the consistence of the cataract. Everything of which the lens is made up may be found—normal lens fibres, whole or broken cataractous lens fibres, myelin globules, fat, cholestearine crystals, and lime salts; all of which are incapable of further development, hence they act as a foreign body. As we have seen, the lens fibres possess the peculiar quality of swelling up to an enormous size, so that their presence may greatly endanger the further existence of the eye. Aside from this, not infrequently after an operation, this capsular epithelium begins to undergo a hyperplasia, and then take an active part in the formation of the secondary cataract and the crystalline pearl.

If the extraction is made so as to remove the *lens in its capsule* from the eye, as Sharp and Mohrenheim attempted to do, and as Pagenstecher did, the injury will be of a different character. The lens (like an amputated member of the eye) can no longer enter into the consideration of the processes of healing; one must, however, not forget, that the lens could not have escaped from the eye without tearing every single fibre of the zonula zinii. This operation has been practiced by Beer, Richter, Sperino Macnamara and Andrews. (Uber Staar Extractionen mit und ohne Entfernung der Kapsel von Herman Pagenstecher, Graefe, Arch., Vol. XXXIV., B. 2, 1888).

After completing the corneal incision, owing to the evacuation of the aqueous and the loss of the greater portion of the contents of the capsule, or of the lens, together with its capsule, the globe loses from $\frac{1}{17}$ to $\frac{1}{14}$ of its volume. Notwithstanding this, as a rule the eye does not become lessened in size, nor does it collapse. By what means is this prevented? It is evident that, whereas in the beginning, aqueous, iris, lens, and vitreous fill out the space, after the operation, this same space is simply occupied by iris and vitreous, where formerly was aqueous and lens. The change of position to which these parts must be subjected, must be considerable. The iris moves forward the depth of the anterior chamber, equal to a distance of three-quarters of a mm. The fossa patellaris, which is still separated from the anterior chamber by the posterior capsule, moves forward ⅛ mm. Such a great transposition of the individual structures can not possibly take place without materially drawing on the structural elements of the iris and *corpus, ciliare,* and, more especially, on the nerves which traverse them. But it is impossible for the vitreous to move forward without the space which it vacates becoming filled in some other way.

In eyes in which the coats are still elastic, these will contract and reduce the volume to a degree equal to the previous tension of the globe. By this means, the most essential portion is compensated for. Hence it follows that where the sclera has lost its elasticity, the cornea becomes wrinkled; or, owing to atmospheric pressure, is pressed, funnel-like, inward.

This, however, is not the only compensation. When the aqueous is evacuated, and, still more so, on evacuation of the lens, the pressure of the blood vessels in the eye must be reduced, to a degree proportionate to that which they were under before the above parts were pressed out, and dependent on the tension of the eye itself. Hence, just at this moment there must take place a sudden and great dilation of all the blood vessels in the eye. It has been a well-known fact for a long time, that in cases in which there existed a pathological increase of intra-ocular pressure, the sudden reduction of this pressure, on opening the anterior chamber, has not infrequently led to the occurrence of hemorrhages into the interior of the eye. In a case, in which I (Becker) punctured the anterior chamber for an embolus of the arteria retinae centralis, with the hope of thereby causing the embolus to change its position, I observed the occurrence of innumerable retinal ecchymoses, though the intra-ocular pressure had previously not been increased. Hence there appears to be no doubt, but that retinal hemorrhages may occur when an extraction is made

From opthalmoscopic examination, we know that where the intra-ocular pressure is reduced, on the use of atropine, hyperaemia of the retina and choroid does take place, together with a dilation of the blood vessels. In favorable cases, one may observe this hyperaemia with the naked eye, by simply watching the change in color which a slightly pigmented iris assumes during an extraction. Finally, Iwanoff's experiments have proven it to be not at all improbable that even in cases of normal extraction, probably during the same, a detachment of the vitreous takes place, so that when the vitreous moves forward a vacuum is produced at the posterior pole, if this is not prevented by an instantaneous transudation. That which has so far been described, can and must occur when an extraction is made, even though an eye speculum is not used, non-fixation of the eye practiced, when a lens is removed, and no special maneuvers are required to bring this about.

Though the greatest care is exercised in inserting and removing the speculum, we do not always succeed in avoiding injury of the cornea. If attention were only directed to this point, frequently after cataract extraction, extensive loss of epithelium would be found. Owing to the great importance which such epithelial losses assume, where infectuous conjunctival secretion is present, it certainly ought to receive the most serious attention.

The iris may be involved in a variety of ways. In every case, the moment the aqueous is evacuated it contracts spasmodically, so that where the pupil is forcibly distended by the passage of the cataract, it must suffer a very considerable bruising and transposition, and not infrequently we find iris pigment adherent to the extracted cataract. Even where the operation proceeds in a perfectly normal manner, the iris is easily pressed into the wound, and then either draws itself back by means of contraction of the sphincter, or the sphincter must be irritated to contract by means of rubbing the lids; or, finally, the iris must be returned to its normal position by means of instruments.

It is entirely irrelevant whether or not we grasp the conjunctiva bulbi alone or together with the tendon of the rectus inferior, in order to fix the eye. Notwithstanding this, not seldom a demonstratable injury is produced. Even where the fixation forceps are used with the greatest care, for days afterward, the points where they grasp the conjunctiva are marked by a suffusion. If the teeth of the forceps are very sharp, and the conjunctiva (as it frequently is in old people) friable, this will lead to hemorrhage, and even to tearing of the tissues. Later on, it will be shown how the sudden occurrence of ciliary injection on fixation may be utilized in determining, whether one should risk or put off the extraction in a case in which cyclitis had supervened after traumatic cataract. In such cases, the simple fixation, in eyes which were previously pale, is sufficient to bring on ciliary injection, and proves that this grasping of the conjunctiva with the forceps, is not such an innocent procedure as one is wont to suppose. (S. Liebreich, 1219).

That which has just been said becomes of even greater importance when the fixation is continued after the eyeball has been opened, and even more so when the operator, after making the corneal incision, in order to be able to excise the iris, leaves the fixation forceps in charge of his assistants, and later again takes charge of them. Since the eye involuntarily rolls upward, a certain amount of force must necessarily be exerted in order to bring the wound into an accessible position. Even in the hands of the most expert operators the tension between the point of fixation and the corneal wound is undoubtedly greater where the closed forceps hanging to the eye is handed over to an assistant. In such cases the cornea will gap wide open, and even fold itself vertically. Just such traction on the cornea, the corpus ciliare and iris becomes the most detrimental factor of an extraction. Depending on the degree to which this second pernicious occurrence is avoided will be found the secret of the great differences in the results of the various skilled operators. Every method and every suggestion which will aid us in lessening this portion of the operative procedure is deserving of the most earnest consideration. Hence, one should choose a pair of forceps which are not too sharp, rather, do not clamp at all, or can be opened every few moments. One should not transfer them closed from one hand to the other, but rather fix them anew, or if it is possible, complete the operation after the corneal incision without fixation. This becomes easier where the operation is made without an iridectomie, or where this has been made in advance of the extraction.

These suggestions were made before the introduction of cocaine, since which time the operation has become a painless one, and the patient can greatly assist the operator by carrying out his orders. Many operators do not fix the eye at all during the iridectomie, but simply tell the patient to look down. Probably the only twitch of pain occurs at the moment the section of iris is being excised.

All pressure on the globe, or displacement of same by means of the lids or instruments, which has as its object the removal of the lens or its remains, is to be looked upon as a part of the general injury. Both may become necessary in perfectly normal operations. Aside from the creasing of the cornea, and the pushing apart of the edges of the wound, the *corpus ciliare* must necessarily suffer.

Finally, the introduction of air into the anterior chamber or the escape of blood may complicate and influence the processes of healing, even where the entire operation was otherwise normally completed. Beer put particular weight on the first-mentioned condition, whereas under normal conditions both blood and air are rapidly absorbed. Nevertheless, such occurrences always call forth a special amount of resistance to injury in such an eye immediately after the operation.

Cataract extraction is not always made without the occurrence of so-called unlucky accidents. These necessarily must exert an influence on the healing process.

I. Aside from an *infection*, the *corneal wound* may be too large or too small. An incision which is too large when the flap extraction is practiced either removes more than half of the base, or at some point approaches too closely to the ciliary body, if it does not strike it either in the middle of the incision, or at the point of exit. In the latter cases, a cyclitis is the unavoidable consequence. The incision can only be too small, relatively speaking, as compared with the size of the cataract. In consequence, the removal of the cataract is made more difficult, and in fact can not be removed without bruising very materially the edges of the wound. In these cases an unnecessary amount of cataractous substance remains behind and can only be removed by resorting to all kinds of maneuvers. In order to deliver the lens, it is necessary to employ a high degree of pressure, and hence the danger of prolapse of the vitreous is correspondingly increased.

II. A PROLAPSUS IRIDIS, occurring during a flap operation, may be cut off, and thus the formation of a staphyloma averted. But it is not always possible to prevent the iris from cicatrizing in the wound in any form of extraction. Even where, at the close of an operation, the iris is left in its normal position, it may, later on, where the wound opens again and the aqueous is evacuated, be washed from its position into the wound and become fixed there.

III. INCARCERATION OF A TAG OF THE CAPSULE. A tag of the capsule may be dragged into the wound by the cystotome, iris forceps, or at the time the lens is delivered. This, owing to its transparency, is apt to be overlooked, and subsequently be the starting point of a series of troubles. It may give rise to cystoid cicatrization, and, as Wagenman has shown, to microscopical fistulous openings, which can give entrance to micro-organisms and the whole trains of symptoms which these produce, even to sympathetic opthalmia. These cystoid cicatrices lead to irregularities of the corneal curvature and consequent irregular astygmatism.

Where simply the iris is incarcerated, the pupil will gradually be drawn to the upper sclero-corneo margin; whereas, if the capsule is involved, irido-cyclitis may be produced. Even glaucoma may supervene, as a result of closure of the filtrating angle.

IV. It is not always possible to completely remove all the visible *remains of a cataract*. From the earliest times, the swelling up of these remains has been looked upon as one of the most detrimental occurrences to a normal process of healing.

V. THE PROLAPSE OF THE VITREOUS is to be looked upon as one of the most important complications of the operative procedure. This may occur before the extraction of the lens, at the same time, or following its removal. The first can only occur, if the operation is not done too roughly, where the vitreous has become fluid, the zonula zinii previously become partially dissolved, and the lens luxated before the operation. It may, however, also be the result of a luxation of the lens, caused by improper use of the cystotome, and the exercise of too much pressure while delivering the lens. The escape of vitreous, together with the lens, or following its delivery, can be avoided by exercising a little care; or it is to be considered as a truly unfortunate circumstance where it follows as the result of a strong muscular contraction on the part of the patient. The escape of vitreous, previous to the delivery of the lens, since it necessitates our going into the eye with instruments, is to be looked upon as a very severe complication.

Ever since the introduction of Daviel's method, the escape of vitreous, as a novel occurrence during cataract extraction, has naturally excited the attention of operators (it even occurred to Daviel and he mentioned it), and has therefore, since that time, been frequently and almost constantly under discussion. It appears that poor results were frequently blamed on this occurrence, and thus sought to be excused. But the most renowned operators, such as Wenzel and especially Beer, opposed this view. The latter even went so far as to declare that one-third of the vitreous might be lost without affecting the favorable result of the case. Even at the present time this question has not been definitely settled. With the introduction of Graefe's scleral extraction, this question again stepped to the front. Von Graefe in his various publications always stated to how great a degree he had reduced the percentage of losses of vitreous. Arlt seems to have followed the proper course (III 1, p. 277), in that he based his prognosis on the cause of the prolapse of vitreous. The prognosis seems to be more favorable, where there has existed a previous fluidity of the vitreous or luxation of the lens, than where, owing to a mistake or an unfortunate circumstance during the operation, vitreous of a normal consistence is lost. In these cases it is more apt to lie in the wound, prevent perfect closure, and since it extends into the conjunctival sac, where this is not perfectly free from pathogenic germs, become infected. The vitreous is one of the best soils known for the growth of micro-organisms, and where the vitreous once becomes infected the fate of the eye is sealed; panopthalmitis is sure to follow, and sympathetic opthalmia is not an unheard-of occurrence.

VI. As a rare occurrence during extraction, *intra-ocular hemorrhages* do occur, even in the simple Daviel method. This, it appears, was first described by Wenzel in 1779. Beer states that he is acquainted with such cases, and says that he only operates such patients at their earnest solicitation, and then only in the presence of witnesses. However, it is not clear how he could foretell the occurrence of such hemorrhages. Arlt was of the opinion that this occurrence could be prevented, if we would refuse to operate an eye, which showed any evidence of increased intra-ocular tension, without having made an iridectomie at least one week in advance. *The cause of such a hemorrhage might, however, be found in the condition of the blood vessel walls.*

Becker states that in 1864 he was a witness to an operation which Arlt made on an amaurotic eye, in which he extracted a calcareous lens which had fallen into the anterior chamber. Immediately on completion of the corneal incision, an enormous hemorrhage took place from the interior of the eye, so that the blood trickled from the corneal wound. It did not come from the iris, but rather from the *corpus ciliare*, from the *retina* or *choroid*, for after the hemorrhage was controlled, one could see a clot protruding from the pupil. In the following few days, this hemorrhage repeated itself, and caused the corneal wounds to reopen again. The eye, however, was saved, and retained its form. This case was a particularly interesting one, because the patient had a very extensive flat teleangiektasie on the whole half of the face. Hence, it is to be presumed that the blood vessels in the eye were likewise varicose.

There are but few cases reported in literature in which, during the operation or immediately following it, an extensive hemorrhage took place from the choroid, and thus instantly and forever destroyed the function of the eye; possibly this is due to the fact that but few men care to report their poor results. As has, however, been personally communicated to me by a colleague, and who by the way is a very busy man, this does occur. He operated an aged physician for cataract, who since early youth had been myopic to a high degree. Immediately following the delivery of the lens, which took place without the occurrence of any mishap, the vitreous, accompanied by a dazzling sensation and violent pain, was extruded through the wound as a globule. The hyaloidea did not rupture, though blood did not escape from the eye, it could be seen through the vitreous. At the same time the eye became as hard as stone, and the sensation to light was instantly abolished. The protruding vitreous was cut off. Phthisis bulbi followed without a corneal ulceration. *Even in such cases the cause of the hemorrhage is no doubt due to a diseased condition of the vessel walls of the choroid.*

Dr. J. A. Spaulding [4] reported such a case, together with a very complete literary review of this subject, but has evidently overlooked the above remarks of Becker, which appeared almost twenty years ago. Practically, his statements agree with those of Becker. He states, "In conclusion, it would seem that hemorrhage from the choroid after extraction, and occasionally after iridectomie, is by no means so rare a complication as one would think. Numerous cases have been reported, and there can hardly be a doubt that many remain unpublished in the dread of publishing what may seem to be a badly performed operation. But where we read the names of the surgeons to whom the accident has occurred, it is plain that the misfortune is due solely to a diathesis of the patient. This being once established, we shall probably hear in the future of many more interesting cases of the sort. The chief cause is undoubtedly atheromatous condition of the vessels, and an abnormal tension of the eyeball suddenly reduced by the incision in the cornea and the outflow of aqueous. When it occurs, the best treatment is to raise the patient's head; to relieve the pain, and to watch the eye carefully, prepared to perform enucleation at the soonest possible moment. Where the accident has occurred in one eye, it is likely to occur in the other, and pressure on the carotids and ergotine is indicated. It does not appear that extraction with iridectomy is more frequently followed by choroidal hemorrhage than simple extraction. The accident can not be foreseen, but may be looked for with increased tension; also in the decrepid and those advanced in years." In this same paper he reports the statement of Da Gama Pinto (Revue de General d'Opth., 1884, p. 97), who witnessed two such occurrences in Becker's clinic.

---

[4] A case of Choroidal Hemorrhage following Extraction. Archives of Opthalmology, January, 1896, p. 92.

Sattler [a] has drawn attention to the fact that the largest number of cases of retro-choroidal hemorrhage have been reported since cocain has come into use. He has attempted to explain this by the assumption, that after the effect of the cocaine, which causes contraction of the vessels, has worn off, an excessive dilatation follows, which in cases where a predisposition exists, is followed by rupture.

In a recent publication, Salina Bloom [b] critically analyzes all the views held as to the cause of this baneful occurrence. In succession are set aside as causes, the loss of vitreous, separation of choroid from sclera, predisposition to hemorrhage, sudden reduction of intra-ocular pressure and its effect on arterial vessels, arterio-sclerosis, increase of arterial blood pressure, as result of psychic excitement, vomiting, coughing, etc., condition of posterior ciliary arteries. "Anatomical examination has shown that the hemorrhage is always *intra-choroidal*, and that the predisposing cause is a *phlebitis or peri-phlebitis of the choroidal veins*. Depending on the degree and stage of this inflammatory process, and the time when the intra-vascular pressure occurs, it is evident why this deplorable disaster may take place in persons apparently healthy—may occur in one eye and not the other."

VII. HEMORRHAGES WHICH ARE RESTRICTED TO THE ANTERIOR CHAMBER have an entirely different significance. As a rule, they only occur where an iridectomie is made at the time of the extraction. They occur, however, more seldom than one would imagine. One must rather wonder, that on making such an extensive wound in the iris, that there is not always sufficient blood lost to make it perceptible to the naked eye.

The causes here are the same as where a simple iridectomie is made. Just as we observe that there, where the instantaneous contraction of the blood vessels at the surface of a wound prevents a large escape of blood, likewise here, if the iris is healthy and moves so far forward as to touch the posterior surface of the cornea. But if the globe has suffered in its elasticity, so that a reduction of pressure exists in the anterior chamber, this may become filled with air or blood. As a rule the blood comes from the vessels of the iris. But the simultaneous presence of air would lead one to believe that the blood had been aspirated from the conjunctiva, and is derived from the conjunctival vessels cut during the operation. Such a hemorrhage may greatly increase the difficulties of the completion of the extraction, because one is not always successful in removing the blood. The operator finds himself necessitated to open the capsule and deliver the lens, so to say, in the dark. The presence of blood in the anterior chamber does not, however, prejudice the prognosis for the worse.

[a] Beriche uber die 25th Versamulung der Opthalmogischen Congress in Heidelberg, 1896, p. 211.

[b] Uber die Retro-choroidealblutung nach Staar extraction. Graef Arch., Vol. XLVI, Part, I, p. 184. 1898.

The same may be said of the presence of air bubbles in the anterior chamber. Only theoretical considerations could have lead so experienced a practitioner as Beer to take the position that the mere contact of the iris with air is to be looked upon as dangerous.

Finally, one must draw attention to the influence which is exerted on the entire surgical procedure by the insertion of instruments into the eye, especially such as are used for pulling or exerting tension.

Since the use of sterile instruments the fears which formerly existed in the minds of even the best operators, regarding the evil effects of the introduction of instruments into the interior of the eye, such as the mere entrance of a cataract knife, the use of the cystotome or the entrance of the iris forceps, are of but historical interest.

It is interesting to note. however, that in the sixties Luer (the instrument maker) advised that a cataract knife should never be used immediately after testing it on the drum leather. He believed that some deleterious matter contained in the alum tanned leather might cling to the knife, and thus be brought into the eye.

Attention was also drawn to fine threads of linen which might be carried into the eye by the iris forceps or cystitome. Hence, all instruments should be held up to the light and carefully examined before using them, to see that no linen threads derived from the cloth on which the instruments are wiped, are not still adherent.

The dangers are greatly increased where one is necessitated to deliver the lens, by getting in behind it with some variety of spoon, Weber's loop or hook (Pagenstecher). It is more apt to occur, since where it is indicated there is already a *prolapsus corporis vitrei*, and it is impossible to avoid destruction of the vitreous, bruizing of the iris, and rough contact with the posterior surface of the cornea. If by simply using the cystotome or iris forceps we are apt to produce a traumatic irritation of the endothelium of the descemetis, how much greater must be this injury where the lens is pressed against the descemetis by a constant pressure from behind the lens.

Irrigation of the anterior chamber, or intra-capsular injection, is a method which has been practiced by various operators. But it does not appear to be entirely free from danger. In an exceedingly interesting paper on this subject Dr. Hugo Magnus [5] gives us a complete historical review of this subject. He tells us that the ancients considered the aqueous as the only nutritive fluid of the eye that once lost it could not be renewed, and that its loss was followed by blindness. This theory was in vogue until the seventeenth century, when it was refuted by Haller,[6] who reviewed all the ancient history. St. Yves was the first to practice irrigation. It was not only used after cataract extraction to remove cortical re-

[5] Zur Historischen Kentniss der Voder Kammer Auswashungen. Graef Arch., XXXIV, Vol. 2, 1888.

[6] Elementa Physiologiae Corporis Humani. Lausanne, 1763, Tom. V.

mains, but to remove inflammatory products in the anterior chamber, and also to press the cornea back into shape, and give it its former curvature after it had collapsed subsequent to an extraction. Its application to cataract dates back to the latter part of the eighteenth century. In the beginning an ordinary syringe was used, and a stream of water forced into the anterior chamber. Florenze was the first to attempt to improve this method.[7] He used an Anel's Syringe. Mannoir and St. Yves simply put luke-warm water in the conjunctiva, held the wound open, and allowed the fluid to enter the anterior chamber. Cassamanta tells us how Feller[8] washed out the anterior chamber with water and spiritus after cataract extraction. Beer, however, who lived in the early part of the nineteenth century, does not mention this method. It was again recommended by B. Benedict.[9] Pauli[10] considers this procedure "an insult to the eye," and Himly[11] calls it "poor practice." This method was dropped during the middle half of the century, and has been totally ignored by the greatest authorities. It has, however, been recommended by McKeown,[12] Wiecherkiewiez and Pannas.[13] Pannas claims that "strict aseptic practice has set the dangers of this method aside," and after removing all blood, pigment, capsular shreds and air from the anterior chamber, he washes out the anterior chamber with a 0.005 per cent. solution of biniodide of mercury. This method, however, has not found general favor, and is but seldom practiced.

Sterile 1-10.000 sublimate solution of atropine or eserine are well borne in the eye.

THE RESULTS OF CLINICAL OBSERVATION. Beer laid down the rule that nature alone would heal simple wounds made with a clean, sharp knife more quickly and more securely than with the assistance of the surgeon; hence, he criticized every ingenious effort made to assist the healing of a corneal wound. All the surgeon has to do is to remove every obstacle in the way of a normal process of healing.

---

7 Observations sur une Cataracte, etc. Actes de la Societe de Medicine Chirurgie et Pharmacie etablie a Brussels. Tom Primier Deuxiene Partie, p. 11. Brussels, 1799.

8 De Methodis suffusionem oculorum curandi a Cassamata et Simoni cultis. Lipsiae, 1782.

9 Handbuch der Praktische Augenheilkunde. Leipsig, 1824. B. 4, p. 231.

10 Uber den Grauen Star, etc. Stuttgart, 1824. p. 137.

11 Die Krankheiten und Missbildungen des Auges und derer Heilung. Zweiter Theil, Berlin, 1843, p. 280.

12 British Medical Journal. January 28, 1888.

13 Des Denier progres realises dans operation de la cataract par extraction, January 5-11, 1886.

In all that has been previously stated, the endeavor has been made to demonstrate that the extraction does not consist solely of a corneal wound, but that even in the most favorable cases in which, after an extraction, no signs of reaction set in, this simply goes to show that under certain conditions; absolute cleanliness, rest, absence of light, and all external pernicious influences; even so complicated an injury will heal.

Naturally, as long as the eyes were kept bandaged for days, the external phenomena which are the result of the process of healing could not be observed. Beer, who in the beginning only removed the bandage on the eighth day, finally shortened the time to four days. After his time the old custom again came into use, and though Arlt and Von Graefe gradually returned to five days, and even three days, they both for a long time warned against doing this earlier than the third day. Jacobson was the first who had the courage to overcome this prejudice, for he not only removed the bandage at the end of the first day, but even from that time on did so every twelve hours, and by focal illumination examined the surface of the wound. As a result of his observations and those of others we have finally gained a knowledge of those changes which can be observed with the naked eye, and which take place in cases where everything progresses in a perfectly normal manner. It must, however, be stated that Bowman had previously very carefully studied on the living all these changes, since in his lectures (p. 28) we find a true description of all those changes which take place during the healing process of a corneal wound, and in such a way as could only have been the result of personal observation. True, ample opportunity is given to study all these processes, in cases of discission, paracentesis of the anterior chamber and simple iridectomies, and cases of non-complicated punctured and incised wounds.

a. If we examine a punctured wound of the cornea a few minutes after a discission, it will appear as a sharply-defined, grey round spot. In the course of a few hours this saturated round spot is less sharply defined externally, and gradually becomes fainter, and is lost in the surrounding tissue, usually about 1-1½ mm. from the periphery. If the wound is aseptic, no more violent reaction follows, and in the course of a few days all that will remain will be a grey spot marking the point of puncture. Its diameter will always be equal to about twice the diameter of the instrument used, and can often be found unchanged years afterward, by focal illumination.

b. Where a simple iridectomie or a simple linear extraction is made, the edges of the wound will become agglutinated more quickly, the more the line of incision falls in the radii of the circle of the corneal surface. The anterior chamber may be restored before sufficient time has elapsed to apply a dressing. In such a case, a grey line marks the site of the wound, and by the time of the evening visit this will be found to have become wider. Where no infection takes place the reaction will be extremely slight, or the edges of the wound may swell up slightly. In more severe cases a gutter-like depression may develop, the mode of healing of which will be presently described.

c. The condition of flap wounds located in the cornea has been experimentally studied by E. Neese.[14] He states that it was immaterial whether a Graefe's knife or a Beer's knife was used. In his examination, made on rabbits, he found during the first hour after the incision the epithelium sharply defined and the cut edges gaping: by the fourth hour, the epithelium in its entirety has surrounded both edges of the wound; by the tenth hour, the epithelium is found descending the edges of the wound, and by the twelfth hour it has descended half way; by the fifteenth hour, the epithelium from the two sides has come together, forming a sort of bridge, and epithelial pearls begin to develop in the depth of the wound. During the next twenty-four hours the depth of the wound fills up with epithelial cells, which gradually reach the surface.

Following an incision the various corneal lamellae contract, those only toward the center coming in close apposition, so that two triangles are formed, with their apices in apposition. As is well known, in making the incision, the plane of the same is changed, it forming either a curve or an angle, and the depth to which the epithelium will descend will depend on the height at which the plane of incision is changed. (Even a more complicated condition develops where the modified Graefe linear extraction is made.) Where the wound gaps wide open, the interspace is first filled with transudated fluid from the corneal lamellae, and exudate from the aqueous and iris, until finally a coagulated fluid closes the gap into which the cells begin to dip from above, and the processes of restitution follow. Active karyokinetic processes set in, in the epithelium, as far back as the limbus, and during the first hour the cells close to the margin of the wound are pushed down into the wound. After a time these latter cells also undergo karyokinetic changes, and this process continues until the entire wound is filled. This is but a provisional process, for after the third day a rich supply of round cells surround the wound, and the real inflammatory reaction does not follow until the fourth day, as a result of which the epithelial indipping is again pushed out by the connective tissue cells. At this time the inter-lamellar spaces are widely dilated, filled with round and spindle cells, which are looked upon as derivatives of the fixed corneal cells. These spindle cells become elongated, assume a more dense consistence, and are more closly packed together. As a result of this partial fibrous condition and contraction of the spindle

---

[14] Uber das Verhalten des Epithels bei der Heilung von Linear und Lanzen messer wunden in der Hornhaut. Graefe Arch., Vol. XXXIII, Bd. 1, 1887.

cells, a certain degree of pressure is exerted on the epithelial indipping; the lower portion is simply cut off and later on atrophies; the upper part is gradually lifted up, as the edges of the wound are brought closer together. The upper portion is raised above the general niveau, degenerates and is cast off. After three weeks it is scarcely possible to follow the entire course of the wound. In the central portion 'there is an uninterrupted continuance of lamellae, only here and there does one see obliquely arranged long drawn out fibres. Toward the surface, the membrane descemeti is wanting, and an indipping of epithelium marks the line of incision. Internally the conditions are relatively the same; Bowman's membrane does not close again.

d. Where there is a sclero-corneal wound, the conditions are more complicated, since we have here a wound of cornea, sclera and conjunctiva. The conjunctival wound soon becomes agglutinated, so that the sclero-corneal wound heals under the conjunctival flap. With perfect asceptic precautions there is scarcely any hyperaemia or swelling of the conjunctiva, and in a few days there comes into view a blueish scleral cicatrix, which, if the case progresses favorably, become paler, until finally it will no longer be discernible by the difference in color. (Jacobson.)

At both the inner and the outer segment of Jacobson's flap, to which no conjunctival flap remains attached, there at once follows a hyperaemia of all the vessels which enter the limbus, and soon this edge of the flap becomes cloudy for a distance of 2-4 mm. The cloudiness is in the neauveau of the vessels, but lies immediately beneath the epithelium. This is to be looked upon as the expression of a reaction, the result of a traumatic "Rand keratitis," which is necessary in order to bring about a proper healing of the wound. (Jacobson.)

On the corneal side, one can always detect a faint greyish infiltration, depending on the degree of irritation to which the entire eye is subjected. On focal illumination one can always discern that the corneal tissue is permeated by greyish white striations, nearly all of which are vertically arranged, extending far into the cornea. The width and the extent of these striations stand in a relative proportion to the amount of reaction. Where an iritis or an irido-cyclitis complicates the case, horizontal striations will be added, and the extent of the network so formed, and its density, will act as a gauge, by which we judge of the seriousness of the process. A cornea, however, which has become opaque in this manner may again become totally clear and transparent, and give us optically a perfectly satisfactory result.

This striated condition of the cornea subsequent to cataract extraction was formerly supposed to be due to a swelling or loosening up of the corneal tissue. Heyman believing that this was due to an injection of the normal lymph channels of the cornea. Dr. Carl Hess,[15] as the result of both clinical and experimental observations, contends that this appearance is due purely to mechanical causes. The essential anatomical changes being a folding of the deep layers of the cornea, the expression of which is found in the wavy condition of the deep layers. This folding being due to the great difference in tension between the vertical and horizontal meridian, after the incision, and in consequence of which the cornea is compressed from side to side.

"After the globe has been incised, the vertical meridian of the cornea becomes very great as compared with the horizontal, which remains almost stationary. The truth of this can be proven by the use of the keratoscope. The first few days subsequent to an operation one finds the circles elongated vertically to an astonishing degree. As a result of the difference in the corneal tension in its vertical and horizontal meridian, the cornea is compressed from side to side, and it is this pressure which in certain cases is sufficient to lead to the corneal striations, and accounts for the wavy contours of the deep layers. It would hardly seem necessary to state that in some corneae more than others, there is some peculiar condition present, which acts as a predisposing cause for the occurrence of these folds."

This striated keratitis should not be confounded with the isolated irregular greyish lines which give to the cornea an appearance very much like the irregular tears and splits in the corneal surface observed in superficial keratitis without the formation of blood vessels. These markings are not observed before the second day, and as a rule disappear in a short time, or they form the starting points for small ulcerations on the inner surface of the cornea. Jacobson believed they were due to injuries of the inner surface of the cornea, received at the time of the extraction. Attention is once more called to the erosions of the epithelium on the surface of the cornea, at the time of the operation. It is also stated that where the bandage has not been removed for a number of days, and the wound is healing without the slightest irritation, the epithelial covering along the entire extent of the flap, and even beyond it, suddenly splits up and is cast off in large shreds, only to be regenerated in the course of a few days. An aetiological impetus could not be found in the operation. This description coincides very much with that of a form of regular remitting

[15] Klinische und Experimentelle Studie uber die Entstehung der Streifen Hornhaut trubung nach Staar Extraction. Graefe Arch., Vol. XXXVIII, B. 4. 1892.

.type of painful keratitis, which, though seldom seen, may follow intermittent fever, and this was even described by the ancients; but concerning this form modern authorities are absolutely silent. (Becker states that he has never seen such a case.)

Not long after the introduction of cocain, operators began to observe a new form of, until then, unknown cloudiness of the cornea, and especially after cataract extractions, and in cases which showed no signs of irritation. This subject has given rise to a great deal of speculation, investigation and discussion. Dr. Carl Mellinger,[16] after reviewing all the literature on this subject, gives us the results of his experimental investigations, made to determine whether it is the cocain or the sublimate solution which gains access to the corneal tissue, and thus produce the cloudiness. He concludes:

"1. Sublimate solution in concentration of 1-5000 causes, where present but a short time in the anterior chamber, a passing parenchymatous cloudiness of the cornea. But if present for a length of time a more intense, or even parenchymatous cloudiness results.

"2. The cocain alone does not cause a corneal cloudiness; its presence, however, in the anterior chamber assists in bringing on the sublimate cloudiness. This is due to the fact that cocaine so affects the epithelium as to make it permeable to fluid in the anterior chamber, and thus opens the door for fluids to reach the corneal parenchyma; further, it reduces the intra-ocular tension; it seems to induce collapse of the cornea, and thus makes easier the entrance of sublimate fluid which has remained behind in the anterior chamber.

3. The passing sublimate keratitis is due to the swelling up of the lymph space system of the cornea. The endothelium being lost, the corneal tissue takes up the aqueous and sublimate solution. A permanent cloudiness follows where the sublimate comes in direct contact with the corneal parenchyma. Practically which solution is to take the place of 1-5000 sublimate has not been definitely decided. The best found is a 3 per cent. boracic acid solution, or a $\frac{1}{2}$ per cent. Na Cl solution. These have no effect on the cornea."

Not infrequently after the evacuation of the aqueous, the cornea is filled with creases, vertically arranged to the direction of the incision, or the center of the cornea becomes depressed at the site of the pupil and its immediate periphery, so that aside from the vertical folds, there will be a

16 Experimentelle Untersuchungen uber die Entstehung der in letzer zeit bekannt gewordenen trubungen der Hornhaut nach Staar Extraction. Graefe Arch., Vol. XXXVII, B. 4, 1891.

number of concentric grooves of greater or less depth. In exaggerated cases the peak of the cornea will be depressed funnel-like, so as to become the deepest point of the corneal surface, whereas the periphery is still supported by the iris. In such a case, if the lens is now removed, not only the entire cornea, beginning at the limbus, but also the iris sinks backward into the fossa patellaris.

In the less serious cases, the curvature of the cornea will be restored by the accumulation of the aqueous, without any further sequelae. The formerly depressed place will still remain visible for a few hours, owing to the increased reflex. (Jacobson.) Whereas, a complete collapse will leave for days a faint grey cloudiness, intersected by many furrows, which will correspond to the previous folds. It is not at all an infrequent occurrence that the cornea will remain depressed funnel-like for hours, and I (Becker) have observed a case where this condition persisted throughout the second day. The cornea remains deprived of its natural glossiness for several days, the cloudiness of its substance lasts longer, without the case taking an unfavorable turn. Subsequent to an injury with extensive loss of vitreous, we not infrequently meet with this condition; likewise in cases in which prolapse of the vitreous takes place during an extraction.

The cause for this greater or less degree of collapse of the cornea is not to be sought alone, in the peculiar condition of the same. The folding and collapse always occur to a greater extent where, on evacuation of the aqueous, and the removal of the lens, the space thus evacuated is not at once compensated for by an increased fullness of the vessels, and a moving forward of the vitreous. But as has already been explained, the latter can only occur where the sclerotic, owing to its inherent elasticity, is able to draw itself together to a smaller volume, and the vitreous is not obstructed in its forward movement by a pathological diaphragm, taking its origin from the ciliary body. Hence, the cornea will always sink inward, when the sclera has lost its elasticity, and becomes rigid, or where the vitreous is held fast by cyclitic bands. If the cornea is not supported from behind, it is not able to withstand the atmospheric pressure. From this collapse we can not conclude that there is a general marasmus of the eye, but rather that the sclera is rigid, or that adhesions have formed between the iris and the capsule of the lens, together with the formation of cyclitic bands.

Since the pressure of the external muscles of the eye and the orbicularis act in the same sense as does the elasticity of the sclera, they may, to a certain extent, replace the latter, and this will explain how they facilitate the pressing forward of the vitreous, the moment the anterior chamber is opened and the lens extruded; whereas, when this factor is eliminated by chloroform narcosis, we more frequently meet with a collapse of the cornea. As has already been pointed out, the same causes which lead to the collapse of the cornea, also lead to the entrance of blood and air into the anterior chamber from the conjunctival sac. The attempt has been made to explain these two occurrences by saying that they result *"ex vacuo."*

This wrinkling up and collapse of the cornea does not only occur after a flap or Graefe's extraction, but even after a simple linear extraction or an iridectomie. If one were to choose the proper case, one would find that after a paracentesis the aqueous would not escape without the application of some pressure to the eye. The difficulty experienced in removing blood from the anterior chamber is due to this lack of vis a tergo.

This view of the subject is further supported, as even Jacobson observes, by the fact that *collapsus corneae*, in all its various gradations, occur more frequently where the operation is done under chloroform narcosis. It is well known that an eye which is normally distended will become relaxed, after the mere entrance of the knife or lance, so as to very much increase the difficulties of the operation. Hence I (Becker) do not entirely agree with the views of Jacobson or Arlt.

"Frequently the view is met with, that there must be a peculiar formation of the cornea, an abnormal thinness, a senile marasmus of the same, which is the only or important cause of the *collapsus corneae*, and the attempt is often made to explain the loss of an eye as the result of a really observed or supposed collapse of the cornea. They even went so far as to declare that a tender and finely folded skin on the hands and chin would indicate a similar condition of the cornea, and owing to this condition make a bad prognosis. I will not deny that in old people the cornea may deviate from the normal and have a reduced thickness. Just as we may determine the thickness of the skin by the thinness or thickness of its creases or folds, so likewise can we observe that the thickness of the folds in the cornea vary, and hence are justified in reaching a similar conclusion, just as in respect to the skin. Becker has found by direct measurement that there may be a reduction from the normal equal to 0.25 mm. In specially selected cases, which have for a long time been subjected to increased intra-ocular tension, not only the cornea but also the sclera is thinned. As a matter of course, a thin, marasmic cornea would be less able to withstand the atmospheric pressure. Hence, when there is an abnormal cornea a collapse would naturally follow much easier. In other cases, where the surface of the cornea has its normal curvature, we do see some cases in which air enters the anterior chamber. Here undoubtedly the external and internal pressure acting on the cornea must be equal, and the bubble of air which enters the anterior chamber fills up the vacuum, and thus prevents the collapse of the cornea. It is also possible for blood instead of air to occupy this space.

"Though I do not believe that collapse of the cornea is something to be wished for, still I do believe that its dangers have been greatly overrated. It is not because the cornea is marasmic, and but poorly disposed to such activity, as is required for the formation of a cicatrix; that the collapse of the cornea is followed by such evil consequences, but one must rather look upon these folds and creases of the individual tissue elements as an additional complication of the trauma produced by the wound. That a collapse of the cornea may last for quite a long time without causing any evil results is attested by the fact that I (Becker) once observed a case in which the cornea remained depressed funnel-like for three days without the slightest sign of an iritis, and went on to perfect restitution."

ABNORMAL CONDITIONS DEVELOPED DURING THE PROCESS OF HEALING.

Clinical observation teaches us that the healing of a sclero-corneal wound may take an abnormal course in a three-fold manner, in that either the cicatrical tissue which binds together the edges of the wound gives way before the intra-ocular pressure, and in this manner brings about the so-called *cystoid cicatrix*, or the iris, or a tag of the capsule, becomes imbedded in the wound, and is held fast in the cicatrix.

a. CYSTOID CICATRIZATION. Whereas, as a rule, subsequent to a linear incision made with a lance or Graefe's knife, a narrow, dense, homogenous cicatrix follows, in exceptional cases it does occur, that the apparently reunited edges of the wound separate again from each other, and in the connective tissue which thus remains loosely connected for a long time, is developed an ectatic condition.

In the beginning the process of healing may go on so devoid of all irritation, that one does not observe the split in the wound, through the conjunctiva. But if the examination is made with a magnifying glass, one will observe that though a number of dense strands of connective tissue do cross the wound transversely, still between the strands one will see only a very thin transparent membranous substance filling out the wound. At these points, possibly in a few days, in other cases after a week or two, the wound begins to give to the intra-ocular pressure. It occurs at times that the process develops gradually, after the patient has been discharged from the hospital. The thin, transparent, membranous substance which closes up the interspaces between the strands is pressed forward; hence, the situation of the wound seems to be filled up with a number of transparent vesicular prominences. Generally this interstitial substance ruptures, and in this manner the aqueous humor is permitted to escape beneath the conjunctiva, which then seems to be raised up by a serous fluid from the sclera. This may take place many months, even years after the operation.

The above has been taken almost verbatim from Graefe's description of cystoid cicatrization, in his first report of sequelae of glaucoma operations, and it is quoted here because later on he declared, that all that he had there said was also true of the scleral extraction.

The vesicular prominences, which are the result of the cystoid cicatrization, may, under certain conditions, attain the size of a pea. The opening which forms the point of communication between the anterior chamber and the vesicle is always very small. When they have existed for a long time, they widen at their base so as to extend over on to the cornea as well as into the episclera, so that it no longer can be looked upon as an almost closed vesicle with a very fine stem, but rather as one situated over a wide opening, which is simply covered by the most superficial layers of the corneal tissue, which undoubtedly takes its origin at the limbus, in the conjunctiva and episcleral tissue.

A cystoid cicatrix does not occur when a clean corneal incision is made, and in fact has only been known to occur since Graefe commenced treating glaucoma by making the iridectomie incision in the limbus. Jacobson never observed this occurrence when he made his incision for an extraction at the edge of the sclera, and Graefe mentioned its occurrence for the first time in his second treatise concerning the modified linear extraction. In this Graefe says: "The injury at the edge of the sclera only then leads to cystoid cicatrization when the intra-ocular pressure is increased. This abnormal healing of the wound has lately been used as a weapon against this operation, especially by the French opponents of the Graefe operation. (Fano, 1259.)"

Becker says: "From my own experience I can support Graefe's view, as I only had a cystoid cicatrix follow in a single case, and in this case I made the operation when Basedow's disease was present. All the other cases which are known to me are taken from Arlt's practice, and that of my predecessor Knapp, and in none of these did intra-ocular tension exist before the operation. By this I do not wish to deny that it is possible for an increased intra-ocular pressure to have existed and still have been overlooked."

"Though Graefe does state, that where cystoid cicatrization is present, and the anterior chamber has been restored, the globe is always soft, hence he assumes that the aqueous humor must escape possibly through the membrane. My experience has been quite the contrary, at least in long-standing cases, for I have always found the globe to be quite tense. Here I will not entirely overlook the fact that such a cystoid cicatrix may for many years rupture periodically."

b. CICATRIZATION OF THE IRIS IN THE WOUND. Very probably Von Graefe separated the cystoid cicatrix from all those anomalous changes which arise in consequence of incarceration of the iris in the wound.

Just as in any iridectomie, some of the iris pigment may be brushed off and remain in the wound. Such a pigmented cicatrix is frequently seen after an iridectomie, more frequently where the puncture is made more peripheric, in the limbus or beyond it. The more peripheric the wound, the easier does the prolapse of the iris follow, and owing to the involvement of the conjunctiva the channel of the wound is deeper, and consequently pigment is more easily contained in the cicatrix. Hence, we can understand how it happens that, after an extraction at the sclero-corneal edge, the cicatrix so much more frequently is pigmented. This can be avoided where the wound is carefully cleansed; the enclosure of pigment, however, is not detrimental in any way.

Especially during the first few years after Graefe introduced his operation, it frequently happened to him and to other operators, that the iris prolapsed into the wound, and became fixed there during the process of healing. During the process of healing one would then observe in one or both angles of the wound, a small blueish-black spot, which either lay exactly on a level with the cicatrix and remained there, or it gradually became prominent, like a small button, and at times protruded as a vesicle of not inconsiderable dimensions. Hence, even in favorable cases, the process of healing was considerably prolonged. After the cessation of all signs of irritation, we had before us a picture such as we are wont to see after glaucoma operations, especially where the operation was made for acute glaucoma.

Naturally, the peripheric position of the incision favored the prolapse of the iris; hence, Graefe advised that the excision of the iris should be made without going into the anterior chamber with the iris forceps, but simply to grasp the prolapsed portion of the iris, and where a prolapse did not occur, this was to be induced by pressing on the sclerotic with the forceps. He lays down the rule that, we should only cut off as much as has prolapsed, and to desist from any effort to draw the iris out of the wound, and that that which does not easily fall forward into the wound will easily draw back again, but for my part (Becker) I will admit this to hold good only in cases where there is reduced, or at least no increased intra-ocular tension. In such eyes, in which the corneal incision is followed by a sinking in of the cornea, a cicatrization of the iris in the wound never follows. If the eye has a shining, tense appearance after the operation, so that the iris is pushed against the posterior surface of the cornea with a certain amount of force, or if increased intra-ocular tension was diagnosticated before the operation, one may surely count on the iris healing in the wound, if one does not carefully excise it along the entire length of the wound. One can choose but one alternative in such a case, either to make a wide coloboma, or to find the iris cicatrized in the wound. Aside from the already mentioned prolongation of the period of healing, a cicatrization of the iris in the wound, has the further injurious effect of causing not only a greater or less disfigurement, but it becomes a source of continuous irritation, the extent of which will be proportionate to the extent of the prolapse.

Though no prominent iris vesicle may form, the simple fixation of the iris in the cicatrix is sufficient to cause the pupil to be drawn toward the wound. Further, one will, from the contour of the pupil, where one can not detect both edges of the cut sphincter of the iris, by this condition alone determine that there is a cicatrization of the iris in the wound, even where this can not be determined externally.

As a matter of course, the cicatrization of the iris in the wound must exert an influence on the curvature of the neighboring corneal tissue, and hence influence the amount of vision after such an operation. Since a pupil which is drawn to the periphery falls in the area of a less regularly curved portion of the cornea, and hence is less favorably situated for good vision, hence, under all circumstances the cicatrization of the iris in the wound must be looked upon as detrimental to the sight on the operated eye.

Owing to the more peripheric position of both Jacobson's and Von Graefe's incision, the almost unavoidable occurrence of an iris prolapse lead these operators to make the excision of the iris, before opening the capsule, one of the integral steps of the operation of extraction. Even in the old flap operation, *if the incision lay too far in the periphery*, or even where only a part of it was so located, or where the globe was too tense, not infrequently *prolapsus iridis* followed. Already Wenzel incised the iris, starting from the pupillary edge, where the escape of the cataract through the pupillary area was connected with great difficulty. Maunoir incised the iris vertically in cases which he found it impossible to replace the prolapse, and by this means found that it drew back of its own accord. In cases in which the lens pushed the iris pouch-like before it, Pourfoor du Petit, and later Carron de Villards, excised a piece of the iris with a scissors, and thus made an artificial opening for the escape of the lens. The occasional excision of the iris after the extraction of the lens was practiced by Von Graefe and Jacobson. In all these cases the iris lays itself with its surface in contact with the wound, so that the iris, like a cloth, is plugged into the wound from within. Under certain conditions the aqueous continues to press it more and more into the wound, until finally it extends beyond the external level of the wound. It may, however, become fixed at any point along the channel of the wound, at its inner opening, along the channel of the wound, at its outer opening, or finally it may be pushed forward like a vesicle beneath the conjunctiva. In the last case, the *prolapsus iridis* is covered externally by the conjunctiva. This finally is forced apart, and we find an atrophic iris tissue, and finally we have a diverticulum of the anterior chamber, which is connected by the latter by a very minute fistula.

This surface cicatrization is to be differentiated from the cicatrization of the stump of the excised portion in the wound. As a rule, this latter condition can not be diagnosticated during life. This form of cicatrization occurs more frequently than at the edges of the wound. If during the operation the iris is transfixed by the knife, it may happen that a shred of iris will remain in the center of the wound. Here, then, one is given the opportunity of studying this form of healing of the iris in the wound. Aside from a pronounced pigmentation of the cicatrix, no other evil results of this mode of cicatrization has as yet been noted. However, this cicatrization of the iris may become the starting point of other pathological changes. It appears that just the minute degrees of this condition are the frequent cause of chronic recurring iritis and irido cyclitis, and may even become the cause of a sympathetic opthalmia.

The cause of this recurring chronic iritis, irido-cyclitis and sympathetic opthalmia has, since the above was written, been explained by Leber,[17] who demonstrated that where the iris, ciliary body, or even the capsule of the lens, cicatrized in the wound, they gave rise to slight differences in the niveau, the formation of slight nodules, and the epithelial covering of these is very apt to be stripped off. Now should a microbic infection take place, the condition is produced which leads to inflammation. This has been conclusively proven by the further investigations of Wagenmann,[17a] who has shown that microbes gain entrance along fistulous tracts years after an apparently successful operation. Here then are the conditions which lead to sympathetic opthalmia, and no plea (for great care in the mode of making the incision, the strictest care in the toilet of the wound, in seeing that the edges are free of coagula, that the iris is free and in its proper position, and that its edges where an iridectomie has been made are not lying in the wound, that no shreds of capsule are lying in the wound) could equal in impressiveness a careful study of the above quoted investigations. They will elucidate a whole train of evil results and where the admonitions are observed will to a very large extent, if not absolutely, prevent their occurrence. *Strict asepsis during an operation is one thing, but who can watch the progress of cases years after an operation*

---

17 Uber die Intercellular Lucken des vodern Hornhaut Epithels in normalen und Pathologischen Zustande. Graefe Arch., XXIV, p. 24. 1878.

17a Uber die operationsnarben und vernarbte iris falle ausgehende glaskorper elterungen. Graefe's Arch., XXV, B. IV, p. 110. 1889.

*and prevent subsequent infection, especially where the conditions of the cicatrix
of the wound offer an opportunity for infection.*

Where these staphylomatous vesicles become very pronounced, it often becomes necessary to excise the cyst walls. Though this procedure may seem a
very simple one, it can not, however, be undertaken without observing the
very greatest care. Though pressure by means of a bandage may be applied
for a long time (Von Graefe), the result is not certain, in that frequently at the
point where the iris cyst formerly existed, there develops afterward a cystoid
cicatrix. As stated in the beginning, as much as I agree with Von Graefe in
separating the cystoid cicatrix from the cicatrization of the iris in the wound,
likewise of the capsule, it nevertheless does occur that we find all these processes developing one next to the other in the same eye. The iris or capsule, or
both, which become fixed in the wound, are the cause, that adhesion per primam
does not follow, and consequently the tissue which is necessary to fill up this
space becomes predisposed "to give," and form an *ectasie.*

Though at the close of the operation the iris may not be found in the
wound, still it is possible that in cases where the aqueous later on forces the
wound open again, the iris may later on be washed into the wound, and this is
more apt to occur where there is increased intra-ocular tension.

c. HYPERAEMIA OF THE IRIS. Only those phenomena will be
considered which can not be looked upon as the results or complication of
pathological processes occurring in other parts of the eye. The first
changes in the iris show themselves even during the operation. After the
evacuation of the aqueous, but more so after evacuation of the lens, the
iris assumes, just as it does in many cases of iritis, a darker color, and at
the same time a slight discoloration. The latter changes become more
apparent when the iris has a light rather than when it has a dark color.
Both conditions are due to a violent injection of the ciliary vessels, which
must necessarily follow as soon as the pressure on the tissue is removed.
At times some of the blood vessels of the iris suddenly become visible, or
slight hemorrhages take place in the tissue, or in the anterior chamber.
If no complications are present this soon disappears after restoration of
the anterior chamber.

d. SIMPLE TRAUMATIC OR ADHESIVE IRITIS. Where atro-
pine is dropped into an eye, one almost invariably finds that its action is
entirely abolished at the time of or during the first few hours after an
operation. Only gradually, do we notice, that it begins to exert its influence again, and even then not along the entire extent of the old pupil and
its coloboma. The two sides of the coloboma seem to offer the greatest
resistance. In favorably progressing cases, we notice, on making our evening visit or the following morning, that the pupil and coloboma are dilated
regularly. In other cases adhesions are noted. This can only occur where

the capsule of the lens and the edges of the pupil touch each other. Hence, the less complete the evacuation of the lens has been, and the longer the time elapsed before the anterior chamber is restored, the more easily will this occur. These observations indicate that but a very short time subsequent to the operation is sufficient for an adhesive iritis to develop along the edges of the wound, in the new pupil, and at single points along the old, and this manifests itself by the early adhesions between the wounded iris surface and its closest neighboring tissue (be this a shred of the capsule or minute intra-capsular remains or blood clots). (Jacobson.)

If we desire to prevent seclusion of the pupil, active use of atropine is indicated. Such synechia, if once formed along the edges of the new pupil, can not, in most cases, be broken up again.

e. PLASTIC IRITIS is to be differentiated from the adhesive variety. This likewise sets in soon after the extraction, often with but slight subjective symptoms, even when the flap wound has healed normally, and characterizes itself in that, to begin with, there is little cloudy aqueous, yellowish flakes appear in the pupillary area which do not sink to the floor, but retain their original position, and very soon form adhesions with the edges of the pupil, and later on also form demonstrable attachments behind the iris. Such yellowish deposits may develop inside of twenty-four hours on the anterior surface of the iris, and in the aqueous without the formation of a fluid pus. (Jacobson.)

Occasionally one observes a jelly-like, yellowish exudate, like the spawn of frogs, which first appears between the edges of the wound, and finally gets into the anterior chamber. It may accumulate to such a degree as to fill out the entire anterior chamber, at the same time showing such a slight cloudiness as to still permit one to distinguish the finer lines on the surface of the iris, so that one inclines more to the belief that one is dealing with a very faint cloudiness of the cornea, rather than an exudate on the iris. Only when this begins to contract, and the periphery of the iris becomes clear, does it become evident as to just what we are dealing with. This jelly-like mass continues gradually to contract more toward the edges of the artificial pupil, and at times is so completely resorbed that aside from a perfectly transparent membrane in the pupil (capsular thickening), and a few synechia, nothing remains.

Becker states that he observed this form of plastic iritis twice in diabetic patients, and in fact only where the cataract was tumescent. It seems most probable that the intensely swollen condition of the lens is the main cause of the chronic irritation of the iris and the iritis. Chemosis and swelling of the lids is still to be mentioned as occasional occurrences, but to only a moderate degree; but true ciliary pain and purulent conjunctival secretion are entirely wanting. In these cases a true hypopyon never occurs (when it does the diagnosis is *infection*).

f. After the original sclero-corneal wound has closed, after the second or third week, a form of iritis may still develop, which is characterized by its persistence and relapses. Up to this time the process of healing may have appeared to be perfectly normal. The only change seems to be, that the eye appears injected, and the iris assumes a darker color or a slight discoloration. Without any change in the form of the pupil, ciliary injection sets in, together with irritability to light, tearing and pain. It is not necessary for vision to be reduced, and we suddenly find a slight hypopyon, which at times disappears and suddenly appears again. If the patient lies on his back, the hypopyon disappears, whereas, as soon as he moves about it develops again. This may continue for days, even months. This peculiar form has been observed in cases in which the capsule was removed, together with the lens. The final result may be a perfectly good one.

Owing to the fact that the iris shows no visible changes, that the hypopyon disappears when the patient lies on his back and develops again when he moves about; and finally, that it develops even when the capsule is wanting, and also owing to the pain in the ciliary region, it is possible that the ciliary body is involved; hence, it would probably be more correct to designate this form as a *relapsing irido-cyclitis*. All therapy seems to be useless.

The above description is undoubtedly that of an infection.

g. A few hours after an operation one may perceive changes in the pupillary area, which will indicate if at the completion of the procedure we will get a black pupil or not. Not infrequently it happens, that though at the close of the operation the pupillary area appears perfectly black, we are surprised at our evening visit to find the pupillary area "filled with a considerable amount of cloudy cataractous remains." Though the pupil appears black at the close of the operation, this does not indicate that the entire lens has been removed. If the examination made previous to the operation proved the anterior lamellae of the lens to be still transparent, these will remain adherent to the capsule at the time of the operation, and later on became cloudy. But it is likewise possible, though all the anterior layers be cloudy, for some of the posterior to have been transparent, and these will remain adherent and unnoticed after an extraction. True we term as *cataracta matura*, a lens system which has become completely cloudy, and this cloudiness has extended to the anterior chamber. Just as it is possible for the posterior cortical substance to remain cloudy for years, in the so-called *choroideal cataract*, the anterior portion remaining clear, likewise, it is possible for the same condition to occur in just opposite form. However, we do not as yet possess the means of making a diagnosis of such a condition. This condition does exist, for in a number of cases Becker found the regular radiating arrangement of the cloudy remains of lens substance when the examination was made at the evening visit.

Frequently cataractous remains came into view, which at the time of the operation were hidden behind the iris. After the wound is closed and the anterior chamber restored they may, owing to their tumescence, appear in the pupillary area, or where an iridectomie has been made in the area of the coloboma.

Not infrequently it is impossible to get the pupil entirely clear. Even in these cases, on making the first visit, the quantity of cataractous mass remaining seems increased, undoubtedly due to the action of the aqueous in causing it to swell up.

The general course of the operation largely depends on the amount of cataractous substance retained. Nevertheless, it is very difficult to determine just how much cataractous mass, if left behind, can become an element of danger. Hence, one of the principal objects in every extraction must always be to remove as much lens substance as possible. According to many operators, the condition of the cataract is not entirely without its influence. At times a certain variety, a sticky (pasty) consistence of the cortical substance in *cataracta nondum matura*, at times the pasty mass of an overripe cataract, is said to be especially dangerous. There does not appear to be a uniform agreement of opinion on this point. But as there is undoubtedly a chemical action, taking place in the secondary disintegration of the cataractous mass; hence, *a priori* we must admit, that the remains of an overripe cataract may act in a detrimental way, owing to its chemical constitution.

As a rule, cataractous remains, even when present in considerable amounts, in and of themselves do not cause a reaction which will end disastrously to the eye. The main danger undoubtedly lies in the fact, that these cataractous remains may become a very detrimental complicating factor, where other portions of the eye are not well disposed. In this manner the attempt has been made to explain the bad prognosis in cases of unripe, especially tumescent cataracts. In these cases, even before the operation, the iris is irritated by the swollen lens, and from this, the active reaction sets in.

Undoubtedly the most frequent sequelae of cataractous remains are posterior synechia. Aside from these a *cataracta secundaria* nearly always develops. Cases do occur in which the pupil remains free and totally black, and in which after complete healing, even on focal illumination, one can only detect a somewhat opalescent membrane, the posterior capsule, but they are exceedingly rare. They can only be explained by supposing that immediately after an operation, the edges of the capsule draw back far into the periphery, so that only the posterior capsule, entirely free of lens substance, remains in the pupillary area. The remains of lens substance left in the equatorial region, are at once shut off, hence, can not swell up and therefore give rise to no further trouble.

h. If one waits a certain length of time before applying the bandage, or if from any cause it becomes necessary to remove it, one will at times note how very quickly the anterior chamber is restored. For this to occur the entire length of the wound must become agglutinated, and further, to have attained a certain amount of security. If at the next visit the condition has remained unchanged, it becomes very probable that this closure following the operation will remain a permanent one.

Paracentesis of the anterior chamber has taught us, that a very few minutes are sufficient to permit the accumulation of a requisite amount of aqueous. If the anterior chamber is punctured so as to evacuate the aqueous at regular intervals, so as to ease pain in the eye, it will be found necessary to repeat this procedure every four or five minutes.

In most cases this closure of the wound does not follow so quickly subsequent to an extraction, or at least is not of a permanent character. Though we do frequently find the anterior chamber restored on making our evening visit, still one may expect it to open again several times before it finally becomes securely closed. Patients state that after they have experienced a slight increase of tension in the eye, they suddenly experience a stinging pain, following which the pressure seems to be removed, and at the same time they experience a feeling as though something were flowing out of theye. The aqueous which reaccumulates must reestablish the intra-ocular pressure, and unless the wound closes securely, must necessarily rupture it again.

As has been said, in exceptional cases the wound does not close on the first day, so that on making our visit we still find the anterior chamber abolished. I have seen such a condition, which is generally recognized as following glaucoma operations, follow a cataract extraction, and continue for four or five days, and in cases where everything seemed to be progressing in a perfectly normal manner. Jacobson reported cases in which the closure did not take place during the first few weeks (l. c., p. 194). During this time, the eye must not necessarily show any sign of reaction, and the result without exception is a good one. One must not imagine that the entire surface of the wound remains open, but there is possibly a very minute point, somewhere, at which the aqueous is continually evacvating itself, or there is possibly a valve-like closure which periodically permits the aqueous to escape. Where a conjunctival flap has been made this escape of aqueous may be recognized by the conjunctival oedema. Where a purely corneal incision is made, this condition is always entirely absent, even where there is a late closure. It is possible for the anterior chamber to be restored, even where this conjunctival oedema is present. This takes place when the pressure of the aqueous beneath the conjunctiva is at least equal to that of the intra-ocular pressure. If in such a case one punctures the conjunctiva, the anterior chamber will be abolished.

That the entire extent of the wound does not remain open is attested by the fact, that it presents all those conditions which have above been described as being present where the progress of the case is a normal one. True one would suppose that the point where the wound has not closed would be indicated by a circumscribed area of reaction, still I (Becker) have never been able to find one.

The cause of a late closure may lie in the peculiar formation of the incision, as where this is jagged, and hence but an incomplete apposition of the edges of the wound follow. More frequently, however, it will be found that remains of lens substance or a shred of the capsule of the lens has gotten in between the edges of the wound, and is keeping the two surfaces separated, and thus making it possible for the aqueous to escape. These cases, which terminate favorably, have nothing in common with those cases in which a delayed closure is caused by an increased intraocular tension. Here we would be dealing with a very dangerous complication, which had been overlooked. Such eyes, if they heal at all, do so only under the most difficult conditions. Indeed, one ought to be glad if they heal at all, even with an ectatic cicatrix. Here the same conditions exist as they do in glaucoma, even though the anterior chamber is abolished, the tension of the globe will still remain increased, vision remains reduced, and the result, as far as vision is concerned, is exceedingly doubtful.

I may here remark, that so long as the aqueous escapes it is impossible for an increased intra-ocular tension to develop. It seems most probable, that the increased tension which arises as a result of operative procedure, must be a most detrimental factor in cases which do not progress favorably. Hence, such an opening in the wound may be looked upon as a regulator of this dangerous intra-ocular tension.

i. One must not confound abolition of the anterior chamber with the condition following iritis or the swelling up of the remains of lens substance, which in the first few days following an operation make the anterior chamber very shallow. Here one will find the signs of an iritis or swollen up remains of lens substance. The aqueous is found to be especially cloudy. The anterior chamber is not narrow because the aqueous is being constantly evacuated, but because the iris and the capsule of the lens are pressed forward.

On the other hand, an unusually deep anterior chamber may develop shortly after an operation. The aqueous may remain perfectly clear, the iris lie somewhat deep and tremble markedly. Focal illumination will then show a very considerable space existing between capsule and iris. Such eyes heal without any posterior synechia, and good vision is obtained. In old people, on whom flap operations are made without iridectomie, in most cases the pupil is narrow, perfectly round, and only the practiced eye can distinguish the trembling of the iris, which lies deeply and in a perfect plane behind the cornea, and owing to the fresh, clear appearance of the eye, recognize that he is not dealing with a case of luxation of the lens, but with a case of *aphakia*, following extraction.

If the iris lies deep, the pupil wide, and the aqueous from the beginning abundant and cloudy, one will observe movable opacities in the anterior portion of the vitreous, and a characteristic blueish red peri-corneal injection. At the same time the globe is tense. Jacobson observed this condition in hydropthalmic eyes. This is explained by the fact that owing to the altered conditions of intra-ocular tension subsequent to extraction, a profuse exudate follows from the dilated vessels of the distended anterior segment of the eyeball. Such a hypersecretion of humor aqueous is said to interfere more with the firm healing of a flap wound than with the final general result. Puncture of the anterior chamber would eventually be indicated in such a case.

PROCESSES OF HEALING WITH INCOMPLETE RESULTS.

Since the object of an extraction is to remove the interference with sight, which is located in the cloudy lens, hence, all final results which interfere with the perfect attainment of this end must be designated as incomplete results. We must, however, differentiate between those cases which are improved by a second operation and those which are to be looked upon as lost, so far as sight on the eye is concerned. In such cases the second operation is always made for secondary cataract (*cataracta secundaria*). Such a cataract may exist without a complication, or *it is adherent to the iris*; hence, at the same time a *cataracta accreta*. A secondary cataract may be complicated by other changes which may occur after an operation, such as the formation of cyclitic bands and detachment of the vitreous. But since operations made on these complicated cases, as a rule, are not followed by good results, hence it is advisable not to count these cases in with those of secondary cataract; so that in speaking of secondary cataract (Nachstaar), only those cases are included which are operable.

a. The pure secondary cataract is only the result of the sequence of changes which takes place during and after an extraction within the capsule of the lens, and is confined to those portions of the lens substance which are not evacuated. Hence, if one may so express it, this is the product of a pure phakitis.

Every one can observe how the lens substance which escapes from the interior of the capsule, but is retained within the anterior chamber, swells up and is absorbed. Every oculist should see to it that the iris is well dilated, so as to prevent the possible formation of synechia. If they are not formed, one will be enabled to see at a recognizable distance behind the pupil, a grey, membranous-like cloudiness, which is more or less transparent, and dependent on the degree of its non-transparency vision will be proportionately impaired. If the pupil is dilated one can easily see that this cloudiness increases toward the periphery; hence, the portion which is hidden behind the iris is more saturated than the portion in the pupillary area. The secondary cataract is thickest in the equatorial region of the lens. (The reason for this has been explained in the third part of this work.) In the pupillary area this thickness is a variable quantity. In isolated spots this secondary cataract may be entirely wanting. At times such a small opening is sufficient to enable one to obtain sufficient vision.

The changeable appearance of the secondary cataract in the pupillary area is characteristic of the pathological changes which take place in the remains of the lens substance.

The duration of the phakitis is variable. True, we discharge a cataract patient as well, when the eye looks pale and the pupil relatively clear. Weeks or months later the patient returns, and we find the pupil occulated by a thick secondary cataract. Years may elapse without any change taking place in the degree of vision, without our being in a position to determine whether or not any change has taken place in the secondary cataract. Then suddenly the patient notices a gradual diminution in the amount of vision, whereas the accompanying symptoms, the irritability to light, the pain, the tearing and ciliary injection, may be so slight as to be scarcely noted by the patient. If such a patient comes under observation at this time, one can see a punctate, striated, or spotted cloudiness gradually developing in the pupil. As a rule, this cloudiness begins near the point of incision, and gradually extends toward the center At the same time the iris may apparently be uninvolved. (This is the picture of the tension of the cicatrized iris or capsule in the wound, possibly a secondary infection along a fistulous tract.)

There is a peculiar form of "drusige" hyaline thickening of the originally clear capsule, which can lead to a very material reduction of vision.

On use of the refracting opthalmoscope one can discern these warty excressences, and on moving the mirror they give a shiny reflex, but are otherwise transparent. Repeated examination will show that these exist in numbers. These conglomerations cause considerable interference with vision, but Becker states that he has never seen them change to total opacities. That the processes which take place in a pure secondary cataract are confined to the capsule of the lens and those lens cells which remain behind, is attested by the fact that the neighboring tissues are not involved in this inflammatory (?) process.

A secondary cataract always forms where the capsule is not extracted. The slightest folds in the capsule cause reflexes, hence, it becomes self-evident, that there must nearly always be an improvement in vision where the cause of these reflexes is removed. But whether a patient will desire a second operation will depend largely on how much he will need his eyes. The amount of vision which ought to be attained will be considered later on. Speaking in a general way a secondary operation is indicated when vision is reduced to 6-60. If during extraction the vitreous puncture (Hassner) is made, and no reaction follows, vision will not only be good, but seldom will this later be diminished.

COMPLICATED CATARACT. PHTHISIS BULBI AND PANOPTHALMITIS.

These are conditions which are but rarely met with at the present day, and only occur when an infection takes place.

A complicated cataract may be the result of an iritis. As has already been mentioned, its slightest forms occur very frequently, and do not always lead to a secondary operation. But the more intense the reaction, the thicker will be the secondary cataract. Just as soon, however, as the symptoms of wound reaction set in, at the sclero-corneal wound, on the iris, in the pouch of the capsule or in the ciliary body, the active development of a secondary cataract will go on, and finally lead to *occlusio pupillae.* According to the extent of the general reaction this can be divided into a number of clinical forms of disease. However, where this process reaches a certain intensity, all those tissues which were involved in the incision will be affected. Depending on the extent of the general reaction, this will lead to an *iritis with occlusion of the pupil,* an *iridocyclitis with occlusion of the pupil, together with the subsequent shrinkage of bands of connective tissue in the vitreous,* a *purulent inflammation of the vitreous, ending in phthisis bulbi,* and finally, to *panopthalmitis,* the greatly feared total loss of the entire eyeball, or a *suppuration of the cornea.*

1. Let us first examine the changes which take place in the cornea. All the processes of wound reaction described above are intensified, and we find the edges of the wound suppurating. While suffering from tearing and irritability to light, the patient complains of pain, the conjunctiva in the neighborhood of the wound, and the edges of the wound themselves swell up. From the second day on, the grey striations in the cornea increase, assume a more yellow color, and finally either a circumscribed portion or the entire length of the wound becomes infiltrated with pus. Having reached this stage of development, this process may come to a standstill on the third or fourth day, gradually retrogressing again, and leave the greater portion of the cornea transparent. Here we always find the iris, the capsule sac, and very often, also, the corpus ciliare in the neighborhood of the wound involved. Depending on the degree of the process we always assume the involvement of the above structures; this, however, can never be determined until the cornea has commenced to clear up. To combat this suppuration the best method is to immediately cauterize the corneal wound along its entire extent with a galvano cautery. The anterior chamber should, if not completely open, be reopened and washed out with a corrosive sublimate solution. As a final result, one always finds the sclero corneal cicatrix drawn in, and a thick secondary cataract, which in its entire extent, is everywhere adherent to the periphery of the iris. Owing to the gradual shrinkage of this secondary cataract, which is connected with the cicatrix of the wound, the iris is gradually drawn toward it. As the pupil now gradually becomes smaller at the sides, the secondary cataract likewise appears to grow smaller, and shows vertical striations, which seem to be continuous with the striations of the iris, giving us the picture resembling the arrangement of the ribs in a large palm-leaf fan. The iris presents in miniature the picture of the so commonly used Japanese fan.

Weeks and months may pass before this process has run its course. All this time, however, the tension of the globe remains normal.

2. If the corneal infiltration does not remain restricted to the immediate vicinity of the wound, on the second or third day one will observe an extension of this striated keratitis, until the entire cornea may finally become infiltrated in a tongue-like manner. There can be no doubt now as to the involvement of the inner portions of the eye. This can be determined by the extensive chemosis and the plastic oedematous swelling of the entire conjunctiva bulbi. The subjective phenomena are also very much increased. It is not necessary that this should lead to complete suppuration of the globe, but it always leads to the formation of an opaque corneal cicatrix, which is intimately connected with the iris, and to a

thick cyclitic membranous cataract. If after months the process finally becomes quiescent, the globe may retain its general form, but its intra-ocular tension will be found to be reduced. Notwithstanding the fact that the light sense may still be present, this flattening of the cornea, *phthisis corneae*, will cause every operation to be without result.

3. This tongue-like infiltration of the cornea seldom leads to suppuration of the same. But one must always be prepared for such an occurrence, and on the third or fourth day there may develop, $\frac{1}{2}$ mm. removed from the corneal edge and concentric to the same, a saturated yellow ring-like cloudiness which is very pronounced (ring abcess of Von Graefe). Such a picture seldom develops without causing a necrosis of the entire cornea, and the much feared panopthalmitis. An ill omen which appears at the same time, together with a flabby oedematous swelling of the con-junctiva, is a very profuse blenorrhoeic secretion from the same. Naturally, such a profuse purulent infiltration of the cornea is from the very be-ginning associated with a purulent inflammation of *the iris, the corpus ciliare, the choroid, the retina, the vitreous,* and even *the sclerotic.* We, how-ever, only make a diagnosis of *panopthalmitis,* when a *protrusio bulbi,* a slight exopthalmus is added. This latter condition is the symptom which tells us, that the purulent inflammation has extended beyond the borders of the eyeball, and that it has invaded the lymph sac of Tenon's capsule, and possibly has extended into the orbital tissue.

Von Graefe (l. c., p. 189) has given us the following classical description of the symptoms which a case of panopthalmitis presents: "After a more or less indifferent course of twelve to eighteen hours, seldom thirty hours, a gradually increasing swelling of the upper lid, together with the formation of a consider-able quantity of thin, dirty, yellowish pus develops. This latter consists less of the secretion of the tear glands than of a transudation from the conjunctival surface, which, together with the epithelial detritus and pus cells, forms a some-what even emulsion. There may be but little pain at this time, and this may depend on the faint reduction of the general sensibility in such patients. If one separates the lids at the very beginning of the disease, a portion of the secretion which was hidden beneath the lids will well forth. At this time neither corneal wound nor pupil show any particular anomaly. However, the entire anterior surface of the eye has a most peculiar yellowish color, due to the excessive filling of the lymph spaces in both conjunctiva and cornea. The general swelling of the former, and the adherence of the "liquid mass" to its surface, gives the eye the ominous "washed out" appearance. The yellowish discoloration of the cornea is due to the filling up of its lymph spaces with a yellowish material. Although these "tubes" seem to be filled with purulent matter in the most pregnant manner, nevertheless, in the beginning this is a very thin layer, so that on throwing the light on the cornea, this has a "steaming" appearance. Even with this condition present the anterior chamber may be fully restored, for truly this is usually the case; but there may still be a fistulous opening. Whether the one or the other condition is present depends largely on the intra-ocular pressure; partly, also, on the condition of the surface of the wound. Where this infiltration develops suddenly and intensely on the edges of the sclero-corneal wound, and also in the sub-conjunctival portion, this will lead more easily to closure of the anterior chamber; whereas, if the process spreads more rapidly along the surface, the anterior chamber will not be so easily resored, and will soon lead to a culminating point."

4. At times one can discover important phenomena on the iris before the cornea is involved, or shows any signs of cloudiness. In the beginning the aqueous is cloudy, the iris discolored, and shows signs here and there of yellowish spots, and finally hypopyon develops, a true acute suppurative iritis. Later on the cornea becomes cloudy in its entire extent, but necrosis of the same seldom follows. Frequently the wound which has closed opens up again, and a drop or two of pus will be found exuding from the wound.

It is possible for a case of suppurative iritis to heal with a perfect retention of form, normal tension of the globe, light sense retained and good projection. But nearly always there is developed a thick secondary cataract, in the formation of which the ciliary body participates; still, I have seen cases attain perfect restitution of sight without undergoing a second operation.

It goes without saying that the capsule plays a very important role in the entire process. It depends entirely to how great a degree the ciliary body is involved, how thick the cyclitic bands behind the lens are, whether the vessels in the same will become obliterated, and whether the vitreous body will shrink, what degree of benefit operative interference would give to the patient. An estimate concerning these conditions in an eye may be formed by testing the tension of the globe. Whether an eye can be made to see or not, depends on these factors.

5. Cyclitis assumes an important role, and in the cases in which keratitis and iritis are most pronounced, the prognosis largely depends on the development of this complication. But cyclitis may disclose itself as the primary and most important symptom, and in a very severe form.

In such a case, during the first few days, neither cornea, iris or pupil will show any suspicious signs. It is only after one believes that all the danger is past, that on the fourth or fifth day the eye becomes reddened. Whereas the cornea appears clear, the iris begins to take on a darker color, and the pupil begins to show a tendency not heretofore observed to cataract, and the subjective symptoms irritability to light, spontaneous pain and tenderness to pressure begin to develop. To this may be added a gradual hyperplasia of the cells in the capsule, and even to a greater formation of flakes in the vitreous; likewise, an exudation in the anterior chamber, as well as a simple cloudiness of its contents, to which may be added pus and blood.

The characteristic feature of this process is its exceptional obstinacy. Notwithstanding all this, it may cease after months, leaving but a very delicate secondary cataract, which even in a case where exceptional requirements are made of the eye, would not require a subsequent secondary cataract. On the other hand, it may lead to a thick secondary cataract, adherent to the iris and cyclitic bands, and even finally result in *phthisis bulbi*. This latter condition even develops very late. Such a result is to be feared where tenderness to pressure will not cease. This process may be complicated by detachment of the retina and internal hemorrhages, thus finally necessitating enucleation.

6. The vitreous body may become primarily affected without either iris or cornea being primarily affected. This, as a rule, occurs when there has taken place a prolapse of the vitreous. Becker states that this has occurred in cases in which the hyaloidea had not ruptured, and the vitreous had simply been exposed as a vesicle in the wound. Such a *hernia corporis vitrei* can only occur where a tear in the zonula has taken place. On the second day one can see yellowish grey shreds extending from the pupil into the vitreous. The wound gaps and flakes of pus exude. In a short time the entire pupil is filled with pus, the iris discolored is pressed forward, and the conjunctiva is chemotic. It is a very noteworthy fact, that though the cornea may be pressed forward to such an extent, by the pus in the anterior chamber as to form a perfect angle, it nevertheless retains its transparency except along a narrow edge, along the line of the incision, so that it is possible to observe accurately and follow up the gradual vascularization of the pupillary edge of the iris, and also the development of blood vessels in the purulent mass in the pupillary area. Naturally, swelling up of the lids and plastic chemosis are present, but only to a moderate degree. The globe, however, under all circumstances, retains its mobility, and a *protrusio bulbi* never occurs. Sensation to light may be retained for a few days, but disappears on the fourth or fifth day.

It is possible for such a purulent inflammation of the vitreous to be followed by total retention of the form of the globe of sensation to light, and even normal tension. In these cases the wound closes toward the end of the second week without the development of increased intra-ocular tension. In these cases one is justified in the belief that the process was restricted to the anterior half of the vitreous. As a rule, in course of time diminished intra-ocular tension develops.

If this discharge of pus continues for any length of time, sensation to light will be totally abolished, even before the wound closes, more frequently, however, after it has closed. During this time the eye has a hard peculiar increased resistance to the touch. It does not feel hard, but gives one the impression that its coats have lost all their elasticity.

The further course continues but slowly. The pains, which have never been severe, after the wound closes become markedly increased. As a consequence, the general health of the patient does not suffer, and the absence of pain helps to keep up his hope. When the last exacerbation of pain ceases, the swelling of the lids disappears. The infiltration of the conjunctiva continues, although the oedema disappears. Gradually the anterior chamber is restored, the vessels of the iris and pupillary area are no longer visible, the tissue which occludes the pupil gradually assumes a grey color, and is reduced to a small, vertical band. From now on the tension of the globe gradually diminishes, and *phthisis corneae* and *bulbi* develop. Six to eight weeks elapse before the recti muscles begin to leave their impress, and months pass before the process of shrinkage comes to a close. During all this time the eye is moderately sensitive, the conjunctiva especially around the cornea is deeply injected, and as a rule the palpebral fissure is kept closed.

7. Hemorrhages which occur during the process of healing are to be differentiated from those which have already been mentioned. They have never been observed following a flap extraction unless associated with a rupture of the wound or due to a trauma. Hence it seems we must seek their cause in the peripheric position of the incision and the iridectomie. This same occurrence has been noted where a simple iridectomie is made. Not unfrequently they pass off without any evil consequences, especially when the hemorrhage has been a slight one, but where this has been severe it is nearly always followed by iritis (Snellen). But if hemorrhages which appear to be very severe recur, they may lead to very unpleasant results.

As a rule, these hemorrhages take place in the anterior chamber, much less frequently do they occur as minute or large ones into the vitreous. The prognosis becomes all the worse, the more reason one finds for their not being the result of trauma. It can not be doubted, that especially during sleep, patients unconsciously rub the healing eye. At times they admit it. If we will eliminate these cases, the following cause may be enumerated with more or less certainty:

(1) Repeatedly have such hemorrhages been observed where the anterior chamber was suddenly restored, after having been abolished for a

considerable length of time. The hemorrhages were never great, and never were followed by evil consequences. It seems probable that the tension which is exerted on the iris, where, owing to the accumulation of aqueous, it is forcibly pressed backward, one of the new formed blood vessels is ruptured, and thus gives rise to the hemorrhage. The patients always state that they felt a sudden pain.

(2) If at times, or shortly after the hemorrhage, an iritis develops, it is more than likely that the hemorrhage is the result of a previous hyper-aemia of the iris, especially since cases of iritis have been observed in which hemorrhages did occur when no operation had been made. Owing to the great rarity of spontaneous hemorrhage in iritis following extraction, one must assume as a second cause diseased friability of the blood vessels of the iris.

(3) Together with Knapp (A. f. A. and O., I, p. 54) Becker considered a predisposition to hemorrhage as the main cause of those hemorrhages which are restricted to the anterior chamber, and which become danger-ous, owing to their recurrence, and which may likewise take place in the vitreous. Those cases of cloudiness of the vitreous reported by Knapp (l. c., p. 57), are most easily accounted for in this manner. According to Knapp such hemorrhages offer a very bad prognosis. The cause, most certainly, is a diseased condition of the vessels which existed before the operation, and this can not always be diagnosticated. The final result need not always be a sad one, as was demonstrated to me (Becker) in a case in which, on the fourth day, a large hemorrhage took place in the vitreous and in the anterior chamber, accompanied by the most violent pains, without a rupture of the wound taking place, and only a quanti-tative perception of light remained. The blood in the anterior chamber soon disappeared, though the resorption of the blood in the vitreous re-quired months; nevertheless, finally a very satisfactory amount of vision was restored. In operating on the second, a preliminary iridectomie was made, and the eye healed without an accident.

The opinion has been expressed personally to me (Becker), that the venous plexus of Leber is incised during the operation, and that the hemorrhage may arise from this cause. However, I have never found such a condition present as would warrant such a conclusion in the innumerable microscopical sections which I have examined.

8. The relative frequency of the above described processes of healing, especially those in which a good result is not attained, is dependent to a large degree on the manner of procedure during the operation; hence, to speak more plainly, on the operator himself. In no department of opthal-mology does the difference between the master and the novice become more

apparent than in the operative, and here, above all, in the performance of a cataract extraction. But even in the hands of the most skillful all cases which have apparently had a similar result, after being operated according to the same method, do not attain a similar final result. Different individuals after undergoing a similar operation react differently. This idea has already been expressed, where it became necessary to separate the simple from the complicated cataracts. Likewise, the fact deserves mention here, that the second affected eye offers a better prognosis than the first affected. In many cases the individuality of the operated eye is responsible for a poor result.

Becker, as the result of the microscopical examination of human eyes which had been operated on for cataract, and also of pigs' eyes, on which he had experimentally operated, makes the following important observations:

Accurate measurements regarding the position of the various forms of incision in the edge of the cornea have shown very interesting differences between the Daviel and the Graefe's incision. In making a *flap extraction*, the outer edge of the wound should not touch the limbus. In three eyes examined the wound lay 1 mm. from the limbus; the inner edge of the wound, therefore, lay 2-2.25 mm. distant from the insertion of the iris. This is about the condition which should exist where the operation is made according to the rule laid down. In the *Graefe extraction*, where the outer edge of the wound falls in the limbus, one is less in a position to measure its distance from the edge of the cornea. The mean distance of the inner edge of the wound from the iris is equal to about 1.25 mm. If a so-called negative incision is made, it is found to lie anterior to the limbus, in the cornea, and in carrying out this method the inner edge of the wound is farther removed from the insertion of the iris.

Frequently a glance at the corneal cicatrix will suffice to show us the method which was employed in operating. A flap extraction made with a Beer knife goes through a line which forms an angle, of varying degree, with the radius of the cornea, hence has an oblique direction, and is considerably broader than the thickness of the cornea. It lies in a single plane, and in transverse section shows that it does not change its direction. However, in the Graefe operation, after making the contra-puncture, the knife must be turned so that the cutting edge looks anteriorly. In doing this it is not always possible to do so without changing the direction of the cutting edge of the knife several times. On section we get an angular cicatrix, if the section is taken from the point where puncture or counterpuncture was made. But we can even recognize a Graefe incision in the section, where this is taken from the center of the line of incision, because this is always more perpendicular to the surface of the cornea.

An angular condition of the incision must, under certain conditions, act as a hindrance to an exact adaptation of the two surfaces of the wound.

The tendency of a corneal wound to open again is dependent on the height of the flap. This tendency, however, is increased by the fact that the two surfaces where these lie in a single plane glide past each other more easily, and give more easily to the intra-ocular pressure than where the two surfaces fit into each other by means of an angle. *This tendency of the corneal portion to glide past the scleral, exists both in practicing the Daviel, and the Graefe method of extraction.* But under like conditions this gliding past each other seems to be greater where the flap extraction is made, than where a peripheral linear incision is made. According to measurements, this difference varies from 0.12 to 0.30 mm. The younger the individual, and the more recent the cicatrix, the greater will be the dislocation; but it appears that in course of time, this may equalize itself again. The astygmatism which develops after an extraction depends partly on this fact. But the most inconsiderable thickening of the corneal tissue along the line of the wound is not without its influence. Both have a tendency to grow less in the course of a few months. In cases where the capsule of the lens, or the iris, cicatrize in the wound, the corneal tissue undergoes greater reaction, and the curvature of the cornea may be considerably altered.

IRREGULAR HEALING OF THE WOUNDS. The normal processes of healing of a corneal wound, may be modified or interfered with by the entrance of foreign substances between the surfaces of the wound. This is aided by the peripheral position of the wound, and the combining of the operation of iridectomie with that of extraction. As a rule, such a wound heals slower, and though the final amount of vision may be good, still during the first few months this acquired asymetry of the cornea will make itself very evident to the patient by its interference with sight. In such a cicatrix we must seek for the causes which produce signs of irritation, which may not begin to manifest themselves until long afterward, and which, together with other pathological conditions which may follow in their track, may finally become fatal to the existence of the eye, and even threaten the other eye.

1. *Pigmentation of the Cicatrix.* In every case where an iridectomie is made, in drawing out the iris and cutting it off, some of the pigment is brushed off in the wound, cicatrized there, and these pigment cells begin to undergo a hyperplasia. Even where a flap extraction without iri-

dectomie is made, the iris may prolapse, thus necessitating its replacement, hence the pigmentation where no iridectomie has been made.

Where the process is in other respects perfectly normal, the pigment is found as small, black granules in the cicatrix; not only in the intracellular substance, but within the cells themselves. Hence, it can not be surprising if isolated granules, carried by the lymph stream, are found in the corneal substance itself. This pigment does not in any way interfere with the perfect healing of the wound.

2. *Cicatrization of the iris in the wound.* The more peripheric the incision, the more apt is this to occur. Becker states that in seventeen anatomical examinations of eyes operated by the flap method, the iris was held in connection with the cicatrical tissue of the cornea but three times, whereas in fifteen peripheral linear extractions, this condition was met with ten times. The manner of its enclosure may be a three-fold one.

In both methods it is possible for the iris to prolapse into the wound and cicatrize there. It will then depend on the extent of the enclosure and the depth to which the iris fills out the wound, how great the interference with the normal processes of healing, and how great will become the density of the new-formed interstital tissue. Ever since extraction has been practiced, has the attempt been made, to avoid the formation of staphylomata. Hence the necessity for making a clean-cut excision of the iris; a care to prevent this cicatrization of the iris in the wound. The frequency of this latter condition is shown by anatomical examination to be very great.

CONDITIONS OF THE CAPSULE. Immediately after an extraction, the incised anterior capsule, in the pupillary area, is in contact with the posterior surface of the cornea, whereas in the periphery it is in contact with the posterior surface of the iris. Being separated only from the anterior capsule by the lens substance which has remained behind, the posterior capsule is forced against the anterior, by the vitreous which presses forward. The posterior capsule, which formerly was convex on its posterior surface, now is convex anteriorly. This must likewise be the case with the hyaloidea. In place of a *fossa patellaris*, we now have a *colliculus*. From now on, the radius of curvature coincides almost with that of the posterior surface of the cornea.

These conditions are all changed as soon as the corneal wound heals, for the aqueous, as it accumulates, pushes the iris and capsule backward again. If finally, in the strict sense of the word, a simple secondary cataract (see page 339) forms, this will be found removed about 1 mm. posteriorly from the posterior surface of the iris. The capsule of the lens, owing to the loss of its contents, and which gave it support, will appear folded.

Owing to the insertion of the zonula fibres, the so-called fixed points can not alter their position; or if they do this, they approach each other and cause folds. This folding will be more apparent in the pupillary area than in the region of the crystalline pearls.

Owing to the incision of the anterior capsule, its condition is a complicated one. This condition assumes great importance when we bear in mind that a piece of the anterior capsule may cicatrize in the corneal wound.

In order to prevent this, some idea should be had as to the proper position of incising the capsule, which is only reached under difficulties. Gayet attempted to solve this question in an experimental way, and Becker states, since he could not obtain a copy of this work he made similar experiments, using pigs' eyes (as fresh as possible). Extractions were made according to the various methods, and using various instruments to open the capsule. The eyes were then hardened in Muller's fluid and then examined.

All varieties of the cystotome were used, and on making a simple movement, merely a jagged angular wound was made, the base of which is perpendicular to the position in which we permit the instrument to act on the capsule. Per example—If the instrument is passed through the corneal incision directly to the opposite side of the pupil, and the incisions made exactly upward, we will find that we obtained a triangular flap with its base horizontally placed. If the lens is now extruded through this three-cornered opening, the base will become enlarged, the flap turns over outwardly and is in great danger of remaining in the wound. If, on the contrary, the instrument is passed horizontally across the capsule, we get a three-cornered flap with its base vertically placed. If the lens is now extruded, the capsule will be torn vertically to the corneal incision, consequently this flap will be pushed to one side and will not be able to get into the wound. One can judge how much depends on the sharpness of the cystotome from the fact that it can be felt to take hold and let go of the capsule several times before it finally penetrates and tears it.

From such incisions and tears as have been described, one can easily see that these flaps have a tendency to turn over outwardly. If, instead of a single incision or tear, a number are made, these can, without difficulty, be brought in connection with the number, form and condition of the flaps. In general, however, the relationship is the same; the flaps are turned outwardly and show frequent and irregular folds.

All the statements regarding the cicatrization of the capsule in the wound were substantiated by the experimental investigations made on pigs' eyes.

Adam Weber's and A. W.'s experiments are to be mentioned here. They removed entire pieces of the anterior capsule from the eye, before delivering the lens. In cases of so-called thickened capsule, this can be done without any great difficulty. At times this will lead to the desired end.[18]

THE COMPLICATED SECONDARY CATARACT. (CATARACTA SECUNDARIA ACCRETA.)

Strictly speaking, a single synechia between the edge of the pupil or the side of the coloboma, and the secondary cataract, is sufficient to bring the latter within this class, though in every other respect this is a simple secondary cataract so far as the processes within the capsule are concerned. Such a synechia may influence the position and the form of the secondary cataract. The frequency of the adhesion between iris and capsule is well known to all observers. As has already been repeatedly stated, frequently the capsule cicatrizes in the corneal wound, and thus complicates not only the wound, but the cataract. In most of these cases, the stump of the iris is likewise involved, and in these cases the enclosure of iris and capsule are responsible for the increased reaction which leads to the formation of a cicatrical secondary cataract, which takes its origin either in the cornea or iris. In some cases the ciliary body is likewise involved in this low grade inflammation, which leads to the formation of connective tissue bands, which are stretched across the eye posteriorly to the posterior capsule and connected with the same.

Owing to the involvement of the cornea, iris, ciliary body and the capsule of the lens, in such a secondary cataract, one can easily comprehend why it is that such an inflammatory process will only cease after weeks, or even months. The more complicated the structure which takes part in the formation of the cicatrix, the more intense will be the shrinkage which will follow, and it is possible for the secondary cataract which is cicatrized in the wound, to be drawn *in toto* to the side of the wound, so that "Petit's Canal" may be widened to an extreme degree on the side directly opposite the wound. This will explain the fact, why it happens, that at times, where a complete occlusion of the pupil, following a cataract extraction, exists, and a coloboma is made diametrically opposite the original incision, a space will be found which is entirely free of the secondary cataract.

---

[18] Nagel's Yahresbericht, 1870, p. 393.

Histologically, these complicated secondary cataracts are made up, not only of the products of lens substance, but of those of iritis, cyclitis and keratitis. Hence it is evident, why in such secondary cicatrical cataracts, aside from the elements described as occurring in simple secondary cataract, we here find connective tissue, pigment, blood vessels, even new-formed bone.

SEQUELAE OF TENSION AND SHRINKAGE OF THE CATARACTA SECUNDARIA ACCRETA. The evil results of a secondary cataract, which is attached to neighboring structures, are not alone confined to interference with vision. Only too often do we find, in this attachment, and shrinkage of this cicatrical tissue, which in course of time must follow, the destructive element which in course of weeks not only threatens to destroy the perception of light, but which leads to recurring inflammation which may finally totally destroy the shape of the eyeball. And, what is still worse, the painful signs of irritation which are the result of the shrinkage of the secondary cataract, which may lead to sympathetic irritation of the second eye.

A single simple posterior synechia changes the normal position of the secondary cataract, in that it is drawn forward. In its turn, this causes the formerly perfectly flat anterior surface of the vitreous to become more or less convex. The vitreous, however, may form a slight convexity in the *fossa patellaris*, even where no adhesions have formed, and in cases in which the crystalline pearl is very thick.

If the secondary cataract is very thick and posterior synechia exist, the iris may be drawn, funnel-like, backward—a condition which is met with at times.

The greater the amount of new-formed tissue in this secondary cataract, the greater will be the extent of its shrinkage, and the longer will the irritation continue, which will be exerted on the ciliary body. In the fewest cases will this irritation be ended at the time the patient is discharged from the physician's care. Though accommodation no longer exists after a cataract extraction, nevertheless, the muscular contractions of the ciliary body undoubtedly go on, when an attempt is made to see objects distinctly which are close by; hence this will also explain the evil results which may be exerted as a result of stopping the use of atropine too soon; likewise, by permitting the patient to use his cataract glasses too soon.

In complicated cataracts, the conditions are still more unfavorable. since the *ciliary body* not only draws on the corneal cicatrix, through the medium of the zonula, but also by means of the iris attached to the capsule. Hence in such cases the indications are to leave the eye at rest as long as possible.

CYCLITIS. The products have already been considered in speaking of complicated cataracts. Here we must differentiate between the direct influence of those lighter forms involved in the formation of secondary cataract and those severe forms due to infection which lead to purulent degeneration of the vitreous and panopthalmitis; and, further, those changes which are due to the shrinkage of these cyclitic products and lead to detachment of the ciliary body and detachment of the retina.

DETACHMENT OF THE VITREOUS. This may occur in a twofold manner; it may be acute or primary, chronic or secondary. Iwanoff found in quite a number of cases which seemed to have healed under perfectly normal conditions, twelve to twenty days after extraction, a detachment of the vitreous from the retina equal to several millometres in the region of the posterior pole. It seems easy to attribute this to the sudden escape of aqueous and lens, at the time of extraction. This detachment was found to be greatest in eyes examined soon after the extraction. If this detachment occurred at the moment of extraction, one can not very well understand why a hemorrhage did not occur more easily; since, however, this did not occur, it is more probable that the detachment resulted from the gradual contraction of the vitreous, which was greatly distended at the time aqueous and lens were evacuated.

A great deal more is known concerning the cause of detachment of the vitreous, as a result of the contraction of new formed cicatrical tissue and blood vessels which are found in the anterior half of the vitreous. Here, again, we are dealing with the results of the contraction of the infiltrated vitreous, subsequent to inflammatory processes.[19]

DETACHMENT OF THE CILIARY BODY. This likewise is due to the contraction of the cyclitic bands, which extend across the eye from side to side posterior to the capsule.

DETACHMENT OF THE RETINA. It has been abundantly proven that these cyclitic bands likewise lead to detachment of the retina.[19a]

GLAUCOMA.

Cases of glaucoma may develop immediately after a cataract extraction, during the healing of the operative wound, and it is not possible in every case to give a satisfactory explanation as to its cause. Rumschewitsch [20] states that these cases are not as rare as one would suppose, and he reports three cases, in one of which the lens was removed in its cap-

[19] See Iwanoff Arch. f. Opth., XV. 2, p. 59-60.
[19a] Erik Nordenson. Die Netzhaut ablosung. Wiesbaden, 1887.
[20] Zur Casuistick des Glaucoma nach Staar Operationen. Zehender's Monatsblatter, June, 1896.

sule. H. Pagenstecher [21] states that this condition usually follows in the first few days, subsequent to the use of atropine; hence great care in the use of this mydriatic is indicated. Such eyes may never have shown signs of hypertonia, but *frequently in eyes which have had former attacks of glaucoma.*

It may occur in eyes which up to the third or fourth week have shown no sign of hypertonia. Here the swelling of the cortical remains may be the cause, but even this condition has been shown to follow when the lens has been extracted in its capsule.

As we have seen, as long ago as 1869 Von Graefe observed cases of acute glaucoma supervene after a discission. Here the swollen lens substance pressed the iris against the filtrating angle, thus closing it off. Priestly Smith [22] reports the case of a child in which, seven years subsequent to a discission, high tension developed. This was found to be due to an annular synechia, which had united the pupillary margin of the iris with the capsule, locked up the posterior chamber, and thus caused a bulging of the iris, with closure of the filtrating angle. A small iridectomie gave exit to the fluid retained behind the iris; the iris retired from the cornea; the eye recovered with normal tension. He shows that not infrequently the pupillary margin is adherent throughout to the remains of the lens-periphery. The pupil may not appear to be blocked by any visible false membrane, still this membrane opposes the free escape of fluid from behind the iris. Priestly Smith states (page 59): "High tension may set in years after a good result. Natason (Uber Glaucom im Aphakischen Augen. Mattieson. Dorpat, 1889) showed that immunity from subsequent glaucomatous complication is not insured by any particular operation. Glaucoma may occur after the flap operation without iridectomie, after iridectomie with variously placed incisions, after an extraction preceded by a preliminary iridectomie, and after extraction in the capsule. They show that in the majority of cases there was some visible complication involving the iris or the capsule, or both, namely, iritis or irido-cyclitis, with occlusion of the pupil, prolapse or adhesion of the iris at the wound, or a similar entanglement of the capsule. This cicatrization of the iris or the capsule of the lens in the wound was likewise demonstrated by Stolting [23] and Hosch.[23a] In some cases, on the other hand, the eye appeared

[21] Glaucom nach Staar Extraction. Zehender's Klin. Monatsblatter, May, 1895.

[22] The Pathology and Treatment of Glaucoma, London, 1891. p. 57.

[23] Glaucom nach Linear Extraction. Graefe Arch., Vol. XXXIII, B. 2, 1887.

[23a] Glaucomatose und Atrophische Excavation in einem aphakichen Auge. Arch. für Augenh., XXVIII, 3. S. 311.

to be quite free from any complication of the kind. This negative evidence is, however, not quite conclusive, for slight adhesions of the kind in question may be quite undiscoverable in the living eye, and that they are frequent, even in satisfactory cases, has been proven by Becker. Becker examined with the microscope thirty-eight eyes from which cataracts had been extracted, and in only one-third of these was the iris free from the scar, although thirty-two of the thirty-eight eyes were removed, not on account of any trouble during life, but after the death of the patient. He expressly states that minute adhesions of the iris or capsule may be quite invisible in the living eye.

"It is obvious that an entanglement of the iris or the lens capsule in the wound may lead to a closure of the filtrating angle in its immediate neighborhood, but this does not suffice to explain the occurrence of glaucoma. We can not assume that obstruction of the filtrating angle, confined to a small part of the circle, is sufficient to cause high tension; on the contrary, we know that such entanglements after cataract extraction are common, while glaucoma is rare."

"Treacher Collins' microscopical examinations [24] give more positive evidence as to the cause of the glaucoma. In nine of the ten eyes examined by him the capsule was adherent to the scar; in the remaining one from which the lens had been removed in its capsule, the hyaloid was adherent in the same manner. The filtrating angle was closed in the neighborhood of the scar in every case; moreover, it was closed at the opposite side of the eye also, and probably throughout the whole of the circle, in seven out of the eight cases; and in those in which it was not closed by apposition of the iris and cornea, it was blocked by exudation."

"In the living eye, also, we can sometimes, I think, make out the cause of a glaucomatous complication after cataract extraction. In some cases the iris and posterior capsule, being united and coated by inflammatory exudation, appear to form an impermeable or insufficiently permeable diaphragm across the eye, which checks the passage of fluid from the ciliary processes into the aqueous chamber. An excess of fluid becomes imprisoned behind this diaphragm. This may happen although a good iridectomie has been made. In a case of this kind, on the eighth day after extraction, and in the presence of acute iritis, with free exudation into the aqueous chamber and very high tension, which had twice rapidly returned after paracentesis of the aqueous chamber, I made an iridectomie downward, tearing completely through the adhering membranes, and ob-

[24] Trans. of Opth. Society of the United Kingdom, Vol. X, p. 108.

taining for the moment a jet black pupil. The eye recovered normal tension and good vision, which are still retained after thirteen years."

"It is not easy, even with the help of pathological specimens, to explain the occurrence of glaucoma after a long interval of time, during which the eye has enjoyed useful vision. It appears probable, however, that a transparent membrane, stretching across from the ciliary processes on the one side to the cicatrix on the other, may in course of time undergo some slight contraction, which draws the processes forward so as to compress the filtrating angle. Or such a membrane may become less permeable than at first. In this way, or perhaps through some 'change in the intraocular fluid itself, filtration from the vitreous to the aqueous itself is checked. This is not mere conjecture. In an, elderly lady I performed a preliminary iridectomie, and later an extraction, apparently with complete success. A few months later an insidious glaucoma began, which at first yielded to eserine, but later became persistent. The field contracted, the disc became cupped. Sclerotomy with a Graefe knife was performed in the region of the extraction wound. On the withdrawal of the knife, hardly any fluid escaped, and the iris applied itself closely to the cornea, showing that fluid was imprisoned behind the aqueous chamber. The point of the knife was then passed in again through the same wound, and through the coloboma into the vitreous. A gush of fluid escaped, the iris retired from the cornea and the globe became slack. The eye recovered with normal tension. Curiously enough, I operated later on the fellow eye of the same patient, and encountered almost exactly the same sequence of events. In some cases of this kind the high tension may be banished by passing a cutting needle through the area of the pupil, so as to divide the posterior capsule and the anterior of the vitreous.'

"With regard to glaucoma following cataract extraction, we can, therefore, assert that there is usually a closure or blockage of the filtrating angle, although we can not in every case ascertain the precise manner of its production. The point of practical importance is, that such an obstruction can be remedied only while it is recent; and when the base of the iris has become adherent throughout to the periphery of the cornea, the glaucoma is incurable."

The warning can not be stated too emphatically to beware of maturing posterior cortical cataracts, and then extracting, without first investigating as to the probable cause of this condition. These cases are always secondary to disease of the uveal tract, and the possibility of a second attack of glaucoma subsequent to extraction should not be forgotten.

Finally, the fact can not entirely be set aside, that the arthritic or gouty diathesis may be the prime causative factor in the production of glaucoma in an aphakic eye, which in this case is independent of any pathological changes attributable to the operation. Dr. David DeBeck has recently illustrated these facts by some very instructive case reports. (The Ohio Medical Journal, Vol. IX, Nos. 4 and 9, 1898.)

CHAPTER IV.

Paradoxical as it may seem, the after treatment begins before the operation, and is not finished when the patient is dismissed from the hospital or the personal care of the physician.

THE MATURATION OF CATARACT. THE ARTIFICIAL RIPENING OF CATARACT.

Formerly months and even years were required before a cataract was considered as operable. Owing to a large quantity of cortical substance which remains behind when a cataract is operated before it is ripe, and the detrimental influence which a large quantity of cortex may cause, operators have always been fearful of extracting an unripe cataract. One can only understand what a ripe cataract is where we take into consideration how it has developed.

Celseus was the first to give a more exact description. "One must wait (before operating) for a kind of ripening of the cataract (maturitas), until it is no longer fluid, but has rather acquired a certain hardness as a result of coagulation." According to Beer,[1] a grey cataract is ripe when it is not possible for it to undergo further development. The expression "ripe cataract" has been handed down to us; but our understanding of the pathological changes has been radically changed, and has been fully considered in the second part of this work.

It certainly does not appear wise nor humane to cause a person afflicted with cataract to pass an indefinite period, waiting for the cataract to reach maturity. Where there is disease of the one eye, the other still having good vision, we may leave it to the discretion of the patient, as to whether he will undergo an operation or not. But where the other eye is also affected, and the patient can no longer follow his vocation, it certainly seems no more than proper that we should do all in our power to both assist him in regaining his sight and hasten the ripening of the cataract. We certainly would err greatly if we would permit those advanced in years to pass the few remaining years of their life in the useless waiting for a cataract to ripen, simply because the ancients imagined that cataract was an excretion, or to wait for the cataract to harden.

At the present day we know that a ripe cataract can easily be ex-

[1] Augenkrankhelten II. 316. Wien., 1817.

tracted from its capsule. Professor Schweigger[2] does not believe that it is necessary to cause an artificial ripening, after the time when physiological changes in the lens have done away with the act of accommodation; that is, toward the fifties and surely after the sixtieth year. He believes that every cataract may be extracted as soon as the interference of sight demands the operation, even if the greater portion of the lens is still clear.

"An equal degree of cloudiness in a young individual would designate an unripe cataract. In a young individual, accommodation is still present, the cortex of the lens still consists of a tenacious sticking mass, which adheres to the capsule, and if now such a lens extraction is made the nucleus still escapes, but the cortex remains behind adherent to the capsule. Though the pupil appear black in the beginning, it will soon become cloudy, owing to the saturation with aqueous; the changes here are simply those following discission. Generally speaking, after the fortieth year, every human lens contains a hard nucleus. If the corneal wound is of sufficient size, and the capsule is properly opened, the cataract can be delivered on the slightest pressure, and it is immaterial whether it is ripe, partially ripe, entirely ripe, or over-ripe. Alfred von Graefe[3] certainly did a great thing when he declared operable the brown, posterior cortical, and the punctate striated cataract." Schweigger declares that for some years past he has handled the subject in a purely practical manner. He operates all patients past the fiftieth year as soon as the senile cataract interferes greatly with the patient's vision, "so that life ceases to be a pleasure to him, and he becomes unable to be self-sustaining, and the doctor may hope that by the removal of the lens vision may be materially improved. It is immaterial whether a greater or less portion of the lens is still clear."

Schweigger seems to believe that all methods of artificial ripening of hard cataract, which have as their object the shortening of the time of blindness, can be dispensed with. He considers them purposeless.

He states: "To my mind it is antiquated to teach the practicing physician how to diagnose a ripe cataract. It is useless to make four operations on one eye. (1) The preparatory iridectomie; (2) The trituration; (3) The extraction through a small opening; (4) A subsequent secondary operation. By a single operation we not only reach the same end, but do it more quickly and better."

It had been observed long since, that where the capsule of the lens was accidentally touched; during an operation either on the iris or opening of the anterior chamber, that a subsequent cloudiness of the lens followed.

[2] The Extraction of Unripe Cataract, Berlin Med. Society, July 2, 1890. Hirschberg's Centralblatt, p. 206.
[3] A. f. O., XXX, 4, 225. 1884.

It was supposed that here the contact between the instrument and the capsule of the lens caused a disturbance, either in the epithelial cells lining the capsule, or a dislocation of the fibres immediately beneath the epithelial cell; as a consequence, interference with the proper nutrition and the regular arrangement of the lens fibres followed, with the further result of cataract formation. Foerster believed that there was a mechanical destruction of the lamellae between capsule and nucleus, and to him is due the credit of having first utilized this fact in hastening the ripening of cataract. He originally made the preparatory iridectomie, and then gently massaged the external corneal surface by means of a strabismus hook, and in the course of four to eight weeks the cataract was ready for extraction. The difficulty in doing this operation has always depended on estimating the requisite amount of pressure to be applied; since if this be excessive the zonula is easily ruptured, and with the result of loss of vitreous at the time of the extraction. This method of ripening has been widely employed. Some bolder operators of the present day even entering the anterior chamber with a small spatula, and triturating the lens direct.

The artificial ripening of cataract has been the subject of considerable experimental investigation by Hellferich,[4] Oettinger [5] and finally by Schirmer.[6] Schirmer experimented on fifty-two rabbits in exactly the same manner as Foerster did, without, however, making an iridectomie. He found that the earliest cloudiness set in in one or two hours after trituration, which could be defined as a series of very fine striations on focal illumination. In the course of a few hours this had advanced toward the equator until a circumference of this cloudy area about the size of a moderately dilated pupil. In forty-six cases a decided cloudiness followed; in ten a total cataract. On microscopical examination he found that as the result of mechanical pressure of the strabismus hook, the capsular epithelial cells undoubtedly degenerate. The nuclei of the cells show considerable resistance, with at first formation of vacuoles, until finally these were pressed out of the shrinking chromatin net-work, which forms a bright halo around them. The chromatin finally splits up in fine granules.

Immediately after the operation the superficial fibres are separated from each other, and spindle-shaped interspaces are formed. These spaces soon increase and are filled with granular substance. The fibres of the superficial layers swell up into vesicles, burst, and their contents exude under the capsule This disintegration is undoubtedly hastened by the

[4] Uber kunstliche reifung des staare. Sitzungs Berichte der Wurtzburger Phys. Med. Gellschaft, 1884, p. 115.

[5] Uber kunstliche reifung des staares. Inaugural Dissertation, Breslau, 1885.

[6] Experimentelle Studie uber die Forstersche Maturation der Cataract. Von Dr. Otto Schirmer Graefe, Vol. XXXIV, B. 1, 1893.

entrance of aqueous into the capsular sac. As a result of this disintegration of lens fibres, the processes of diffusion set in between the lens and
humor aqueous, just as in other forms of cataract, and since the fibres
possess a different coefficient of refraction, this zone becomes non-
transparent to rays of light, and hence will appear white. But if the fibres
disintegrate, and a more homogenous mass is formed, the substance may
be carried out of the capsule to such an extent as to cause small indentations on the surface of the anterior capsule. Meanwhile, the lens continues to grow at the equator, and the new fibres extend immediately beneath the epithelium toward the pole, so that the entire detritus may be
surrounded by new formed lens fibres.

In every case where we expect a successful maturation the massage
must be exerted to an equal degree on all fibres, in order that we may produce an equal destruction, and thus lead to a total cataract. The fibres
can only be destroyed where the tension within the capsule is increased.
"This pressure causes a dislocation of the various lamellae, and the formation of interspaces in which fluid stagnates, thus setting up an abnormal process of diffusion and a subsequent disintegration of the lens fibres."

THE AFTER TREATMENT.

Sufficient has already been said concerning the preparatory treatment.
If necessary the patient's general health should be cared for, examination
of the lungs, the presence of an aggravated bronchitis, should be alleviated as much as possible, in order to prevent coughing spells during the
time the patient must be quietly on the back, and the urine should always
be examined, and finally, the bowels should always be thoroughly evacuated before the operation. The conjunctiva should be thoroughly cleansed
with antiseptic solutions before the operation.

At the present day neither atropine nor eserine are used previous to
an operation. Becker, however, gives us special indications for their use,
which are likewise applicable today. He tells us, "In performing the flap
operation the right eye was brought fully under the influence of atropine.
The idea being to lessen the chances of the iris coming in contact with
the knife, and at the same time facilitating the exit of the lens." We believe
the observation is correct, for though the pupil contracts the moment the
aqueous is evacuated, the iris is more easily dilated by the lens after opening the capsule of the lens, when the eye has been previously atropized.
For the time being, the action of the atropine is overcome by the induced
spastic contraction of the sphincter, without this action being of a lasting
character. In the course of a normal healing, one will find that the pupil

which at the time of the operation was contracted, will in the course of a few hours become fully dilated again.

Likewise, in the beginning atropine was used in the Graefe operation. Eduard Meyer, however, suggested that its use previous to the operation be abandoned, and this suggestion has found general favor. The belief was expressed that cicatrization of the iris could be avoided in many cases, since, if we did not paralyze the sphincter previous to the operation, the iris would contract after the escape of aqueous, and thus permit the iris from becoming involved in the wound."

For the same reason DeWecker, in making his operation without excision of a piece of the iris, goes a step further, in that, at the conclusion of the operation, he drops a drop of sulphate of eserine ($\frac{1}{2}$ per cent. solution) into the eye, and thus by contraction of the pupil draws the iris out of the wound. Instead of a mydriatic he uses a myotic.

It is a matter of special importance to carefully examine and watch the conjunctiva before the operation. A host of observers have shown us the effect of an infected lachrymal secretion. The deleterious effects of a tear sac blenorrhoea have been recognized for a long time, and one would hardly expect to find an operator at the present day who would perform an operation without first healing the latter condition.

The same is true, though to a lesser degree, of all forms of conjunctival disease. A chronic catarrh should be suppressed as much as possible, and one should not forget that after an operation, owing to pressure of a bandage, the secretion may rapidly increase again. This should diligently be watched, the conjunctival sac kept clean, and thus the accumulation of the secretion prevented.

It is a peculiar circumstance that trachoma, granular conjunctivitis (chronic blenorrhoea of Arlt, opthal aegyptica), is not to be looked upon as a contra-indication to the performance of an extraction. At least this is true where pannus has developed, for the vessels in the cornea lead to a rapid and fortunate healing of the corneal wound.

THE AFTER TREATMENT. Von Graefe warned us against a certain indifference which even men of the greatest ability have been guilty of, as soon as the process of healing takes an anomalous course. He says: "True, owing to inability to explain in every case the cause of the intense reaction, one easily falls into the fatal error of simply laying one's hand in one's lap just as soon as the pain, active secretion, redness and swelling of the conjunctiva, uncleanness of the wound, cloudiness of the cornea, hypopyon, or hemorrhage into the anterior chamber set in. True, at the suggestion of a more experienced colleague, one tries one thing then another, but since no one method seems to avail in all cases which present the same symptoms, we become dissatisfied, and at times desist from any further attempts. Thus we turn from one mode of treatment to another, and finally we become completely skeptical, since no form of treatment is uniformly followed by favorable results."

This was written before the study of bacteriology had assumed its present important position, and before the full extent of the action of micro-organisms, in the production of inflammation was recognized. Today we know that all pathogenic germs may and do lead to destruction of the eye. Prevention of an infection is the watchword, for after the interior of the eye is once invaded, we may as well stand by, for we are helpless to stay the inflammation. All we can do is to alleviate the pain, meet complications as they arise, and eventually enucleate to prevent infection of the other eye.

The first symptom which demands attention is pain. Since the normal course of healing is accompanied by pain, it would certainly seem important to fix a border line where this becomes pathological. This, however, is impossible, since some patients are more sensitive than others. This pain is usually described as a burning pain. This never increases, but usually continues during the first few hours, gradually growing less. After five or six hours there should no longer be a continuous pain. From time to time the patient experiences a slight sensation of pressure. This is followed by a short, pricking sensation, followed by a sensation as though something were flowing from the eye. This sensation is due either to the accumulation of tears in the conjunctival sac, which in cases where the margins of the lids have become agglutinated together, can only escape when the pressure of the accumulated tears forces the lids apart. Or the pressure and the pricking pains are due to the accumulated aqueous forcing the edges apart, and thus escaping, either beneath conjunctiva or into the conjunctival sac, and then finally escaping between the edges of the lids.

These sensations can not be included with those of active reaction. As soon as the pain becomes paroxysmal, or changed from a burning to a tearing, lancinating, boring or thumping, it is to be alleviated by any method possible.

The bandage should be removed, the wound carefully examined and carefully cleansed. If the pain continues, cold applications and a hypodermic injection of morphia are indicated. Under all circumstances the patient should have a good night's rest. If necessary bromide of potash and chloral are indicated.

In normal cases, all signs of wound reaction disappear between twelve and twenty-four hours. Becker warns us that the very worst forms of disease begin to manifest themselves toward the close of the first night. The bandage should at once be removed and the wound examined, and if there is no tearing or swelling of the lids, the simple application of a fresh dressing, together with the usual washing off of the edges of the lid, will be sufficient. If, however, the linen pad which covers the eye is wet and covered with purulent secretion, we know that we are dealing with an infection. Von Graefe advised, after carefully cleansing the lids, that we touch the entire surface with nitrate of silver and then thoroughly neutralize the same. In robust individuals he even practiced venesection. Today use of antiseptics is called for, and as has already been stated, many operators cauterize the edges of the wound, and the anterior chamber is washed out with an antiseptic solution. If this does not stay the inflammatory process the eye is lost.

MENTAL DERANGEMENTS AFTER CATARACT EXTRACTIONS. It is customary to bind up both eyes during the first four or five days subsequent to an extraction, and during this time acute delirium has been known to develop. While in this state patients tear the bandages from their eyes, and thus forever destroy the results of what might otherwise have been a successful operation. Cases are recorded in which the wildest mania developed, and in which it was impossible to restrain the patient. Parinaud and Sichel believed this to be a cerebral disturbance, due to the removal of light and the restricted diet subsequent to the operation. Grandelement, Galezowski, Salvator, Angela Ledda, as due to use of atropine, Chibret to alcoholism; whereas Borreli believed this to be due to a predisposition to mania. Swanzy believes that it is due to the quiet and exclusion of light, following a period of some anxiety and excitement. He believes that permission to sit up in bed, with the admission of some light, will speedily restore the mental equilibrium. Therapeutically, sulphonal, chloral and the bromides are useful.

Patients should never be left alone, even during the night. They may unconsciously disarrange the dressing, and thus infect the wound. In restless patients, it is even advisable to tie the hands. Many a successful operation has been brought to naught by the patient sticking his hand or fingers against the bandage with sufficient force to rupture the wound, which has closed leading to prolapse of iris or vitreous, even to an intraocular hemorrhage. Many operators today have the nurse tie the patient's hands at night, or an electric bell is within reach, so that the nurse may be called at any moment.

DISCHARGE OF THE PATIENT FROM THE PHYSICIAN'S CARE. It is certainly not only a matter of interest to the patient who longs to return home, but also to the physician who may desire (in hospital practice) the bed for other patients, that the patient be not detained a single day longer than is absolutely necessary. Already Beer stated that the average time for a normal healing was about fifteen days. Later operators placed this time, including cases in which the processes of healing was not perfectly regular, at three weeks.

It is certainly not without interest to note that Gussenbauer fixed the time of a normal healing after an extraction at seventeen days; that is, that a total restoration of the connection between the divided corneal fibres was established in that time. Hence we must assume that the injury to other structures, iris, capsule, etc., does not in any way interfere with the timely healing of the cornea. But it is quite a different matter as to how soon, in the individual case, a patient can be discharged and released from the observation of the physician. It is customary to be guided by the condition of the conjunctiva bulbae. On the one hand, we meet with cases in which this does not become injected; whereas, on the other this injection may simply be the result of a conjunctival catarrh, without a more serious cause. But just for this first class it is of great importance to be able to fix the time of observation, since, according to Gussenbauer's anatomical investigations, it would be wrong, even in the most favorable case, to let a patient go before the beginning of the third week.

True, patients have left the clinic as early as the sixth and eighth day, without suffering the slightest detriment from this cause. Others, again, released on the twentieth day, returned a short time afterward, either with a corneal infiltration, hemorrhage into the anterior chamber, iritis or irido-cyclitis. Hence, it seems but proper that the patient should be kept under observation as long as possible, even though the process of healing has been a normal one. For where is the operator who will be willing to assert in any special case that the pathological changes which have been started in the iris and capsule have entirely ceased?

A still more fatal error is to permit the patient to begin the use of his glasses too soon. Though it is true, that owing to the loss of the lens, the eye has lost its power of accommodation, still we must not assume, that the ciliary muscle does not contract when an effort is made to accommodate, especially in cases in which the other eye still performs its functions, and the attempt is made to see objects near by. As a result of every such accommodative effort, a certain traction on and displacement of the zonula fibres follows. As long as the processes of proliferation are still going on in the secondary cataract, even in the simple secondary cataracts, these apparently unimportant movements may be sufficient to reawaken these processes of new formation, and thus lead to a greater thickness and density of the secondary cataract. But if this secondary cataract has already closed, it will then depend entirely on the extent of the cicatrization, and the structures which have taken part in its formation, what the character of the induced sequelae will be. We have already seen how the shrinkage of the complicated secondary cataract may become the cause of long-continued signs of irritation on the operated eye, and how this condition may induce sympathetic irritation; so likewise, the early use of cataract glasses, owing to their inducing efforts at accommodation in the operated eye, are only too often the indirect cause of iritis and cyclitic irritation which develops later on. Many a case of cicatrization of the iris and capsule, which would not have given rise to any trouble, take a fatal termination as the result of the early use of glasses.

It is not an easy matter to make a general statement as to the time after which the use of glasses can no longer be looked upon as detrimental. This depends on the mode of healing. The older physicians were correct when they laid down the rule that cataract glasses should not be used until months after an extraction.

THE SECONDARY OPERATIONS. In the broad sense of the term, these ought to be considered a part of the after treatment, since both the simple and complicated secondary cataracts may give rise to occasion for practicing these secondary operations. Whether the amount of vision obtained after a cataract operation will be sufficient or not does not alone depend on the degree of vision attained, but also on the demands which the patient makes on his eye. A farmer or a day laborer will be well satisfied if he can read medium-sized print; whereas, one who follows intellectual pursuits will require more vision, and request a secondary operation.

Since a secondary cataract may also result from injuries of the lens system, and since the difference between secondary cataract subsequent to an operation for cataract and traumatic cataract is really only one of degree, hence the treatment of both will be considered together.

The therapy of injuries of the lens, and of traumatic cataract, as well as the prognosis of these injuries, and the character of operation to be made, depends entirely on which other portions of the eye were injured, and what the condition of the eye is after the injury has healed.

TREATMENT OF RECENT INJURIES. Traumatic cataracts, in which there has been no injury other than of the capsule, do not require, during the period of their formation, any other treatment than that which any other disease process present at the time may require. Use of atropine prevents iritis and breaks up any possible synechia already present. It is dependent on other circumstances whether the cataract will remain partial or become complete.

If only the capsule of the lens has been involved, and no foreign body has remained in the lens, which is only possible where the wound in the capsule is a small one, the pupil is to be widely dilated by atropine, and then await developments and see whether the wound in the capsule heals, or if the tumescent lens substance is extruded into the anterior chamber. If the corneal wound heals, and no signs of a violent reaction develop during the first few days, which may result from the most trivial solutions of continuity, owing to increased tension in the eye, the same regulations are to be followed as in cases of discission. Simultaneous injury of the iris will not call for any special therapeutic procedure. Often the involvement of the iris is the cause of a more rapid healing of the wound in the capsule. Under certain circumstances a cut in the sphincter of the iris may assume the role of a prophylactic iridectomie.

One of the evil results of the above conditions may be a swelling up of the lens substance. As a result of his painstaking observations of traumatic discissions, Von Graefe restricted the indications for discission to the young. This swelling lens substance may lead to *secondary glaucoma* in the aged, and at times even in the young. In younger eyes the elasticity of the outer coats is greater; hence, a passing intra-ocular tension is more easily borne, until finally disturbance in the circulation sets in, and permanent increase of tension sets in. Hence, in the aged, owing to the greater rigidity of its walls, glaucoma and excavation of the papilla set in much sooner, the conditions being the same. Not infrequently we see the eyes of children under the influence of traumatic cataract for weeks and months, and in a condition of increased intra-ocular tension, without the optic nerve suffering in any way. Whereas, in old people we find the most insignificant swelling of isolated pieces of lens substance lead to glaucoma. This has been shown to be due to pressure on the root of the iris. This presses against the filtrating angle in the anterior chamber, and thus excluding a part of the filtrating angle, leads to interference with the outflow of fluid, and thus causes glaucoma.

If it is evident that glaucoma is about to set in, or if it is already present, one should not delay. The pressure phosphenes are especially valuable in testing the field of vision, since the tumescent lens substance materially affects, owing to the diffusion of light, all tests for projection. The indications seem to be divided between simple iridectomie, cataract extraction, or a combination of both methods. In young children one would make an extraction of the lens by a simple linear extraction, or by modified extraction in use today. If violent symptoms have developed, and call for interference, the lens will always be found to be so intensely swollen as to escape at once on making the incision. If the individual is older, and the increased intra-ocular tension is due to but slight swelling which is pressing on the posterior surface of the iris, the entire lens not being swollen, a simple iridectomie at the place where the pressure is exerted, would give by far the best results, and if necessary one would later on make a much better cataract extraction. If the patient is past the years of adolescence, and the lens is swelling, one will find the greatest relief follow a linear incision.

In the above described cases it frequently happens that the injury to the lens is the smallest part of the injury to the eye. This is always the case when the corpus ciliare is injured, be this ever so slight. The fatal influence which a shrinking cicatrix of the ciliary body exerts, not only on the injured but on the second eye, is too well known. Likewise, where a foreign body is in the vitreous, be it ever so small, the injury to the lens becomes a matter of secondary consideration.

Very broad incised or punctured wounds, as well as total destruction of the form of the globe are, as a matter of course, complicated by injuries to the lens.

After the signs of inflammation have disappeared, one must take into consideration the volume of the traumatic cataract before deciding on the method to be employed. If the difference of volume from a normal lens is but slight, one will be called upon to make a regular operation. The more the volume is reduced the more nearly will the cataract come under the same variety as the secondary cataracts.

TRUE TRAUMATIC CATARACT. If the traumatic cataract differs but little in volume from the normal lens, vision may be totally restored by performing a technical cataract operation. And since such traumatic cataracts usually develop as soft cataracts, a linear extraction is indicated. Notwithstanding the fact that synechia are frequently present the performance of the extraction is not, as a rule, connected with any difficulty; the results, however, are not very encouraging, depending largely on the further injury to other parts of the eye at the time of the accident, and the possible infection at that time.

In all these cases one should not forget, before operating, to test the light sense and the projection.

As has already been said, the operation offers no special difficulties. It is only where there is a capsular cataract present, or where the capsule has cicatrized in the cornea, iris, or ciliary body, that it does not give easily to slight traction; hence, one should not attempt to draw it out of the eye by force, though it does interfere with sight. *Violent traction, especially on the ciliary body, will be followed by the most detrimental results.* Even where such difficulties are not encountered, frequently the most violent reaction follows. The operative procedure leads to a recurrence of the cyclitis, which had but recently subsided.

Naturally the irritability of the eye decreases, the longer the time elapsed since the accident, and we may assume that a period is reached in every eye, at which time no evil consequences as a result of the accident will exert their influence on the proper healing of the operative procedure. Hence, it would be advantageous to fix a time when it would be well to interfere. It has been said that a traumatic cataract should not be operated earlier than the sixth or eighth week. Such a rule has no value, since under strict asceptic precautions the operation can not of itself induce any further injury to the eye. But where the case is complicated by iritis, cyclitis or choroiditis, it certainly would not be wise to undertake an operation. During this time Becker laid great stress on the circumcorneal injection, and laid down the rule, that the time for operating had arrived as soon as the pericorneal injection ceased to appear in grasping the conjunctiva with the forceps.

Seldom do we meet with a membranous cataract, (*cataracta membranacea*), or a secondary cataract (*cataracta secundaria*), without finding the iris bound down to the capsule in one or more places. Especially in cases of traumatic cataracts do we find broad adhesions. This is explained by the fact that during the period of swelling or immediately following the operation, the iris, for a considerable period of time, remains in contact with the capsule. Frequently, however, the iris receives a direct injury, or at least is irritated. Thus, depending on the character of the injury or the processes which have taken place subsequently, will we find a simple adhesion, a broad adhesion, or a proliferation of cells from the iris into the capsule. A deep anterior chamber, the irregular form of the pupillary edge of the iris which is adherent, the processes of an opaque membrane in the pupil, pigmented here and there, possibly vascularized, are all landmarks for the diagnosis of the above condition. If a piece of the iris has been excised at the time of the operation, one can also observe how the cloudy membrane gradually is lost in the cicatrix after the operation. In such a case, the secondary cataract usually lies far forward, adherent to the iris, or the cicatrical tissue in the cornea.

In the simple non-complicated secondary cataracts a *discission* with one or two needles will bring about the desired result, and with a high degree of safety and efficiency. This operation of *discission* after extraction is not without its dangers, which, according to Knapp,[1] causes *glaucoma* in from 1-2 per cent. of aphakic eyes. He believes that the *character* of the secondary cataract, and the *manner of attacking* the same, are the main

_____

1 Archives of Opthal., Vol. XXVII. No. 5.

factors. The reaction—glaucoma and cyclitis—being due to the traction on the cicatricial bands stretching to the ciliary body.

If the secondary cataract is fixed in the wound by cicatrical tissue, one frequently meets with success by making an iridectomie in the opposite direction, and thus regain a satisfactory amount of vision; since in such cases the greatest portion of the secondary cataract is drawn toward the wound. Frequently, however, the largest pupil fills up again, so that even a second iridectomie is without result. This usually is the case where the vitreous is detached and changed to connective tissue, and takes part in the formation of cicatrical bands. Such a result can not be foretold with certainty before an operation, but its occurrence is to be feared in all cases in which the cicatrix is drawn inward, and the tension is reduced, when the iris is discolored, and the membrane in the pupil appears to be vascularized. Both of the last symptoms are indicative of abnormal circulatory conditions. In consequence, during the operation, the anterior chamber becomes filled with blood, which is only absorbed after many days or weeks. When one finally does get a good view of the conditions present, one finds the pupil, which had again been made, filled up with new formed tissue. The operative procedure has awakened anew the formation of the cyclitic bands, and the momentary result of the operation has been brought to naught.

For this reason other operative procedures have been introduced to take the place of the iridectomie. It was advised that the cornea be severed by a 3 mm. wide two-edged knife; then go in with a pair of forceps and cut out a large piece of the iris, so as to lessen the chances of the space filling up again. (Agnew A. Weber.) Later on DeWecker favored the iridectomy (Annal. d'Ocul., Tom. LXX, p. 123). The advantages of the iridectomie which he makes with the lance-knife, and his "Pince-Ciseaux." lie in the fact that his operative procedure does far less injury, because the iris is not drawn out to be excised; but since it is held tense, he simply incises it and allows it to retract. Mooren followed this suggestion. Kruger advised cutting out a piece of the membrane with a scissors-like punch (Klin. Monatsblatt, 1874, p. 429).

Owing to the influence which everything which causes tension on the ciliary body exerts in causing cyclitis, it must be apparent that a secondary operation will be more certain of bringing about a good result, the more the above circumstances are avoided. With this object in view the two following operations were introduced:

BOWMAN'S METHOD. Two discission needles are employed; one is passed through the inner quadrant of the cornea and through the center of the opacity; the second needle is passed through the outer quadrant of the cornea, and into the opacity close to the first. The points are then separated, and thus a hole is made in the membrane.

NOYES' METHOD. A puncture and counter puncture is made with a Graefe knife in the horizontal meridian of the cornea, and as the knife is withdrawn it is made to puncture the secondary cataract. Two blunt hooks are now entered through the original corneal punctures, and the points passed through the openings in the membrane. By traction the opening is enlarged without any dragging on the iris or ciliary body.

THE THERAPY OF LUXATION OF THE LENS.

The treatment of luxation of the lens, just as that of cataract, be this of traumatic, spontaneous or consecutive origin, can only be considered prophylactically. This, however, has but little practical value, owing to the rarity of traumatic luxation, and because it occurs even less frequently as the result of certain occupations than the traumatic cataract, which is the result of accidental or designed injury of the eye.

The attempt was made a few times (Hornig, 1160a) to replace in the fossa patellaris a loosened or even a partially or totally dislocated lens by therapeutic measures, and thus to bring it back into its normal position. Eduard Meyer (1160b) reports a case in which a lens which was dislocated upward and inward returned again to its proper position in the pupil, notwithstanding the dislocation on the other eye increased. However, it did not remain fixed in its position, but moved about when the eye was moved about violently.

No cases are reported in which it has been possible to stop this increasing ectopia. Here, just as in cases of spontaneous sinking down of the lens, one can not hope for relief until we have discovered the cause. For though we accept Schirmer's idea, that the failure of the lens to grow during the time the remaider of the eye is growing, as the cause of the increasing dislocation in cases of ectopia, still one can not understand how the lens is to be urged on, or the remainder of the eye retarded in its growth. Similar reasons are given for the cases of spontaneous luxation following fluidity of the vitreous.

If the dislocated lens is still partially in the pupillary area and transparent, either myopic astygmatism or double refraction will ensue. The interference with sight may then be partially or totally relieved by glasses. If, however, the lens is cataractous, the interference with vision may be overcome by an iridectomie, very much in the same manner as has been advised in cases of zonular cataract. Knapp was the first (965) to advise iridectomie in cases of luxated cataractous lenses, which still occupied the pupillary area. Naturally, a permanent result only is to be expected, where the dislocated cataract has become fixed. Knapp's case was a dislocated traumatic cataract which had formed adhesions with the iris. Since in cases of shrunken traumatic cataract, the *zonula zinii* is frequently drawn to one side, and the interspace found considerably wider; so an iridectomie properly made will aid us in restoring a very considerable degree of vision.

Von Graefe was the first to practice iridectomie in cases of zonular cataract in 1855.

Though we might look upon the spontaneous sinking of the cataractous lens out of the pupillary area as an *auto-cure*, it may, nevertheless, if it is free in the eye, at any time give rise to secondary glaucoma. This is more apt to occur when a freely moveable transparent or cloudy lens gets in the anterior chamber. The extraction becomes a necessity in both cases.

PART V.

THE APHAKIC EYE.

DEFINITION AND DIAGNOSIS OF APHAKIA. According to the suggestion of Donders (Ametropie en hare gevolgen, Suermann en Donders, 1860, p. 87), we designate that condition in which the lens is absent from the dioptric system of the eye by the term *Aphakia* (a privativum and *φακή* the lens or bean).

Aphakia may be produced by different causes. It occurs most frequently as a result of operation for cataract or of an injury. In both ways the lens may either be removed from the eye at once, or after opening of the capsule be resorbed in the eye, or simply be depressed in the vitreous. Under the latter condition the lens is still in the eye, and may even remain transparent for a long time. We are, however, justified in designating this condition as aphakia, since the lens can no longer influence the direction of the rays of light. In cases of incomplete luxation (be this traumatic in its nature or spontaneous, or as in cases of *ectopia lentis*, in which not infrequently part of the pupil is free, whereas in the other portion of the pupil the rays of light as they enter are acted on by the lens), there exists a double condition of refraction. As a rule, myopia and hypermetropia are present at the same time, and we have before us a case of monocular diplopia. The myopia is due to the increased curvature of the surface of the luxated lens, and hence in an emmetropic eye this does not become very great. Whereas, the hyperopia differs in no way from the refractive condition of a completely aphakic eye.

It is not always an easy matter to determine the presence of aphakia at first sight. The appearance of the eye depends largely on the method of operation employed, the kind of injury produced, and the manner in which the process of healing progressed. In the foregoing chapters all those symptoms have been enumerated which could serve to aid us in making the diagnosis in every possible case.

Whether the operation or the injury has been followed by an occlusion of the pupil, one can judge by the external appearance of the eye. Where the operation was combined with an iridectomie, or the lens has escaped from the eye, in consequence of a rupture of the sclera, the coloboma of the iris, or the displaced pupil, will lead us to investigate the condition, and lead us to determine whether or not the lens is present. But if we are dealing with a case in which a successful extraction was made without an iridectomie, or a case of simple discission, a reclination or a spontaneous sinking of the lens in the depths of the eye, the aphakia will be characterized by a deep anterior chamber, the presence of iridodonesis, the absence of the Purkinje figures of the lens, and by the high degree of hyperopia.

This abnormal depth of the anterior chamber will be all the more apparent the older the individual, and consequently the shallower the anterior chamber on the non-operated eye. In cases of luxation of the lens, or ectopia, it is the unequal depth of the anterior chamber which directs our attention to the proper diagnosis.

Iridodonesis alone is not positive evidence of the absence of the lens, since peripheric tremulousness of the iris has been observed in cases of high myopia; also in cases of fluidity of the vitreous, without the lens being luxated. Trembling of the iris is not seldom wanting in cases in which the lens is absent, as per example, in cases in which the iris is bound to the capsule by synechia, but also where it is entirely free. It is possible that this is due to the development of an enormous crystalline pearl. This trembling of the iris becomes more noticeable, in cases in which either the lens moves about freely, or in which the vitreous which contains the lens has become fluid.

Parenthetically it may be here stated, that often in old people, where the iris has not been excised, the reaction of the pupil is not only as it should be, considering the age, but frequently is more active, and even in cases in which a coloboma has been made, the iris reacts to light.

The presence of the reflected pictures on the surface of the lens in doubtful cases, decide the presence of the lens in the pupillary area. Frequently on focal illumination, especially when an additional lens is used to enlarge the images, can the arrangement of the lens fibres be detected, or at least can we recognize its presence by the grey reflex of its substance. If this experiment gives us a negative result, we can only be positive of the absence of the lens, when aside from the reflected picture on the cornea, there still remains a second in the pupil. For since in most cases, even when the operation has been perfectly successful, the posterior capsule remains in the pupil, this can always give rise to a reflected image. This, however, as a rule, owing to the folds in the capsule, its want of curvature is exceedingly large, indistinct and distorted; nevertheless, I have repeatedly been able to observe a reflex moving in the same direction as the source of light. Woinow[1] has convinced himself, that this is an upright image, and he concludes that this reflecting surface

[1] A. f. O., XIX, 3, p. 110.

must have been slightly convex anteriorly. He even went a step farther and noted that these pictures grow smaller in looking at near objects. However, the images were too indistinct to be measured with the opthalmometer.

Even after an extraction in which the capsule is also removed, one can frequently demonstrate a reflecting surface, posterior to the plane of the pupil. In the case of a woman, 36 years of age, from both of whose eyes Becker removed shrunken congenital cataracts, and in which the microscope had given the absolute certain diagnosis that the entire capsule had been removed, this reflecting surface could not only be plainly recognized, but on dilating the pupil and using the opthalmoscope, one could see, most distinctly, the radially placed torn fibres of the *zonula zinii*.

The degree of hypermetropia is of itself, in cases of emmetropic and hypermetropic eyes, sufficient to make a diagnosis of aphakia, for it is a very exceptional thing to find a hyperope of $\frac{1}{3}$ or $\frac{1}{4}$, in a case where the lens is still present.[a] Degrees of $\frac{1}{8}$ to $\frac{1}{4}$ are very seldom due to a short axis. The diagnosis of aphakia in cases of high myopia, however, can not be determined optometrically.

THE OPTICAL SYSTEM IN APHAKIA. "Owing to the removal of the lens, the complicated dioptric system which exists under normal conditions in the eye, now becomes the simplest of which it is possible for us to conceive. Notwithstanding its different histological structure, we may look upon the cornea as having an index of refracting about the same as that of the aqueous humor. The very slight difference which was found in the coefficient of refraction, was determined by measurements made on the dead cornea. If we examine a living cornea in the aqueous, as is well known, differences will only begin to manifest themselves after a time, and these are to be looked upon as due to a gradual death of the tissue. Hence, during life the cornea is not only to be looked upon as homogenous, but as optically like the aqueous."

"Likewise, there is scarcely any optical difference between *humour aqueous* and *corpus vitreum*. Already the younger De la Hire found (1707), at the time he was called upon by the Akademie to answer the new teachings of Brisseau, contrary to what he had believed, that a mixture of aqueous and vitreous, taken from a pig's eye, remained perfectly clear, and thus proved that these two fluids neither exerted any chemical change on each other, nor did they have a different coefficient of refraction. All later investigations have simply further proven, that both not only possess the same index of refraction, but that this is the same as that of distilled water."

---

[a] In order to translate the inch scale to the Dioptre, multiply the fraction by forty. Thus, $\frac{1}{4} \times 40 = \frac{40}{4} = 10$ D.

"If we will simply consider the results of the investigations of the four last investigators, Helmholtz, Cyon, Fleischer, and Hirschberg, we will see that they respectively place the coefficient of refraction at 1.3365, 1.33532, 1.3373, 1.3374, and that of the vitreous at 1.3382, 1.33566, 1.3369, 1.3360, and we will further see that all these figures only differ in the third decimal place. And further, if we will take into consideration that Cyon made his calculations on the ox's eye, and that though Helmholtz and Hirschberg have found differences between aqueous and vitreous, which exceed somewhat 0.001, which however, may be ignored, we certainly can not go amiss if we accept as a basis for our work the figure attained by Fleischer. But since Fleischer has drawn attention to the fact, that owing to the increased temperature of the blood in the living eye, we will have to reduce the refracting indices of aqueous and vitreous about C. 0.001; hence, since our calculations are to be made for the living eye, we may place the index of refraction of the fluid media of the eye in aphakia—1.3360, which agrees almost exactly with the index of refraction of distilled water as determined by Brewster—1.3358."

"According to Listing it is not the surface of the cornea but rather a capillary surface of tears which is to be looked upon as the refracting surface. Hence, Hirschberg had a happy thought when he determined to estimate the index of refraction of the tears. This equals 1.33705, and hence only differs in the third decimal place. Hence the cornea, the center of which only comes under consideration here, is to be looked upon as a perfectly parallel surface, placed between two fluids of equal indices of refraction, and hence it can not exert any dioptric influence."

The same may be said of the capsule when this has been retained in the eye after a cataract operation. It may be folded, and reflect the light and contain cloudy masses here and there, absorb the light and cause dispersion, but it can never act as a refracting medium.

"This capillary sheath of tears, which fills out all the uneven places on the corneal surface, and which is to be looked upon as the true refracting surface, is dependent for its form, as a matter of course, on its underlying structure, the cornea. Its curvature is determined by its catoptric effect; that is, by the size of its images, and its power of refraction depends on this curvature and the coefficient of refraction (1.336) of the transparent media. Though the cornea is not spherical, but has rather an ellipsoidal curvature, one may ignore this departure from the globular form; since in the first place, at that point in the center of the cornea where the visual line cuts the same, this departure in a single meridian is exceedingly slight; and secondly, because in making the optometric examination of the refractive condition of the aphakic eye, in order to prescribe cataract glasses, we only make use of spherical glasses, and the choice of the same is nearly always confined to the condition of the refraction of the horizontal meridian. Hence, for the present we will not consider a congenital or acquired asymetrie in the curvature of the cornea. (Astygmatism.)"

"The simple dioptric system of the aphakic eye, which we shall take as our model for all our future considerations, consists of a spherically-curved refracting surface and two refracting media, the atmosphere which has an index of refraction 1.000, and the fluid media of the eye, which have a refractive index 1.336."

"If we now also know the radius of curvature of the refracting surface, we can easily determine the cardinal points of the system, according to Helmholtz's simplified formula of Gauss, and we can easily determine the interesting equations as to the length of the axis of an aphakic eye of known refractive condition, and *vice versa*, given the length of the axis; also concerning the size of the images at a given distance, and *vice versa*; also concerning the enlargement on combining the cataract glasses with the aphakic eye."

Owing to the great simplicity of such a formula, as compared with that of the complicated system of a complete eye, Listing came upon the idea of substituting the dioptric strength of his average schematic eye by a refracting surface; however, retaining the position of the posterior nodal point, and thus he constructed his so-called *reduced* eye.

"However, notwithstanding the analogy which exists between the reduced and the aphakic eye, they differ in that in the latter case we are always in a position to measure the curvature of the cornea with the opthalmometer, so that we are no longer dealing in the abstract, but are met by a condition of affairs which really exists."

"Hence, in arriving at the following general formulas we need not confine ourselves to the computations of Listing and Helmholtz in their schematic eyes. This is the result of the work of Donders (l. c., p. 258, Eup. Translation, 1864, p. 310), in that he does not use the average radius of curvature of the cornea of the aphakic eye, as computed by Listing and Helmholtz, 8 mm., but he uses the results of his own measurements, made on eyes of old men, the average of which he placed at 7.7 mm."

"Under these conditions the average measurements of the aphakic eye will be as follows: Corneal radius, 7.7 mm.; index of refraction of the media of the eye, 1.3360. The anterior focal distance, $\varphi^1 = 22.91$ mm. The posterior focal distance, $\varphi^2 = 30.61$ mm."

"From this we see that the visual axis in a case of normal curvature of the cornea must have a length equal to 30.61 mm., in order that parallel rays of light may come to a focus on the retina in a case where the lens is wanting. But since the length of the axis is almost always much shorter, hence in general we find the aphakic eye hyperopic to a high degree. From now on I shall designate the hyperopia as *aphakic hyperopia*."

"In order to find the degree of aphakic hypermetropia, with a given length of the visual axis, we need only calculate to what point behind the cornea the incidental rays must converge, in order after refraction by the cornea, to unite on the retina. This is done according to Helmholtz's formula (l. c., p. 44).

$f_{\prime} = \frac{F_{\prime} f_{\prime\prime}}{f_{\prime\prime} - F_{\prime\prime}}$ and $f_{\prime\prime} = \frac{F_{\prime\prime} f_{\prime}}{f_{\prime} - F_{\prime}}$, in which $f_{\prime\prime}$ the length of the visual axis and $f_{\prime}$ the point sought behind the cornea.

According to the same formula we can also determine the length of the visual axis, when the focal distance of the glass which corrects the hypermetropia and its distance from the center of the cornea are known. Accordingly, as this glass is held at a greater or less distance from the eye, eyes with varying lengths of the visual axis can see in the distance."

EMMETROPIC APHAKIA. "The finding of the proper glass with which an aphakic eye can see in the distance is practically a matter of experiment. In order to do this, we either follow the suggestion of Donders, using a luminous point; or we use the Snellen's test types, such as are usually employed in testing cases of refraction. By this means we at the same time gain an idea as to the acuity of vision."

Experience has taught us that a glass which has a focal length of more than 3.5" (+11 D), will be required in order to see distinctly in the distance. In the last hundred cases operated, thirty-five received glasses of $\frac{1}{3\frac{1}{2}}$, (+11 D); fifty-two glasses ranging between $\frac{1}{4}$ (+10 D) and $\frac{1}{3}$ (+11 D). Aside from this twenty-four glasses No. $\frac{1}{4}$ (+10 D); so that by adding these together, we find that seventy-six, about three-quarters of all those, received cataract glasses of $\frac{1}{4}$ to $\frac{1}{3\frac{1}{2}}$. Only eight patients saw distinctly in the distance with stronger glasses, and sixteen with weaker glasses. The weakest glass which I ordered was for $\frac{1}{12}$, the strongest $\frac{1}{3}$ This agrees with Snellen's statements, who gave a glass of $\frac{1}{3\frac{1}{2}}$ in 65 per cent. of cases; in 11 per cent. stronger, and in 24 per cent. weaker glasses. (If Westhoff doubts these figures for acquired H, this must evidently be a clerical error for Donders, from whose reports the above statements are taken, is likewise of the opinion that in the majority of cases a glass of $\frac{1}{3}$ to $\frac{1}{3\frac{1}{2}}$ (+10 D to +11 D) will be necessary to see distinctly in the distance.) The conditions are confirmed by all reports.

"If we assume the average distance at which a cataract glass is placed from the cornea, equal to 0.5", we would still find, taking into consideration the distance of the nodal point from the cornea, in the majority of cases after the cataract operation, the acquired H would equal $H \frac{1}{2.65}$ the radius of cornea being 7.7 mm; the length of the optical axis being 23.86 (7) mm."

"(In the case of the schematic eye, the radius of the cornea would be 8 mm., and the length of the optic axis would be 24.5 mm., which would be more than above.) Hence such an eye, having a corneal radius of 7.7 mm., an index of refraction of 1.3360, and an optical axis of 23.86 (?) mm., may be looked upon as an emmetropic eye. We therefore call it *the emmetropic-aphakic eye*."

"Very frequently, however, the distance of the center of the glass is farther removed from the center of the cornea than 0.5". Where the distance of the glass is 0.75", the length of the optic axis is reduced (7.7 mm. radius) to 23.39 mm. Hence, it is still considerably greater than is the case in Helmholtz's schematic eye (22.23). If we will now assume that most cases of senile cataract occur in eyes which were emmetropic before they became cataractous, and became affected with senile hypermetropia, we come upon a contradiction between the average length of the optical axis as determined by Helmholtz, and ourselves, after cataract operations, and according to optometric examinations."

In any special case, we need not satisfy ourselves with the average length of the radius of the cornea after a cataract operation, for we can obtain this accurately by measurements made with the opthalmometer. Here assuming that the index of refraction of the vitreous has not changed, we can obtain the exact length of the axis. In the following table I have taken those in which the corneal radius was measured in the horizontal meridian with the opthalmometer before the operation by Reuss and Woinow. Since the distance from the eye is not stated, I have taken this to be in one case 0.5"; in another as 0.75". From these tables it also becomes evident, that the average length of the axis, without exception, is greater than is the schematic eye."

Hence, it follows, that not only the corneal radius given is too great, but that also the refractive strength of the lens, be this the result of improper position or a too great absolute strength, has been assumed too great.

TABLE VII.

NAME.	ρh.	Focal Distance of the Glasses Ordered for Distance.	$f_1 = -$	H aph.	Length of the Visual Axis $f_u =$	$f_u = -$	H aph.	Length of Axis $f_u =$
Pischinger . .	8 0780	9."5	9."00	$\frac{1}{8.65}$	29".38	8."7	$\frac{1}{8.40}$	26."80
Nitsch	7.9275	6.00	5.5	$\frac{1}{5.15}$	27.10	5.25	$\frac{1}{4.90}$	26.66
Werhotta . . .	7.7282	4.5	4.0	$\frac{1}{3.65}$	25.20	3.75	$\frac{1}{3.40}$	25.70
Pohlhammer .	7.4954	3.75	3.25	$\frac{1}{2.90}$	24.84	3.00	$\frac{1}{2.65}$	24.86
Donabaum .	8.1794	3.5	3.00	$\frac{1}{2.65}$	24.86	2.75	$\frac{1}{2.40}$	24.34
Furtlehmer . .	7.8976	"	"	"	24.20	"	"	23.70
Karger	7.6108	"	"	"	23.71	"	"	23.04
Leisser	7.4155	"	"	"	23.05	"	"	22.60
Dolak	7.8740	3.25	2.75	$\frac{1}{2.40}$	23.68	2.5	2.15	23.17
Matcheky . . .	7.5862	"	"	"	23.07	"	"	22.54
Fisher	7.8544	3.00	2.5	$\frac{1}{2.15}$	21.93	2.25	$\frac{1}{1.90}$	21.34

ρh=Radius of horizontal meridian of cornea ; f, as in formula on page 376. H. aph, aphakic hypermetropia ; f, as given on page 376, f determined length of axis.

MYOPIC AND HYPERMETROPIC APHAKIA. "If the eye was myopic previous to the operation, it will require weaker glasses after the operation. And likewise, where an eye requires a weaker glass after operation to see in the distance, we conclude that the eye must have been myopic. We can then also approximately judge the degree of myopia. Donders reports a case in which an aphakic eye was not improved, either by use of a plus or minus glass. In this case the visual axis of an eye which had become emmetropic by aphakia, must have had a length of 30 mm., and from this we may draw the deduction that as long as the lens was present in the eye there must have existed a myopia of about ⅛ (—10 to —11 D). A glass of ⅕ (+ 5 D) or less is now sufficient to see in the distance, and not infrequently patients state that they now see better with a + 4 D, or + 5 D, or less. than they formerly did with the myopia of ⅛ (—8 D) or more."

"Donders, who drew attention to the fact that zonular cataract, as a rule, is associated with myopia, was given the opportunity to measure the radius of curvature of the cornea in three cases, which were myopic before and hypertropic after the operation, and from this he determined the length of the optic axis. Table VIII shows their length. It happens that in the first case the axis of curvature of the cornea is somewhat shorter, and in the two latter somewhat longer than usual. Hence, from the length of the visual axis one can determine the degree of myopia."

TABLE VIII.

AMETROPIA.		CURVATURE RADIUS OF CORNEA.	CALCULATED LENGTH OF THE VISUAL AXIS.
Before the Operation.	After the Operation.		
M=1:6	H=1:5.12	7.6	25.96
M=1:8.5	H=1:4.5	7.92	26.89
M=1:24	H=1:8.2	8.04	25.02

"We find that congenital hyperopia acts in exactly the opposite manner. However, Donders declares that one seldom finds an aphakic H > 1:2.5. I do not remember that I even prescribed a stronger convex glass than ¼. In the two hundred cases reported by Snellen, I find only two cases in which 2¼ was prescribed. One of these cases had been previously operated on (iridectomie) for glaucoma, and with success."

AVERAGE MEASUREMENTS OF THE EMMETROPIC EYE. "Based on the values given for the emmetropic eye in the foregoing paragraph, we can construct an absolutely emmetropic average eye, if we will reconstruct the lens within the same. Of this lens we neither know its focal distance nor the position of its principal points; however, we do know, that it must fulfill certain conditions, namely, to cause rays of light which enter the aqueous converging, so as to meet at 30, 61 mm. behind the cornea, to so alter their course as to come to a point at 28.36 mm. To this problem there are an indefinite number of solutions, in that the focal distance of the lens is dependent on the position of the principal points, and *vice versa*. The calculation has shown, that a lens having the focal distance, as in the schematic eye (43.707 mm.), answers the above condition when its conjoined principal point is 9.754 mm. posterior to the cornea. According to our anatomical knowledge such a position of the lens is an impossibility. However, if we will calculate the focal distance of a crystalline lens, the optical center of which shall be in the nodal point of the aphakic eye (7.7 mm. behind the center of the cornea), and which shall answer the above conditions, we will obtain a value of 54.84 mm. Such a position of the lens is a possibility, though it has not been anatomically proven. Since following an operation we desire to calculate for the aphakic eye what the previous refractive condition was, we must determine, as has already been explained, what the true conditions are in the emmetropic eye, and to do this the schematic eye does not suffice; hence, I give below the calculation made for an average emmetropic eye."

$r=7.7$ mm., $e=1.3360$, $f_1=23.86$ mm., focal distance of the lens $=54$ 84 mm. and position of the same $=7.7$ mm., $F_1=16.15$ mm., $F_3=21.59$ mm. Position of $H_1=2.25$ mm., $H_3=2.28$ mm., $K_1=7.68$ mm., $K_3=7.71$ and finally the position of $F_1=-(16.16-2.25)=-18.90$ mm., and the position of $F_3=23.87$ mm.

Finally, it is interesting to note that according to Helmholtz the focal distance in the air of the lens in his schematic eye is 8.9 mm.; whereas, according to ours this has fallen to 11.16 mm."

"In the construction of our average emmetropic eye we have made two assumptions. It is only an assumption, and has not been proven that an aphakic eye, which has its H. neutralized by a lens of 3.5" focal distance, placed at 0.5" distance from the centre of the cornea, must have been emmetropic before the operation. Owing to the very great importance of the propositions which must follow, it is a matter of the greatest importance, and its value can hardly be estimated, if it were to become possible to determine the aphakic H. exactly, in eyes in which the condition of refraction is known. The second assumed factor is the position of the the lens. If it should ever happen that we should be enabled to make an extraction on an eye which, before becoming diseased, had been under observation, and in which we had estimated the refraction, the corneal curvature, the depth of the anterior chamber, and the curvature of the anterior surface of the lens; and again, after the extraction, estimate its refraction and its corneal curvature, this would certainly materially aid us in our estimates, concerning our knowledge of the lens system in the living human eye. As this would also aid us in determining the index of refraction of the lens and its individual lamella, the only fact still remaining unknown would be the form of the posterior surface of the lens, and on which the thickness of the lens depends. Under these existing conditions it seems proper that the following figures should be stated as having a direct bearing on the question.

TABLE IX.

NAME.	AGE.	NON-OPERATED.			OPERATED.				
		EYE.	R.	ρh.	EYE	OPERATION.	H aph.	ρh.	LENGTH OF AXIS.
Schweller ..	11	L.	$-\frac{1}{36}$	7.74	R.	Discission	$\frac{1}{2.4}$	7.526	23.086
Weiss.....	11	L.	$-\frac{1}{36}$	7.87	R.	{ Discissio modificato	$\frac{1}{2.7}$	7.66	23.787
Hilbert....	40	R.	$-\frac{1}{36}$	7.6414	L.	Graefe's Ext.	$\frac{1}{3.17}$	7.024	22 779
Kircher ...	68	L.	$+\frac{1}{9\frac{1}{2}}$	7.2828	R.	"	$\frac{1}{4.22}$	7.247	24.456

"The above table contains a series of figures bearing on the condition found existing in four individuals, in each of whom an eye had been operated on for cataract; whereas the other eye still had a transparent lens, and in which the refractive condition could be estimated by the test types and the opthalmoscope. An exact inquiry into the history of the case showed that previous to the disease the patient had seen equally good with both eyes. In order to determine the length of the axis of the aphakic eye, the distance between the glass and the cornea, was estimated as nearly as possible. Though the radius of the cornea may be diminished in its horizontal meridian as a result of the operation, this will not shorten the length of the axis of the eye. Hence, one may safely transfer the investigation of this point to the sound eye. In the fourth case the length of the axis appears relatively short, owing to the abnormally increased corneal curvature; especially if one will compare this case with an analogous one, case 2, in table VIII. In that case the corneal radius was abnormally large, here it is abnormally small. The minimum measurement, according to Donders, of 7.28 mm., coincides exactly with the radius of Kircher's case. A portion of the myopia hence is dependent on the cornea, and in this case we are dealing with one of corneal myopia."

"Conditions which exist between aphakic H., length of the optic axis, and also the R. previous to the operation. In preparing the following table, which shall serve to illustrate the mutual dependence between the degree of H. aphakia and the length of the optical axis, I have started with the express value of F. The value of f. was obtained from the well known formula, $f_{\iota} = \frac{F_{\iota} \cdot f_{\mu}}{f_{\mu} - F_{\mu}}$ and according to which this table has been estimated. On these values, taking into consideration the distance of the glass from the center of the cornea and the nodal point in the aphakic eye, the values of the correcting glass and the aphakic H. are dependent."

TABLE X.

f_u—Mm.	f_i—		H acquisita. (Distance from K—7 7.)	Correcting Glass when Distance from Eye.		R.
	Mm.	P. Z.		13.54 Mm.—0 5 P.	20.31 Mm.—0 5 P.	
30.61	∞	∞	$\frac{1}{\infty}$	0	0	$-\frac{1}{2.5}$
29.56	649.92	24	$\frac{1}{23.65}$	$\frac{1}{24.5}$	$\frac{1}{24.75}$	$-\frac{1}{8}$
28.58	324.65	12	$\frac{1}{11.65}$	$\frac{1}{12.5}$	$\frac{1}{12.75}$	$-\frac{1}{3.5}$
27.24	216.64	8	$\frac{1}{7.65}$	$\frac{1}{8.5}$	$\frac{1}{8.75}$	$-\frac{1}{4\,6}$
26.81	163.48	6	$\frac{1}{5.65}$	$\frac{1}{6.5}$	$\frac{1}{6.75}$	$-\frac{1}{5.7}$
26.16	135.30	5	$\frac{1}{4.65}$	$\frac{1}{5.5}$	$\frac{1}{5.75}$	$-\frac{1}{6.4}$
25.75	121.86	4.5	$\frac{1}{4.15}$	$\frac{1}{5}$	$\frac{1}{5.25}$	$-\frac{1}{7.6}$
25.25	108.82	4	$\frac{1}{3\,65}$	$\frac{1}{4.5}$	$\frac{1}{4.75}$	$-\frac{1}{10.0}$
24 68	94.78	3.5	$\frac{1}{3.15}$	$\frac{1}{.4}$	$\frac{1}{4.25}$	$-\frac{1}{1.75}$
23.86	81.24	3	$\frac{1}{3.65}$	$\frac{1}{3.5}$	$\frac{1}{3\,75}$	$\frac{1}{\infty}$
23.40	74.47	2.75	$\frac{1}{2.40}$	$\frac{1}{3.25}$	$\frac{1}{3\,5}$	$+\frac{1}{27.7}$
22.87	67.47	2.5	$\frac{1}{2.15}$	$\frac{1}{3}$	$\frac{1}{3\,25}$	$+\frac{1}{12.0}$
22.24	60.98	2.25	$\frac{1}{1.90}$	$\frac{1}{2.75}$	$\frac{1}{3}$	$+\frac{1}{7.1}$
21.51	54.16	2.0	$\frac{1}{1.56}$	$\frac{1}{2.5}$	$\frac{1}{2.75}$	$+\frac{1}{4\,6}$

The last column of figures requires an explanation. It is designated R. (refraction). The reciprocal values which they represent are, according to Zehender's suggestion, the various grades of hypermetropia where they are minus, and the various grades of myopia when they are positive, and emmetropia is designated by $\frac{1}{\infty}$. All these values have been estimated according to the formula: $f_i - F_i = \frac{F_i F_u}{f_u - F_u}$ [1]). Helmholtz, l. p. 49, 7[a].

Since f,—F. represents the difference of position between the retina of the emmetropic and the ametropic eye, hence it became necessary in the foregoing paragraph to determine for the emmetropic eye the length of its axis, and for this reason it was given in the one table as 23.86 mm."

"As a matter of course, this table only contains the average values. A comparison of this table with the foregoing one will serve to clear up all the causes of all individual differences."

ACCOMMODATION OF THE APHAKIC EYE. "The eye does not desist from making accommodation efforts after the loss of the lens. The subjective sensation of accommodative effort on which Donders, and so correctly, lays such great stress, is very evidently present. Not only do patients who have been operated on one eye or both, without any knowledge of the subject, express themselves very plainly, stating, that notwithstanding every effort, they are not able to see; but in those cases where the one eye is aphakic while the other is still in possession of its accommodation, intelligent patients state, that they are made aware of the well-known sensation in the operated eye."

"Under like conditions, in cases where no iridectomie has been made, and in which no muscular insufficiency is present, the aphakic eye will follow the accommodative effort of the other eye, by making the correspondent movement of convergence, and likewise the pupil will undergo contraction or dilation. Hence, there can be no doubt, that in both eyes the muscle of accommodation has a similar innervation, and is likewise incited to contract. This view is further strengthened by a series of pathological experiences which have already been referred to. These accommodative efforts, however, have no result. *With the loss of the lens every trace of accommodative power passes away.* Donders has given us the proof of this axiom."

1. "A youthful individual was successfully operated on both eyes for *congenital cataract.* By using glasses $\frac{1}{3}$ (+7.5 D), 5" from the eye, he saw a luminous point, perfectly round and sharply defined. A screen was placed between the one eye and the luminous point, and now in converging so as to cause the visual axis of both eyes to be directed to this screen, this luminous point still appeared unchanged, or at most somewhat smaller and more sharply defined. If now this lens before the eye was only moved forward, (10 mm.), this luminous point in distance ceased to be so sharply defined, and seemed to be elongated in the opposite direction. This visual line became slightly shorter on converging, without, however, becoming merged into a single point. This shortening, as well as the diminution in size of the point which had been so sharply defined, seemed to depend on the narrowing of the pupil during the act of convergence. 2. In a second cataract operation, made on a very intelligent young man, Donders was further enabled to determine, that where a point of light could be sharply seen by using a certain lens, the addition of a lens of light could be sharply seen by using a certain lens, the addition of a lens of $+\frac{1}{180}$ or $-\frac{1}{180}$ would materially change the sharpness of the image. In a third case this difference was noticeable on the addition of a $+\frac{1}{300}$. Invariably the patients state, by the addition of a $+\frac{1}{180}$, the image becomes

drawn out vertically, and by the use of a $-\frac{1}{130}$ in the horizontal direction. Whereas, by converging of the visual line, in making his experiment, so as to see near, was not followed by the slightest effect on the form of the images. If one will make an exact examination of the amount of vision ($V=\frac{d}{D}$) in an aphakic eye, for some particular point, for which the eye is equipped with a certain glass, and will then further examine the amount of vision which the eye possesses for points lying either in front of or behind the selected point, one will find the vision becomes reduced in both directions. From this it must follow, that the eye does not possess any accommodation, for if it did the amount of vision would either remain the same, or in cases of positive accommodation, owing to the object being brought closer to the eye, and the moving forward of the second nodal point, even became somewhat greater (Coert over de scynbare accommodatie by aphakie). The truth of these experiments, undertaken at the suggestion of Donders, became all the greater, since it was further shown that the circles of dispersion, the pupils being of equal size, became larger instead of smaller in cases in which there was an aphakic dioptric system."

"During the previous century, this question of the accommodation of the aphakic eye (see Donders, 1526) was the subject of very extensive investigations, carried on especially by English physicians and investigators in natural sciences. Hunter attempted to prove the correctness of the theory which had been accepted since the time of Leeuwenhoek, namely, that the lens was made up of muscular fibres, and that by means of their contraction and relaxation we were enabled to accommodate for various distances. His successor, Home, hit upon the lucky idea of deciding this question of accommodation by making his investigations on the aphakic eye. In this work he sought the assistance of Ramsden, and both came to the conclusion that even without a crystalline lens there existed considerable accommodation. They, however, made no further investigations after they found that Benjamin Clark, who had been operated on for cataract, and on whom they made their investigations, could read at different distances with the same glass. Home then conceived the idea that the cornea changed its form during the act of accommodation. In investigations made in this direction, they distinctly saw the cornea advance further forward, and from this they concluded that the cornea became more convex on accommodating for near. On November 27, 1800, Thomas Young appeared before the Royal Society, and opposed both of these statements of Ramsden and Home, and proved in the most convincing manner that in seeing near objects neither the cornea became more convex nor did the visual axis become elongated, and aside from this he proved, not only by exclusion, but by the most positive facts, that the seat of accommodation could only be found in the lens itself.

"Assisted by his friend Ware, he likewise examined a series of cases of aphakia. In doing this he employed Porterfield's optometer, which is based on the principle of Scheiner's experiments, and he convinced himself that the points of intersection of the threads across the image always are seen exactly in the same position. Wherever a slight difference occurred, he could always find that a corresponding change in distance between the eye and the glass was to blame. Young further found that in making the Scheiner's experiment, if small objects were seen double the patients were not able, by exerting any degree of effort, to bring the objects closer together. Though he stated that his results were only "tolerably satisfactory," nevertheless this seems really to have settled the question. It is a well known fact that these investigations of Thomas Young, "On the Mechanism of the Eye," had long been forgotten; hence, it can not be so much of a surprise to find such men as Arlt and others ascribing to the aphakic eye a slight degree of power to adapt itself to various distances. The question again became an important one after Kramer, in 1852, had given us the direct proof that the lens becomes more convex during the act of accommodation. Since it was exceedingly difficult to prove that these images on the lens diminished in size to a degree proportionate to the extent of accommodation as measured by the optometer, hence they tried to positively settle the question by determining whether a trace of accommodation still remained after loss of the crystalline lens. The first investigations made in this direction by Von Graefe did not clear up this subject. (Beobachtungen uber die Accommodation bei Linsen defect u. s. w. Arch. fur Opthal., II, 1. p. 187. 1855). Graefe verified Ramsden's experiments. "Only lately I examined a patient who had undergone an operation for cataract on both eyes but four weeks previously, and he could read medium sized print (No. 77 Yager's test types) with a -|-3 convex, at a distance of 6" to 20". But since only a short time previous to this he himself had explained why eyes with high degrees of hypermetropia are better able to distinguish small objects, notwithstanding the increased size of the circles of dispersion, when they bring the object much closer to the eye; hence, he was admonished to be careful, and thus was enabled to express the opinion, 'that shortly after a cataract operation there was either none whatever or possibly only a trace of accommodation left. And where he says that the amount of adaptability in the operated eye, as compared with that existing under normal conditions is exceedingly slight, his doubt as to the remnant of accommodation left is of such a character, that he sought for a means to explain this."

"The cause for these unsatisfactory results was owing to the fact that the idea of 'width of accommodation' and 'amount of vision' had not yet been so accurately determined. After Helmholtz had expressed himself, 'in order to prove that accommodation is still present, the patient must be able to distinguish an object at a given distance distinctly or indistinctly, even after he has attempted to see an object at the same or at a greater distance,' it still remained for Donders to give us the accurate proof, that an aphakic eye possessed absolutely no power of accommodation. (See text.) Hence, it will be a matter of the greatest surprise to learn that in 1872 Foerster (Klin. Monatblatt. p. 39. Accommodations vermogen bei Aphakie) expressed himself, that accommodation was present in eyes devoid of a lens. Foerster has nothing further to offer us than the Home-Ramsden experiments, and he even neglected in the single case which he examined to make an accurate test of the refract on, to give the amount of vision for distance, the size of the test type used, and to inform us whether or not care was taken to see that the lenses were properly centered, so as to coincide with the visual axis. Hence, it seemed hardly necessary to reply to his paper. Nevertheless, it called forth a mass of refutations. Mannhard re-repeated Ransden's experiments, using the Snellen test type and Burghardt's dotted tests. The more delicate the object used the more delicate these tests for amount of vision and distance became; the more this apparent width of accommodation shrank together. I was enabled to get the same mentioned colleague and make these experiments on him, and I also used the rodoptometer, the apparent width of accommodation equaled with $+\frac{1}{2}$ and Sn No. $1\frac{1}{2}$ about $\frac{1}{10}$, with Burghardt's dotted tests No. 3, less than $\frac{1}{5}$ and with the rodoptometer, less than $\frac{1}{100}$. The use of this rodoptometer, which was not used by Foerster, appears to me to be the most conclusive of all the tests for vision. Above all, to make these tests properly, the patient should be a scientifically educated as well as an honest man. Above I have already mentioned the investigations of Coert, made under the supervision of Donders. Wolnow sided with Foerster to a certain degree. He placed a piece of cobalt glass in a slit and illuminated this from the rear, and then found that in his own atropized eye, simply moving the instrument 2-3 mm. nearer to his eye was sufficient to cause the edges of the split to be bordered with colors. He however found that those who had undergone cataract operation could see this slit at a more variable distance without the appearance of this border, so that in intelligent patients with a vision equal to or less than two-thirds, he could find a remnant of accommodation of about $\frac{1}{10}$.

THE ACUTENESS OF VISION IN APHAKIA. "Strictly speaking, every cataract operation has attained an optical result, in which vision is better after, than it was before an operation. For example, if fingers could no longer be counted before the operation, and if this has become possible afterward; or if fingers can be counted at a greater distance than before the operation, one surely would not say that the eyesight has not been improved by the operation. However, neither patient nor physician would be satisfied with such a result. Both have acceded to the operation with the hope, that a useful degree of vision would be restored, and only if this is attained, as compared with an insufficient or partial restoration, can one speak of a satisfactory result."

"Since one meets with every degree of vision, from counting of fingers up to $\frac{20}{15}$, hence repeatedly in compiling statistics, the want of a sharp line to guide our results has made itself apparent; but such does not exist. In special cases this depends entirely on the requirements which the patient demands from his eyes."

"But seldom does the acuteness of vision of the aphakic eye equal that of the normal eye. This is determined by the Snellen type, always, however, bearing in mind the age of the patient. However, as Donders pointed out, owing to the magnifying power of the cataract glasses, we must make a slight correction."

"Owing to the fact, that either convex glasses of varying strength are required to see at the various distances, or the glasses must be adjusted at varying distances from the eye; hence, the acuity of vision, where this is simply determined by convex glasses, will show great differences for the various distances. Equal values can only be attained, if one will multiply these with the corresponding so-called (verkleinerungs zahlen) reduced figures."

"If we will now consider those cases of aphakia which have been corrected for distance by spherical glasses, we must look upon the attainment of an acuity of vision of 20-70 as the average amount following a successful cataract operation. But in many cases $V=\frac{20}{100}$ or $\frac{20}{100}$ for distance, answers all requirements, which are needed for near work. If one will now classify the results following the operation into losses, partial and total good results, we must look upon all as belonging to the first class, in which vision is less than $\frac{1}{10}$ at twenty feet. And all belong to the third class, in which vision is $<\frac{1}{10}$."

Knapp states: "Considering V $\frac{20}{100}$ to $\frac{20}{70}$ as a good result, $\frac{11}{100}$ to $\frac{1}{100}$ as a moderate result, mere perception of light and blindness as failure, the visual results in 1,000 successive cases, 1866-1888, were, good 85.4 per cent., moderate 8.3 per cent., failure 6.3 per cent.; loss from suppuration 4.2 per cent., loss from all causes 2.1 per cent.

From June 10, 1886, to June, 1897, I have practiced the simple extraction as a rule. In 300 simple extractions, good, 96.33 per cent.; moderate, 2.66 per cent.; failure, 1.01 per cent.[a]

"Those cases deserve especial attention in which $V=\frac{20}{10}$. Such a result is entirely wanting in Knapp's and Snellen's cases, the former having but one case in which vision reached ½, and the latter but six cases in which vision equaled ½, but in not a single case did vision equal 1. Compared with these statements, I wish to mention one made by Weber, who passingly (1117, p. 190) says, that according to the method employed at present, hardly in ⅙ of the cases does vision equal 1. Such a statement is hard to understand, unless one assumes, that he determined vision in a manner entirely different from the method laid down."

CAUSES FOR THE DIMINUTION OF THE ACUITY OF VISION IN APHAKIA ASTYGMATISM AS A RESULT OF THE OPERA-

[a] Norris and Oliver. System of Diseases of the Eye. Vol. III., page 818.

TION. That normal vision, according to the Snellen idea, is so seldom attained after a cataract operation, so long as we confine ourselves to the use of spherical glasses, demands an explanation, especially since Weber has definitely stated that 'the moving forward of the nodal points, should justify us in theoretically expecting an acuity of vision much greater than normal, after a cataract operation.' "

"Let us only consider the senile cataract, and we will find one cause for this at once in the fact, that according to the investigations of DeHaan, in the sixtieth year vision sinks to $\frac{4}{4}$; that is, to $\frac{20}{28,5}$. Aside from this opacities in the pupillary area are supposed to be the main cause of the reduction in the vision. Surely we have already dwelt sufficiently on the fact that even in cases of simple secondary cataract, the folds in the capsule, and the slight cloudy spots in the same, give us the anatomical basis for the increased reflection and dispersion of light. In consequence of this, not only are the retinal images less brightly illuminated, but likewise, as a result of the dispersion of light, the images are less sharply defined. The influence of a secondary cataract, becomes most evident, for in cases of a very dense secondary cataract, vision may be exceedingly good, if there is but a small opening, and at times this is proven by the extraordinary influence which a discission of a secondary cataract exerts on vision. But even after such a procedure, or after the extraction of a cataract in its capsule, even after making a vitreous puncture, we but seldom attain a result in which vision equals $\frac{4}{4}$. Since the curvature of the surface which separates the vitreous from the aqueous has no influence on the sharpness of the retinal images, and since an immovable pupil or even a large coloboma (at least as it is associated with direct seeing) is without influence on the acuity of vision, hence the main cause for the diminution of vision in the successful cases of cataract operation must be sought in *the changed curvature of the cornea*, which is the most important of all the refractive surfaces."

"Donders (Eng. Edit., 1864, p. 315) in 1864 drew attention to this fact. It appears that Javal (Klin. Monatsblatt., 1865, p. 339) was the first to really measure the amount of astygmatism in those who had undergone cataract operation. In one case, by using a cylinder of $\frac{1}{16}$, the acuity of vision was increased from $\frac{1}{4}$ to $\frac{3}{4}$; whereas, by the most careful selection of a proper spherical glass, this could only be increased to $\frac{1}{2}$. Graefe likewise expressed himself, that the cause of this astygmatism which appears after cataract operations in a good many cases, is due to a less perfect cicatrization, which leads to this cylindrical curvature of the cornea. But if vision was normal before the formation of the cataract, and if after the operation vision is very materially improved by the use of a cylindrical glass, this could be explained by assuming that in the former integrity of the lens system the degree of corneal and lens astygmatism exactly compensated each other, and later on when aphakia had set in, the corneal astygmatism still remained. Whereas, in such cases the conditions remain totally stabil; still, under the first named conditions these gradually become changed to the advantage of the patient. Haase (Wiesbaden Klin. Beobachtungen, III, p. 116) then more fully examined into the causation of this astygmatism which develops after cataract operations. He found that in cases in which the incision was made exactly in the horizontal meridian, one would always find the meridian which refracts most strongly exactly horizontal. If the direction of the incision was slightly changed, then likewise also the direction of the most strongly refracting meridian. During the process of healing of a flap incision, the intra-ocular pressure will constantly press the edge of the wound, which still gives apart. By this means the curvature of the cornea becomes flattened in its vertical meridian; whereas, the curvature of its horizontal meridian will be increased. In cases of abnormal healing, as in *prolapsus iridis*, the astygmatism is so irregular that a good correction can not be obtained by use of cylinders. In the six cases of flap extraction which he reports, the astygmatism varied from ⅙ to ½."

"Reus and Woinow (1167) have collected the largest amount of material having a bearing on this subject. They were enabled to make opthalmometric examinations in thirty-one patients who had been operated for cataracts. Of these twenty-three had been measured before the operation. From this they were enabled to determine how much of the astygmatism had developed in consequence of the operation. If we will now consider those twelve cases (1, 3, 5, 8, 10, 13, 15, 17, 18, 24, 28 and 31) in which the principal meridian was exactly vertical and horizontal, both before and after the operation, we find in only eleven cases an increase in the curvature; that is, a shortening of the corneal radius in the horizontal, and only in ten cases is there a diminution of curvature; that is, an increase of the corneal radius in the vertical meridian. In the other cases the result was directly opposite. And in fact, both forms occur as well after flap extractions as after the corneal extraction."

"Hence, it seems quite evident that the degree of astygmatism after an operation depends very materially on the degree present before the operation, and also on the direction of the same. One can not, however, in any given case, determine from the degree of astygmatism present after an operation which method of operation would have given the best result."

"This much, however, is certain, that in the twelve mentioned cases, the particular condition was produced by the operation. Reuss is very careful in making his statement, and merely says, that the astygmatism is caused by the cicatrix, and its degree is largely dependent on the more or less perfect processes of healing. More exactly stated, always dependent on the kind of astygmatism present before the operation. The direction of the acquired astygmatism is always dependent on the position of the incision, its extent, on the perfect healing, and its regularity depends on whether or not the iris and capsule become cicatrized in the wound."

"Although we must acknowledge that we do not as yet possess any positive anatomical explanations for those cases in which the vertical meridian has an increased curvature, and the horizontal a diminished curvature after the operation; nevertheless, in all of the thirty-one cases measured by Reuss and Woinow the corneal astygmatism was changed as the result of the operation. Hence, Reuss is correct when he considers the above second explanation of Von Graefe as only correct for those eyes which were operated by discission or reclination, but not for those in which the lens was removed from the eye by an excision. Now, in what manner does this cicatrix bring about this acquired astygmatism? Concerning this point, up to the present time there have existed but suppositions. After such data as can be gleaned from our knowledge concerning the cicatrix following cataract extraction, and according to the facts which have been given us as a result of the experimental investigations of Gussenbauer and Guterbock, there can scarcely arise any question as to the influence of an intercalar substance in cases of perfect cicatrization, since this was found to be but 0.02 mm. in width. However, the inclosure of foreign substance, especially of the capsule or the iris, where this has taken place to a large degree, must exert an influence on the conditions of curvature of the cornea. Even in cases in which a perfect cicatrization has taken place, it does occur that the lip of the corneal wound becomes displaced toward the sclera, and in five cases I (Becker) have been able to measure this exactly. This varied from 0.12 mm. to 0.3 mm. It appears (if the number of these observations can be looked upon as sufficient from which to draw conclusions) to be larger after flap extraction, ceteris paribus, than after the scleral extraction, and aside from this is favored by the enclosure of foreign substance in the cicatrical tissue. And finally I (Becker) was enabled to prove that the portions of corneal and scleral tissue close to the cicatrix were very much increased in thickness, in abnormal cases as much as 0.5 mm. Beyond a doubt this is due to infiltration and oedematous swelling of the tissue, and hence can not be considered as an increase in the amount of tissue laid down in the direction of the corneal lamellae, that is perpendicular to the direction of the wound, without a simultaneous swelling being present."

"We must, however, call attention to another factor which gives rise to change in the corneal curvature. The clinician, and rightly, too, knows but too well that the drawing in of the extraction cicatrix is but a much-feared symptom of beginning phthisis bulbi. Aside from this I have repeatedly drawn attention to the great tension which the contraction of secondary cataracts, which have cicatrized in the wounds, exert while shrinking, on the *corpus ciliare*, the vitreous, etc. Now, there can be no doubt but that even where this exists to a slight degree in eyes which can see, the shrinking of this secondary cataract by its tension will draw the cornea backward. By this means the curvature of the cornea will become increased vertically to the direction of the incision; and hence, the cornea is given a more cylindrical shape, and the curvature of the horizontal meridian will become diminished."

"For the present I must leave unanswered the question as to whether this tension of a secondary cataract can act in just the opposite way, causing an increase of the horizontal and a diminution of the vertical meridian."

"This influence, which the various methods of cicatrization of wound exerts on the condition of the curvature of the cornea, must be entirely different, and makes its effect felt in just the opposite way where the incision is made vertically or obliquely. The pushing more anteriorly of the edge of the corneal wound must necessarily have as its result a diminution of the curvature of the cornea, vertical to the direction of the wound. But if no sliding past each other of the edges of the wound has taken place, and if one can everywhere see the scleral edge of the wound and the underlying edge of the cornea, the swelling of the substance which lies between the edges of the wound, must cause the increase in the curvature of the cornea in the vertical meridian. For if we attempt to introduce the segment of a circle between two fixed points of a segment of another circle, this can only be accomplished by increasing the radius of curvature of the latter."

"The action of a connective tissue mass between the edges of the wound acts differently, depending on whether a sliding past each other of the edges of the wound has taken place or not. If the outer edges of the wound are in exact apposition, owing to the presence of this connective tissue mass, the curvature likewise must become greater. If at the same time this mass causes a forward displacement of the edges of the wound, this flattening action of the cicatrix must be increased. If the incision is made perpendicular to the surface of the cornea, as it is in the ideal Graefe's extraction, such a displacement forward can not occur so easily, and therefore is not so frequently observed as after the flap extraction, in which the incision is made perpendicular to the visual line. In the flap operation there is a greater tendency for the edges of the wound to gap, and this is in accord with the greater frequency and the greater degree of displacement forward. Based on measurements made by me, the amount of flattening which the cornea suffers as a result of displacement after flap extraction can be measured."

"Starting out with the assumption that the cornea has a spherical curvature, a vertical section of the same would be represented by the segment of a circle, the chord of which would be equal to the distance from the upper to the lower edge of the cornea. The length of this segment is calculated by the formula: $\frac{2\,R.\,n.\,\rho°}{360°}$, when $\rho°$ is equal to the angle which the segment of the circle subtends, the radius (R.)—7.7 mm., and the distance from the upper to the lower edge of the cornea equals 10 mm., then the length of this segment of the circle (P.) equals 10.8834 mm."

"The direction which the edge of the corneal wound takes as it moves forward, is determined by the direction of the original incision. If this falls in that of the ideal linear incision, in the direction of its greatest circle, the anterior movement will take place in a iine that is along the radius drawn from the center of the circle toward the upper edge of the cornea. The segment of the circle will remain the same, but the chord which it subtends will have grown larger. If this forward movement equals respectively, 0.12, and 0.15, and 0.3 mm., the radius will be, respectively, 8.0798, 8.1775, and 8.7638 mm. Starting out with the assumption that previous to the operation both the vertical and the horizontal meridian had a radius of 7.7 mm., they will now have a radius respectively of $\frac{1}{17.98}$, $\frac{1}{14.47}$ and $\frac{1}{6.964}$. In making this calculation, the further hypothesis was drawn that this flattening of the corneal surface was equally distributed over the entire vertical meridian. However, in doing this no attention was paid to the fact, and the same was done in the calculation of Reuss and Woinow, that simultaneously with this flattening in the vertical meridian, an increased curvature manifests itself in the horizontal."

"Notwithstanding this, the calculations of Dr. Weiss show, that the average measurement as used by me is sufficient to explain the degree of astygmatism found after an extraction. This increased curvature of the horizontal meridian, which for the time had been neglected, may be assumed to correct the astygmatism which had previously existed in the opposite direction."

"Various observers have noted, that the astygmatism which develops after cataract extraction becomes less as time goes on. This can be explained anatomically by the gradual diminution of the infiltration, and swollen conditions of the area surrounding the wound, and by the gradual contraction to a smaller volume of the connective tissue mass when present, and also by the gradual return of the flap to its normal niveau, where this has glided past its fellow, owing to the tense drawing together of the interstitial tissue. This can not be absolutely proven, since it is not possible to make anatomical examinations of the same eye at various periods. But these conclusions are justified, and may be assumed to be facts, as the result of anatomical examinations of various eyes made at different periods after operations. Hence, the astygmatism must gradually diminish in both directions."

"I (Becker) owe special thanks to Dr. Roder, of Strassburg, for the personal communication of a case which clinically is of the very greatest interest. He noted that the astygmatism following an operation suddenly became less after the making of an iridectomie for secondary cataract. The horizontal incision made with the lance, made to relieve the secondary cataract, must for the time have relieved the tension which this exerted at the sight of the original wound. Hence, if the curvature of the cornea perpendicular to the direction of the incision before the irdectomie was greater, one must certainly be able to see that the cutting through of the capsule would have released and equalized this; but since likewise a less degree of curvature in the vertical and an increased degree in the horizontal should likewise be abolished by an iridectomie, we must also seek part of the explanation for this in the vertical incision of the capsule, made with the pinceciseaux. But since this fact has not as yet been as well proven as could be desired, it would hardly seem necessary to seek for an anatomical basis for the same as yet. But if this should be proven to be true, it certainly would become a matter of unusual interest. There would then appear to be a way in which to cure, by operative means, astygmatism which results from operation."

"Although the measurements of Reuss and Woinow made on the living, and my (Becker) measurements made on anatomical preparation, coincide exactly with the results obtained by Haase, namely, that corneal astygmatism is greater after the flap extraction than after the linear extraction, one must nevertheless be careful and not accept this as an absolutely established fact. Haase undoubtedly picked out the most pronounced cases, since during an entire year he only measured the astygmatism in six cases of all those operated by Pagenstecher; whereas, among Reuss' and Woinow's thirty-one cases, there are but five flap extractions, and of these but in three cases was the cornea measured before. In addition to this, I find that the greatest degree of astygmatism noted, $\frac{1}{5.94}$, did not occur after a flap operation, but after a linear extraction. Nevertheless, the subject is certainly deserving of every consideration, and as early as 1867 Weber drew attention to the fact, that the various operations exerted a varying influence on the methods of healing and the subsequent astygmatism. And it can not be denied, that if it should finally be shown that one operation is more responsible for this condition than the other, this factor would certainly weigh heavy in the balance against it. Dr. Weiss has lately taken up these investigations again, and I may state, that five cases which were measured before and after operation by the Weber's method, in three cases change in form were found after the operation, which had an astygmatism of 1:11.2, 1:15.4, 1:27.3; whereas, in two cases which were operated by Weber, the astygmatism was $\frac{1}{6}$ and $\frac{1}{9.08}$. The influence which the subsequent correction of the acquired astygmatism following cataract extraction has on the acuity of vision of the aphakic eye, is shown by the following investigations of Reuss and Woinow. In twenty-nine eyes which were subjected to a thorough examination by the use of spherical glasses, four acquired $V = \frac{20}{200}$, four $V = \frac{20}{100}$, thirteen, $V = \frac{20}{80}$, six, $V = \frac{20}{70}$, two, $V = \frac{20}{50}$. But where these same eyes were corrected by a combination of spherical and cylindrical glasses, there was but a single case in which $V = \frac{20}{200}$, which could not be improved. In the others, however, vision was raised four times to $V = \frac{20}{70}$, three times to $\frac{20}{50}$ seven times to $\frac{20}{40}$ ten times to $\frac{20}{30}$ and four times to $\frac{20}{20}$. The last figures are especially interesting, because once vision of $\frac{20}{100}$, twice vision of $\frac{20}{70}$, and once vision of $\frac{20}{50}$ was raised to this high degree."

The above statements have been verified by Adolph O. Pfingst. He draws attention to the literature on this subject, Laquer,[2] Chimemi,[2a] Burnett.[3]

He states: "We know that in the majority of cases the addition of a cylinder to the spherical lens improves the vision. As the cornea gradually assumes its original or almost original shape by the contraction of the cicatrix, the cylinder glass frequently ceases to be of benefit. To avoid the expense of a new glass after this contraction has taken place, we are, and especially in hospital practice, often called upon to prescribe at once the lens which we consider best for ultimate use." He gives the following interesting tables:

A.—CASES WITH COMPLICATED HEALING OF WOUND.

Extraction of Irideetomy. W. R.—with the Rule. Ag. R.—against the Rule.

No.	Astig. before operation.	Astig. 2 wks. after opera.	Astig. 6-10 weeks after operation.	Astig. 4-6 months after opera.	Astig. 6-10 months after opera.	REMARKS.
1	1.0 D. W. R.	9.5 D. Ag. R.	6 weeks, 3 5 D. ag. R.	6 mon., 2.5 ag. R		Slight incarceration of iris in middle of section.
2	1.0 D. W. R.	10.0 "		4½ month, 2 0 ag. R.		Iris drawn upward, and slight a d hesion to middle of section.
3		18.0 "				Prolapse of iris, abscised 14 hours later.
4		13.0 "	.	:		Prolapse of small head of vitreous. Small incarceration of iris.
5	1.75 D. W. R.	12.0 "				Patient ruptured wound 3 times. Adhesion of iris to middle of sec.
6		17.0 "	6 weeks, 1.90 ag. R.			Large incarceration of iris in middle of section.
7	0.75 D. Ag. R.	6.0 "	8 weeks, 6.5 ag. R.			Prolapse of iris, abscised 8 hours later.
8	0.5 D. W. R.	12.0 "				Iris adherent to middle of section.
9		22.0 "				Iris adherent to section in its entire extent.
10	0.5 D. W. R,	7.0 "				Incarceration of column or iris in wound, on nasal side.
11		12.0 "		6 month 6.0 ag. R.		Prolapse of iris, abscised 12 hours later.
12		17.0 "				Adhesion of iris in entire length of wound.
		155.5				Average. 12.9 D.

[2] Arch. fur Opthalmol., XXX., 1884.
[2a] Annales di Ottal., 1890.
[3] A Treatise on Astygmatism, p. 129.

B.—CASES WITH UNCOMPLICATED HEALING OF WOUND.

No.	Astig. Before Operation.	Two Weeks After Operation.	6-10 Weeks After Operation.	4-6 Months After Operation.	6-10 Months After Operation.	REMARKS.
13	0.5 D W. R.	7.0 D. Ag. R.	10 whs., 3.0 Ag.R.	6 mo., 1.5 D. Ag. R.	10 mo., 1.5 Ag. R.	
14		2.5 "	6 " 2.0	4 " 1.75 W. R.	10 " 1.75 W. R.	
15	Em.	6.0 "	9 " 2 0	4 " 12.5 Ag. R.	6½ " 1.25 Ag. R.	
16	0.75 W. R.	4.5 "	8 " 2.0	5 " 1.5 "	7 " 1.5 "	
17		3.5 "	8 " 1.25	6 " R.		
18		11.0 "	7 " 3.0	6 " 1.0 Ag. R.		
19		3.5 "	9 " 2.5	6 " 1.75		
20	0.5 W. R.	8.0 "	6 " 2.5	4½ " 2.0		
21	3.0 W. R.	3.5 "				
22	Em.	7.5 "	10 " 3.0	4½ " 3.0 "		
23	0.5 W. R.	7.5 "	6 " 2.0	4 " 0.75 "		
24		7.5 "	8 " 3.0	4 " 1.75 "		
25	0.75 W. R	15.0 "	6 " 3.5	4 " 2.0 "		
26	0.75 W. R.	3.75 "	6 " 2.0			
27		8.5 "	7 " 1.0	4 " 0.5 W. R.		
28		5.0 "	8 " 2.0			
29		5.5 "	6 " 2.5	5 " 2.25 Ag. R.		
30		1.75 "	10 " 1.75 W. R.			
31	0.5 Ag. R.	6.5 "	6 " 2.0 Ag. R.			
32		9.0 "	9 " 2.25 "			
33	1.0 W. R.	7.0 "	8 " 1.25 "			
34	4.5 W. R.	8.0 "	5 " 6.0 "			
35		10.0 "	6 " 2.25 "			
36		10.0 "	9 " 2.25 "			
37		1.75 "	10 " 1.75 W. R.			
38	Em.	13.0 "	6 " 7.0 Ag. R.			
39		6.0 "	8 " 2.5 "			
40	0.75 Ag. R.	2.5 "	8 " 1.25 "			
41	Em.	5.5 "	6 " 2.0 "			
42-59		118.5 "				Represents 17 cases, which were only examined once.
		299.75				Average, 6.40 D.

Total number of cases, 59. Total astygmatism, 455.25 D. Average of astygmatism. 7.7 D.

From these he draws the following conclusions:

"Briefly recapitulating, we see: (1) That two weeks after the flap extraction of cataract, there is corneal astygmatism, varying from 1.75 D with rule, to 20.0 D, against rule. (2) That the greatest amount of this astygmatism disappears in the following four to six weeks. (3) That it is absolutely reduced in six months, after which it seems there are no further changes."

"Bearing these facts in mind it is evident that an accurate estimation of the ultimate glasses can not be made at the end of two weeks. The rule among opthalmologists is to give a temporary glass for three to four months, and allow cicatrical contraction to take place before deciding on the final glass. But even in selecting this temporary glass, being governed by our table, we may select it so as to do for permanent use. In cases with less than 5.0 D of astygmatism, which in four months is generally reduced to 1 or 2.0 D, we have usually prescribed the spherical lens which gave the best vision, even though the addition of a cylinder lens was of benefit at the time. In cases with more than 5.0 D, and especially in those in which the wound had healed with complications, we added 2.0 D cylindrical, with axis indicated by the opthalmometer and the test glasses, provided the vision was improved. By putting together a sufficiently large number of cases, at least with those in complicated healing, we may be able to arrive at a conclusion as to the changes to be expected in each individual case. The subject would, I think, furnish a field for further investigation."

THE APPARENT AND REAL ACUITY OF VISION IN APHAKIA. Vision in the aphakic eye is seldom brought up to 20-20, either by use of spherical glasses or when they are combined with cylinders; and this certainly must become a very striking fact, if we stop to think, that the retinal images in the aphakic eye are, in all those conditions in which they are sharply defined, larger than in the emmetropic eye.

"By larger I mean the condition of the retinal image as compared in the two eyes. In a case of hypermetropia, one compares the image produced in the corrected eye, both with the image in the same eye during accommodation, as also with the image which would appear in an emmetropic eye. But since there is no accommodation in the aphakic eye, hence the first mentioned image used for comparison can never be a sharply defined one. It certainly is less a matter of interest in any special case how large the image will be, or how large it would be in the emmetropic eye, than what is the average size of the image. Hence, for comparison we will again use the average eye which we used in constructing our emmetropic eye. Since the posterior nodal point almost exactly coincides with the nodal point of the emmetropic, aphakic eye, hence we can use the same figures in tables XI, XII and XIII, showing the enlargement and diminution for both cases."

"This enlargement is due to the fact, that the second nodal point of the combined system *under all circumstances* (see Mauthner. Vorlesungen uber die Optischen Fehler des Auges, p. 192 and 193), moves in front of the nodal point of the *aphakic*, and therefore, also in front of the second nodal point of the emmetropic eye. Hence, the retinal images of objects observed at equal distance, are to each other, as the distance of the second nodal point of both systems from the plane of the image, which, when seen distinctly, exactly coincides with the retina. Hence we may place them in relation with the distance, instead of the size of the image. (See Mauthner, l. c., p. 175.)"

"Above it was stated, that in a case of hyperopic aphakia, it would be impossible to obtain a sharply-defined image without a correction. There is a single exception when the retina lies in the second principal focal plane of the aphakic system. If an aphakic eye is 30.61 mm. long, then parallel rays of light will come to a point exactly on the retina; that is, will form sharply-defined images of objects placed at infinity. This image will be, as compared with an emmetropic eye, very much enlarged. If we will now designate the size of the image of an accurately seeing aphakic eye by B_2, that of the emmetropic eye as B, further the distance of the nodal point from the retina in the former by K_2n, and of the latter by Kn, hence the relation will be $B_2 : B = K_2n : K_n$. If we will now substitute for the second side of the equation their values, it will be

$$B_2 : B = 30.61 - 7.7 : 23.86 - 7,7.$$
$$= 22.91 : 16\ 16.$$
$$= 1.417 : 1.$$

and it will then be 1:1, 417=0, 705:1; hence, B2=1.417B, and the amount of *vision* thus obtained by the optometric measurement of the aphakic eye is to be multiplied by 0.705, so as to be comparable with the emmetropic eye."

Thus, if we found that vision in an aphakic eye 30.61 mm. long was equal to $\frac{20}{20}$ we would have to multiply this result by 0.705 in order to obtain the actual degree of vision, as compared with retinal image of equal size, or expressed differently $V = \frac{20}{20}$ would be the *apparent* degree of vision, and $V = \frac{20}{20} \times 0.705 = V = \frac{14.1}{20}$, or $V = \frac{20}{28.36}$ would be the *actual acuity of vision* in an aphakic eye 30.61 mm. long, without any correction for the distance. If we will now place before the aphakic eye a convex lens of $\frac{1}{10}$ at a distance of 0.5" from the cornea, and make the calculations for this combined system, we will find that $K_2n = 29.58$ mm. Comparing this with the emmetropic eye, we will find that the increase $= 29.58:16,16 = 1.830$; whereas the diminution equals 0.546. From this it follows that this enlargement is must greater, when, as in the case where a convex glass of $\frac{1}{10}$ is placed before the eye, "the eye is accommodated for a distance equal to 10.5."

The apparent acuity of vision is determined by the following:

$$V\ \frac{20}{20} \times \frac{1.830}{1.417} = \frac{20}{20}.\ \ 1.290 = \frac{20}{15.50},$$

and this in its turn again, multiplied by the amount of diminution 0.546, give us the actual degree of acuity of vision."

$$= \frac{20}{15.50} \times 0.546 = \frac{20}{28.36}.$$

"In this single instance, in which an aphakic eye is enabled to see images perfectly distinctly, we can compare the acuity of vision of the aphakic eye for near and far. The figure representing the enlargement of the image, where we artificially produce accommodation for 10.5" distance equals 29.58:22.91=1.290. By this means, just as for near

$$V = \frac{20}{20} \times 1.290 = \frac{20}{15.50}.$$

"The enlargement or the apparent acuity of vision is dependent where the focal strength of the convex lens remains the same, on its distance from the eye, and where the distance from the eye remains the same, on the focal strength of the glass chosen. If one will at the same time so change both factors, so that the focal strength of the glass, less the distance (f-x) always remains the same, there will likewise take place a very considerable movement anterior to the second nodal point. All three methods are important in general practice. By means of the last mentioned method one can very materially, one might almost say at one's pleasure, increase the size of the retinal image for a specified distance, and at the same time the apparent acuity of vision will be greatly increased. The first two methods, as we shall see, serve to take the place of the lost accommodation, and hence we must try to compare these methods with that which gives an apparent enlargement, to see which gives the greatest advantages. Tables XI to XIII are designed to give a general idea of these conditions. Each one shows six or seven complete calculations of the combined systems. In all three I (Becker) started with the above totally emmetropic aphakic eye, which resulted from the removal of the lens from an emmetropic eye. Its values are therefore found in the first column of each table."

"In table XI, using the same eye, instead of beginning with $+\frac{1}{8.5}$, this is combined with $+\frac{1}{4}, \frac{1}{4.5}, \frac{1}{5}, \frac{1}{7}$ and at the respective distances $1'', 1.5'', 2'', 3'', 4''$, from the eye. The individual columns contain the values of the separately calculated combined systems."

"From the first column we at once learn the very important condition of this combined system; namely, that the second principal point and the second nodal point move anterior to their respective first points; so that the value of H_1 H_2 K_1 K_2 becomes negative. Whereas there is a rapid increase for the values of the anterior and posterior focal points, and also for the distance of the principal and nodal points from each other, the position of F_2; that is, the position of the posterior focal point, remains unchanged.

TABLE XI.
The Emmetropic Aphakic Eye.

The correction for distance	$\frac{1}{85}$	$\frac{1}{4}$	$\frac{1}{4.5}$	$\frac{1}{5}$	$\frac{1}{6}$	$\frac{1}{7}$
The distance from centre of cornea	$0.''5$	$1.''0$	$1.''5$	$2.''0$	$3.''0$	$4.''0$
Anterior focal point F of the combined system	20.84	23.82	26.80	29.88	35.74	40.73
Posterior focal point F_2	27.84	31.83	35.81	39.79	47.75	55.71
Distance from F_2	23.867	''	''	''	''	''
Distance from H_1	-1.22	1.09	6.90	16.25	55.10	88.82
Distance from H_2	-3.97	-7.94	-11.91	-15.91	-23.87	-31.88
$H_1 H_2 = K_1 K_2$	-2.75	-9.03	-18.81	-32.16	-78.97	-120.65
Distance for K_1	5.78	9.07	15.91	26.15	67.11	108.80
Distance for K_2	3.03	0.04	-2.90	-6.01	-11.86	-16.85
$K_2 n$	20 83	23.85	26 80	29.88	35 74	40.73
Kn	16.16	''	''	''	''	''
Enlargement $K_2 n : Kn = ^1$	1.289	1 432	1.658	1.849	2.212	2.520
Diminution figure $Kn : Kn$	0.775	0.698	0.603	0.540	0.453	0.396

"That is to say, in all six columns the calculations are made with the glass placed at the distance from the eye as designated above. By comparing the figures which represent the degree of enlargement we learn that the selection of a weaker glass is followed by an enormous enlargement of the retinal image. If we select a glass with a focal length of 1" instead of 2.5, this enlargement is doubled. And if we used a $+\frac{1}{14}$ the patient would see the object seven times enlarged. Vision is about the same as though one placed before an emmetropic eye a $-\frac{1}{2}$, and then in front of this, at a distance of 11" from the eye, place a convex glass with a focal distance of 14". This combination being about the same as that of a Holland or Galileo's telescope. The aphakic eye, like every highly hypermetropic eye, can be made to simulate the action of the telescope by the use of a simple convex lens of from 10-2" focal distance, under which circumstances the hypermetropic eye takes the place of the ocular. An aphakic eye can be corrected for distance by any convex glass, whose focal length is greater than the correcting glass placed at the shortest possible distance from the eye. During this procedure, the enlargement of the image grows rapidly. However, as the distance of the glass from the eye increases, the field of vision contracts, so that after all, such a combination, just as is the case with the opera glass, is only used occasionally."

ARTIFICIAL ACCOMMODATION IN THE APHAKIC EYE.

"Strictly speaking, an aphakic eye ought to have a separate pair of cataract glasses for every distance at which one is desirous of obtaining a sharp and distinct image. If one starts out with the assumption that the distance of the glass from the eye remains unchanged the above statement becomes a fact. But the same effect can be produced by changing the distance of the glass from the eye. So that, beginning with a certain glass, which gives the proper correction for distance, every aphakic eye in a two-fold manner may be made to see objects placed at a shorter distance. Both methods coincide, in that the position of the posterior principal focal point becomes gradually farther removed from the retina of the aphakic eye; that is, removed more anteriorly. The relation of the retina of the aphakic eye, is to the principal focal point in the new system, as the retina in the myopic eye, or as the principal focal point in the accommodating eye, is to the retina of the emmetropic eye; hence, the conjugate anterior focal distance lies at a definite distance in front of this system. Hence, the conjugate anterior focal distance lies at a definite distance in front of this system. As the second nodal point of this combined system, also simultaneously becomes farther removed from the retina in the aphakic eye; hence under both conditions the size of the images will grow."

"But these two methods of accommodation do not give similar values. By increasing the distance of the glass, as has already been indicated, the enlargement of the image rapidly increases; but since at best this removal of the cataract glasses from the eye can not be farther than the length of the nose will permit, hence the usual reading distance can not be arrived at by this means. True, by choosing a stronger glass, placed at the ordinary distance from the eye, this enlargement takes place less rapidly than in the former case; however, there is no reason why a glass should not be chosen, by means of which objects can be sharply discerned at a distance of 8-10", or a little farther. For this reason this latter method finds more general approval. Tables XII and XIII explain this under all possible conditions. Both tables start out with the emmetropic average eye which has become aphakic."

TABLE XII.

The Emmetropic Aphakic Eye, combined with $+ \frac{1}{8.5}$ with distance from the centre of Cornea.

	0."5	0."75	1."00	1."25	1."5	1."75	2."00
Anterior focal distance F_1	20.84	22.29	23.96	25.89	29.08	30.88	34.18
Posterior focal distance F_2	27.84	29.78	32.91	34.60	37.64	41.26	45.69
Distance from F_2	23.86	23.40	22.87	22.25	21.51	20.68	19.60
Distance from H_1	-1.22	-0.56	-1.24	3.22	9.34	16.50	26.64
Distance from H^2	-3 97	-6.88	-9.14	-12.85	-16.18	-20.68	-26.09
$H_1H_2=K_1K_2$	-2.75	-5.82	-10.38	-15.57	-25.47	-37.13	-52.78
Position from K_1	5.78	6.98	9.29	11.90	20.25	30.11	42.41
Position from K_2	3.03	1.11	-1.09	-3.67	-5.22	-7.02	-10.82
K_2n	20.84	22.75	24.95	27.53	29 08	30.88	34.18
Kn	16.16	"	"	"	"	"	"
$K_2n:Kn=_1$	1.289	1.407	1.543	1.703	1.799	1.910	2.115
$Kn:K_2n=_1$	0.775	0.710	0 648	0.587	0.555	0.524	0.472
F_1' { Mm	} ∞	1465.88	789.68	579.05	4.6577	400.90	374.12
{ P. Z.		54.1	29.1	21.8	17.8	14.8	18.0

NOTE.—In this and the following table F_1 equals the anterior focal distance of the aphakic eye in its proper relation to the retina, or is equal to distance for which the eye is accommodated, by placing before it a convex glass, calculated just as R in table X.

TABLE XIII.

The Emmetropic Aphakic Eye, with the glass at 0.5″ distant from the Cornea centre.

Combined with +	$\frac{1}{8.5}$	$\frac{1}{3}$	$\frac{1}{2.75}$	$\frac{2.5}{1}$	$\frac{1}{2.25}$	$\frac{1}{2}$
Anterior focal distance F_1 . .	20.84	20.54	20.84	20.12	19.95	19.;8
Posterior focal distance F_2 . .	27.84	27.44	27.18	26.86	26.58	26.(9
Position from F_2	23.86	22.82	22.24	21.49	20.64	19 55
Distance from H_1	−1.22	−1.41	−1.52	−1.55	−1.81	−:.00
Distance from H_2	−3.97	−4.58	−4.94	−5.87	−5.89	−(.54
$H_1 H_2 K_1 K_2$	−2.75	−3.17	−3.42	−3.72	−4.08	−4.54
Distance from K_1	5.78	5.45	5.82	5.09	4.87	4.56
Distance from K_2	3.03	2.28	1.90	1.37	0.79	0.02
$K_2 n$	20 84	21.59	21.97	22.50	23.08	23.85
Kn	16.16	″	″	″	″	″
$K_2 n : Kn =_1$	1.298	1.347	1.353	1.392	1.422	1.475
$Kn : K_2 n =_1$	0.775	0.742	0.739	0.711	0.703	0.677
F_1 in $\begin{cases} \text{Mm} \\ \text{P. Z.} \end{cases}$ . . .	$\begin{matrix} \infty \\ 20.7 \end{matrix}$	562.91 13.6	369.29	249.79 9.2	184.64 6 8	139.75 5.1

In table XII the glass of $\frac{1}{3.5}$ has been removed from the eye from ¼ to ¼″ up to 2′. But even by bringing about the furtherest possible distance from the eye, the artificially produced near point could only be brought up to 13″ from the eye. Nevertheless, the enlargement grows until it has doubled itself. In table XIII the various glasses, ⅓, $\frac{1}{2.75}, \frac{1}{25}, \frac{1}{2.25}$, ½ are all placed at an equal distance. On using $\frac{1}{2.25}$ the aphakic near point reaches 9″ distant from the eye. With ½ the eye can see distinctly at 5″. Whereas, by such an excessive accommodation, the enlargement only becomes one and one-half times enlarged.

THE SELECTION OF SPHERICAL GLASSES. "In practice, as a rule, we begin to seek the proper correction for distance by use of a +¼ (+·10 D), and where we do not get the requisite amount of vision we move the glass either a little nearer or a little further away from the eye. If in the latter position sight is improved, we take a stronger glass and continue this procedure. In this manner we soon arrive at the glass which gives the best result. In the other case we go from ¼, ⅕, ⅙, etc. After having in this manner arrived at the proper glass for distance, we can in like manner arrive at the proper correction for reading. However, one will save time if one will bear in mind, that to the glass which gives a proper correction for an infinte distance, should be added the glass having the reciprocal value for a distance; thus, if the correction for infinity is $\frac{1}{85}$ to accommodate for a distance of 20″, we would have $\frac{1}{3.5} + \frac{1}{2.0} = \frac{1}{8}$ (exactly $\frac{1}{2.97}$), for 10.5″ would be $\frac{1}{3.5} + \frac{1}{10} = \frac{1}{2.5}$ (exactly $\frac{1}{2.59}$), etc. Naturally, one does not have all the lenses corresponding to these fractional figures the result of calculation, so one uses the lens which comes nearest to it in the test case, and we correct the slight difference by the distance at which the glass is placed from the eye. Any one who must frequently prescribe strong glasses for distance, soon learns to give the proper correcticn for near."

"The dioptric system now being in use, having once found the correction for distance, the glass for near is very easily found by adding to this the glass which would represent the amplitude of accommodation up to the point at which the patient wishes to read. Thus, if this be 25 cm. $\frac{25}{100}$ 4 D, then if glass required for distance is 10 D for near, 10 +- 4 D = 14 D would be required; if this is 12 D for near, 12 +- 4 D = 16 D would be required."

In order to see a point distinctly, which is at a distance Y removed from the lens, the rays of light which emanate from it, after they have passed through a lens having a focal length of F_2, which is accommodated for near, must converge to the same point, as do parellel rays after they have been deflected by a lens F_1, which is the proper correction for distance. This mutual dependence of Y and F2 is expressed (by the conjugate focal distance) in the following equation: $\frac{1}{y} + \frac{1}{F_1} = \frac{1}{F_2}$.

"By calculating the value of y we get the point at which distinct vision is possible in front of the lens. To get the exact distance at which distinct vision is to be obtained in front of the cornea or the nodal point of the eye, this distance from the lens from these points is to be added."

Having found the correcting glass for distance, it becomes a matter of interest to know with exactly which glass placed at the same distance, it would become possible to see distinctly at 10" or 8" from the eye. Thus, if $F^1 = \frac{1}{3.5}$ and y=10," then $\frac{1}{F_2} = \frac{1}{10} + \frac{1}{3.5} = \frac{13.5}{35} = \frac{1}{2.59}$. Now, if we retain the value of F^1, and if y=8", then $\frac{1}{F_2} = \frac{1}{18} + \frac{1}{3.5} = \frac{11.5}{28} = \frac{1}{2.43}$.

Hence, one would see distinctly at a distance of 10, 5" with a lens $\frac{1}{2.59}$ at a distance of 0.5" from the eye, and distinct vision at 8.5" with a lens $\frac{1}{2.43}$, 0.5" from the eye. Since both of these glasses are not found in the test case, one chooses the nearest glass, $\frac{1}{2.5}$, and if the distance of the glass before the eye is not changed, accurate vision will be attained, at 8.75" from the glass, 9.25" from the cornea and at 9.60" from the nodal point of the eye.

"Now, if one will look in table XIII and find the distance for which an aphakic eye is focus when armed with a convex glass of $\frac{1}{2.5}$ focal distance, placed at 0.5" distance, one will find that this is given in the fifth column as $\frac{1}{9.2}$ which coincides with our second value, 9.25. At the same time we discover that the degree of vision for near objects is much greater than for distance would have led us to expect. The reason for this is, as has already been indicated, due to the increase in size, owing to the strength of the convex glass used."

If the degree of vision attained is not sufficient to answer the requirements of the patient, we have another means at our disposal to enlarge the retinal images, and thus to increase the apparent degree of vision, one either removes the glass further from the eye or one uses a stronger glass. But in both cases, as can be seen from tables XII and XIII, the object must be brought nearer to the eye. The patient then sees, if one may use the expression, as if he were looking through a Galileo's telescope, or is using a lens to enlarge images.

From all that has been said it will be seen, that no statistical results are of any value, in which simply the number of the Snellen or Yager's test type read are given, only then do they give a correct idea as to the degree of vision attained, when, at the same time, the distance at which they are read is also stated. But even then the most tiresome calculations are necessary, since the smallest test type of Yager and Snellen, in cases of normal vision, must be read at a much greater distance than is the usual reading distance."

THE CYLINDRICAL CORRECTION. "Just as soon as one finds that the amount of vision attained for either distance or near does not equal the average degree which ought to be attained by the use of spherical glasses, the attempt should be made to improve this by the use of cylinders. Reuss and Woinow have demonstrated to us, that in most cases this procedure will be successful, if there is not a very large secondary cataract present. If we have found the cylindrical correction for distance, we simply add this to the spherical combination for near."

"The above named authorities claim to have found, that in the aphakic eye, at times when looking at near objects, the degree and position of the meridian in which the astygmatism lies is changed; however, this observation has never been corroberated by any other observers."

"As a rule, the number of the cylindrical glass is found by experiment, but in order to save time one may start out with the average degree ($\frac{1}{12}$ to $\frac{1}{14}$), and place it in the well-known direction of least curvature which appears after cataract operations. A very valuable control experiment is that of measuring the corneal curvature with the opthalmometre. Since when we have arrived at the corneal astygmatism, we have at the same time arrived at the total astygmatism of the entire eye."

"Reuss and Woinow have advised the use of a cylinder, as found by opthalmometric examination; but still, since following this examination, one must still test to see how much vision is attained, one can not see why this procedure is to be preferred."

"Thomas Young showed that by placing a spherical convex lens obliquely, the homocentric rays of light which fall on it do not exactly come to a point, but come together in two lines placed vertical to each other, so that we can produce a similar effect by placing the glass somewhat obliquely to the line of vision, thus producing an effect analogous to the combination of a spherical and cylindrical lens. And it is well known that those who wear glasses often unconsciously correct slight degrees of astygmatism by bending, moving forward, or displacing their spectacle frame."

"We often find patients who have undergone cataract operation place their glasses in an oblique position. Every beginner often is very much confused to find the patient state that at times he sees better, at times worse with the same glass, or is unable to explain this condition satisfactorily to himself; or in other words, that he can see better with his spectacles than he can with a glass of the same focal strength, which the physician places in front of his eye. Both conditions are explained by the cylindrical action of a glass held obliquely. That which the patient often does unconsciously is often a valuable aid in the hand of the physician, who in this simple manner can increase the degree of vision. Donders drew attention to the fact in 1864, and Javal used it in 1865, and I believe that in many cases one can avoid giving a cylindrical correction by employing this means. Unfortunately as yet we have no scientific explanation for this practical and important subject."

THE INFLUENCE WHICH GLASSES EXERT ON THE VISION OF APHAKIC EYES.

a. CONTRACTION OF THE FIELD OF VISION. From time immemorial it has been customary to prescribe large round glasses for cataract glasses. It was supposed that by this means we could increase the size of the field of vision. Many patients, however, remonstrated against such glasses, because the weight often became a burden, and frequently the patients would go and have them cut oval. By doing this they did the proper thing in more ways than one."

"Already Thomas Young had shown that rays of light passing through a bi-convex lens placed obliquely, did not come together at a single point, but in two focal lines at a certain focal distance. This departure from the regular refraction increases with the size of the exposed surface of the glass, and with the angle at which the glass is placed, and with its curvature. As a result, when looking through convex glasses, objects in the periphery of the field of vision look distorted. To overcome this evil effect Wollaston constructed his periscopic glasses; whereas several practical opticians of his time advised glasses of a smaller diameter, since they started out with the assumption, that the outer portion of the retina is less sensitive, hence, could well get along without an optical correction without any evil effects. The advantage which Wollaston hoped to get from periscopic glasses has not been practically realized, at least for convex glasses. Since it was shown that the so-called prismatic displacement, at least for the periscopic glasses, is just as great as it is with bi-convex or plain convex glasses."

"When weak convex glasses are used, this disturbance, so far as the excentric vision is concerned, is not very great. But if, as is the case with those who have undergone a cataract operation, strong convex glasses are exclusively used, we find, as Berlin showed, that it is not a matter of distortion, but a zonular, concentrically-defined defect in the periphery of the field of vision. Even when the large round circular cataract glasses are used, the outer periphery of the retina receives its light direct, without passing through the cataract glasses. Owing to the highly prismatic action of the edges of the cataract glasses, light does not reach the pupil from a not inconsiderable zone of the field of vision. And since a total reflection also takes place from the edges of the cataract glasses, Berlin especially draws attention to the fact, that this zone is not sharply outlined in any direction as a result of the action of this total reflection. Since the outer limits of the field of vision are more dependent on the size of the glass, by making these smaller we can at least limit this eccentric loss of the peripheric field of vision. Hence, I see no reason why we should prescribe large, heavy, and therefore very uncomfortable cataract glasses instead of the oval glasses, when at the same time we desire the benefit of a diminution of the peripheric distortion, and loss of the excentric portion of the field, especially above and below."

"For the upper half of the field, the advantage certainly would not be of any great importance, but when glancing downward the condition of affairs certainly assumes great importance. Only too often do cataract patients complain of defective ability to exactly locate objects. In walking, especially in going up or down stairs, they are frequently impeded, so that many, especially when they have a slight myopia, prefer to walk about without their glasses. On using the oval glasses this defective power of locating objects is at once corrected. Undoubtedly the patients receive inaccurate images of the floor on which they are walking, but at the same time they do not receive interrupted or distorted retinal images."

"Owing to the highly prismatic deflection which all the rays of light receive, except those which traverse the centre of the glass, we must be especially careful to see that in cases where both eyes have been operated, the glasses are perfectly centered. Otherwise, very annoying diplopia or asthenopic trouble will arise."

"If only the one eye has been operated, and the other can no longer be used to see with, the glasses for distance and near may be put in one frame, with a neutral nose piece, if a high bridge on the nose does not veto such a procedure."

"Hence, the field of vision of the aphakic eye extends over as much space as does a complete eye. Only the former can not see so well, in the periphery as in the center, even when provided with glasses, owing to the distortion of the images. And this inconvenience is increased by the cataract glasses. This contraction of the field, as a result of the use of the convex glasses, becomes increased when the distance of the glasses from the eyes is increased. Hence, owing to these conditions, accommodation can be accomplished by the use of stronger glasses. Naturally, the increase in the apparent acuity of vision for distance suffers also where there is a very large contraction of the field of vision. Hence, it is almost impossible to wear continuously in front of both eyes glasses far removed, notwithstanding the pleasure which such patients may derive from wearing their simple opera glasses."

EXACT CENTERING. "In the selection of cataract glasses more depends on the selection of a proper frame than on any other condition in which glasses are required, for on this is dependent the fact whether the eye and the glass will be properly centered. For instance, the prismatic deflection when using a $+\frac{1}{3.5}$ at 1 mm. distance from the center is as great as in a $+\frac{1}{12}$ at 3 mm. distance from the center (1° 15′). By this means not only is there a very perceptible distortion of objects, and the arrangement of the same, brought about in the periphery of the field of vision, but light is broken up into its various colors, which becomes very annoying to the patient. Hence, no one who is necessitated to wear glasses, worries himself so long and so persistently, so as to get them in a proper position in front of his eyes, as does the patient operated on for cataract."

"As long as only one eye has been operated on, we may permit the patient to worry himself in getting his glass properly centered. But in prescribing cataract glasses for both eyes, other factors come into play, such as the occurrence of diplopia, and we must take into consideration the muscular condition of the eyes, and then it becomes the physician's duty to see that the glasses have a proper position, in their relation to the eyes, according to the general fundamental rules. If, as is usually the case under such circumstances, we prescribe separate glasses for distance and near work, we must at least approximately take into account for each special case, the angle which the lines of vision must make with each other, and aside from this we must see to it that the glasses are so bent as to form an obtuse angle, open anteriorly."

FEW PECULIARITIES OF APHAKIC VISION. *a*. Entopic Vision. It would hardly seem necessary to state, that in consequence of loss of the lens, all entopic phenomena which arise in the lens system are wanting, if it were not, that at times during the formation of a cataract, these phenomena force themselves to the attention of the patient in the most disturbing manner.

In aphakia the patient becomes aware of opacities in the vitreous under entirely changed optical conditions. Since the entire vitreous has moved perceptibly away from the focal plane; hence, where no cataract glass is used, every cloudiness in the same must cast a shadow on the retina, and since the power of accommodation is wanting, hence all vitreous opacities will at once be recognized, as soon as an eye equipped with cataract glasses directs its attention to any object which is at a distance equal to that for which the glass is intended.

ERYTHROPSIA. A peculiar ~~subjective~~ phenomenon of the aphakic eye is the sudden occurrence of red vision, of which the patients not infrequently complain, and which frightens them greatly the first time it occurs. It occurs suddenly; at times it lasts but a few minutes; in other cases, hours and even days. It always disappears gradually. Since all patients who observe this are sure to relate it to their physicians, hence it can be stated with certainty that it occurs in from 3 to 5 per cent. of all cases.

Since no evil results have ever been observed following its occurrence, one is justified in quieting the fears of the patient by making a good prognosis. Becker had the opportunity repeatedly to examine, with the opthalmoscope, such a patient during an attack, and believed that he might safely state, that he did not observe a hyperaemia, either of the retina or the optic nerve.

Erythropsia has been the subject of considerable investigation by Hirschler, Dimmer, Purtscher, Meyerhauser, Steiner, Benson and many others.

Dr. Hirschler has been the subject of this peculiar phenomena himself, and has given us a graphic description of his sensations.

He states 4 that he had always been very near sighted (M. 1-10, suffered from mouches volantes, and frequently scotoma scintillans fugax). Strong light always caused trouble, and frequently caused "nachbilder." In 1878 his left eye became diseased, and in 1880 cataract developed in his right. In 1882 a Von Graefe extraction with a broad coloboma. With the exception of micropsie, the process of healing and convalescence was perfect. Notwithstanding astygmatism with a $+ 5\frac{1}{2}$ V $\frac{2.0}{7.0}$, and with a $+ 3\frac{3}{4}$, read Y 1. The peculiar phenomena

--- --- --- --- --- --- --- --- --- --- --- ---

4 Zum Rothsehen der Aphakischen. Weiner Med. Wochenschrift, 4, 6, 1883.

of erythropsia began the fifth month after the operation. As soon as evening approached the entire firmament appeared red, whereas all terrestrial objects were red through the reflection of the red light from above. This phenomenon was also present indoors, but only on looking toward the windows. This continued regularly for about one hour, gradually disappearing. During the continuance of this phenomenon the acuity of vision was not reduced. Even on cloudy days this red discoloration of the firmament did not fail to appear, even if the rain was coming down in torrents. This phenomenon never occurred during the day. However, if the eyelids were brought sufficiently close together this red discoloration could be made to disappear during the evening. However, closure of the right cataractous eye did not exert the slightest influence on this phenomenon. Towards the fall of the year the erythropsia disappeared just as suddenly as it had come. He seeks the cause in the large iris colobom, not as a result of the colored rays of dispersion, but rather as a result of the intensity of the light which, falling on the peripheric portions of the retina, caused there an unusual degree of irritation. This excessive irritation is followed by exhaustion. In this case, the peripheral portion of the retina being so exhausted that light at twilight was not strong enough to arouse sensation to its fullest degree. This exhaustion must manifest itself for rays of light which have higher indices of refraction, whereas the sensitiveness for the red rays is still present, as a result of which the field is colored red. The results of experiments with stenopaic glasses verifies this.

Purtscher[5] investigated this subject, drawing the following conclusion:

1. *That erythropsia is not an optical phenomenon.* Dispersion of colors could not be thought of, because then only the edges of objects would be colored.

Two causes might be thought of, cloudiness of media or hemorrhages in the vitreous, but both can be set aside because if present they could be detected with the opthalmoscope. Further, there is no reduction of acuity of vision during the time everything appears red to the patient.

2. *The occurrence of erythropsia in aphkia is not dependent on the presence of a coloboma.* In his own case of traumatic cataract, likewise in Dimmer's case, there was no coloboma.

3. *An explanation on the basis of contrast in colors can not be brought in accordance with the facts.* Though it has been supposed that after remaining for a long time where everything is green, the complimentary color red will appear. One fact mitigates greatly against this assumption, for in many cases the red appeared at once on waking in the morning.

---

5 Zur Frage Erythropsia. Centralblatt fur Praktischer Augenheilkunde. Juni. 1883.

4. *Hirschler's explanation has a physiological basis for it. He explains the erythropsia as due to fatigue of the retina, which becomes most evident in the evening, and manifests itself mostly for the more highly reflective rays, whereas, the rays of less refractive power can still act.*

Aubert [6] states that sensitiveness for blue or green is lost in ten minutes, when dark blue or dark green glasses are worn; whereas, red can still be seen after several hours. One might suppose that a retina which becomes fatigued very rapidly (for colors), would lose its sensitiveness for refractive rays of diffuse light much sooner than its sensitiveness for the less highly refractive red rays.

Further, one ought not forget the fact that among pigments *red* can still be recognized where the intensity of the light is reduced, after all other colors can no longer be seen. Hence, it would seem that the conditions for the recognition of red rays are more favorable when the intensity of the illumination is reduced.

This fact becomes still more important where, in a fatigued eye, hemeralopia also is present (as Hirschler states of his own case), and which he assumes to occur generally in aphakics, where coloboma has been made.

5. *This phenomenon of seeing everything red is purely a subjective one, and has its seat in the sensitive apparatus which receives the rays of light. It is partly direct, partly indirect, depending on nervous influences.*

For the former, one can assume, that a retina which had been shielded for a long time from the more intense impression of light by a developing cataract, would certainly be more sensitive to the action of light after the obstacle had been suddenly removed. Likewise, the tendency to fatigue would be greater.

He gives a series of cases and further investigations,[7] and after reviewing all the literature, reasserts all the above, and finally concludes:

"This phenomenon of seeing red is purely a subjective one, due to irritation, or finally, a fatigue of the visual apparatus—the result of partly direct, partly indirect, nervous, special and vaso-motor influence. Individuals of a naturally nervous disposition and aphakic—possibly more correctly, those who have suffered from cataract—are predisposed. This predisposition is, in all probability, heightened by coloboma."

Immediately after delivery of the lens, patients not infrequently see everything in a color other than normal, as per example, the finger looks

---

6 Graefe Saenisch H., II, 2, S. 557.

7 Foerster Beitrage zur Frage der Erythropsie. O. Purtscher Centralblatt fur Augenheilkunde. February and March. 1884.

blue. One looked upon this as a contrast action; for as we stated, an intense yellow color of the nucleus influenced the perception of colors in the cataract patient. Under such circumstances we would expect this phenomenon to disappear a certain length of time after delivery of the lens, and ought to be entirely wanting in soft cataracts, which have a yellow nucleus. Both, however, are not true; it can, however, be shown that this phenomenon is due to particles of lens substance left behind in the aqueous, and to very finely diffused blood. This blue discoloration always disappears as soon as the lens substance is absorbed. At times simply permitting the aqueous to be evacuated a number of times by separating the edges of the wound, is sufficient to cause the finger held before the eye to again assume its normal color.

Fuchs [a] has given us the most exhaustive exposition on this subject, and has shown that erythropsia may occur in normal eyes. He came to the conclusion that the cause must be sought in some direction other than in the illuminated field. He found that erythropsia ensued even when colored glasses were used, and concluded that the erythropsia is entirely independent of the color of the light. Finally, he sought its origin in the color of the visual purple of the retina, which begins to regenerate every time the eye is removed from the influence of the light. He, however, indicates that he can not explain why at times the red seeing is preceded by green.

Snellen [b] believes that this is a contrast phenomenon. The portion of the eye which had been exposed to the bright light will appear red, whereas the portion which has been protected (being in the shadow), by contrast will appear green. Finally, he points to the fact that a very thin, transparent lid, owing to its great vascularity, a strong light passing through it into the eye, on trans-illumination, will appear of a purple color.

b. OPTHALMOSCOPICAL EXAMINATION. "As is well known, in the emmetropic eye, the entire curvature of the retina lies in the focal plane of the dioptric system. According to Thomas Young this is supposed to be due to the lamellar formation of the lens. Helmholtz agrees with the idea, and more recently, owing to this property of the concentric arrangement in layers of lenses, Ludimar Herman has applied to them in a somewhat different sense the name "periscopic." It is a fact, that in making the direct examination, even those points in the periphery, even where it is still possible to get a view of the fundus, do not give us distorted pictures. But I can not agree with Donders when he states that we can see the various portions of the retina without changing our accommodation. The former is caused by the lens, which seems to be shown with

a Über Erythropsie. Graefe's Arch., XLII., Part 4. 1896.
b Erythropsie, Graefe's Arch., XLIV., Part I. 1897.

a certain degree of certainty by the fact, that in aphakia we can only recognize the periphery of the fundus in variously distorted pictures. However, we can not draw any certain conclusion from this, because on the one hand we know that the curvature of the cornea suffers, as a result of the operation, and because on the other hand the capsule which is folded and left behind under all circumstances, causes an irregular astygmatism, which becomes more manifest in the periphery than in the center."

"Donders quite to the contrary saw the periphery of the fundus much more distinctly when the lens was absent than when it was present. And since, in the former case, the peripheral images are also properly projected, he assumes that in aphakia the indirect examination is so changed, that the form of objects in the retinal pictures are now better seen with the opthalmoscope, and hence are less properly projected by the eye."

c. BINOCULAR VISION IN APHAKIC EYES. "Up to the present time binocular vision in aphakic eyes has not been adequately investigated. For the little which we do know we are indebted to Von Graefe (807). The question becomes pre-eminently a practical one, where we are to decide whether or not we shall operate when a cataract is present on only one eye. The question must be answered variously, depending on the fact whether the other eye is still intact, hence able to see, or whether the second eye is already attacked by cataract, but is still in a condition to see. Aside from this, we must take into consideration whether or not the eye to be operated on promises a satisfactory result as to vision. If this is not the case, the operation is to be made for cosmetic reasons, and it would seem hardly necessary to state here, that everything depends on whether it would be practical to operate or not under such conditions.

"In those cases in which the second eye is already affected, it is not difficult to come to a decision. Nevertheless, experience has taught, that where two eyes see under such different conditions, they disturb each other very much during the act of seeing. Each eye blends the other. As long as the non-operated eye answers all the special demands for seeing on the part of the patient, he prefers to use the non-operated eye, especially for near work; and at times even when the degree of vision on the operated eye is greater. This is explained by the fact, that in the operated eye much illy-refracted light enters the eye, which blends the distinct picture of the other eye, always assuming that the secondary cataract is not a large one, causing an enlarged retinal image, which without a correction is a very indistinct one; and hence, the patient finds himself in a position similar to that of anisometropie, however, receiving rather less diffused light than the non-operated eye."

"If the non-operated eye no longer suffices for seeing, this over-blending will still take place. But it loses its disturbing qualities the more the cataract progresses. Hence, we can often answer complaints with this consolation, if we do not prefer to cut off the eye entirely from the act of seeing by placing an opaque disc before it. Notwithstanding all these drawbacks, no one should ever hesitate to operate a ripe cataract because the other is not yet ripe. And indeed *the time for an operation has arrived, when the second affected eye begins to fail in its service.* Hence, we save the patient, short as this might be, time of enforced idleness. One ought, with Graefe, to wish every person without exception, who is affected with cataract, a successive development of the trouble on both eyes."

"If we are dealing with a cataract on the one eye, where the other eye shows no sign of becoming affected in the same way, as in a case of *cataracta traumatica* or *complicata*, one must consider, that after even a successful operation, the patient will have a high degree of anisometropia during the rest of his Lfe. In a certain proportion of these cases of acquired anisometropia, and as it occurs in congenital cases, the image on the operated eye is suppressed. As a result no absolutely sharp fixation on the operated eye takes place during the act of accommodation and the associated movements. Likewise, by the use of prisms, one can neither bring about the perception of double images nor a deviation of the visual line. (V. Graefe.) Investigations have not as yet been made to find out whether or not these occur in eyes which before the cataract operation had perfect binocular vision. In another percentage of cases Von Graefe found that true binocular vision did occur, without causing the patient any particular annoyance, notwithstanding the enormous difference in the refractive condition of the two eyes. If the fixation is absolutely correct, the eye will turn inward in using an adducting prism, and it will turn outward behind an abducting prism. Stereoscopic vision is present, and distance can be properly judged."

"Up to the present time I have only had one patient under observation who could be used for making these experiments—the young colleague whom I have so repeatedly mentioned. I can positively assert, that during complete and accurate fixation he was not disturbed in the least by the difference in the size of the images. The use of prism gave the same results, and he was not aware of any difference in his ability to judge distances and in looking at stereoscopic pictures. I regret, however, that I have not been enabled to make any more exact experiments. Hence, this very interesting subject is still to be investigated."

"Though such successful cases are to be looked upon as exceptional, one must nevertheless emphasize the fact, that no disadvantage has as yet been absolutely proven against such an operation. True, we have stated, that the other eye is blended. Even in those cases in which it is present, the patients become accustomed to it, in the course of a few weeks. It is said that not infrequently strabismus appears on the operated eye. This does occur, but it certainly is dependent on a disturbance of the muscular balance which must have existed before the operation. If it should occur, a tenotomie will correct it. Finally, the cry against a one-sided operation is raised, of the occasional occurrence of diplopia, a condition which, according to Von Graefe, is but exceedingly seldom noted."

"After all this, there can be no real disadvantage. If we will but for the time set aside those exceptionally successful cases, in which a really binocular vision is attained, a mere cosmetic result ought to favor the operation; but above all, *the enlarging of the binocular field of vision on the side of the operated eye.* Firstly, the latter at least prevents the development of the pathognomic one-eyed position of the head. (That is, a turning of the head toward the side of the blind eye, and the eye turns toward the side of the seeing eye.) Secondly, the patient preserves the power of locating objects correctly. Since in binocular vision, with two healthy eyes we only obtain very imperfect retinal images, outside of the horopter, hence in acquired anisometropia the inaccurate pictures in the periphery of the retina suffice to permit us to exercise proper judgment as to the relative lateral displacement and depth of surfaces; notwithstanding the fact that the retinal images in both eyes do not fall upon identical points."

d. AMBYOPIA EX ANOPSIA. "An interesting fact is brought to our notice, when a cataract which has existed for a long time is finally extracted. Graefe relates a case in which an operation was finally made after a cataract had existed for sixty years, and in which excellent vision was attained. Becker operated a woman 68 years of age, who had a *cataracta traumatica accreta*, which had existed since her third year. The operation was done after the other eye had been lost, as a result of hypopyon keratitis, and the vision attained was exceedingly satisfactory; the woman was able to pray again, hence read in her prayer book. Analogous cases certainly come under the observation of every operator."

"The cases in which such good results are attained are usually cases of traumatic origin. As is well known, vision is nearly always very much reduced in cases of congenital cataracts, especially when they are complicated by nystagmus."

An interesting study, is *the education of sight* in those congenitally blind from congenital cataract. Here, after a successful operation, the patient sees, but can not recognize the objects seen until after sight has been educated by the employment of the senses, such as touch. Thus, the patient is shown a key—sees it plainly, but does not recognize the object— but let him touch it, and he will at once say, that is a key. The object once recognized by the aid of other senses, is ever after recognized on sight.

LITERATURE.

1532. 1. Arlunus, J. P., De suffusione, quam cataractam appellant. Mediolani.

1574. 2. LeGrand Nicol., et Lambert, Nicol., Non ergo suffusionum omnium eadem est curatio. Paris.

1600. 3. Laurentius, Andr., Discours de la conservation de la vue. Paris. (Handelt vom grauen Staar.)

1601. 4. Moller, S., Diss de suffusione. Francof. ad Viadr.

1649. 5. Fienus, Th., De praecipuis artis chirurgicae controversiis. Lib. II. De cataracta. Francof.

1664. 6. Rolfink, Werner, Disp. de cataracta. Jena.

7. Bartholinus, Th., De oculorum suffusione epistola. Hafniae.

1670. 8. Friderici, J. A., Disp de suffusione. Jenae.

9. Meibom, J. H. (J. G. Rose), Disp. de cataracta. Helmstadt.

10. Anonym., Lettre sur une nouvel le opinion au sujetde la cataracte. Rouen.

1675. 11. Harder, M., Disp. de cataracta. Basil.

1672. 12. Niemand, H., Disp. de suffusione. Argentorati.

1684. 13. Sperling, P. G., Aeger suffusione laborans. Jenae.

14. Papelier, J. E., Aeger suffusione laborans. Argent.

1688. 15. Fehr, J. L., Cataractae depositio in utroque oculo feliciter celebrata. Misc. Ac. Nat. Cur., Dec. 2.

1691. 16. Pechlin et Drelimour, Verknocherte Linse, in Pechlin observ. phys. med., p. 296. Hamburg.

17. Schelhammer, G. C., Disp. de suffusione. Jenae.

1695. 18. Albinus, B., resp. L. D. Gosky, Disp. de cataracta. Francof. ad Viadr. und Lugd., Bat. 1738. Halleri Bibl. Chirurg., I, p. 450 u. Halleri Disp. Chirurg. select. tom. II. Lausanae, 1755.

1700. 19. De la Hire, Phil., Tract de cataracta. Parisiis. (?)

1704. 20. Schacher, P. G., Diss. de cataracta. Lipsiac.

1706. 21. Wedel, G. W., Disp. de cataracta. Jenae.

22. De la Hire, Phil., Tr. de cataracta. Paris.

23. Brisseau, P., Traite de la cataracte et la glaucoma. Tournay.

24. Histoire de l'Acad. Royale des Sciences. (1) De la Hire, Sur les cataractes des yeux, p. 12. (2) De la Hire, Sur la nature des cataractes qui se forment dans l'oeil, p. 20

25. Lang, C. J., Diss. de cataracta. Paris.

1707. 26. Maitre-Jean Antoine, Traite des maladies des yeux. Paris.

27. Hist. de l'Acad. Roy. des Sciences. (1) Sur les cataractes des yeux, p. 32. (2) Mery. Si le Glaucoma et la cataracte sont deux differentes ou une seule et meme maladie, p. 491. (3) De la Hire le fils, Remarques sur le cataracte et le glaucoma, p. 550.

1708. 28. Histoire de l'Acad. Roy. des Sciences. (1) Sur les cataractes des yeux, p. 39. (2) Mery de la cataracte et du glaucoma. p. 241. (3) De la Hire le fils, Remarques sur la cataracte et le glaucoma, p. 245. (4) Saint Yves, de la cataracte, p. 501.

29. Jacobi, L. Fr., Disp. de cataractae nova pathologia. Giford.

30. LeFrancois, Alexander et J. N. de la Hire, Ergo potest stare visio absque crystallino. Paris.

31. Brisseau, P., Suite des observations sur la cataracte. Tournay.

1709. 32. ———, Traite de la cataracte et du glaucome. Paris.

33. Mery, Jean, Observation sur un glaucoma cru cataracte. Histoire de l'Acad. Royale des Sciences.

1710. 34. Dieterichs, G. A., De cataracte. Vesel.

1711. 35. Lusardi, Dissert sur l'opacite du cristallin et sur l'operation de la cataracte. Gand.

36. Chapuzeau, A. L., Disput de cataracta. Leidae.

37. Camerarius, E., De nova cataractae theoria. In epistolis Taurinensibus. Tubingae.

1712. 38. Stephan, Dissert de lente cristallina ocul. hum. Lips.

39. Laurentius, Heister, De cataracta in lente crystallina. Diss. tres. Altorf, 1711, 1712. 1743, resp. Widman, Vogt et Pauli.

40. ———, De cataracta et de mira paralysi. Ephemer. Ac. nat. Cur. Cent. 1 et 2, 1712.

41. ———, De cataracta quadam lactea rara et singulari in dissecto oculo observata. Ephemer, Ac. Nat. Cur. Cent., 4 et 5, 1715.

42. ———, Tract. de cataracta, glaucomate et amaurosi. Altorf, 1713; ed. sec. ib., 1720.

43. ———, Apologia systematis sui de catar., glaucom. et amaurosi contra objectiones Woo'housis et Parisiensis medicorum dianci. Altorf, 1717.

44. ———, Vindicia sententiae suae de cataracta. Altorf, 1719.

1713. 45. Gakenholz. A.Chr., Disp. de visione per cataractam impedita. Helmst.

1714. 46. Woolhouse, J. Th., Epistola inter additamenta Maitre Jeanii. Leidae.

1715. 47. Vater, Ch., Disp. de suffusione oculorum. Wittebergae.

48. LeCerf, Chr., Probestucke in Augenkrankheiten des Hrn. Woolhouse. Jena. (Handelt besonders vom Staar.)

1717. 49. Woolhouse, J. Th., Dissertations scavantes et critiques sur la cataracte et le glaucome de plusieurs modernes. Frankfurt, 1717 u. 1730. Lateinisch von Christ. le Cerf u. d. T., Dissertationes de cataracta et glaucomate contra. systema Brissaei, Antonii et Heisteri. Francof, 1719.

1718. 50. Woolhouse, J. Th., Observation sur des cataractes membraneuses. Memoires de Paris.

51. Gastaldus, J. B., An cataracta vitium lentis. Avignon.

1719. 52. ———, Quaestio medica, an cataracta a vitio humoris aquei vel crystallini oriatur, an a glaucomate differat et aliter quam operatione chirurgica curari possit. Paris.

1719. 53. Heisterus, L., Epistola qua sententiam suam de cataracta a cavilla-
tionibus et objectionibus qui busdam defendit atque illustrat. Act.
Erudit. Lips.

54. Sincerus Fidelis, Kurze Critik uber des Oculisten Woolhouse Lugen
und Sschandschriften, zur Defension Herrn Heisters. Leipzig.
(Handelt hauptsachlich vom grauen Staar.)

55. LeCerf, Chr., An Licht besehener Staar oder pasquillantischer Criti-
cus Sincerus F'delis. Leipzig.

56. Wiedeman, Fr., Bericht vom Stein auch Bruchen zu schneiden und
Staar zu stechen. Augsburg.

1720. 57. Bianchi, O. S. oder Plancus, Lettera intorno alla cataratta. Rimini.
58. Lichtmann, J. M., Beschreibung des Staars. Nurnberg.

1721. 59. ———, Geschickter Augenarzt, Beschreibung des Staars und Hirn-
fells. Nurnberg.

60. Freitag, J. H., Dissert. medica de cataracta. Argentorati. Auch in
Haller, Disp. Chirurg. sel. tom. 2. Lausannae, 1755.

61. Cocchi, A. G., Epistola ad Morgagnum de lente crystallina oculi humani, vera suusionis sede. Romae.

1722. 62. Bianchi, Lettera esaminando una lettera del Cocchi gli monstra alcuni errori; tragli altri esser falso che l'umor cristallino sia sem-
pre la vera sede della suffusione. Rimini.

63. Benevoli, Ant., Lettere sopra due osservazioni fatte intorno alla cataratta. Firenze.

64. ———, In Ephemerid, naturae curios. cent. II, IV u. VII. Beobachtungen von Heister, Thomasius und Sproegel.

65. St. Yves, Traite des maladies des yeux. Paris.

66. Roberg, L., Disp. de cataracta. Upsal.

67. Pinson, Observations sur la cataracte et le glaucoma. Dictees a Mr.
de Woolhouse. Journ. des Scavants. Juillet, p. 42.

68. Deidier, Lettre ecrite a Mons. Woolhouse, ibidem, p. 36. (Beschreibt
darin eine cataracta membranacea accreta.)

69. Sauveur Morand, Observations sur la cataracte des yeux. Mem. de
Paris.

1724. 70. Antonio Benevoli, Nuova proposizione intorno alla caruncula dell'
Uretra e della cataratta glaucomatose. Firenzi.

71. Molineux, Sectio oculorum duorum cataracta affectionum, Philos.
Transact., 1724.

72. John Rauby, On occount of the dissection of an eye with a cataract.
Philos. Transact., 1724.

1725. 73. Woolhouse, Th., Disp. de cataracta. Trivult.

74. Francois Pourfour du Petit, Dissertation sur l'operation de la cataracte. Memoires de Paris.

1726. 75. ———, Memoire dans lequel on determine l'endroit, ou il faut piquer
l'oeil dans l'operation de la cataracte. Memoires de Paris.

1727. 76. Doebel von Doebeln, J. Jac., De cataracta natura et cura. Lordir.

77. Petit, Diss. sur une nouvelle methode de faire l'operation de la cataracte. Mem. de Lit. et du P. des Molets, III. Paris.

78. Wigelius, Canutus, Disp. de cataracta. Upsal.

79. Ribe, Diss. de cataracta. Upsal. •

1728. 80. Grateloup, B. Fr., De cataracta. Theses medico-miscellaneae. Argent.

81. LeMoine, Anton, Quaestio med.-chir., an deprimendae cataractae exspectanda maturatio. Paris, und in Haller Disput. chirurg. sel. 2, 1755.

1729. 82. Duddel, Treatise on disenses of horny coat, etc. London.

83. Hofmann, Fr., Disp. de cataracta. Hallae.

84. Henrici, M. H., Disp. de cataracta. Leidae.

85. Hecquet, P. H., Lettre sur l'abus des purgatifs et des amers. Paris. Von demselben, 1730, 5 Briefe uber den grauen Staar.

86. Petit, Fr., Lettre, dans laquelle il demontre, que le crystallin est fort pres de l'Uvee et rapporte de nouvelles pruves, qui concernent l'operation de la cataracte. Paris. Halleri Disp. chir. sel., V. 370.

1730. 87. Adam, Aeg. et L. P. Lehoc, Ergo praecavendae cataractae oculi paracentesis. Paris.

1731. 88. Fizes, Ant., Disp. de cataracta. Monsp.

89. Magnol, Ant. et Laulanie, An cataractae confirmatae operatio chirurgica unicum remedium. Monsp.

1732. 90. Ferrein, Ant., Quaestio medica, quinam sint praecipui, quomodo explicentur et curentur lentis crystallinae morbi, quae est duodecima quaestio inter eas, quas defendit. Monspelii.

91. Benevoli Anton, Manifesto sopra alcune accuse contenute in uno certo Parare del S. Pietro Paoli. Firenz.

92. ———, Giustificazione delle replicati accuse del S. Pietro Paoli. Firenz. (Beide Schriften beziehen sich auf den grauen Staar.)

93. Petit, Fr., Reflexions sur ce que Mr. Hecquet a fait imprimer sur les maladies des yeux. Paris.

94. ———, Lettre contenant des reflexions sur les decouvertes faites sur les yeux. Paris. (Beide Schriften handeln vom grauen Staar.)

1733. 95. Franken, J. H., Over het stryken van verschiedene cataracten. Amsterd.

1736. 96. Taylor, J., New treatise on the diseases of the crystalline humor of the eye, or of the cataract and glaucoma. London.

1738. 97. Juch, H. P., Disp. de suffusione. Giford.

1739. 98. Vallisnieri, Historie von der Erzeugung der Menschen. Lemgo, p. 297. Doppelte Linse in einen Auge.

1740. 99. Col. de Villars, A. F. Leo et Le Hoc, An oculi punctio cataractam praecaveat. Diss. Parisiis und in Haller, Disp. Chirurg. selectae. Tom., II.

100. Roscius, J. J., De vera cataracta crystallina lactea. Regiom.

1741. 101. De la Faye, G., Ergo vera cataractae sedes in lente. Paris.

1742. 102. Elias Col. de Villars, Ergo vera cataractae sedes in lente. Paris.

1743. 103. De la Soue, J. M. Fr. et Arcelin, Disp. starene potest visio absque crystallino. Paris.

1744. 104. Henckel, J. F., Diss. medica de cataracta crystallina vera. Francof. u. Halleri Disp. Chir. sel., II, p. 85.

1745. 105. Anonym., Treatise on cataract and glaucoma. London. Auch in Haller. Biblioth. Chir., II, p. 278. (Von einem Schuler Woolhouse's.)

106. Trew, Chr. Jac., De cataracta. In commercio litterario. Norici, 1, 136.

1748. 107. Daviel, Jacques, Sur une nouvelle methode de guerison de la cataracte par 15 extraction. (Auch in Memoire de l'Acad. de Chirurg. II, p. 337, 1853.) Mercure de France, 1748. (?)

108. La Faye, Ibidem, p. 563.

109. Quelmalz, S. Th., Progr. depositionis cataractae effectus exponens. Lipsiae.

110. De la Faye, G., Memoire pour servir a perfectionner la nouvelle methode de faire l'operation de la cataracte. Mem. d'Acad. de Chir., II, p. 563.

111. Roscius, J. Jac., Diss. de vera cataracta lactea crystallina. Regiom.

112. Nannoni, Angelo, Della cataratta. In dessen dissertazioni chirurgiche. Parigi. Andere Ausgabe. Firenz. 1751.

1749. 113. Reghellini, Janus, Lettera chirurgica sopra l'offesa della vista in una donna, consistente nel raddoppiamento degli oggetti, segnito dopo la depressione delle cataratta. Venezia.

1750. 114. O'Halloran, S., A new treatise on the glaucoma or cataract. Dublin, und Haller, Bibl. Chir., II, 345.

115. Palucci, Histoire de l'operation de la cataracte faite a six soldats invalides. Paris.

116. ———, Description d'un nouvel instrument, propre a abaisser la cataracte avec tout le succes possible. Paris. (Beide Schriften Deutsch. u. d. T. Beschreibung eines neuen Instruments, den Staar mit allem nur moglichen Erfolg niederzudrucken, nebst einer Nachricht von den Operationen, welche damit bei 6 Invaliden u Paris unternommen worden, von dem H. Palucci. Leipzig, 1752. Mit Kupfer.)

117. Guntz, J. G., Animadversiones de suffusionis natura et curatione. Lipsiae und Haller, Disp. Chir., sel. II, p. 105.

1751. 118. De Vermale, Lettre sur l'extraction du cristallin hors du globe de l'oeil, imaginee par Daviel. Paris. Journ. de Med., II, p. 418.

119. Andre, Lettre sur l'extraction du cristallin hors du globe de l'oeil, nouvelle operation imaginee par Mr. Daviel.

120. Palucci. Precis de la methode d'abattre la cataracte. Mem. de Paris.

121. Rathlauw, J. P., Traite de la cataracte. Anst.

1752. 122. ——, Verhandeling van de cataracta derzelve vorzaaken kentekenen en gevolgen en inzonderheit de manier der operatie. Amsterdam. Haller Bibl. Chir., II, 290.

123. Siegwart, Diss. de extractione cataractae ultra perficienda. Tubingae, Halleri Disp. Chir., sel. II, und Reuss, Diss. Med. Tub., Vol. III.

124. Palpucci, Methode d'abattre la cataracte, Paris, (Gegen die Extraction).

125. Thurant, J. B., De Jussieu, M. Anton, Ergo in cataracta potior lentis crystallinae extractio per incisionem corneae, quam depressio per acum. Paris und Halleri Disp. Chirurg., sel. II.

126. Gentil, C. J. et Pousse, Fr., Quaestio med.-chir. an in deprimenda cataracta ipsius capsula inferne et postice imprimis secanda est. Paris.

127. Hope, Thomas, Letters concerning Daviel's method of couching a cataract. Philos. Trans.

1753. 128. Morand et Verdier, Rapport des operations de la cataracte par l'extraction du cristallin, faites devant les Commissaire de l'Academie par M. Poyet. Mem. de l'Acad. de Chir., II, 578.

129. Froschel, G. H., Buchner, Disp. de cataractae omni tempore deponenda. Halae.

130. Sharp, Samuel, A description of a new method of opening the cornea, in order to extract the crystalline humor. Phil. Trans.

1754. 131. Daviel, H. et Le Bas, Ergo cataractae tutior extractio forficis ope. Paris.

131a. Deidier, Antoine, Consultations et observations. Paris. Beschreibt den Krystallwulst nach Reclination. Die Linse war vollstandig aufgesogen.

132. Warner, J., Cases in surgery, with introductions, operations and remarks. London. Second edition.

133. Hoin. Sur une espece de cataracte nouvellment observee. Paris. (Handelt vom Kapselstaar.)

1755. 134. Daviel, Jacques. Von einer neuen methode, den Staar durch Ausziehung des krystalls zu heilen. In den Abh. der k. par. Ac. d. Chir. Bd. 2, Ins. Deutsche ubersetzt. Altenburg. (Enthalt die Geschichte und Beschreibung der von D. erfunden operation.)

135. La Faye, Abhandlung, welche die neue methode, die operation des Staars zu machen, zu verbessern dient. Ebend. (Beschreibt ein neues Instrument zum Oeffnen der Hornhaut.)

136. Morand und Verdier, Bericht von den operationen des Staars durch Ausziehung des krystalls, die im beisein der Commission der Academie von H. Poyet gemacht worden. Ebend. (Bezieht sich auf Daviel's methode.)

1756. 137. Taylor, J., Erorterung uber die kunst das verlorene gesicht wieder herzustellen, so durch krankheit der krystallinischen feuchtigweit verloren gegangen. Pesaro.

1756. 138. Daviel, Jacques, Journal de Medicine. Fevrier, p. 124.

139. ——, Henry, Lettre addressee a Mess. les auteurs du Journal des Scavans sur les advantages de l'extractio de la cataracte. Nouvelle methode inventee par Mr. Daviel. Journ. des Scav. Fevrier. p. 375.

140. Wahlbom, J. G., Bemerkungen uber das staarstechen. Abhandlungen der Schwedischen Akademie.

1757. 141. Acrell, Olaus, Vergleichung zwischen den vortheilen und unbequemlichkeiten, welche jeder art des staarstechens begleiten, durch eigene versuche und bemerkungen unterstutze. K. Sw. Wet. Acad. Trim., III; auch in Schriftwaxling om alle brukelige satt at operum Staaren pa agonen. Stockholm, 1766.

142. Tenon. Theses ex anatomie et chirurgia de cataracta. Paris.

1758. 143. Theronde de Vallun, C. F. A. J., Descemet. Non E. sola lens cataractae crystallinae sedes. Paris.

144. Lander, Diss. de cataracta. Edinburg.

1759. 145. Sabatier, B. R. et Martin, P. D., Theses de variis cataractam extrahendi methodis. Parisiis.

146. Daviel, Jacques, Von zwei angebornen Staaren, welche er auszog. Koningl. Swel. Wet. Acad. Trim., I.

147. Morand, J. Fr. Cl., Lettre concernant quelques observations sur divereses especes de cataractes. Mercure de France. Aout.

148. Holn, J. J. L., Lettre concernant quelques observations sur diverses especes de cataractes. Merc. de France. Aout; auch in Janin, p. 169.

1760. 149. —— (on Morand). Seconde lettre a Mr. Daviel sur la cataracte radiee, la convexite du chaton du cristallin apres l'extraction de celui-ci, et une cataracte fenetree. Merc. de France. Mars.

150. Schurer, J. L., Quaestio, num in curatione suffusionis lentis crystallinae extractio depressioni sit praeferenda. Argentorum.

151. Daviel, Jacques, Mercure des France. Janier. Antwort auf einen Brief von Holn.

1761. 152. Ten Haaf, G., Korte verhandeling uspens de nieuwe wyze van de cataracta to geneezen door middel van het crystalline vocht nyt het oog te neemen. Rotterdam.

1762. 153. Demours, Petrus. Sur une maladie des yeux ou l'on indique la veritable cause des accidents qui surviennent a l'operation bien faite de la cataracte par extraction et l'on propose un moyen pour y remedier. Journal de Medicine. XVI, p. 49.

154. Cantwell, Andrew. Account of t he success of Daviel's method of extracting cataracts. Philos. Transact.

1763. 155. Palucci, N. J., Descriptio novi instrumenti pro cura cataractae nuper inventi et exhibiti. Wien. (Zur Extraction.)

1764. 156. Reghellini, Janus, Osservazioni sopra alcuni casi rari medici e chirurgici Venez. (Betrifft vornehmlich die Staaroperation.)

1764. 157. Taylor, J., Lettre a Mrs. de l'Acad. de Chir. sur l'art de retablir la vue obscurie par la maladie connue sous le nom di cataracte ou l'on demontre les dangereuses consequences de l'operation de la cataracte par extraction. Paris, 1764. Seconde lettre ohne Jagreszahl.

1765. 158. Colombier, J., Diss. nova de suffusione seu cataracta oculi anatome et mecanismo lucupletata. Paris. Auch in Sandifort thes. diss., Vol. 3, 1778. (Geschichtliches und Vorschlag zur Abenderung der Daviel'schen operation.)

1766. 159. Schaeffer, J. G., Geschichte des grauen Staars und der neue operation, solchen durch Herausnehmung der Krystallinse zu heilen, nebst daraus gefolgerten und erorterten Fragen. Regensburg.

160. Jericho, F. W., Diss. sistens modum sectionis in cataracta instituendae, variasque circa opthalmotomiam cautelas. Traject. ad Rhenum.

161. Martin. R., u. Wahlbaum, Abhandlungen in Schriftwaxling om alle brukelige satt at opera on Starrin Stockholm.

162. Richter, A. G., De variis e xtrahendi cataractam modis. Goettingae.

163. Astruck, J. A. (Elias de la Poterie), Ergo incisioni corneae in curatione cataractae praeferenda est embroche. Paris.

1767. 164. Reichenbach, Cautelae et observationes circa extractionem cataractae, novam methodum synizesin operandae sistentis. Tubingae. Auch in Reuss, Diss Med. Tub., Vol. III, und in Sandfort Thesaur. Diss., Vol. III, 1778.

1768. 165. Le Vacher et Contouly, De cataracta nova ratione extrahenda. Parisiis.

166. Colombier, J. et d'Onglee, Ergo pro multiplici cataractae genere multiplex. Paris.

167. Richter, A. G., Operationes aliquot, quibus cataractam extraxit. Goettingae.

168. Ronnow Casten, Om en ben och stenartig Staar wid hela om kretsen of uvea fast wuchsen som lyckeligen blifwit med. nalen nertrykt. Stockholm.

1769. 169. Hoin. Von einem stralichten Staare. Memoires de l'Academie de Dijon. I.

1770. 170. Janin, J., Lettre sur les cataractes a M. Palletier. Journal de Medicine, XXIV, p. 374.

171. Henkel, J. F., Vom grauen Staar. Chirurg. Operationen, I. Stuck, 95.

172. Richter, A. G., Observationum chirurgicarum fasciculus, continens de cataractae extractione observationes. Gott.

1772. 173. Van der Steege, De suffusionem methodis Wenzelii et Contii extrahendi. Groningae.

174. Rosenthal et Mayer. Examen quarandum optimarum cataractam extrahendi methodorum imprimis Wenzeliance. Gryphiswald.

1772. 175. Janin, Memoires et observations sur l'oeil. etc. Lyon.

176. Berner, G. E., De cataracta oculi dextri in puero quatuordecim mensium feliciter curata et discussa. Acta natur. curious, III, obs. 26.

177. Marx, M. J., Observ. quaedam medica cum fig. aeneis. Berol. (Durch Arzneimittel geheilter Staar.)

1773. 178. Richter, Abhandlung von der Ausziehung des grauen Staars. Gottingen.

1774. 179. Hellmann, J. C., Der graue Staar und dessen Herausnehmung nebst einigen Beobachtungen. Madgeburg.

180. Szen, Car., D. inauguralis de cataracta ab effluviis aquae fortis nata. Jenae.

181. Pellier de Quengsy, Observ. sur l'extraction d'une cataracte singuliere. Journ. de Med., XLII, p. 79. (Es war eine sog. cat. chorioidealis.)

1775. 182. Chandler, G., A treatise of the cataract. Its nature, species, causes and symptoms, etc. London.

183. Pott, Percival, Chirurgical observations relative of the cataract, the polypus of the nose, etc. London. (Gegen die extraction.)

184. Borthwick, Treatise upon the extraction of the crystalline lens. Edinburgh.

185. DeWitt Gisbert, Vergleichung der verschiedenen methoden den staar auszuziehen. Giessen. Auch u. d. T.: Des Herrn de Witt neueste methode den Staar Auszuziehen. (2) Aufl. Giessen, 1777. Abhandlung von Ausziehung des Staars. Marburg, 1794.

186. Odhelius, J. L., Ammerkingar wid stare operationen den sinkans Skotsel Jereften. Stockholm.

1776. 187. Mejan, Th., Diss. de cataracta. Montpellier.

188. Pellier de Quengsy, Observ. sur une cataracta regardee de mauvaise espece, qui guerit neanmoins par l'extraction. Journ. de Med., XLV, p. 355.

189. Buddeus, Disp. an cataractae depressio cum capsula praeferenda extractioni.

1777. 190. Omeyer, Verhandeling over een nieuwe manier van operatie van de cataract. Amsterdam. (Vom grauen und weissen Staar, der in acht Fallen angeboren gewesen.)

2191. Olof Acrel, Chirurgische Vorfalle. Uebers. v. Murray. Gottingin. Bd. I, p. 105.

191a. ———, Ueber einen steinartigen Staar. Abhandlungen der Schwedischen Akademie (1778), und Chir. Vorf., Bd. I.

1778. 192. Lorenz Odhelius, Synizesis pupillae an beiden Augen mit festgewachsenen Staaren, deren einer Steinhart war; glucklich operirt. Ebenda.

1779. 193. ———, Cataracta membranacea, von einer gewaltsamen Ursache; glucklich operirt. Ebenda.

1779. 194. Wenzel, Sohn, Diss. de extractione cataractae. Paris.

195. Panajota, Nicolaides, Diss. Antylli ta biphana. Halae.

196. Boettcher, Diss. de suffusione. Halae.

197. Cusson, Remarques sur la cataracte. Montpellier.

1780. 198. Nannoni, L., Dissertazione sulla cataratta. Milani.

1781. 199. Mohrenheim, J., Abhandlung vom grauen Staare. Wienerische Beitrage, I. Band.

200. Bartolazzi, G., Dissertazione sopra una cieca nata guarita in noi
trattasi di una rara specie di cataratta connata. Verona. Uebersetzt. Leipzig, 1784.

1782. 201. Petit, Remarques sur l'operation de la cataracte par extraction.
Mercure de France. Avril.

202. Mursina, Vom grauen Staar und dessen Ausziehung. Medic. Chirurg. Beob. Berlin.

203. Sigerist, Franz, Beschreibung und Erklarung des Staarnadelmessers
und Gegenhalters. Gratz und Wien.

204. Feller, Chr. Gotth., Diss. de methodis suffusionem oculorum curan-
dis a Cassamata et Simone cultis. Lips.

1783. 205. Butter, A new propos for the extraction of the cataract. London.

206. Pellier de Quengsy, Recueil de memoires et d'observations sur les
maladies qui attaquent l'oeil. Montpellier.

207. Ludwig, Ch. F., De suffusionis per acum curatione. In exercita-
tionibus academicis, 1790. Lipsiae.

1784. 208. Marchand, Memoire et observations sur un nouveau moyen de prevenir l'aveuglement qui a pour cause la cataracte. Nisme.

209. Demours, fils, Ant. Pierre, Memoire sur l'operation de la cataracte.
Paris.

210. Chaussier, Observation sur une cataract, compliquee avec la dissolution du corps vitre, Nouv. Memoires de Dijon.

1785. 211. Hildebrand, C. W., De accuratiore cataractae deponendae methodo.
Francof.

212. Willburg, Betrachtung uber die bisher gewohnlichen operationen
des Staars, etc. Nurnberg.

1786. 213. Wenzel, Traite de la cataracte avec des observations, etc. Paris.
Uebersetzt Nurnberg, 1788.

214. Wathen, J. Th., A dissertation on the theory and cure of the cataract, in which the practice of extraction is supported, and that
operation in its present improved state is particularly described.
London. Vertheidigt. die extraction.

215. Odhelius, J. L., Versuche uber venerischen Staar und dessen operation. Neue Abhandlungen der konigl. Schwed. Akad. der Wissenschaft. Uebersetzt von Kuntner und Brandis.

216. Gleize, Nouvelles observations sur les maladies de l'oeil. Paris.
(Handelt vornehmlich von grauen Staar.)

1787. 217. Brunner, E. A. L., Diss. inaug. de cataracta. Goettingae.

218. Sparrow, J. R., Vom erfolge der Ausiehung und Niederdruckung des Staares bei der namlichen person. London Medical Journal, IX. London.

219. Schaffer, J. C., D. inaug. de cataracta membranacea. Cum figuris. Marburg.

220. Zirotti, Giambattista, della cataratta e sua depressione. Como.

221. Warner, Jos., Vom grauen Staar, in dessen chirurg. vorfallen und Bemerkungen. Aus dem Engl. Leiplg.

222. Kite, Charles, Heilung des grauen Staars durch die elektricitat. In ausererlesene Abhandlungen z. Gebr. pr. Aerzte, Bd. 12. Leipzig.

223. Tenon, J. R., Theses et Anatome et Chirurgia de cataracta. Paris.

224. Lucas, Ueber den grauen Staar, aus dem Engl. ubersetzt. Altenburg.

1788. 225. Overkamp, C. W., Argumenti chirurgici scorsim opthalmologici, libellus, etc. Gryphswaldis.

226. Weidinger, De praecipuis morbis oculi interni. Franc. ad Viadr.

227. Ziehenhagen, Uebersetzung von E. A. L. Brunner, Diss. inaug. de cataracta. Gottingae.

228. O'Halloran, Sylvester, A critical and anatomical examination of the parts immediately interested in the operation for a cataract; with an attempt to render the operation itself, whether by depression or extraction, more certain and successful. Transact. of the Irish Acad. (Besonders abgedruckt, London, 1790.)

1789. 229. Knox, W., Von einem durch die elektricitat in beiden Augen geheilten Staar. Med. Commentarien der Gesellschaft der Aerzte in Edinburg. Uebers von Diel. Altenburg.

1790. 230. Buchner, F., Verhandeling over de voortreffelykheid van de operatie der cataract, volgens de manier der ondere. Amsterdam.

231. Richter, A. G., Anfangsgrunde der Wundarznelkunde, Bd. III, p. 240. Gottingen. Extraction.

232. Rowley, Treatise on 118 principal diseases of the eye. London.

233. Habermann, G. F., D. med. chir. sistens historiam cataractae in puella annorum septem observatae. Jenae.

234. Mesplet, Bemerkungen uber die Staar operation. Journ. de Med. Juillet.

1791. 235. Jung, Methode de grauen Staar auszuziehen. Marburg.

236. Hofer, Eine merkwurdige Staar geschichte. Salzburger Zeitung, 4 Bd., p. 158.

237. Beer, J. G., Praktische Beobachtungen uber den grauen Staar und die Krankheiten der Hornhaut. Wien.

238. Conradi, Chr., Bemerkungen uber einige Gegenstande der Ausziehung des grauen Staares. Leipzig.

239. Sparrow, J. R., Ueber das Ausziehen des Staares mit Praktischen Bemerkungen. Medic. faits and observations, Vol. I. London, 1791,

1792. 240. ——, Ueber vier durch die Ausziehung gemachte gluckliche Staar operation. Repertor. Chir. u. Med. Abhandlg.. 1 Bd. Leipzig,1792.

241. Wardenburg, Dissert. de methodo cataractae extrahendae nova. Gottingae.

242. Van Wy, Gerrit, Jan, Nieuwe manier van cataract of staarsnyding beneffens. Heel en Vradkundige Waarneemingen. Arnheim.

243. Assalini, Discorso sopra un nuovo stromento per l'estrazione della cataratta. Pavia.

244. Peacock, H. B., Observations on the blindness occasioned by cataracts, showing the practicability and superiority of a method of cure without an operation. London.

245. Conradi, G. Chr., Ein paar worte uber die diat nach den operationen, insbesondere des grauen Staares. Salzburger Zeitung, 4 Bd., p.818.

246. ——, Dissertazione chirurg. sulla cataratta coll' agiunta di varie osservazioni Genua. Anonym.

247. Verschiedene Staar operations geschichten.

1793. 248. Bishoff, A treatise on the extraction of the cataract. London.

248a. Hildebrandt, Fr., Einige Beobachtungen uber den grauen Staar. Loder's Journal fur Chir., I, p. 102 u. 226.

1794. 249. Sattig, Samuel Godefroy, praes. Reil, J. Chr. Diss. de lentis crystallinae structura fibrosa. Halae. (Bezieht sich auch auf Cataract.)

250. Ware, James, Ein merkwurdiges Beispiel von einer Herstellung des Gesichtes durch Zertheilung einer cataract. Abhandlungen der Med. Gesellschaft in London. Aus dem Engl., 1794.

1795. 251. Santerelli, Richerche per facilitare il cateterismo e l'estrazione delle cataretta. Vienna.

252. Ware, J., An inquiry into the causes which have most commonly prevented success in the operation of extracting the cataract. Dasselbe Deutsche von Leune. Leipzig, 1799.

1796. 253. Loder, J. Chr., Progr. de curatione externa post cataractae extractionem. Jenae.

254. Schiferli, R. A., Diss. inaug. de cataracta. Jenae.

1797. 255. ——, Abhandlung vom grauen Staar. Jenae.

256. Barth, Etwas uber die Ausziehung des grauen Staars. Wien.

257. Conradi, Vorschlag einer einfachen methode den Staar zu stechen. Arnemann's Magazin, Bd. I, p. 61.

258. Beer, G. J., Einige praktische Bemerkungen uber des Staares betreffend. Ibidem, Bd. I, p. 284.

259. Arnemann, J., Einige Bemerkungen die operation des Staares betreffend. Ibidem, p. 340.

260. Hildebrand, Einige Beobachtungen uber den grauen Staar. Loder's Journal, Bd. I.

261. Ebert, Phil. Jac., praes. Reil, J. Chr., Diss. de oculi suffusionum curationibus et antiquis et hodiernis. Halae.

1799. 262. Beer, G. J., Methode den grauen Staar sammt der Kapsel auszuziehen. Wien.

262a. Sybel, De quibusdam materiae et formae oculi aberrationibus a statu normali. Halae.

262b. Beer, Praktische Bemerkungen uber den Nachstaar. Salzburger Med. Chirurg. Zeitung. V. Beilage.

1800. 263. Earle, James, An account of a new method of operation for the removal of the opacity in the eye, called cataract. London.

1801. 263a. Himly, Chr., Ist es rathsam, die Staar operation zugleich auf beiden augen vorzunehmen. Opthalmol. Beobachtungen und Untersuchungen. Bremen u. Opthal. Bibliothek v. Himly, I, p. 160.

263b. ——, Ueber den schwarzen ring im umfang des harten staars. Ibidem, I, p. 92.

264. Vorfall der krystallinse ohne aussere ursache. Ibidem, p. 105.

265. ——, Schwierigkeiten bei der Willburgischen Art den Staar niederzudrucken. Ibidem, p. 145.

266. ——, Soll man den Staar nicht operiren, so lange der kranke noch mit dem andern Auge gut sieht? Ibidem, p. 148.

267. ——, Soll man bei der Staar operation das andere verbinden? Ibidem, p. 154.

268. Schmidt, J. A., Ueber Nachstaar und Iritis nach Staar operationen. Wien.

269. ——, Pruefung der von Beer bekannt gemachten methode den grauen Staar sammt der kapsel auszuziehen. Loder's Journal fur Chir., III.

270. Jacobi, Theoret. Praktische Grunde gegen die Anwendbarkeit der von Beer vorgeschlagenen methode den grauen Staar sammt der kapsel auszuziehen. Wien.

271. Scarpa, A., Saggio di osservazione e di esperienze sulle principali malattie degli occhi. Pavia.

272. Homuth, B. G., praes. Kreysig, F. L., Diss. continens observationes de cataracta. Viteberg.

273. Wardenburg, J. G. A., Neuigkeiten aus der Staar operation. Gottingen.

274. Ware, James, Case of a young gentleman who recovered his sight when seven years of age, after having been deprived by cataracts before he was a year old; with remarks. Philos. Transact.

275. Martens, Fr. H., Et was uber die methode Beer's, den grauen Staar nebst der kapsel auszuziehen. In dessen Paradoxien, Bd. 1.

276. Redlich, W., Ueber Jacobi's Widerlegung der Beer'schen methode den grauen Staar auszuziehen. Ebenda, Bd. 1.

1802. 277. Beer, G. J., Antwort auf Schmidt's aufsatz in Loder's Journal. Ebenda, Bd. 3.

278. Schmidt, J. A., Entgegnung auf Beer's antwort. Ebenda.

1802. 279. Weidmann, J. P., Ueber die Ausziehung des Staars und eine leichtere und sichere methode derselben; dem Nationalinstitut in Paris vorgelegt. Himly und Schmidt. Opthalmol. Bibliothek., Bd. 1.

280. Carre, P. L., Essay sur la cataracte. Paris.

281. Kirby, Jeremiah, Diss. de lentis caligine. Edinb.

282. Lichtenstein, G. J. A., De situ lentis crystallinae cataracta afflictae vario, methodi extractoriae modificationes indicante. Helmstad.

283. Flander, J. Fr., praes. Plonquet. G. C., Meletemata circa cataractam. Diss. Tub.

284. Scarpa, Traite pratique des maladies des yeux. Paris.

285. Siebold, Ein grauer Staar, der sich von selbst senkte; nebst kurzen Bemerkungen uber die Depression. Himly und Schmidt. Opth. Bibl., Bd. 1, p. 137.

1803. 286. Hey, W., Practical observations in surgery, illustrated with cases. London, und in Langenbeck's Bibl., Bd. 1, 1806.

287. Hintz, J. A., Uebersicht der bis jetzt offentlich gewordenen Verhandlungen uber die von Beer wieder angeregte extraction sammt der kapsel. Opthalm. Bibl. v. Himly u. Schmidt, II, 1, p. 104.

288. Siccovon, Ens, Historia extractiones cataractae. Worcumi Frisiorum.

289. Fleury, J. B., Diss. sur la cataracte. Paris.

1804. 290. Mayer, Ph., Diss. novam cataractae extrahendae methodum describens. Gott.

1805. 291. Elsasser, Ueber die operation des grauen Staars. Strassburg, 1804.

292. Cooper, Samuel, Critical reflections on several important practical points relative to the cataract. London.

293. Pfotenhauer, A. Fr., praes. Seiler, G., Diss. sistens cultrorum ceratotomorum et cystitomorum ad extrahendam cataractam historiam. Vitebergae.

1806. 294. Buchhorn, Dissert. de keratonyxide. Halae.

295. Wardrop, Practical observations on the mode of making the incision of the cornea for the extraction of the cataract. Edinb. Med. and Surg. Journal, V, January.

296. Langenbeck, C. J. M., Ueber die Staar operation. Bibl. f. Chir., t. 1.

297. Himly, Allegemeine Regeln zur symptomatischen Untersuchung kranker Augen. Opth. Bibl. v. Himly u. Schmidt, III, 2, p. 23.

298. Guerin, J. B., Diss sur l'operation de la cataracte. Paris.

1807. 299. Home, Everard, An account of two children born with cataracts in their eyes. Phil. Transact.

1809. 300. Weinhold, Carl Aug., Anleitung den verdunkelten Krystallkorper im Auge des Menschen jederzeit bestimmt mit seiner Kapsel umzulegen. Ein versuch zur Vervollkommnung der Depression des grauen Staares und der kunstlich en Pupillenbildung. Meissen.

301. Beauhene, M., Diss. de l'organisation de l'oeil et sur l'operation de la cataracte, appliquee au traitment des animaux domestiques. Paris.

1809. 302. Brouard, Rapport des operations (des cataractes par extraction et par depression) de Forlenze. Annuaire de la Societe de Med. de Depart. de l'Eure.

1810. 303. Gouliart, Brouard et Maheux, Memoire sur les operations de la cataracte et autres, faites par Forlenze a l'Infirmerie des prisons. Ebenda.

304. Buchhorn, De keratonyxide, nova catar. aliisque oculi morbis med. method. Madgeburg.

305. Santerelli, Delle cateratte. Forli.

306. Walther, Th. Fr., v., Ueber die Krankheiten der Krystallinse und die bildung des grauen Staares. Dessen Abhandlungen aus dem Gebiete der Prakt. Medicin. Landshut.

307. Bruckmann, Wahrnehmungen bei einer Verdunkelung der Krystallinse; ein autonosographischer Versuch. Holn's Archiv. f. Med. Erfahrungen, 1810 und 1812.

1811. 308. Buchhorn, Die Keratonyxis, eine gefahrlose methode. Madgeburg.

309. Langenbeck, Pruefung der Keratonyxis, einer neuen methode, den grauen Staar durch die Hornhaut zu recliniren oder zu zerstuckeln. Gottingen.

310. ——, Zur Prufung der Keratonyxis Bibl. f. Chir., T. IV.

311. Gibson, Practical observations on the formation of an artificial pupil in several deranged states of the eye, to which are annexed remarks on the extraction of soft cataract, and three of the membranous kind through a puncture of t he cornea. London, 1811, and the New England Journal of Medicine and Surgery, 1, III, n. I-IV, 1819.

312. Sporl, J. F. E., praes. Graefe, C. F., Dissert. de cataractae reclinatione et de keratonyxide. Berol.

313. Scheuring J., Parallelle der vorzuglichsten operations-methoden des grauen Staares. Bamberg.

1812. 314. Montain, Traite de la cataracte. Paris.

315. Jaeger, Fredericus, Dissert. de keratonyxidis usu. Viennae. Auch in Radius Script. Opth. Minor., Vol. I.

316. Gibson, B., Practical observations. Manchester.

317. Benedict, T. W. G., Kritik der Weinholdschen Staarnadelscheere. Beitrage fur Prakt. Medic. u. Opth., I.

318. Ware, James, On the operation of largely puncturing the capsule of the crystalline, in order to promote the absorption of the cataract. London.

319. Partra, A. E., De l'operation de la cataracte. Paris.

320. Muter, R., Practical observations on various novel modes of operating on cataract. and of forming an artificial pupil. Paris.

1813. 321. Haan, Diss. sur la keratonyxis. Paris.

322. Faure, J. N., Observation d'une operation de la cataracte, faite par la keratonyxis. Bullet. de la Fac. de Med. et de la Soc. de Paris.

1814. 323. Benedict, Zur Prüfung der Keratonyxis. Neue Bibl. f. Chir., t. 1.

324. Edwards, Discres. sur l'inflammation de l'iris et la cataracte noire. Paris.

325. Benedict, F. W. G., Monographie des grauen Staars. Breslau.

326. Reisinger, Fr., Bemerkungen über die keratonyxis, die vorzüglichste operations methode des grauen Staars. Beitrage z. Chir. u. Anat. Gottingen.

327. Travers, Further observations on the cataract. Medico-chirurgical observations of London, Vol. V, p. 406.

328. Wardrop, Sketch of life and writings of the late Benjamin Gibson. Edinburgh Med. and Surg. Journal, Vol. X.

1815. 329. Langenbeck, Zur Prüfung der Keratonyxis. Neue Bibl. f. Chir., t. 1.

330. Fleischmann, Leicheneroffnung. Erlangen, p. 202. (Verknocherte Linse.)

331. Sciege, J. A., Diss. quaenam in operatione cataractae methodus sit optimi. Berol.

332. Evans, Observations on cataract and closed pupil. London.

1816. 333. Scarpa, Trattato delle princip. malatti degli occhi. Pav.

334. Mensert, W., Verhandeling over de keratonyxis. Amsterdam.

335. Betz, J. G., Diss. de amovenda cataracta per keratonyxidem. Jenae.

1817. 336. Adams, A practical inquiry into the causes of the frequent failure of the operations of depression and of the extraction of the cataract, as usually performed. London.

337. Beer, Lehre von den Augenkrankheiten. 1, II. Wien.

1818. 338. Langenbeck, Beschreibung seines Keratoms zur Zerstuckelung des Staars. Ibid., t. 1.

339. Gendre, J. a., Diss. sistens diversarum cataractae operandae methodorum inter se comparationem. Landish.

340. Guille, Nouvelles recherches sur la cataracte et la goutte sereine. Ed. 2, Paris.

341. Onsenoort, A. G. van, Verhandeling over de graauwe Staar, den kunstigen Oogappel, etc. Amsterd.

1819. 342. Kirchmayer, Dissert. de cataractae extrah. methodis. Landish. Bibl. f. Chir., t. III. Hanover.

344. Canella, G., Riflessioni critiche ed esperienze sul modo di operare la cataratta col mezzo del cheratonissi. Milano.

345. Faure, N. J., Memoire sur la pupille artificielle et la keratonyxis. Paris.

346. Adams, Treatise on artificial pupil. London, p. 94. (Verknocherte Linse.)

347. Schindler, H. Br., Diss. de iritide chronica ex keratonyxis suborta. Vratislav.

348. Bieske, O. L., Animadversiones de cataractae genesi et cura. Erlangae.

1819. 349. Lusardi. Traite de l'alteration du cristallin, suivi d'un extrait d'un memoire inedit sur la pupille artificelle. Paris.

350. Baerens, B. Fr., praes. Gmelin, F. G., Diss. sistens lentis crystallinae monographiam physiologico-pathologicam. Tubingae. (Radius, Script. Opth. Min.)

1820. 351. Heilbrunn, Dav.. Diss. de variis cataractae curandae methodis. Berolinae.

352. Andreae, A., Uber die Lehre vom grauen Staar und die methoden, denselben zu operiren. Graefe u. Walther, Journal, Bd. I.

353. Langenbeck, C. J. M., Ueber die keratonyxis und die operation des grauen Staars durch Versigen der Linse und Zerstuckelung. Neue Bibl. f. Chir. u. Opth., Bd. 2.

1821. 354. Lachmann, Instrumentorum ad corneae sectionem in cataractae extractione perficiendam descriptio historica. Gotting.

355. Ammon, A., v., Opthalmoparacenteseos historia, etc. Gotting.

356. Travers, Synopsis of the diseases of the eye and their treatment. London.

357. De la Garde, P. C., A treatise on cataract. London.

358. Pacini, Diss. de keratonyxide. Lucca.

359. Hannath, John, Diss. de cataracta. Edinb.

1822. 360. Giorgi, Memoria sopra un nuovo strumento per operare la cataratta et per formare la pupilla artifiziale. Imola.

361. Pugliatti, O., Riflessioni di ottalmiatria prattica, che comer nono la pupilla artifiziale e la cataratta. Messina.

1823. 362. Haertelt. Dissert. extractionis cataractae praestantis, etc. Vratisl.

363. Jaeger, C., Dissert. exh. fragmenta de extractione cataractae et experimenta de prolapsu artificiali corporis vitrei. Vind.

364. Catanoso, N., Osservazioni cliniche sopra l'estrazione della cataratta. Messina.

365. Molinari, J., Commentat. de scleronoxydis sequelis earumque cura. Ticin. Reg. (Radius, Script. Opth. Minor.)

366. Bowen, J., Practical observations on the removal of every species and variety of cataract, by hyalonyxis or vitreous operation. London.

1824. 367. Gurlt. Ueber die resorption der kataraktosen linsen in der voderen augenkammer. Reisinger's Annal. Sulzbach.

368. Dieterich, Ueber die verwundungen des linsensystems. Tubingen.

369. Huellverding, S., Dissert. sistens quasdam circa cataractae discissionem observat. Viennae.

370. Ruella, Diss. sur la cataracte. Paris.

371. Stephenson, J., A treatise on cataract and the cure of every species of cataract, by hyalonyxis or vitreous operations. London.

372. Gorgone, G., Considerazioni pratiche sull operazioni della cataratta. Napoli.

1824. 373. Reisinger, Fr., Eine neue Staarnadel zur keratonyxis. Baier. Annalen. Sulzbach.

1825. 374. Zenschner, F. A., Mein verfahren bei der ausziehung des grauen Staars. Rust's Magaz. f. d. ges. Heilkunde, Bd. 19.

375. Pamard, De la cataracte et de son extraction par un procede particulier. Paris.

376. Gondret, L. Fr., Mem. sur le traitement de la cataracte. Paris et Montpellier.

377. Schreyer, Grundriss der chirurg. operationen. Nurnberg, Th. 1, p. 399. Werkzeuge zur Kapseleroffnung.

378. Cocteau et Leroy d'Etiolles, Experiences a la reproduction du cristallin. Acad. de Med. de Paris, 10 Fevrier. Journal de Physiologie par Magendie, VII, p. 30, 1827.

1826. 379. Grossheim, E. L., Ueber Jaeger's methode der Staar extraction mittelst des Hornhautschnittes. Graefe u. Walther, Journal, Bd. IX.

380. London, Short inquiry into the principal causes of the unsuccessful termination of extraction by the cornea, with the view of showing the superiority of D. Jaeger's knife of the single cataract knife of Wenzel and Beer. London.

1827. 381. Ritterich, Bemerkungen uber die operation des grauen Staars. Beitrage ur Vervollkommnung der Augenheilk. Leipzig, I, 1.

382. Lusardi, Memoire sur la cataracte congenitale, etc. Paris.

383. Parfait-Landran, Mem. sur un nouveau procede a introduire dans l'operation de la cataracte par extraction. Paris.

384. Conaud, These de la cataracte et de son traite ment. Paris.

385. Backhausen, P., Diss. de regeneratione lentis crystallinae. Berol. in Radius, Script. Opth. Min., Vol. III, 1830.

386. Schwarz, Doppelte Linse. Gemeins. Deutsche Zeitschrift fur Geburtskunde, I, p. 521.

1828. 387. Sommering, W., Beobachtungen uber die organischen Veranderungen im Auge nach Staar operationen. Frankfurt a M.

388. Ammon, A. v., Ueber die angeborene cataracta centralis. Graefe u. Walther, Journ. f. Chirurg. u. Augenheilk. t. IX.

389. Seliger, Uebersucht der verschiedenen Staar ausziehungsmethoden, nebst prakt. Belegen uber die Wesentlichen Vorzuge des Hornhautschnittes nach oben. Wien.

390. Appiani, Dissert. de phacohymenitide. Fienni.

391. Breton, Bericht uber die bei den Eingebornen von Ostindien gebrauchliche Operationsweise des grauen Staars. Transact. of the Medical and Physical Society of Calcutta, Vol. II, 1826. Hecker's Annal. d. Heilkunde, Bd. 11.

392. Placer, J., Diss. de cataracta et nonnullis eam extrahendi methodis. Berol.

1828. 393. Gondret, L., Mem. sur le traitement de la cataracte. Bd. 3. Paris.

1829. 394. Nieberding, F. A., Diss. de diversarum cataractae curandae methodorum indicationibus. Berol.

395. Meyer, H., Diss. sistens cataractae operationem perficiendi meth-
oduum, qua ulitur C. Himly. Rostock.

396. Ott, F. A., Diss. de nova Jaegeri cataractam extrahendi ratione.
Straubing.

397. Bancal, Manuel pratique lithotritic, suivi d'un memoire sur la cataracte. Pavia. Auch in Graefe u. Walther Journal, Vol. No. 25,
1837.

1830. 398. Frey, J. M., Diss. de cataracta. Berol.

399. Closset, G. A., Diss. sistens quaedam de praecipuis morbis, qui post
opera+ionem cataractae oriri possunt. Berol.

400. Rosenmuller, F. A., Diss. de staphylomate scleroticae nec non de
melanosi et cataracta nigra nonnulla adhibens. Erlangae.

401. Rosas, Handbuch der Augenheilkunde, 1, III. Wien.

402. Bech, Dissert. de cataracta centrali: Lips.

403. Ammon, v., Ueber den krankhaften consens der Hornhaut, der krystallinse und ihrer Kapsel. Z. f. d. O., I, p. 119.

1831. 404. Schmidt, J. A., Von der cataracta v. Ammon's Z. f. d. O. I, p. 850.

405. Schon, Ueber den marasmus senilis der kapsel und linse im menschlichen auge. Ibid.

406. Lechla, Wutzer, Jahn, Ueber Coloboma iridis mit gleichzeitiger cataracta lenticularis und uber die Genesis der Irisspaltung. Z. f. d.
O. I., p. 253.

407. Ammon, v., Spontaner Vorfall einer Krystallinse in die vodere
augenkammer. Z. f. d. O. I., p. 260.

408. Gescheidt, Colobomo iridis mit Partialtrubung der Linse (c. L. centralis). Z. f. d. O. I., p. 549.

1832. 409. Warnatz, Dissert. de cataracta nigra. Lips.

410. ——, Die schwarz gefarbte anderen ahnlichen augenkrankheiten.
Z. f. d. O. II, p. 295.

411. Ullmann, Spontaner Vorfall einer Augenkammer und entfernung
derselbe durch die extraction. Z. f. d. O. II, p. 129.

412. Ammon, v., Zur pathol. Anatomie der Fossa hyaloidea im menschlichen Auge. Z. f. d. O. II, p. 388.

413. ——. Prof. Rosas' Ansichten uber die Sehversuche gleich nach voll-
zogener Extraction des Staares. Z. F., d. o., p. 400.

414. Dupuytren, Bemerkungen uber den grauen Staar. Mitgetheilt von
Behr. Z. f. d. O. II, p. 460.

415. Arnold, F., Anatom. Untersuchungen uber das Auge des Menschen.

416. Schmidt, Aemil, Diss. de Keratotomia sursum vergente secundum
Jaegeri methodum. Berol.

417. Carron du Villards, Ch. J. F., Lettre a Mr. Maunoir sur un nouvel
instrument destine a rectifier ou aggrandir l'incision de la cornee
dans l'operation de la cataracte par extraction. Paris. Graefe u.
Walther Journ., Vol. XXIII, 1835.

434

1832. 418. Ammon. v., Verdickung und Verwachsung der Art. centralis oculi als Ursache des Centralstaars der Kapsel und Linse, und zur Lehre der cataracte centralis überhaupt. Z. f. d. O., p. 485.

1833. 419. Beck, De oculorum mutationibus, quae cataractae operationem sequuntur, observatio, adnexis corollariis. Freib. Deutsch von Beger in von Ammon's Zeitschr., f. d. O., Bd. 4.

420. Ammon, v., Der angeborene Staar in path., anat., in pathogen, und in operativer Hinsicht. Z. f. d. O. III, 70.

421. ———, Operation des grauen Staars an einem Albino. Z. f. d. O. III, p. 116.

422. Beger, Ueber die Verwundbarkeit des Auges und seiner Haute. Z. f. d. O. III, p. 145.

423. Heidenreich, Schwarze cataracte mit weissem exsudate auf der kapsel. Z. f. d. O. II, p. 205.

424. Werneck, Zur Aetiologie und Genesis des grauen Staars. Z. f. d. O. III, p. 473.

425. Mannoir, Th., Essai sur quelques points de l'histoire de la cataracte. These. Paris.

426. Rast, De variis cataractae operandae methodis. Solinb.

427. Bergeon, G. C., De la reclination capsulo-lenticulaire, ou nouveau procede d'abaissement de la cataracte avec aiguille nouvelle. These. Paris.

428. Lattier de la Roche, Mem. sur la cataracte et guerison de cette maladie sans operation chirurgicale. Paris.

1834. 429. Deutsch, u. d. T., Beobachtungen und Erfahrungen uber die Heilung des grauen Staars ohne chirurg. operation, etc. Ilmenau, 1834.

430. Carron du Villards, Recherches pratiques sur les causes qui font echouer l'operation de la cataracte suivant les divers procedes. Paris.

431. Kyll, Geschichte einer freiwilligen Zerreissung der Cornea und Heraustreten der Linse. Z. f. d. O. IV, p. 157.

432. Starrhetti, Partieller Vorfall einer durchsichtigen Krystallinse. Z. f. d. O. IV, p. 463.

433. Dupuytren, G., Von der Cataracta. Klinisch-chirurg. Vortrage für Deutschland bearbeitet von Beck u. Leonhardt, Bd. 1. Leipzig.

434. Rinecker, Fr., Entzundung der Gefass, Nerven und Glashaut des Auges und ihr Ausgang in das hintere Elterauge, in Folge der Niederdrückung des Staars. Inaug. Wurzburg. Auch. Z. f. d. O. V, p. 358.

1835. 435. Warnatz, Resorptio cataractae spontanae. V. Ammon's Z. f. d. O., V, p. 49.

436. Lorch. Von einigen durch Naturhulfe gehobenen Augenkrankheiten. Z. f. d. O. IV, p. 38.

437. Schon. Marasmus senilis der Kapsel und der Linse. V. Ammon's Z. f. d. O. IV, p. 73.

1836. 438. Kollar, J., Diss. de praecipuis morbis post cataracta operationem secudariis. Vratislav.

439. Becker, Th., A. F., Diss. de ambigue quorandum recentiorum keratotomorum praestantia. Lips.

440. Reute, Verbessertes Verfahren bei der Scleroticonyxis. Holscher's Ann. f. d. Gesammte Heilkunde, t. III.

441. Unger. Ausziehung zweier Cataracten aus amaurotischen Augen. Z. f. d. O. V, p. 357.

442. Jaeger (Rinecker), Geschichte einer Entzundung der Ader-Nerven und Glashaut und ihres Ausganges in das hintere Eiterauge in Folge der Niederdruckung des Staars, nebst anatomisch pathologischer Untersuchung des Auges. Z. f. d. O. V, p. 358.

443. Comperet. These sur la cataracte, Paris.

444. Unger, Operation einer Cataract bei gleich zeitig bestehender Harnruhr, z. f., d. o. v., p. 356.

1837. 445. Sichel, Traite de l'opthalmie, la cataracte et l'amaurose. Paris, in 8o, p. 750.

446. Carron du Villards, Recherches medico-chirurgicales sur l'operation de la cataracte, les moyens de la rendre plus sure et sur l'inutilite des traitements medicaux pour la guerir sans operation. Paris, in 8o, p. 423.

1838. 447. Burkhardt, Appreciation physiologique de deux cas de luxation du cristallin. Ber. der Naturf. Ges. in Basel u. Ann. d'Ocul., XXX, p. 114.

448. Onsenoort, van Gesch, der Augenh. als enleitung in d. Studium derselben. Deutsch von Wutzer.

449. Pauli, F., Sublatio cataractae, eine neue methode den grauen Staar zu operiren. V. Ammon, Monatsschr., I, p. 97.

450. Benedict, Bemerkungen uber einige neuere Encheiresen zur Erleichterung der Staar operation. V. Ammon. Monasschr., I, p. 198.

451. Pauli, F., Ueber den grauen Staar und die Verkrummungen und eine neue Heilart dieser Krankheit. Stuttg., in 8o, p. 439.

452. Beck, Ueber die entstehung der cat. caps. anterior. V. Ammon, Monatsschr. f. Medicin. Augenheilk. u. Chirurg., t. II.

453. Stoeber, Observations des cataractes traumatiques, addressees a l'Acad. Roy. de Med. de Paris. Ann. d'Ocul., III. p. 64.

454. Loewenhardt, Resorption d'une cataract au moyen d'un seton passe a travers le cristallin opaque. Ann. d'Ocul., I, p. 20.

455. Cunier, Du displacement spontane du cristallin. Ann. d'Ocul., I, p. 59.

456. Carron du Villards, Du deplacement du cristallin. Ibid., t. I, p. 74.

457. Petrequin, Nouvelles remarques sur l'operation de la cataracte par l'abaissement. Ibid., I, d. 157.

1839. 458. Lombard, Considerations et observations sur la guerison des cataractes et des effections de la cornee transparente par une methode resolutive, etc. Paris, in 8o, p. 86.

436

1839. 459. Furnari, Essai sur une nouvelle methode d'operer la cataracte par
l'extraction par la sclerotique. Paris, in 8o, p. 16.

460. Bron, Traitement homoeopathique de la cataracte. Ann. d'Ocul., II,
p. 218.

461. ———, Cataracte lenticulaire guerie par le cannabis sativa. Ibid.,
p. 181.

462. Pauli, Ein beitrag zur Lehre von der Reproduction der Linse. V.
Ammon, Monatsschr., II, p. 84.

463. Averdam. B. H. J., Diss. de cataracte. Berol.

464. M. X., Quelle est l'influence qu' exerce l'operation de la cataracte
sur la vie de ceux pui la subissent. Ann. d'Ocul., H., p. 57.

465. Onsenoort, van, Deplacement du cristallin suite d'une lesion remarquable de l'oeil. Ann. d'Ocul., II, p. 188.

1840. 466. Stocher, V.,Observations de cataractes traumatiques. Ann. d'Ocul.,
T. 3.

467. Drouot, F., Nouveau traite des cataractes, causes, symptomes, complications et traitement des alterations du cristallin et de la capsule sans operations chirurgicales. Bordeaux.

468. Sichel, Methode simple et facile de faire des cataractes artificielles.
Ann. d'Ocul., IV, p. 147.

469. Tyrell, A practical work on the diseases of the eye and their treatment medically, topically and by operation. London, in 8o, Vol.
II, p. 556.

1841. 470. Hoering, G., Ueber die Dislaceratio capsulae, nach Jager. Wurtemb.
Med. Corresp., B. 1, No. 8.

471. Dittrich, Dissert. sistens conspectum cataractarum, in clinico et con-
signatione opthalmiatrica operatorum. Pragae, in 8o.

472. Sichel, De la cataracte glaucomateuse, de l'inutilite et des suites
facheuses de son operation. Ann. d'Ocul., V, p. 232.

473. Malgaigne, Opinion sur la nature et le siege de la cataracte. Ibid.,
VI, p. 62.

474. Lerche, Ueber die Heilwirkung des Galvanismus in einigen organischen Augenkrankheiten (Cataracta). Zeitschr., d. V. f. Heilkunde, in Preussen, No. 24.

475. Cunier, Compte rendu, XXII. Cataracte verte. Ann. d'Ocul., V,
p. 249.

476. Fahl, G. R. J., Diss. de praecipuis morbis, qui cataractae operationes
sequi possunt. Berolini.

477. Stromeyer, C., Das corektom, ein neues instrument fur kunstliche
pupillenbildung und fur die extraction des angewachsenen Staars.
Allg. Ztschr. f. Chirurg., No. 22.

1842. 478. Guepin, Note sur la nature et la formation des cataractes. Ann.
d'Ocul., VI, p. 203.

479. Serre (de Montpellier), De l'operation de la cataracte sur un oeil,
comme moyen de retablir la vue des deux yeux. Ibid., VI, p. 210.

1842. 480. Hoering. G., sur le siege et la nature de la cataracte. Ibid., VIII, p. 13.

481. Sichel, Etudes cliniques et anatomiques sur quelques especes peu connues de la cataracte lenticulaire. Ann. d'Ocul., VIII, p. 127.

482. Benedict, Einige Bemerkungen uber die aetiologie der cataracta u. s. w., abhandlungen us dem Gebiete der Augenheilkunde. Breslau, in 8o.

483. Textor, Uber die Wiedererzengung der Krystallinse. Wurzb. in 8o.

484. Blasius, Nouveau procede de l'extraction de la cataracte. Ann. d'Ocul., IX, p. 34.

485. Sanson, Traite de la cataracte. Paris, in 8o.

486. Engel. Untersuchung eines kapselstaars. Oesterr. Med. Wochenschr. No. 9.

487. Strauch, Mitthellungen uber den Galvanismus als Mittel gegen den grauen Staar. V. Walther's u. V. Ammon's Journ., I, p. 1.

488. Szokalski, v., Reflexions au sujet de la note de Mr. Guepin, sur la nature et le siege de la cataracte. Ann. d'Ocul., VI.

489. ———, Response to Mr. Guepin. Ebenda.

490. S. van der Porten, Diss. de cataractae extractione adjecta nova extrahendi ratione. Halae.

491. Benedict, F. W. G., Ueber die sog. cat. nigra und deren diagnose. Ueber cataracta gypsae; ueber die behandlung der entstehenden cataract. Abhandlungen a. d. Geb. d. Augenheilkunde. Breslau.

492. Petrequin, J. E., Mem. sur un nouveau procede pour l'operation de la cataracte per extraction. Ann. d'Ocul., VI, p. 193.

493. Bernard, P., Cat. operee par la methode sous-conjunctivale. Ebenda VII.

494. Freund, Die operation des grauen Staars, wie diese gegenwartig von Englands vorzuglichsten Aerzten auzgefuhrt wird. Allg. Med. Centr. Zig., Nos. 67, 68, 69, 78, 79.

495. Mackenzie, W., Cataracte lenticulaire, operee par extraction. Section de la cornee au moyen du couteau-aiguille. Remarques sur les couteaux-aiguilles. Ann. d'Ocul., X, p. 209.

496. Sichel, Lettre sur la nature et le siege de la cataracte. Ann. d'Ocul., VI, p. 64.

497. Leroy D'Etiolles, Lettre sur la nature et le siege de la cataracte. Ann. d'Ocul., VI, p. 70.

498. Heyfelder, Das chirurgische und augenkranken-klinicum der Universitat Erlangen, vom 1 Oct., 1841, bis 30 Sept., 1842. Heidelberger Medic. Annalen, 1842.

1843. 499. Vaillin, Le succes de toute operation chirurg depend autant des soins qui la precedent et de ceux qui la suivent que de l'operation elle-meme; application de ce principe a la guerison de la cataracte. Paris.

438

1843. 500. Duval (d'Argenton), Considerations generales sur la cataracte. Ann. d'Ocul., IX, p. 61.

501. Gulz, Velpeau's extraction des grauen Staars am rechten auge. Oesterr. Med. Wochenschr., No. 39.

502. Quadri, Monographie de la double-depression destinee a detruire la cataracte. Paris.

503. Magne, De la cataracte noire. Ann. d'Ocul., IX, p. 244.

504. Gerhardt, Ueber den Vorfall der Krystallinse im menschlichen auge. Heidelb. Med. Annalen., IX.

505. Barbarotta, Guarigione spontanea di cataratta. Osservatore Med., No. 5.

506. Valentin, Mikroscop. Untersuchungen zweier wiedererzeugter Krystallinsen des Auges. Henle u. Pfeuffer's Zeitschr., f. Rat. Med., I.

507. Travignot, Memoire sur les cataractes secondaires. Paris.

508. Reute, Zur Genese der Cataract und des Nystagmus. V. Walther's und v. Ammon's Journ., II, St. 4.

509. Fronmuller, Sonderbare Entstehung einer Cataract. Ibid., St. 2.

510. Jans, Cataracte operee avec succes chez une femme aveugle depuis vingt cinq ans. Ann. d'Ocul., X, p. 128.

511. Stafford, Cataracte congenitale, operee chez un sujet de 23 ans. Ann. d'Ocul., X, p. 143.

512. Mackenzie. Cataracte lenticulaire, operee par extraction. Section de la cornee au moyen d'un couteau-aiguille, remarques sur les couteaux-aiguilles. Ann. d'Ocul., X, p. 209.

513. Rigler, Note sur l'anatomie pathologique de la cataracte. a propos de la discussion survenue entre Mons. Guepin et Szokalski. Ann. d'Ocul., X, p. 220.

514. Boling, Cataracte operee avec succes sur un vieillard de 110 ans. American Journal.

515. Mannoir. Mem. sur les causes de non-succes dans l'operation de la cataracte par extraction et des moyens d'y remedier. Ann. d'Ocul., II.

516. Boulogne, A., Mem. sur deux instruments nouveaux, destines a l'extraction et a l'abaissement de la cataracte. Marseille.

517. Sichel, J., Etudes cliniques et anatomiques sur quelques especes peu connues de la cataracte lenticulaire. Ann. d'Ocul., VIII. p. 169. (Fortsetzung.)

518. Drauot, Des erreurs des oculistes sur la cataracte, l'amaurose et les traitemens opposes a les affections. Paris.

1843. 519. Gluge. Note sur l'ossification du cristallin. Ann. d'Ocul., X, p. 226.

520. Bonchacourt, Observations sur les concretions calcaires dans l'oeil. Cont. les petrifactions de la lentille. Ann. d'Ocul., X, p. 250.

521. Guepin. Quelle conduite faut-il tenir dans les cataractes etroites. congenitales ou autres? Faut-il dans l'operation de la cataracte presser sur l'oeil pour faire sortir le cristallin? Response a la lettre de Mons. le Doct. Rigler. Ann. d'Ocul., X, p. 291.

1844. 522. Hoering, G., Ueber den Sitz und die natur des grauen Staars. Eine von der Redaction der Annales d'Oculistique Gekronte Preiss-schrift. Heilbronn, 1844.

523. Duval (d'Agentan), De la cataracte secondaire. Ann. d'Ocul., XI, pp. 5, 61, 170 und 209.

524. Fleckles, Heilung einer cataract durch die Carlsbader Heilquellen. Hufeland's Journ., Mars.

525. Sichel. Observations et considerations supplementaires sur le glaucoma et la cataracte glaucomateuse. Ann. d'Ocul., XI, p. 157.

1844. 526. Scott, Cataract and its treatment, comprising an easy method of dividing the cornea for its extraction, etc. London. British et Foreign Med. Review. April.

527. Jager, Eduard, Ueber die Behandlung des grauen Staars an der opthalmol. Klinik der Josephs Acedemie. Wien.

528. Mirault (d'Angers), Sur la cataracte capsulaire secondaire. Ann. d'Ocul., XII. p. 731.

529. Landrun, J. F. P., De la kistotomie posterieure on dechirement de la crystalloide posterieure apres l'extraction, comme moyen de s'opposer aux cataractes membraneuses secondaires. Paris.

530. Pamard, Memoires de chirurgie pratique, conten. la cataracte, l'iritis et les fractures du col de femur. Paris.

531. Duesing, Das Krystallinsensystem des menschlichen auges in physiologischer und pathologischer Hinsicht. Berlin.

532. Pamard, De la cataracte et son extraction par un procede particulier. Ann. d'Ocul., XII, pp. 149, 191.

533. Guepin, A., De la refraction de la lumiere dans l'oeil apres l'operation de la cataracte par extraction. Ann. d'Ocul., VI, p. 12.

534. Guthrie, Observations cliniques sur la cataracte. Med. Times, Oct. et Dec.

535. A. de Grand-Boulogne, Memoire sur deux instruments nouveaux destines a l'extraction et a l'abaissement de la cataracte. Ann. d'Ocul., XI, p. 56.

536. Blasius, Sur une nouvelle modification apportee au couteau-aiguille pour l'extraction de la cataracte. Ann. d'Ocul., XI, p. 135.

537. Lusardi (pere), Response a cette question: Quelle est l'influence qu' exerce l'operation de la cataracte sur la vie de ceux qui la subissent. Ann. d'Ocul., XI, p. 145.

538. Berard, De l'operation de la cataracte faite sur un seul oeil, sans attendre que la cataracte soit formee dans l'oeil opposee. Ann. d'Ocul., XI, p. 179.

539. Sichel, Cas rare d'ossification de la capsule cristalline dans une cataract traumatique. Ann. d'Ocul., XI. p. 223.

540. Szokalski, Operation de cataracte sur un vieillard de 103 ans. Ann. d'Ocul., XI, p. 272.

1844. 541. Abren, Cristallin remonte et passe dans la chambre anterieure, 22 mois apres la depression de la cataracte. Ann. d'Ocul., XII, p. 36.

542. Tilanus, Observation d'irideremie congenitale, compliquee de cataracte. Ann. d'Ocul., XII, p. 43.

543. Abréu, Diss. sur un nouveau procede pour la reclinaison depression de la cataracte et sur les resultats obtenus dans cette operation, a l'institut opthalmique a Bruxelles. Ann. d'Ocul., XII, p. 53.

544. Turnbull, Nouveau traitement de la cataracte et le quelques autres maladies des yeux sans operations chirurgicales. Traduit de l'anglais par lusardi (pere) et Paul Bernard.

545. Textor, De l'operation de la cataracte par keratonyxie. Ann. d'Ocul. XII, p. 212.

546. Fischer, Eclaircissements sur la relation qu' faite Cheselden au sujet d'un jeune aveugle de 14 ans qu'il opera il y a pres de 120 ans. Bericht uber die Verhandl. der naturf. Gesellschaft zu Basel. 1844, VI, p. 111. Ann. d'Ocul., XXX, p. 114.

1845. 547. Stricker, Die krankheiten des Linsensystems nach physiol. Gundsatzen, Frankfurt.

548. Frerichs, Path. Anatom. und Chemische Untersuchungen uber Linsenstaare. Hann. Ann., Nov. u. Dec.

549. Desmarres, De la cataracte pigmenteuse ou uveenne et son diagnostic differential. Journ. de Chirurg. de Malgaigne et Ann. d'Oc., XIII, p. 132.

550. Arlt, Zur Nosogenie der catar. caps. cent. anterior und der catar. pyramidalis. Oesterr. Med. Wochenschr., No. 10 u. 11.

551. Furnari, De la pretendue influence des climats sur la production de cataracte et de l'innocuite de la reverberation directe et de la lumiere sur les milieux refringents de l'oeil. Ann. d'Oc., XIII, p. 158.

552. Christiaen, De l'extraction simultanee du cristallin et de sa capsule. Ibid., p. 181.

553. Guthrie, On cataract and its appropriate treatment by the operation adapted for each peculiar case. London.

554. Sichel, Considerations pratiques sur l'extraction des corps etrangers implantes dans le cristallin. Ann. d'Oc., XIII, p. 193.

555. ———, Etudes cliniques sur l'operation de la cataracte. Gaz. des Hopitaux et Ann. d'Oc., XIV, pp. 75, 111, 155.

556. Roux, Generalities sur les deux procedes d'operation de la cataracte. Ibid., XIV, p. 177.

557. Serre (de Montpellier), Operation de la cataracte selon la methode par deplacement, faite avec succes apres soixante ans de cecite. Ann. d'Oc., XIV, p. 224.

558. Dubois (de Neufchatel), Operation de la cataracte datant de 44 ans, suivie de retablissement de la vue. Gaz. Med. et Ann. d'Oc., XIV, p. 229.

1845. 559. Gerold, Ueber cataracta natatilis und liq. Morgagni. Zeitschr. des Vereins fur Heilkunde in Preussen, No. 25.

560. Cooper, Remarques sur l'extraction de la cataracte. Prov. Journ. Juin.

561. Hervez de Chegoin, De l'operation de la cataracte par elevation. Ann. d'Oc., XIII, p. 37.

562. Pamard, Memoires de chirurgie pratique, compr. la cataracte, l'iritis et les fractures du col de femur. Paris. Ann. d'Oc., XIII, p. 83. (Fortsetzung.)

563. Duval, Quelques reflexions sur les premieres impressions d'un aveugle ne rendu clairvoyant; suivies de considerations sommaires sur la maniere d'operer les cataractes de naissance de differentes ages. Ann. d'Oc., XIII, pp. 97 and 241.

564. Heyfelder, De l'influence de la commotion sur l'oeil. Ann. d'Oc., XIII, p. 145.

565. Vinella, Ossification de la capsule du cristallin. Ann. d'Oc., XIII, p. 279.

566. Vogel, Examen microscopique d'un cristallin opaque. Ann. d'Oc., XIV, p. 29.

567. Debron, Nore sur le passage du cristallin dans la chambre anterieure pendant l'operation de la cataracte par abaissement. Ann. d'Oc., XIV, p. 32.

568. Tavignot, Abaissement en masse du cristallin et de la capsule. Ibid., p. 33.

569. A. G., Operation de la cataracte sur un oeil sans attendre que l'autre oeil soit affecte. Ann. d'Oc., XIV, p. 34.

570. Rub. Ogez., Cataract monocle avec strabisme interne de l'oeil; operations heureuses; guerison. Ann. d'Oc., XIV, p. 134.

571. ——, Cataracte congenitale de l'oeil droit chez une femme de 41 ans ayant perdu l'oeil gauche depuis un an; operation suivie de succes. Ann. d'Oc., XIV, p. 226.

572. Serre, Operation de la cataracte selon la methode par deplacement, faite avec succes apres 60 ans de cecite. Ann. d'Oc., XIV, p. 224.

573. Dubois, Oper. de la cataracte datant. de 44 ans, suivie de retablissement de la vue. Ann. d'Oc., XIV, p. 229.

574. Tavignot, Notes sur les cataractes anciennes. Gaz. Med. de Paris.

1846. 575. Andreae, Grundriss der gesammten Heilkunde. Leipzig. Theil, I, p. 99-118. Cataract literatur.

576. Watson, Historical et critical remarks on the operation for the cure of cataract. Edinburg.

577. Gosselin, Recherches sur l'abaissement de la cataracte. Arch. Gener. de Med. Janv. et Fevr.

578. Sichel, Essai preliminaire de statistique des resultats d'operation de cataracte. Ann. d'Oc., XVI, p. 50.

442

1846. 579. Walther. Cataractologie. V. Walther's u. v. Ammon's Journ.. V. H. 2.

580. Frommuller, Wiedererzeugung der Krystallinse. Ibid., VI, H. 2.

581. Bartes, De la cataracte. La Clinique de Montpellier. Fevr. et Aout.

582. Seidl und Kanka, Bericht uber die Wiener Augenklinik und die mit ihr verbundene Abtheilung des Allg. Krankenhouses. Oestr. Jahrb., 1846.

583. France, J., Cas d'ossification et de deplacement de la lentille cristalline. Gaz. Med. de Paris, No. 4, 1846, et Ann. d'Oc., XV, p. 38.

584. Miguel, Cristallin passe dans la chambre anterieure depuis un an. Emploi de la pomade de Gondret. Resorption. Bulletin Gener. et Therapeutique. Ann. d'Oc., XIV, p. 125.

585. Sichel, De quelques accidents consecutifs a 'extraction de la cataracte et en particulier de la fonte purulente de la cornee et du globe oculaire; des moyens de prevenir ces accidents. Bull. Gener. de Therap. Ann. d'Oc.. XV, p. 128, 180; XX, p. 112.

586. Guerneiro, Compte rendu de la clin. opthal. de M. Ansiaux, pour l'annee, 1845. Ann. d'Oc., XIV, p. 145.

587. Gerster. Reascension d'une cataracte deprimee. Medic. Corresp. B. 1. Bayrischer Aerzte. Ann. d'Oc., XVI, p. 91.

588. Sichel, Double extraction de cataracte, suivie de non succes complet; phthisie de l'oeil droit et atrophie commencente de l'oeil avec obliteration de la pupille. Iridodialysis pratique a trois reprises. chaque fois avec succes immediate sous le rapport de la manoeuvre, non-retablissement de la vision. Atrophie complete de l'oeil un a deux and apres l'operation. Ann. d'Oc., XVI, p. 388.

1847. 589. Stricker, Staar oder Starr. V. Walther's u. v. Ammon's Journ., t. VI.

590. Guepin (de Nantes), Notes sur les resultats comparatifs de l'abaissement et de l'extraction dans l'operation de la cataracte. Ann. d'Oc., XVII, p. 39.

591. Laugier. Nouvelle methode d'operer de la cataracte ou methode par aspiration. Ibid., p. 29.

592. Armati. De l'operation de la cataracte par aspiration. Revendication de priorite en faveur de M. le prof. Pecchioni de Sienne. Ibid., p. 79.

593. Cunier, Nore pour servir a l'historie de la succion de la cataracte. Ibid., p. 85.

594. Sichel, Recherches historiques sur l'operation par succion ou aspi ration. Ibid., p. 104.

595. Magne. Note sur un couteau-aiguille, nouvel instrument pour l'oper ation de la cataracte. Ibid., p. 111.

596. Behn et Ammon, Zur path. anatomie des prolapsus lentis traum. und hydrops tunicae Jacobi. (V. Walther's u. v. Ammon's Journ.. VII, H. 2.

597. Lagoguey, Du traitement de cataractes laiteuses par succion. Gaz. Med. de Paris, No. 47.

1847. 598. Prichard, De la cataracte des jeunes gens. Prov. Journ.. No. 20.

599. Buhrlen, Bemerkungen uber die cataracta capsularis sec. nach reclination des linsenstaares. Wurtemb. Corresp., B. 1, No. 19.

600. Hannover, Quelques observations sur la structure du cristallin des des mammiferes et le l'homme. Ann. d'Oc., XVII, p. 97.

601. Heylen, Cataracte lenticulaire chez une femme de 74 ans. provocation de salivation dans le but de prevenir les accidents inflammatoires. Operation par abaissement. Reussite. Reflexions. Ann. d'Oc., XVII, p. 115.

602. Rivaud-Laudran, Compte rendu de sa clinique a Lyon pendant l'annee, 1846. Ann. d'Oc., XVIII, pp. 3. 12.

603. Magne, De la valeur, de l'operation de la cataracte par aspiration. Ann. d'Oc., XVIII, p. 38.

604. Blanchet, Operation de la cataracte par succion. Ibid., p. 38.

605. Bonisson, Remarques sur l'insuffisance de l'humeur aqueuse qui se manifeste a la suite de l'operation de la cataracte et dans quelques autres cas. Ann. d'Oc., XVII, pp. 61, 108.

606. Sichel, De la delocation et de l'abaissement spontanes du cristallin. Oppenheim's Zeitschr., f. d. Ges. Medicin, 1846. Ann. d'Oc., XVIII, p. 127.

607. Heylen, Nouvelles observations tendant a prouver l'efficacite de la salivation mercurielle, comme moyen de prevenir l'inflammation consecutive a l'operation de la cataracte. Ann. d'Oc., XVIII, p. 244.

608. Magne, Cataracte capsulaire ossifiee, passee dans la chambre anterieure; extraction. Ann. d'Oc., XVIII, p. 271.

609. Velpeau, Emploi de la belladonne apres l'operation de la cataracte. Ann. d'Oc., XVIII, p. 279.

610. Brett, On cataract, artificial pupil and strabismus. London.

611. Malfatti, Neue Heilversuche, I. Gelungene Vertilgung des grauen Staars durch eine aussere Heilmethode. Wien.

1848. 612. Rau, Ueber die Behandlung des grauen Staars durch Pharm. Mittel. V. Walther's u. V. Ammon's Journ., 1, VIII, H. 3.

613. Neil, On the cure of cataract, with a practical summary of the best modes of operating. Liverpool.

614. Rivaud-Landrau, De la kystotomie posterieure, ou dechirement de la cristalloide post. apres l'operation de la cataracte par extraction, comme moyen d'eviter la formation des cataractes capsulaires consecutives. Ann. d'Oc., XIX, p. 54.

615. Marcus, Ueber die Nachbehandlung bei Staaroperationen. Casper's Wochenschrift, No. 49.

616. Sichel, Des principes rationels et des limites de la curabilites des cataractes sans operation. Bullet. de Therap. et Ann. d'Oc., XX, p. 76.

444

1848. 617. Gerold, Elementa photometri ad curam cataractae secund. adhibendi, etc. Madgeburg.

618. Malgaigne, Des divers especes de cataracte. Ann. d'Oc., XXI. p. 234.

Meliori, Cataracta centr. capsul. als Bildungsfehler mit auffalender Kleinheit des Auges und aller seiner Theile. Oesterr. Med. Wochenschr., No. 12.

620. Nelaton, Displacement traumatique du cristallin. Gaz. des Hop., No. 32.

621. Leuw, de, Versteinerung der Linse und ihrer Kapsel. Zeitschr. d. V. f. Heilk. in Preussen, No. 36.

622. Rau, W., Ueber die Behandlung des grauen Staars durch Pharm. Mittel v. Walther's u. v. Ammon's Journ., t. VIII, H. 3.

623. Guepin, Notes sur des operations de cataracte suivies de phenomenes remarquables. Ann. d'Oc., XIX, p. 116.

624. Retzius, Du galvanisme comme moyen du traitement de la cataracte. Ann. d'Oc., XIX, p. 123.

625. Langier, Nouvel essai de l'operation de la cataracte par aspiration ou succion. Ann. d'Oc., XX, p. 28.

626. Boyer, Entrainement des parties anterieures du corps vitre, pendant l'operation de la cataracte par abaissement. Gaz. Med. de Paris; Ann. d'Oc., XX, p. 61.

627. Sichel, Des principes rationels et des limites de la curabilite des cataractes sons operation. Bullet. general de Therapeutique; Ann. d'Oc., XX, p. 76.

628. ——, De la sortie du corps vitre pendant ou apres l'operation de la cataracte. Bull. Gen. de Therap.; Ann. d'Oc., XX, p. 182.

629. ——, Lettre a Mns. Malgaigne en refutation de quelques assertions emises dans l'artide qui precede. Ann. d'Oc., XX, p. 242.

1849. 630. Pauli, Aus der Praxis und am Schreibtische. Med. Corresp., Bl. Bayrischer Aerzte, No. 42.

631. Bowman, Lectures on the parts concerned in the operations on the eye, etc. London, 1849. Auch in London Medical Gazette, 1847 u. 48, und Ann. d'Oc., XXIX-XXXXII.

632. Buzzi, Aiguille pour la cataracte laiteuse. Bolletione delle Scienze Mediche, et Ann. d'Oc., XXI, p. 261.

633. Boyer, Lucien, Deux operations de cataracte executees par un nouveau procede d'abaissement (repulsion anguleuse du cristallin). Ann. d'Oc., XXII, p. 21.

634. Langenbeck, Max, Klinische Beitrage aus dem Gebiete der Chirurgie und Opthalmologie. Gottingen.

635. Werdmuller, Einige kurze Bemerkungen uber die Natur und Entstehungsweise des acquirirten grauen Staars. Schweiz. Centr. Zeitschrift, V. 1, u. Ann. d'Oc., XXX, 103.

636. Prichard, Manque congenital du cristallin. Prov. Journ., No. 8.

1849. 637. Bayard, De la maturite des cataractes et des cataractes secondaires. Gaz. des Hop., No. 87 et 115.

638. Hasner, d'Artha Collodium als Verbandmittel nach der Staaroperation. Prager Vierteljahrschr., 3.

639. Trinchinetti, Observations sur les premieres impressions visuelles percues par deux aveugles de naissance, apres l'operation de la cataracte. Giornale del Instituto Lombardo, 1847. Ann. d'Oc., XXI, p. 259.

640. Duval, Coup d'oeil sur la memoire publiee par Lucien Boyer sous titre: De l'entrainement des parties anterieures du corps vitre, pendant l'operation de la cataracte par abaissement. Ann. d'Oc., XXII, p. 75.

641. Boyer, Lettre en response aux observations critiques qui precedent. Ibid., p. 82.

642. Sauveur, Statistique des sourds-muets et des aveugles de la Belgique. Ann. d'Oc., XXII, p. 86.

643. Tavignot, De l'hydropsia de la capsule du cristallin. Ann. d'Oc., XXII, p. 97.

1850. 644. Nelaton, Parallele des divers modes operatoires dans le traitement de la cataracte. These de Concours, 7. Fevr. Paris u. Onn. d'Oc., XXIV, p. 127.

645. Pilz, Zur Pathologie des Krystallinsensystems des menschlichen Auges nebst praktischen Bemerkungen uber Staaroperation. Prag. Med. Vierteljahrschrift. Jahrg., VII.

646. Brodhurst, On the cristalline lens and cataract. London.

647. Cornaz, E.. Quelques observations d'abnormites congeniales des yeux. Ann. d'Oc., XXIII, p. 47. (Mikropthalmus mit Cataract.)

648. Fronmuller, Beobachtungen aus dem Gebiete der Augenheilkunde. Furth.

649. Rivaud-Landrau, Cataracte capsulo-lenticulaire produite par la foudre un med.

650. Gosselin, Deplacement subit des capsules demeurees dans champ de la vision lors de l'abaissement de cataractes. Arch. Gen. de Med. Juin, u. Ann. d'Oc., XXXV, p. 192.

651. Desmarres, Operation de la cataracte et de la pupille articielle dans un cas de micropthalmos double. Gaz. des Hop., No. 4, u. Ann. d'Oc., XXIII, p. 18.

652. Dyer. Sam., Cataracte hereditaire. Prov. Journ., No. 4.

653. Walton, Cataracte capsulaire. Medical Times, January.

654. Buhrig, Ueber die operation der cataracta. Deutsche Klinik, No. 38.

655. Dieterich, v., Operation der mit dem ganzen umfange der iris verwachsenen cataracta durch centrale Durchbohrung. Med. Zeitung Russland's, No. 20.

656. Wilde, Ciseaux pour enlever la cristalloide opaque et des fausses membranes. Med. Times, Dec.

446

1850. 657. Rivaud-Landrau, Cat. capsulo-lenticulaire produite par la foudre. Ann. d'Oc., XXXV, p. 188.

658. Jungken, Ueber Staaroperationen. Deutsche Klinik. No. 8, 1850, u. Ann. d'Oc., XXXV, p. 189.

659. Beauclair, Recherches et experiences sur la cataracte noire et sur son diagnostic. Ann. d'Oc., XXIII, p. 130.

660. Petrequin, Recherche sur la cataracte noir et sur son diagnostic differentiel. Ann. d'Oc., XXIII. p. 172.

661. Aignie, Tentative de guerison de la cataracte sans operation. Revue Therapeut. du Midi, u. Ann. d'Oc., XXIII, p. 177.

662. Prichard, Absence congenitale du cristallin. Ann. d'Oc., XXIII, p. 74.

663. Rivaud-Landrau, De la luxation et du deplacement du cristallin par une cause traumatique. Ann. d'Oc.. XXIV, p. 74.

664. Barrier. Quelques faits intercessants de clinique opthalmologique (Linsenluxation). Ann. d'Oc., XXIV, p. 83.

1851. 665. Follin, Examen d'un oeil opere de la cataracte par extraction, quinze ans avant le mort du malade. Ann. d'Oc., XXV, p. 1451.

606. Hassner, d'A.. Ueber aetiologie der cataract. Prager Vierteljahrschrift, Jahrg. VIII.

667. ——. Ueber das anatomische verhaltniss der linsenkapsel zum glaskorper. Deutsche Klinik., No. 12.

668. Gerhard. Peut-on prevenir la formation d'une cataracte secondaire dans l'operation par scleroticonyxie? Ann. d'Oc., XXV, p. 1851.

669. Coursserant. De la pre-eminence de l'extraction sur l'abaissement de la cataracte. Avantage de la keratotomie superieure. Ibid, XXVI, p. 160.

670. Ammon, v., Opthalm. Skizzen. Verdunkelung oes Orbiculus capsulociliaris; seine Bedeutung fur die cataractologie. Deutsche Klinik, No. 45; Ann, d'Oc., XXVII. p. 26. 1852.

671. Lebert, Anatomie pathologique et curabilite de la cataracte. Un. Med. et Ann. d'Oc., XVI, p. 192.

672. Gihon, H.. On the cataract. The Philadelphia Lancet, No. 1, January.

673. Balfour, C. W., De la luxation spontanee du cristallin. Med. Times. March.

674. Jaeger. E.. Neuer Opthalmostat. Wien. Zeitschr., No. 6.

675. Jacob, De la cataracte. Dubl. Med. Press., Juill et Aout.

676. Rivaud-Landrau, Cataracte pierreuse luxee dans la chambre anterieure. Gaz. des Hop., No. 118.

677. White. Cooper, Cataract operation an einem Baren. Med. Times, 1850, u. Ann. d'Oc., XXV. p. 86.

678. Ullmann, Aeusserst spat eingetretene Aufsaugung der Theille einer durch Staaroperation zerstuckelten linse. Med. Zeitschr., I, 44.

679. Ansiaux. Clinique du dispensaire opthalmique de Liege, pendant l'annee. 1850. Cataractes. cat. capsulaire secondaire—emploi de la serre-tele de Desmarres: cat. congenita'es; cat. traumatique; cristallin pierreux. Ann. d'Oc.. XXV. p. 63.

1851. 680. Larrey, Luxation du cristallin demeure transparent. Ann. d'Oc., XXV, p. 176.

681. Robert, Lesions traumatiques du cristallin et de sa capsule. Ann. d'Oc., XXV, p. 194.

682. Nelaton, Extraction de la cataracte par la keratotomie superieure. Gaz. des Hop., u. Ann. d'Oc., XXV, p. 201.

683. Magne, A., Ueber Verbindung der synchisis mit cataracta petrosa. Union, 129.

1852. 684. Sichel, Note sur la pince-tube pour l'extraction scleroticale des cataractes capsulaires et des fausses membranes. Ann. d'Oc., XXV. p. 142.

685. Furnari, Nouvelle invention d'un instrument pour l'operation de la cataracte et la pupille artificielle. Ibid, p. 144.

686. Stellwag, von Carion, Statistische Beitrage zur Lehre vom Staar u. s. w. Zeitschr. d. Wiener. April, Mai, Juni.

687. Blot, Anat. pathol. de la cataracte noire. Gaz. Med. Padis, No. 26, u. Ann. d'Oc., XXXV, p. 188.

688. Davaine, Examen microscop. de deux cataractes lenticulaires. Gaz. Med. Paris, No. 49, u. Ann. d'Oc., XXXV, p. 188.

689. Ammon, v., Zur genesis der catar. centr. pyramid. nach sections resultaten. Deutsche Klinik, No. 9.

690. Laugier, Nouvelle Aiguille a lance mobile pour l'abaissement de la cataracte. Keratotome cache termine par une lance mobile articulee pour l'extraction de la cataracte. Ann. d'Oc., XXVIII, p. 113.

691. Wilde, Cataracta Morgagni. Med. Times and Gaz., October.

692. White, Cooper, Cataractes congenitales. Ann. d'Oc., XXXV, p. 187.

693. Oppolzer, Cataract als complication des diabetes mell. Heller's Jour. f. Psych. u. Path. Chemie., No. 11 u. 12.

694. Chadwick, Luxation du cristallin sons la conjonctive. Lancet, Avril.

695. Comperat, Luxation spontanee du cristallin transparent dans la chambre anterieure. Extraction, guerison. Un. Med., No. 71, u. Ann. d'Oc., XXVIII, p. 138.

696. Larrey, H., Luxation du cristallin transparent. Gaz. Med. Paris, u. Ann. d'Oc., December, 1851.

697. Kanka, Untersuchungen uber den grauen Staar. Ungar. Zeitschr., No. 34.

698. Thompson, H., Cataracte traumatique. Guerison spontanee. Dubl. Med. Press., December.

699. Bowman. De l'emploi des deux aiguilles a la fois dans les operations qui se pratiquent sur l'oeil, et specialement dans la cataracte capsulaire et la formation d'une pupille artificielle. Med. Times and Gaz.; Ann. d'Oc., XXIX, p. 293. 1853.

700. Appia, Notice sur soixante huit operations de cataracte. Ann. d'Oc., XXX, p. 105; Schweiz. Zeitschr., f. Med. Chirurg. u. Geburtshulfe, 1852, H. 505.

.448

1852. 701. White, Cooper, Ueber angeborene cataract. Med. Times and Gaz.
July, 1852.

702. Deval, Ch., Consecutive amaurose nach der Staaroperation. Bullet.
de Therap. Aout.

703. Gerdy, Neue nadel zur depression der cataract. Gaz. des Hop., 91,
u. Un., 93.

704. Ammon, v., Extravasation sanguine dens la capsule cristalline. Note
pour servir a l'histoire de l'hemopthalmie interne et surtout des
vaisseaux de nouvelle formation dans les extravasations sah-
guines. Ann. d'Oc., XXVII, p. 39.

705. Jobert, Operation de la cataracte. Traitement preparatoire. Ann.
d'Oc., XXVII, p. 65.

706. Chassaignac, Nouveau procede pour maintenir la glace en contact
avec l'oeil, comme moyen de prevenir ou de combattre les inflammations oculaires particulierement a la suite des operations de la
cataracte. Ann. d'Oc., XXVII, p. 66.

707. Wedl, De la stase sanguine qui se montre dans les vaisseaux ciliares,
immediatement apres la sortie de l'humeur aqueuse. Zeitschr.
der Ges. der Aerzte in Wien, u. Ann. d'Oc., XXVII, p. 190.

708. Deville, Des cataractes congenitales. Expose de la pratique des
chirurgiens anglais, et en particulier de Mons. W. White Cooper.
Ann. d'Oc., XXVIII, p. 86.

709. Courserant, De la preminence de l'extraction sur l'abaissement de lt
cataracte. Avantages de la keratotomie superieure. Ann. d'Oc.,
XXVIII, p. 107.

710. Charriere, Aiguille-pince pour l'operation de la cataracte. Reclama-
tion Ibid, p. 207.

711. Tavignot, Faut-il employer les collyres irritants dans les conjonc-
tives consecutives a l'operation de la cataracte. Ann. d'Oc.,
XXVIII, p. 208.

712. Dubreuil. Contusion de l'oeil gauche. Hemopthalmie sous-conjonctivale. Luxation du cristallin. Ann. d'Oc., XXVIII, p. 211.

713. Gerdy, De l'emploi d'une nouvelle espece d'aiguille dans l'abaissement de la cataracte. Ann. d'Oc., XXVIII, p. 214.

714. Deval, Amaurose consecutive a l'operation de la cataracte. Ann.
d'Oc., XXVIII, p. 223.

715. Sichel, Ueber eine Rohrenpincette zur extraction der kapselcataract
u. Losung falscher membranen. Ann. d'Oc., Mars. Aout, May,
1853.

1853. 716. Bechler. De dislocatione lentis cristallinae. Lips.

717. Guepin, de Nantes. Des cataractes de naissance et des operations qui
leur conviennent. Ann. d'Oc., XXX. p. 75.

718. Richard, A., Des divers especes de cataracte et leur indications ther-
apeutiques speciales. These de Paris. u. Ann. d'Oc.. XXXI, p. 139.

1858. 719. Dinge, Statistique des resultats de l'operation de la cataracte pratique d'apres les indications rationelles. These de Paris, u. Ann. d'Oc., XXXI. p. 146.

720. Dixon, Observations de cataractes liquides de Morgagni. The Lancet, No. 9.

721. Berghem, Cataracte guerie par un traitement medical. Ann. de la Societe Med. d. Anvers., p. 268, u. Ann. d'Oc., XXXV, p. 189.

722. Lopez, Traitement medicale de la cataracte par l'iodure de potassium et l'ammoniaque liquide. El Porvenir Medico, Nov., 1853, u. Ann. d'Oc., XXXV, p. 118.

723. Desmartis, Cataracte liquide operee par aspiration, description d'un nouvel aspirateur. Revue de Therap. du Midi., No. 9, u. Ann. d'Oc., XXXV, p. 190.

724. Jenni, Inflammation de la capsule cristalloide. Gaz. des Hop., 127; Ann. d'Oc., XXX, p. 87.

725. Kirk, Depots osseux dans la membrane vitreuse et le cristallin. Month. Journ., November.

726. Walton, Haynes, Diagnostic des cataractes commencantes chez les personnes agees. Med. Times and Gaz., October.

727. Gros, Du cristallin et de sa capsule. Ann. d'Oc., XXIX. p. 22.

728. Chassaignac. Catar. corticalis. Extraction, Anwendung der Kalte u. des Eises, schnelle Heilung. Gaz. des Hop., 109.

729. Canton, Ossification du cristallin et de la capsule. Lancet u. Ann. d'Oc., XXIX, p. 51.

730. Follin, Untersuchung der retina und der krystallinse mittelst eines neuen optischen Instrumentes. Rapport daruber von Chassaignac. Memoire de la Societe de Chirurgie, III, 4.

731. Jacob, A., De l'operation de la cataracte pratique a l'aide d'un fine aiguille a coudre introduite a travers la cornee. Ann. d'Oc., XXIX, p. 172.

732. Laugier, Nadel zur suction der cataract. L'Union, 110, u. Ann. d'Oc., XXXIV, p. 36.

733. Follin, Luxation sous-conjonctivale du cristallin. Arch. Gener. de Medicine. p. 210; Ann. d'Oc., XXXIV, p. 39.

734. Trexler, Reascension de cataractes operees a l'aiguille. Ann. d'Oc., XXX, p. 100.

735. Guepin, Connaisons nous bien les fonctions du cristallin? Ann. d'Oc., XXIX, p. 147.

736. Trettenbacher, Statistique de l'hospital opthalmique de Moscou, 1850-53. Ann. d' Oc., XXX, p. 129.

737. Quadri, Intorno all' ernia iride consecutiva all' estrazione anteriore del cristallino.

738. Bosch, De l'opacite de la capsule cristalline. Ann. d'Oc., XXX, p. 225.

739. Alessie, Opthalmostat du Prof. Jaeger modifie. Ann. d'Oc., XXX, p. 229. Nouveau kystitome. Ibid, p. 230.

1853. 740. Herviez, Revue opthalmologique du service de M. Petrequin. Cataracte, cataracte noire. Ann. d'Oc., XXX, p. 249.

741. Burdach, Ueber die Verfettung von proteinhaltigen substanzen in der peritonealhohle lebender Thiere. Virch. Arch., VI. p. 103. (Dorthin gebrachte linsen-verfetteten.)

742. White, Cooper. Du changement de la vue comme signe precurseur de cataractes dures. Associat. Medical Journal. November, 1853.

743. Kletzinsky, Vergleichung der Zusammensetzung der krystallinse und getrockneter cataracten. Zeller's Arch. f. Physiol. u. Pathol. Chemie, 1853, p. 256.

1854. 744. Bowman, Lecons sur les parties interessees dans les operations pu'on pratique sur l'oell. Ann. d'Oc., XXXI, p. 7.

745. Lohmeyer, Beitrage zur Histologie und Aetiologie der erworbenen Linsenstaare. Zeitschr. f. Rat. Med., V. H., 1 u. 2.

746. Donders, Entzundliche cataract. NNederl. Lancet, No. 9.

747. Broca, Memoire sur la cataracte capsulaire, etc. Arch. d'Opth. de Jamain, H., p. 184.

748. Graefe, A. v., Ueber Staaroperationen. Deutsche Klinik., Nos. 1, 2, 4 u. 6; Arch. f. Opthal., Bd. I, 1, p. 323-325.

748a. ——, Cataract mit doppeltem biconvexem linsenkern. A. f. O., I, 1, p. 323.

748b. ——, Extraction einer 60 Jahre reifen cataract. Ibidem, p. 326.

748c. ——, Cataract aus phosphorsauer kalkerde bestehend. Ibidem, p. 330.

748d. ——, Falle von cataracta nigra, mikroscopische untersuchung einer solchen. Ibidem, p. 333.

748e. ——, Zwei falle von linsenluxationen. Ibidem, p. 336.

749. Jaeger, E., Ueber staar u. Staaroperationen. Wien, in 8o.

750. Pamard, De l'operation de la cataracte chez les personnes tres avancees en age. Ann. d'Oc., XXXI, p. 224.

751. His, Mikroscop. Untersuchung eines weichen linsenstaars bei diabetes. Arch. f. Pathol. Anat., VI, p. 561.

752. Carton, De l'operation de la cataracte par keratotomie superieure. These de Paris.

753. Critchett, Cataracte capsulaire congenitale. Dubl. Med. Press.

754. Oettingen, Observationes quaedam de cataractae operatione extractionis ope instituenda. Diss. Inaug. Dorpati.

755. Robin, Ch., Opacite de la capsule du cristallin constatee sous le microscope. Arch. d'Opthalm., II, p. 101.

756. Alessi, Luxation du cristallin. Cataracte capsulo-lenticulaire. Ibid, p. 99.

757. Franchon, Etude sur la cataracte noire. Ibid, p. 161.

758. Cade, A., Memoire pratique sur la cataracte., suivi d'un tableau synoptique des operations de l'auteur. Montpellier, in 8o.

759. Taire, Quelques considerations sur l'operation de la cataracte par extraction. Ibid, p. 111.

1854. 760. Anagnostakis, Essai sur l'operation de la retine et des milieux de l'oeil sur le vivant, au moyen d'un nouvel opthalmoscope (cristallin). Ann. d'Oc., XXXI, p. 110.

761. Cornaz, Recherches statistiques sur la frequence comparative des couleurs de l'iris. Ann. d'Oc., XXXI, p. 250 und 276.

762. Jacob, Description du cristallin et de sa capsule. Ann. d'Oc., XXXII, p. 24; Encyclopedie Anatomique.

763. Game, Cataracte congenitale operee avec succes sur un homme de 55 ans. Moniteur des Hopitaux. Juin.

764. Walton, Haynes, Degenerescence cretacee du cristallin et de sa capsule, dans des yeux qui ont subi une desorganization, comme cause de douleur et d'irritation et d'alterations morbides de l'oeil sain, qui imitent l'asthenopie et menacent de cecite. Med. Times and Gaz., p. 154. 1854.

765. Saez, Effect facheux d'un air humide et froid sur les operes de cataracte. La Cronic de los Hospitales, 8 Mai, 1854. Ann. d'Oc., XXXV, p. 190.

1855. 766. Doumit, De l'operatio de la cataract par keratotomie superieure, accidents qui peuvent se presenter, statistique raisonnee, etc. Ann. d'Oc., XXXV, p. 164.

767. Heyman, Classification des cataractes. Schmidt, Jahrb., LXXXV, p. 116.

768. Magne, Memoire sur les hereux effets de la glace appliquee immediatement apres l'operation de l'abaissement. Gaz. Med. de Paris, No. 38-45.

769. Rau. Cataracta nigra u. angeborene cataracte. Arch. f. Opth., Bd. 1, A. 2, p. 167-205.

775. ——, Sectionsbefund nach vorausgegangener reclination. Ibid, p.273.

770. Graefe, A. v., Ueber die lineare extraction der linsenstaare. Ibid, p. 291.

771. ——, Abberration der Augenachse bei der fixation bedingt durch Schiefstellung der linse. Ibid, p. 291 .

772. ——, Ein aussergewohnlicher fall von extraction einer in die vordere Kammer vorgefallenen verkalkten linse. Ibid, Bd. II, A. 1. p. 195.

773. ——, Falle von spontaner linsenluxation. Ibid, p. 250.

774. ——, Notiz von Schichtstaar. Ibid, p. 273.

776. Arlt, Die krystallinse und ihre kapsel, in: Die krankheiten des auges. Prag.

777. Anslaux, J., Luxation du cristallin sous la conjonctive. Gaz. des Hop., No. 24.

778. Malgaigne. Sur le siege et les diverses varietes de cataracte. Rev. Med. Chir., Janv. et Fevr.

779. Sichel, Memoire sur la cataracte noire. Arch. d'Opth., t. IV, p. 31.

780. Faber. Die behandlung der cataracte secundaria zu Paris. Deutsche Klinik, No. 51.

1855. 781. Hayes, J., Aiguille tranchante pour l'operation de la cataracte. American Journ. Juillet.

782. Richard, Ad. et Robin, Ch., De la nature des cataractes capsulaires. Gaz. Hebd., No. 38.

783. Critchett, Operation de cataracte adherente chez un adulte. Med. Chirur. Transact., XXXVIII.

784. France, Luxation du cristallin sous la conjonctive. Guy's Hosp. Rep., 3, Ser. 1.

785. Walton, H., Cataracte noire. Assoc. Journ. December.

786. ——, Luxation spontanee du cristallin. Med. Times and Gaz. Dec.

787. Ritterich, Zur Staaroperation. Deutsche Klinik, No. 50.

788. Testelin, Note sur quelques points de la structure du cristallin et de sa capsule, a l'etat normal et a l'etat pathologique. Ann. d'Oc., t. XXXIV, p. 109, et t. XXXV, p. 61.

789. Taylor, Corps amylaces dans le cristallin. The Lancet, 1855, p. 242.

790. Critchett, Cataracte capsulaire congenitale. Ann. d'Oc., XXIII, p. 94.

791. Doumit, De l'operation de la cataracte par keratotomie superieure. Paris. These.

792. Warlomont, Quelques mots sur la pratique opthalmologique des chirurgiens de Londres. (De l'extraction de la cataracte.) Ann. d'Oc., XXXIV, p. 7.

793. Quadri, Cataracte traumatique guerie par l'application de la belledone. Ann. d'Oc., XXXIV, p. 19.

794. Sichel, Iconographie opthalmologique (cataracte). Ann. d'Oc., XXXIV, p. 53.

795. Nelaton, Operation de cataracte, entropion. serre fine. Journ. de Med. et de Chir. Prat., 1854, p. 113 u. Ann. d'Oc., XXXV, p. 176.

796. Deval, De la luxation sous-conjunctivale du cristallin. Bull. Gener. de Therap., XLVI, p. 451, u. Ann. d'Oc., XXXV, p. 157.

797. Letenneur, Guerison spontanee d'une cataracte traumatique. Compte rendu de la Societe Med. de la Loire-Inferieure, 1855, u. Ann. d'Oc., XLIII, p. 50.

798. Salomon, Degenerescence graisseuse du cristallin, cas dans lequel de nomun cristallin. Assoc. Med. Journ., 1855, u. Ann. d'Oc., XLIII, p. 127.

1856. 799. Muller, E., Cataracta nigra. Arch. f. Opth., Bd. II, A. 2, p. 164.

800. ——, Schichtstaar. Ibid, p. 166.

801. Robin, Anatomie pathologique des cataractes en general. Arch. d'Opth., t. V.

802. Spielmann, De la cataracte. These de Strasbourg.

803. Huge, De la cataracte secondaire et son extraction par la sclerotique. These de Strasbourg.

804. Joseph, Bemerkungen uber krankhafte Vorgange an den Augen Cholerakranker. Gunsb. Zeitschr. f. Klin. Med., t. VII.

1856. 805. Graefe. A. v., Wie Kranke, deren eines auge am staar operirt ist, sehen, etc. Arch. f. Opth., Bd. 2, A. 2, p. 177.

806. Wedl, Untersuchung einer getrubten krystallinse. Zeitschr. d. Gesellschaft d. Wien. Aerzte, No. 47.

807. Critchett, De la facilite de l'extraction de la cataracte dans certains cas de pupille artificielle. Lancet, 25 Juin, et Gaz. des Hop., No.115.

808. Desmarres et Robin, Ch., Structure de la cataracte ponctuee. Gaz. des Hop., No. 64.

809. Desmarres, Extraction lineaire d'une cataracte traumatique chez un enfant. Guerison en 24 heures. Ibid, No. 76.

810. Salomon, Vose, Extraction des cataractes traumatiques recentes comme moyen de diagnostic. Assoc. Journ., Avril.

811. ——, D'un signe caracteristique des cataractes dures. Ibid. Juin.

812. Stellwag, v. Carion, Ein fall von ectopia der normwidrig kleinen krystallinse. Wien. Wochenbl., No. 49 et 50.

813. Peruzzi, Cataracte capsulaire guerie par un traitement mercuriel. Raccogl. di Fano u. Ann. d'Oc., XLIII, p. 58.

814. Tavigot, Nouvelle methode operation de la cataracte par debridement. Academie des Sciences, 19 Mai, 1856.

1857. 815. Prichard, Anatomie, physiologie et maladies de la membrane pupillaire. Etiologie de la cataracte capsulaire centrale, traduit de l'anglais par M. Doumic. Union Med., No. 126 et 128.

816. Muller, H., Ueber die anatomischen verhaltnisse des kapselstaare. Arch. f. Opth., Bd. III, A. 1, p. 55.

817. ——, Ueber den Sitz des Kapselstaars und Mittheilung neuer Falle. Verhandl. d. Phys. Med. Gesellsch. zu Wurzb., t. VIII.

818. ——, Untersuchungen uber die Glashaute des Auges, insbesondere die Glaslamelle der Choroidea und ihre senilen veranderungen. A. f. O., II, 2, p. 1 und loco, p. 231.

818a. Forster, Zur pathologischen anatomie der cataract. A. f. O., III, 2, p. 187.

819. Jordan, F., Furneaux, Rapports de la cataracte avec les maladies du coeur. Brit. Rev., Avril.

819a. Graefe, Ueber verkleinerung des linsensystems mit erhaltung der transparenz. A. f. O., III, 2, p. 576.

819b. ——, Notiz uber entstehung des schichtstaars an dislocirten linsen. Ibidem, p. 372.

819c. ——, Beobachtung einer partiellen dislocation der linse unter die conjunctiva durch ein trauma. Ibidem, p. 365.

820. Nelaton, Cataracte double (tremulante). Un. Med., No. 78.

821. Taylor. R., De la cataracte suivi de remarques sur l'anatomie et la physiologie du cristallin. Med. Times and Gaz. Mai.

822. Williams, De la cataracte zonulaire. Americ. Med. Chir. Rev. Sept.

823. Castorani, De l'etiologie de la cataracte. Gaz. des Hop., No. 82 et Gaz. Hebdom., No. 36.

1857. 824. Desmarres, Operation des cataractes capsulo-lenticulaires adherentes. Gaz. des Hop., No. 106.

825. Valez, Des cataractes artificielles. Journ. de Brux., Juin.

826. Kunde, Ueber kunstliche cataract. Zeitschrift fur Wissensch. Zoologie, VIII, p. 466.

827. Streitfeild, Statistics of cataract. K. L. O. H. Opthalm. Hosp. Rep. I.

828. Bader. Ibid, p. 43, 142.

829. Dixon, Abnormal position of the crystalline lens occurring in four members of the same family. Opth. Hosp. Rep., I.

830. Streatfeild, Six cases of cataract in one family. O. H. R. I., p. 104.

831. Martin, On the operations for cataract among the natives of India. O. H. R. I., p. 161.

832. Hulke, Observations on the growth of the crystalline lens, and on the formation of capsular opacities. O. H. R. I., p. 182.

833. Valenciennes et Fremy, Recherches sur la nature du cristallin dans la serie animale. Bull. de l'Acad. des Sciences. Juin, 1857.

1858. 834. Cooper, White, Des luxations du cristallin. Med. Times and Gaz., 2 Janv.

835. Sichel et Robin, De la cataracte noire. Gaz. Med. de Paris, No. 51.

836. Fenner, C. S., De la cataracte. Amer. Med. Chir. Rev. Janv.

836a. Graefe, Ueber die iridectomie bei spaterer verschiebung der krystallinse. A. f. O., IV, 2, p. 211.

836b. ———, Ueber die mit diabetes mellitus vorkommenden sehstorungen. Ibidem, p. 230.

836c. ———, Verklebung der vordern linsenkapsel mit membrane descemetii und bemerkungen uber gewisse formen von nachstaar. Ibidem, p. 241.

837. Koeberle, de la cataracte pyramidale. Gaz. de Strasb., No. 5, et Ann. d'Oc., XLIII, p. 192.

838. Mahieux, Luxation spontanee du cristallin, utilite de l'atropine pour le reduire. Monit. des Hop., Avril, et Bullet. de Therap., Juin.

839. Salomon, Vose, Cas de cataractes unilaterales, influence de l'operation sur la vision. Brit. Med. Journ., April 17.

840. Geissler, Zur lehre vom grauen staar. Schmidt's Jahrb., t. C, p. 249.

841. Kuhnhorn, De cataractae aquae inopia effecta. Gyrphiae. 1858.

842. Streatfeild, Cataract first affects the right eye or left eye. O. H. R. I, p. 214.

843. Salomon, Vose, The reclination of cataract with two needles. O. H. R., I, p. 218.

1859. 844. France, The cataract in association with diabetes. Opth. Hosp. Rep., I, p. 272.

845. ———, On the use of forceps in extraction of cataract. Ibid, II, p. 20.

846. Hulke, Rupture of the eyeball, with escape of the lens, etc. Ibid, I, p. 292.

1859. 847. Arlt, Ueber cataracta. Spitalzeitung, No. 1.

848. Caffe, Traitement medical de la cataracte. Gaz. des Hop., No. 8.

849. Guepin, Traitement medical de la cataracte. Bull. de Therap., Fevr.

850. Laurence, Z., Luxation traumatique du cristallin. Med. Times and Gaz., 5 Mars.

851. Rohrer, J. S., Cataracte congenitale; operation; guerison. Amer. Med. Chir. Rev., Jan.

852. Robin, Ch., De l'anatomie de diverses formes de cataracte. Bull. de l'Acad., XXIV, p. 843, u. Ann. d'Oc., XLIII, p. 193.

853. Weber, C. O., Vorfall der linse und einheilung eines wimperhaares in der vordere augenkammer. Med. Centr. Zeit., No. 5.

854. Bonafos-Lazermes, De la cataracte. Journ. de Toulouse. Juill.

855. Van Dommelen, Guerison medicale de la cataracte. Nederl. Tijdsch., Juin.

856. Hildige, J. H., Hemorrhagie apres l'operation de la cataracte. Lancet, 12 Sept.

857. Jager, E., Fall von cataract. Wien Zeitschr., No. 31.

858. Bayard, Traitement de la cataracte par la galvanocaustique. Gaz. des Hop., No. 149.

859. Dechambre, De la cataracte diabetique. Gaz. Hebd., No. 51.

860. Desmarres, Curec avec cystotome pour l'extraction lineaire de la cataracte. Gaz. des Hop., No. 121.

861. Joseph, G., Dislocation eines cataractosen linsensystems in folge v. einwirkung vo at pin-eintraufelung. Gunzb. Zeitschr., No. 5 u. 6.

862. Waldhauer, Cataracta centralis. Rigaer Beitr. z. Heilk., IV, p. 100.

863. Walton, Cataracte: position abnormale de l'iris et du cristallin, diabete, operation, succes. Med. Times and Gaz., 12 Nov.

864. Graefe, v., Ueber sehstorung bei diabetes. Deutsche Klinik, 1859, p. 104.

865. Caussade, Recherches pour servir a l'histoire pathologique de la cataracte et de son traitement. These. Montpellier.

866. Lowenhardt, Procede pour l'extraction de la cataracte. Gaz. Hebd., No. 7, u. Ann. d'Oc., XLIV, p. 53.

867. Chassaignac, Resorption de l'iris du cristallin. France Medicale u. Ann. d'Oc., XLIV, p. 53.

868. Zepernik, Meletemata de cataracta. Diss. Dorpat.

1860. 869. Gosselin, Repos absolu des paupieres et du globe de l'oeil apres l'operation de la cataracte. Gaz. des Hop., No. 165.

870. Weber, C. O., Ueber den bau des glaskorpers und die pathologischen, namentlich entzundlichen verwundungen desselben. Virchow's Arch., XIX, p. 367.

871. Leport, Guide pratique pour bien executer, bien reussir et mener a bonne fin l'operation de la cataracte par extraction superieure. Paris, u. Ann. d'Oc., XLIII, p. 200.

1860. 872. Viol, Zuckergehalt des grauen staars bei diabetes. Med. Centr. Zig., No. 51.

873. Wilson, Dislocation of the lens. Opth. Hosp., No. III, p. 65.

874. Graefe, A. v., et Schweiger, Cataracta traumatica u. chronische cho-rioiditis durch einen fremden korper in der linse bedingt. Arch. f. Opth. Bd. VI, p. 134, und ectatische chorioditis mit scleralstaphylom, linsendislocation und excavation des schnerven. Ibid, p. 156.

875. Muller, H., Nachtrage zum kapselstaar. Verhandl. d. Wurzb. Phys. Med. Gesellsch., t. X.

876. Hesser, Faserschichtenstaar. Zeitschr. d. Ges. d. Aerzte z. Wien, No. 23.

877. Mitchell, De la cataracte diabetique, experiences physiologiques. Gaz. Hebd., No. 48.

878. ———, On the production of cataract. Amer. Journ. of Med. Science.

879. Just, Eigenthumlicher kapselstaar, etc., und hinterer polarstaar. Oesterr. Zeitschr. f. Prakt. Heilk., No. 30.

880. Schuft, Die Ausloffelung des Staares. Ein neues verfahren. Berlin in 8o, u. Ann. d'Oc., XLIV, p. 151.

881. Sichel, Extraction de la cataracte. Gaz. des Hop., No. 20 et 32.

882. Graefe, A. v., Ueber die vorsuge eines von Dr. Schuft, erfundenen loffels bei der linearextraction. Arch. f. Opth., Bd. VI, A. 2, p. 155.

883. Mitchell, Cataract bildung durch injection von zuckerlosung ins subcutane zellgewebe. Oesterr. Zeitschr. fur Prakt. Heilk., No. 39. The Amer. Journ. of Med. Sciences, January, 1860. Gaz. Hebdom., No. 48; Ann. d'Oc., XLV, p. 79.

884. Richardson, Ueber kunstliche cataractbildung. Oesterr. Zeitschr. f. Prakt. Heilk., No. 45.

885. ———, Synthesis de la cataracte. Journ. de Physiol., Oct., p. 645.

886. Bouisson, Histoire d'un aliene aveugle qui, apres avoir subi l'opera-tion de la cataracte, a recouvre a la fois le vue et la raison. Montpellier Med., Nov.; Ann. d'Oc., XXXIV, p. 246.

887. Schartow, E., Historia operationum ad cataractae lenticularis san-ationem spectantium. Gryphiae, 1860. Dissert.

888. Bader, Report on cases of cataract treated by "linear extraction," at R. L. O. H., from April, 1857, to May, 1860. O. H. R., II, p. 346.

889. Ammon, v., Acyclia. Irideremia et hemiphakia congenita. Nova acta Acad. Caes. Leop. Carol., t. XXVII, u. Ann. d'Oc., XLIII, p. 282.

890. Cornuty, De la paracentese de l'oeil, 6, Phlegmon de l'oeil a la suite des operations de cataracte. Ann. d'Oc., XLIV, p. 92.

891. Oeil atteint de cataracte double, dite polaire, developpee dans la capsule anterieure, et de cataracte du centre de la lentille cristal-line, avec rayonnement sur la face posterieure du crystallin. Gaz. des Hop., p. 322, u. Ann. d'Oc., XLIV, p. 146.

892. Sichel. Du cephalostat, appareil servant a fixer la tete pendant les operations de cataracte qu'on pratique chez les enfants. Bull. de Ther., LIX, p. 141. u. Ann. d'Oc., LIV. p. 149.

1860. 893. Coursserant, Cataracte; nouveau procede d'extraction. Soc. de Med. Prat., 7 Juin, u. Ann. d'Oc., XXXIV, p. 246.

894. Leport, Fourche a deux branches pour la fixation de l'oeil dans les operations qu'on pratique sur cet organe, in "Guide pratique pour bien executer l'oper. de cat. par extraction." Paris et Rouen. Ann. d'Oc., XLIV, p. 247.

895. Quaglino, Luxation spontanee du cristallin, etc. Giorn. d'Opthalm. Ital. et Bull. de Therap., Avril.

896. Desmarres, Extraction voluminoser cataracten durch den linear-schnitt. Allg. Wien. Med. Zeitg., No. 27.

897. Hogg, J., Luxation du cristallin dans la chambre anterieure par suite d'un eternument prolonge, extraction guerison. Lancet, June.

898. Teisser, Luxation du cristallin dans la chambre anterieure a la suite d'une operation. Rev. de Therap, Med. Ohir., No. 11.

899. Blanc, Questions cliniques relatives a la cataracte. Gaz. Hebd., No. 36.

900. Kuchler, H., Die umlegung des grauen staars durch die sehnenhaut, ihre gefahren und die mittel denselben vorzubeugen. Deutsch. Klin., No. 31, 33.

901. Fano, Luxation sous-conjonctivale du cristallin. Gaz. des Hop., No. 152.

902. Squere, W. J., De la cataracte et de son traitement chirurgical. Brit. Med. Journ., Sept. 15, 22.

903. Desmarres, Fils, amblyopie avec signes de nyctalopie par agenesie incomplete du cristallin, observee chez trois freres. Mon. des Sc. Med., 1138, u. Ann. d'Oc., XLV, p. 196.

1861. 904. Critchett, Practical observations upon congenital cataract. Opth. Hosp. Rep., III, p. 137 and 183.

905. Pagenstecher, Die verlagerung der pupille durch iridodesis. Arch. f. Opth., t. VIII, A. 1, p. 192.

906. Muller, E., Beitrag zur kehre der spontanen linsenluxation. Ibid, p. 166.

907. Schweigger. Ueber entstehung des kapselstaars. Ibid, p. 227.

908. Heddaeus, Partieller schichtstaar. Ibid, p. 315.

909. Wilde, Congenital diseases and malformations of the dioptric media. Dubl. Quart. Journ., No. 61. February.

910. Hulke, Cases of congenital cataract treated by iridodesis. Opth. Hosp. Rep., III, p. 339.

911. Poland, On the use of forceps in extraction of cataract; France's method. Opth. Hosp. Rep., III, p. 268.

912. Swain, Case of cataract and diabetes. Opth. Hosp. Rep., III, p. 381.

913. Ritter, Folger de reclination und discission. A. f. O., VIII, 1, u. Ann. d'Oc.. p. 323.

914. Lecorche, De la cataracte diabetique. Arch. Gener. de Med., Mai; Ann. d'Oc.. XLVIII, p. 106.

458

1861. 915. Jager, E. v., Spontane heilung von trubungen in der menschlichen linse. Oesterr. Zeitschr. f. Prakt. Heilk., No. 31 u. 32.

916. Tedeschi, Nouveau procede pour operer l'extraction de la cataracte. Un. Med., Avril; Ann. d'Oc., XLV, p. 280.

917. Heymann, Spontane freibeweglichkeit der linse. Zeitsch. der Gesellsch. f. Natur. und Heilkunde. Dresden. u. Ann. d'Oc., XLVIII, p. 189.

918. Fischer, De la luxation spontanee du cristallin. Arch. Gen. de Med., Janv., u. Ann. d'Oc., XLVI, p. 83.

919. Quadri, A., Note sur un cas de traitement de la cataracte sans operation. Ann. d'Oc., XLIV, p. 202.

920. Fano, Sur la sortie premature du niyeau du cristallin dans la cataracta molle operee par extraction. Gaz. des Hop., p. 394, u. Ann. d'Oc., XLVI, p. 220.

921. Rivaud-Landrau, Statistique d'operations de cataracte. Gaz. Med. de Lyon, p. 450.

922. Zehender, Die krankheiten des linsensystems. Handbuch der Augenheilkunde. Erlangen.

923. Saemisch, Zur operation der cataract. Wurzb. Med. Zeitschr., II, p. 272.

924. France, Observations de cataracte diabetique. Med. Times and Gaz., 9 Mars.

925. Cade, Am., Cataract congenitale double operee a l'age de 18 ans. Bullet. de Therap., Juin.

926. Demarquay, Keratotomie superieure, procede sous-conjonctival, keratotomie superieure et iridectomie. Gaz. des Hop., No. 53.

927. Peachy, H. D., Guerison spontanee d'une cataracte. Amer. Med. Chir.urg. Rev., Mars., p. 317.

928 Gouriet, Resorption lente et progressive du cristallin; daltonisme; des diverses methodes de scleronyxis. Gaz. des Hop., No. 113, u. Ann. d'Oc., XLV, p. 166.

930. Giraud-Teulon, Des mouvements de concentration lateral de l'appareil cristallinien pour satisfaire a l'unite de la vision binoculaire, fant lors de l'intervention des prismes ou des lunettes que dans certains cas pathologiques. Ann. d'Oc., XLV, p. 113.

931. Sichel, Materiaux pour servir a l'etude anatamique de l'opthalmie periodique et de la cataracte de cheval. Ann. d'Oc., XLVI, p. 181.

932. Prault, Operation des grauen staars bei einem 12 jagrigen knaben. Allg. Wien. Med. Ztg., No. 37.

933. Serres, Operation modlee de la cataracte. Gaz. Hebd., No. 38.

1862. 934. Meyer, Ignaz, Die kriebel-krankheit als ursache der staarbildung. Wien. Wochenschr., No. 47, 1861, u. Arch. f. Opth., VIII, A. 2, p. 120.

935. Sperino, Etudes cliniques sur l'evacuation repetee de l'humeur aqueuse, etc. Turin, in 8o.

1862. 936. Swain. Case of cataract and diabetes. Opth. Hosp. Rep., No. 17, p. 331.

937. Graefe, A. v., Cystoide vernarbung bei iridectomie wegen glaucom. A. f. O., VIII, 2, p. 263.

938. Alessi, Cause de la cataracte chez les paysans des bords du Don. Ann. d'Oc., XLVII, p. 30.

939. Mooren, Die verminderten gefahren einer Hornhautvereiterung bei der Staarextraction. Berlin, in 8o.

940. Jamin, A., Du broiement de la cataracte. Gaz. des Hop., No. 18.

941. Smith, G., De l'abaissement de la cataracte aux Indes. Edinb. Med. Journ., p. 101. Fevr.

942. Walton, H., Operation pour la resorption de la cataracte dure. Lancet, 14 Avril.

943. ———, De la discission de la cataracte. Brit. Med. Journ., 7 Juin.

944. Browne, Observation de cataracte. Dubl. Journ. Mai

945. ———, Cataracte congenitale. Ibid. November.

946. Stoeber, Cataracte diabetique, extraction lineaire. Gaz. de Strasb., No. 5 et 6.

947. Chausit, A., Luxation sous-conjonctivale du cristallin. Gaz. des Hop., No. 101.

948. Gerardi, Ueber Staaroperationen auf dem Lande. Wien. Med. Halle, No. 40.

949. Hart, E., Deux cas de cataracte et extraction par la section iferieure, etc. Lancet, 5, Avril, Oct. et Nov.

950. Tetzer, Max, Ueber cataracta. Allg. Wien. Med. Zeitg., No. 1-4.

951. Alessi, Resultats des operations de cataracte et relation d'un cas d'extraction, dans lequel la pointe du keratome s'est brisee dans la cornee.

952. Rivaud-Landrau, Statistique d'operations de cataractes (2317). Ann. d'Oc., XLVII, p. 65.

953. Alessi. Un aveugle-ne sourd-muet, gueri de la cecite congenitale. Ann. d'Oc., XLVII, p. 112.

954. Lanne. Pince-aiguille a cataracte. Gaz. des Hop., Fevr., u. Ann. d'Oc., XLVII, p. 109.

955. Coursserant, Incision de l'iris dans la keratotomie superieure. Gaz. des Hop., No. 132.

956. Desormeaux. Blessure du cristallin. Ibid.

957. Hulme. Luxation du cristallin, avec transformation cataracteuse chez neuf membres d'une famille. Lancet, 23 Dec.

958. Nelaton, Cataracte double, extraction lineaire. Gaz. des Hop., No.145.

1863. 959. Jacobson. Ein neues gefahrloses operations verfahren zur heilung des grauen Staars. Berlin, in 8o.

960. Bolling, A. Pope. A case of laminar cataract. Opth. Hosp. Rep., IV, p. 79.

1863. 961. Boulsson, D'un cas particulier de diabete avec cataracte double. Montpellier Med., Janv.

962. Wecker, Iridesis in einem falle von doppelter linsenluxation. Klin. Monatsbl., Marz, u. Gaz. des Hop., No. 22. Ann. d'Oc., XLIX, p. 159.

963. Knapp, Erfolgreiche pupillenbildung bei einer durch einen Stoss dislocirten linse. Ibid. Avril.

964. Graefe, A. v., Extraction bei marastischem auge. umschriebene suppuration. Ibid. Avril, Juin.

965. Hays, Remarks on cataract. Amer. Journ. of Med. Science. Juillet.

966. Sichel, Sur une espece particuliere de delire senile, qui survient quelquefois apres l'extraction de la cataracte. Un. Med., Janv.

967. Borelli, Nouveau cas de delire nostalgique consecutif a l'operation de la cataracte. Giorno d'Opth. Ital.

968. Becker, F. S. v., Untersuchungen uber den bau der linse bei den Menschen. und Wirbelthieren. Arch. f. Opth., IX, A. 2, p. 1.

968. Graefe, A. v., Ueber die zweckmassigkeit einer breiten discissionsnadel bei operation flussiger cataracten. Ibid, p. 43.

969a. ——,Extraction fremder Korper, reclinirter linsen und entozoen aus dem glaskorperraum. Ibid, p. 79.

970. Knapp, Beiderseitige linearextraction eines diabetischen Staars. Zehender Klin. Monats., 168, u. Ann. d'Oc., LI, p. 50.

971. Graefe, A. v., Ueber den druckverband bei augenkrankheiten. Ibid, p. 111.

972. Hildrige, Sur le traitement de la cataracte par l'evacuation frequente de l'humeur aqueuse. Gaz. Med. de Paris, p. 507.

973. Quaglino, Sulla cura medica della cataratta et sugli effecti della paracentesi corneale repetuta, etc. Ann. Univ. di Med. Milano, 181.

974. Masen, Cataracte traumatique, e tc. Bull. de la Societe Medic. de Gand. Mars.

975. Mauduy, De l'operation de la cataracte par extraction lineaire. These. de Paris.

976. Eberhardt, Memoire sur la cataracte lamellaire. Nantes, in 8o, p. 15, Gaz. des Hop., No. 64.

977. Froebelius, Cataractbildung durch vier generationen einer familie hindurch. Petersb. Med. Zeitschr., No. 8 u. 9.

978. Hart, E., Cas d'extraction et de discission de cataracte. Lancet II, 13 Mars et 16 Avril.

979. Schirmer, Ueber spontane luxation durchsichtiger linsen. Greifswalder Beitr., I, p. 77.

980. Lanne, Delire nerveux a la suite de l'operation de la cataracte. Gaz. des Hop., No. 57.

981. Magne, Delire apres l'operation de la cataracte. Bull. de Therap., 30 Mai.

1863. 982. Laugier, Luxation du cristallin dans la chambre anterieure. Gaz. des Hop., No. 87.

983. Carter, Rob, Les nouveaux procedes d'extraction de cataracte. Med. Times and Gaz., 24 Oct.

984. Becker, O., Function der ciliarfortsatze. Wiener Med. Jahrbucher.

985. Laurence, Irrigations apres l'extraction de la cataracte. Brit. Med. Journ. Juillet.

986. Saint-Ildephont, Traitement de la cataracte sans operation. Revue de Ther., No. 15, 402.

987. Warlomont, Cas de mort a la suite d'une operation de cataracte par discission. Ann. d'Oc., LI, p. 239.

1864. 988. Critchett, A case of congenital cataract treated by iridesis, in which some modifications were introduced in the operation. Opth. Hosp. Rep., IV, p. 150.

989. Zehender, Ueber die zweckmassigste schneideform der zur lappen-schnitt extraction dienenden messer. Klin. Monatschr., p. 73.

990. Leuckardt, Ueber die parasiten der menschl. linse. Ibid, p. 86.

991. Melchior, Sur le developpement de la cataracte dans le diabete. Ann. d'Oc., LI, p. 262.

992. Servais, Observations de cataracte produite par la foudre. Recueil de Memoires de Med., de Chirurg. et de Pharm. de Paris, p. 229.

993. Jacobson, Zur lehre der cataract extraction mit Lappenschnitt. Arch. f. Opth., X., A. 2, p. 78.

994. ———. Ueber die cataract operation mit Lappenschnitt. Ibid, IX, A. 2, p. 147.

995. ———, Ueber cataract extraction. Klin. Monatsbl., p. 30.

996. Knapp, Ueber behandlung des grauen Staars. Zweiter Jahresber. Heidelberg.

997. Arlt, Verkalkte linse. Glaskorperblutung. Klin. Monatsbl., 1864, p. 364.

998. Graefe, A. v., Ueber die kapseleroffnung als voract der Staaroper-ation, nebst bemerkungen uber die Wahl des operationstermins. Ibid, p. 209.

999. Manhardt, Ueber extraction unreifer cataracten. Ibid, p. 408.

1000. Bauzon, De l'extraction lineaire. These. de Paris.

1001. Critchett, Description d'un nouvel instrument pour l'extraction de la cataracte. Lancet, et Ann. d'Oc., LI, p. 44.

1002. ———, De l'extraction de la cataracte au moyen de la curette. Ann. d'Oc., LII, p. 115, u. Klin. Monatsbl. p. 349.

1003. Lawson, Traumatic cataract produced without rupture of the external coats of the eye. Opth. Hosp. Rep., IV, p. 179.

1004. Pridgin Teale, A suction curette for the extraction of soft cataract. Ibid, IV, p. 197.

1005. Froebelius, Falle von Staarextraction mit einem vorschlage zur modification derselben. Petersb. Med. Zeitschr., p. 28.

1864. 1006. Hart, E., De la cataracte au point de vue de diagnostic et du traite-
        ment. Lancet, 15 Avril.

1007. Jarjavay, Cataract capsulaire secondaire. Gaz. des Hop., No. 12.

1008. Jouon, Note sur les cataractes strat. et sur leur traitement. Nantes,
        in 8o, p. 11.

1009. Bader, Two cases of diabetic cataract. Opth. Hosp. Rep., IV, p. 288.

1010. Rydel, Luc., Stationaler kernstaar oder schichtstaar. Wien. Med.
        Halle. Nos. 7, 8, 10, 11, 13, 15 u. 16.

1011. Singer, Mat., Zwei falle von pyramidenstaar. Ibid, Nos. 14, 17,
        19 u. 20.

1012. Sichel, Ueber druckverband nach Staaroperationen. Deutsch. Klin.,
        No. 4.

1013. Blessig, Vergleichende casuistik der einfachen und der mit iridec-
        tomie verbundenen Staaroperationen. Petersb. Med. Zeitschr.,
        No. 3.

1014. Lawson, G., De la cataracte congenitale. Brit. Med. Journ., 9 Juill.

1015. Martin, E., De l'operation de la cataracte et du procede oderatoire
        de reclinaison par la cornee keratoyxis. Paris, in 8o, p. 38.

1016. Massol, A., Nouvelle methode de traitement a suivre apres l'oper-
        ation de la cataracte. Paris, in 8o, p. 16.

1017. Walton, H., Cas de cataracte. Brit. Med. Journ., 7 May.

1018. Hunt, Ossification du cristallin. Americ. Journ., Juill. p. 94.

1019. Hasner, d'A., Ueber die glaskorperpunction bei der extraction des
        Staars. Wien. Med. Wochenschr., No. 42.

1020. Mattioli, G. B., Studii che conducono alla possibilita della guarizione
        della cataratta incipiente immature dei giovani, col ridurle a cata-
        ratte traumatiche et far'e absorbire a mezzo della paracentesi
        oculaire. Venezit, in 8o, p. 14.

1021. Taylor, Ch., De l'extraction de la cataracte. Brit. Med. Journ., 12
        November.

1022. Wecker et De la Croix, H., Luxation du cristallin cataracte, obliter-
        ation de la pupille, etc. Gaz. des Hop., No. 8.

1865. 1023. Jacobson, Ueber die zulassigkeit des chloroforms bei Staaropera-
        tionen. Arch. fur Opth., XI, A. 1, p. 114.

1024. Moers, Beitrage zur pathologischen anatomie der linse nach ver-
        suchen an thieren. Virchow's Arch., XXX, p. 45.

1025. Bence, Jones, Proceedings of the Royal Institution of Great Britain,
        Vol. IV, Part VI, No. 42, October. (Experimente uber das spate
        auftreten resorbirter stoffe in der linse, besonders von kohlensau-
        rem lithium.)

1026. Braun, Beitrag zur heilung des harten staars. Ibid, p. 200.

1027. Bessac, J. M., Etudes sur l'etiologie de la cataracte. These. de
        Paris, in 4o, p. 37.

1028. Bonneval, Galigny de, De la cataracte zonulaire et de son traite-
        ment. These. de Paris, in 4o.

1865. 1029. Pagenstecher, C., Ueber verletzungen der linsenkapsel. Klin. Monatsbl., in 4o, p. 71.

1030. Sophus-Davidsen, Zur lehre vom schichtstaar. Inaug. Dissert. Zurich.

1031. Galezowski, Luxation du cristallin sous le conjonctive et de la cataracte par extraction. Ann. d'Oc., LIII, p. 196.

1032. Wecker, Extraction de la cataracte sans ouverture de la cristalloide. Gaz. Hebd., No. 30.

1033. ———, De l'etiologie de la cataracte. Ann. d'Oc., LIV, p. 16.

1034. Guerserant, P., De la cataracte chez les enfants. Bullet. de Therap., 15 Fevr.

1035. Laurence, Z., De l'extraction de la cataracte d'apres Mooren. Brit. Med. Journ., 11 Fevr.

1036. Walton, H., Observations de cataracte. Med. Times et Gaz., 8 Avr.

1037. Zehender, Ueber staarmesserformen. Klin. Monatsbl., III, p. 122.

1038. Stephan, Traumatische luxation de linse mit cataractbildung. Ibid, p. 164.

1039. Berlin, Zur statistik der Jacobson's chen extractions-methode. Wurtemberg. Corresp., B. 1, No. 19.

1040. Critchett, On the removal of cataract by the scoop-method, or the method by traction. Opth. Hosp. Rep., IV, p. 315.

1041. Bowman, On extraction of cataract by a traction instrument with iridectomy; with remarks of capsular obstructions and their treatment. Ibid, p. 332.

1042. Kruse, H., Ueber cataractbildung. Zeitschr., f. Rat. Medic., XXIV, p. 261.

1043. Salomon, Vose. Annular synechia and cataract, etc. Opth. Rev., No. 5, p. 28.

1044. Graefe, A. v., Remarks on traumatic cataract. Berl. Klin. Wochenschr. u. Opth. Rev., No. 6, p. 37. Ann. d'Oc., LIV, p. 270.

1045. Kuchler, Ueber die form der staarmesser; uber nachbehandlung nach der staaroperation. Deutsch. Klin., Nos. 39, 40 u. 43.

1046. Moon, Observations sur l'extraction lineaire de cataracte molle, suivie d'un decollement de la retine. Ann. d'Oc., LIII, p. 256.

1047. Taylor, Cinq cas de cataractes traites par l'extraction suivant la methode de Mooren. Ann. d'Oc., LIII, p. 258.

1048. Holmes, Observations de cataract pyramidal. Amer. Journ. of Opth., II, 14.

1049. Szokalsky, Cristallin luxe sous la conjonctive. Ann. d'Oc., LIV, p. 212.

1050. Wecker, Luxation du cristallin et cataractes reconnues, malgre l'obliteration de la pupille a travers l'iris atrophie. Gaz. des Hop., 8, 29. Ann. d'Oc., LIV, p. 125.

1051. Lawson, F., A case of dislocation of the lens into the anterior chamber; excessive pain two years after the injury and loss of sight; extraction of t he lens followed by immediate posterior hemorrhage. Opth. Hosp. Rev., IV, p. 379.

464

1865. 1052. Prie, Observations de cataracte. Paris, in 8o, p. 11.

1053. Graefe, A. v., Ueber modificirte linearextraction. Arch. f. Opth., X, A. 3, p. 1.

1054. Ullersperger, Kleine mitthellung fur die geschichte der operation des grauen staars. Ibid, XI, A. 2, p. 262.

1866. 1055. Adams, Math., The modern methods of dealing with cataract. Brit. Med. Journ., 13 Janv.

1056. Monte, Michele de, Note sul' inflammatione del cristallino e della sua capsula, 11. Morgagni, I.

1057. Follin, Des diverses methodes operatoires de la cataracte. Arch. Gener. de Med., Fevr., p. 212.

1058. ——, Luxation congenitale du cristallin. Gaz. des Hop., No. 20.

1059. Martin, E., De l'extraction de la cataracte dure au moyen de la curette-erigne. Gaz. des Hop., No. 9.

1060. Paikrt, A., Luxation u. fractur der linse in folge von verletzung. Allg. Milit. Arztl. Ztg., No. 4.

1061. Hart, E., Clinical lectures on cataract, with reference to improved methods of diagnosis and treatment. Lancet, 21 May.

1062. Hasner, d'A., Klinische vortrage uber augenheilkunde. 3, Abth. Die krankheiten des linsensystems. Prag, in 8o, p. 106.

1063. Luca, Dom., De l'extraction de la cataracte capsulaire et capsulo-lenticulaire. Il. Morgagni, No. 2 et 3.

1064. Bowman, Cases of malformed, misplaced and dislocated lenses, in some of which glaucomatous symptoms were developed. Opth. Hosp. Rev., V, p. 1.

1065. Samelson, A., A case of pyramidal cataract, with microscopic examination (by Prof. C. Schweigger) of the lens after extraction. Ibid, p. 48.

1066. Cowell, G., Two cases of traumatic cataract, possessing some interesting points of diagnosis. Ibid, p. 131.

1067. Meckeand, Extraction des cataracte molles par succion. Brit. Med. Journ., 30 Juin.

1068. Testelin, Luxation sous-conjonctivale du cristallin. Gaz. des Hebd., No. 31.

1069. Arlt, Ueber v. Graefe's linearextraction der cataracte. Wien. Med. Wochenschr., No. 24.

1070. Samelson, A., v. Graefe's modificirte linear extraction. Deutsch. Klin., No. 7.

1071. Kuchler, Ueber extraction des staars. Ibid, 37-39.

1072. Classen, Ueber staaroperation. Ibid, No. 43.

1073. Fano, De l'operation de la cataracte. Gaz. des Hop., No. 124.

1074. Sichel, Du mode operatoire qui convient le mieux aux cataractes capsulaires centrales et capsulaires-lenticulaires centrales, etc. Bull. de Therap., 15 Sept.

1866. 1075. Pagenstecher, Ueber die extraction des grauen staars bei uneroff-
neter kapsel durch den scleralschnitt. Klin. Beobacht. aus der
augenheilanstalt zu Wiesbaden, III, p. 1.

1076. Iwanoff, Beitrag zur pathologischen anatomie des hornhaut und
linsenepithels. Pagenstecher. Klin. Beobacht., III, p. 126.

1077. Matrion, G., Des indications de l'operation de la cataracte et du
choix de la methode operatoire. These. de Paris, in 4o, p. 70.

1078. Vitrac, E., Etude sur le traitement de la cataracte par discission.
These. de Paris, in 4o, p. 52.

1079. Arguillo, Marcello, De l'operation de la cataracte par l'extraction
lineaire. These. de Paris, in 4o, p. 36.

1080. Keand, M., Case of extraction of soft cataract in both eyes by suction. Brit. Med. Journ., 30 Juin.

1081. Hutchinsin, Cataracts in childhood fully developed in one eye.
Operation on one eye at the age of fifteen. No sight obtained,
owing to atrophic changes in optic nerve. Pupil of this eye very
active. Opth. Hosp. Rep., V, p. 216.

1082. Newmann, Spontaneous rupture of film of capsule three months
after extraction of lens. Opth. Hosp. Rep., V, p. 223.

1083. Hutchinson, Operations for solution of senile cataracts commenced
at an early period, without allowing the cataract to ripen. Opth.
Hosp. Rep., V, p. 329.

1084. Walton. Haynes. Black cataract. Brit. Med. Journ., 27 January.

1085. Bouyer, Cataracte traumatique avec synechia posterieure. Gaz.
des Hop., No. 118.

1086. Desmarres, A., Des applications de l'iridectomie au traitement de
la cataracte. These. de Paris, in 4o, p. 95.

1087. Tillaux, Luxation sous-conjonctivale du cristallin. Gaz. des Hop.,
No. 127.

1088. Wells, Lectures on cataracts and the modern operations for its
treatment. Med. Times et Gaz., 17 Oct., 10 Nov., 8 Dec. u. 22 Dec.

1089. Graefe, v., Nachtragliche bemerkungen uber die modificirte linear
extraction. Arch. f. Opth., XII, A. 1, p. 150.

1090. ——, Cysticercus in der linse. Ibid, XII, A. 2, p. 191.

1091. Windsor and Little, Th., Cases of flap extraction of cataract under
chloroform. Opth. Rev., No. 8, p. 365.

1093. Dyer, Fracture of the lens of one eye and of the anterior capsule
of both eyes from death by violent hanging. Trans. of the Amer.
Soc., Boston. Juin.

1094. Hirschmann, Luxatio lentis spontanea. Klin. Monatsbl., IV, p. 98.

1095. Borelli, Osservazione di doppia cataratta molle risanta rapidamente
coll' estrazione lineare. Giorno d'Oft. Ital., IX, p. 180.

1867. 1096. Milliot, Memoire sur la regeneration du cristallin. Bull. de l'Acad.
des Sciences, 28 Janv., et Gaz. des Hop., No. 6.

1097. Knapp, Metastatische choroiditis. A. f. O., XIII.

466

1867. 1098. Gourlet, Cas remarquable de luxation spontanee du cristallin et de sa capsule dans la chambre anterieure. Gaz. des Hop., No. 43.

1099. Monoyer, Une extraction de la cataracte dans un cas de luxation spontanee et d'opacification du cristallin, etc. Gaz. Med. de Strasb., No. 14.

1100. Paoli, Cesare, Del metodo operativo preferibili in vari casi di cataratte. Firenze, in 8o.

1101. Simi, A., Supra uno scritto des c. s. Prof. Cesare Paoli intitulata sul methodo operatorio preferibile nel vari casi di cataratta. Lucca, in 8o, p. 9.

1102. Tavignot, Traitement de la cataracte par l'extraction directe. Nouveau procede. Abeille Med., No. 48.

1013. Walton, H., Extraction de la capsule opaque apres la perte du cristallin. Brit. Med. Journ., 2 Fevr.

1104. Stephan, Erfahrungen mit studien uber die staaroperation. Erlangen, in 8o, p. 62.

1105. Rydel u. Becker, Spontane aufhellung der catar. traumat.; cataract. caps. centr. anter. mit cat. nuclearis; zwei seltene staarformen. Voy. Ber, uber die Augenklin. d. Wien. Univers. Vienne, in 8o.

1106. Macnamara, Linear extraction of t he lens. Opth. Rev., No. 11, p.371.

1107. Windsor, Th., A new operation for cataract. Ibid, p. 251.

1108. Quaglino, On scleronyxis. Ibid, No. 12, p. 371.

1109. Little, Cases of flap extraction, etc. Ibid, p. 398.

1110. Williams, H. W., Remarks on the use of suture to close the corneal wound after removal of cataract by flap extraction. Opth. Hosp. Rep., VI, p. 28.

1111. Businelli, Caduta del nucleo del cristallino nella camera anteriore sette anni dopo l'operatione di cataratta per abassamento, etc. Giorno d'Oftal. Ital.. X, p. 153.

1112. Liebeich, Du diagnostic de la cataracte et de l'appreciation des methodes operatoires applicables a ses differentes formes. Nouveau Diction. de Med., VI; Ann. d'Oc., LVIII, p. 103.

1113. Pires, De l'operation de la cataracte par extraction lineaire scleroticale. These. de Paris, in 8o, p. 86.

1114. Knapp, Bericht uber hundert staarextractionen nach der neuen v. Graefe'schen methode ausgefuhrt. Arch. f. Opth., XIII, A. 1, p. 85.

1115. Weber, A., Die normale linsenentbindung der modificirten linear extraction gewidmet. Ibid, p. 549.

1116. Bergmann, Ueber entfernung des grauen staars mit der kapsel. Ibid, XIII, A. 2, p. 383.

1117. Graefe, v., Notiz uber die linsenentbindung bei der modificirten linear extraction und vereinzelte bemerkungen uber das verfahren. Ibid, p. 549.

1867. 1118. Kampf, Traumatische cataracte mit fremden korper in der linse. Oesterr. Zeitschr. f. Pract. Heilk., No. 9.

1119. Kuchler, Ueber die querextraction des staars. Memorabilien, XII, 1.

1120. Magni, De la cataracte, son diagnostic et son traitement. Riv. Clin., VI, 2.

1121. Wells, Soelberg, Lectures on cataract and the modern operation for its treatment. Med. Times et Gaz., 23 et 30 March.

1122. Watson, Spenser, Cas de cataracte traumatique. Ibid, 11 Mai.

1123. Hoering. F., Die modifircte Graefe'sche linearextraction. Wurtemberg Med. Corresp., B. 1, No. 24.

1124. Leudiger-Formentel, Cataracte double chez un enfant de 4 ans, e tc. Union Med., No. 66.

1125. Meyer. Ed., Du nouveau procede de M. de Graefe pour l'extraction de la cataracte. Ibid, No. 99, et 101.

1126. Terson, De la cataracte. Analyze critique et indications des anciens et nouveaux procedes operatoires. Toulouse, in 8o, p. 79.

1868. 1127. Hasner, d'Artha, Dir neue phase der staaroperation. Prag., in 8o, p. 15.

1128. Graefe, v., Ueber v. Hasner's kritik der linearextraction. Klin. Monatsbl., VI, p. 1.

1129. Ritter, Anatomie du cristallin. Wecker, Traite des Maladies des Yeux, 2 e d., II, p. 1.

1130. Mauthner, Lehrbuch der Opthalmologie. Wien.

1131. Schumann, Ueber den mechanismus der accommodation des menschlichen auges. Dresden.

1132. Coccius, Der mechanismus der accommodation des menschlichen Auges. Leipzig.

1133. Rothmund. Ueber cataracten in verbindung mit einer eigenthumlichen hautdegeneration. A. f. O., XIV, 1, p. 159.

1134. Knapp, Bericht uber ein Hundert staaroperation, etc. Ibid, p. 285.

1135. Foucher, Lecons sur la cataracte, in 8o, p. 287.

1136. Kuchler, Die querextraction des grauen staars der erwachsenen. Erlangen, in 8o. p. 37.

1137. Wolfe, J. R., On improved methods of extraction of the cataract. Lancet, 11 April.

1138. Wecker, Des nouveaux procedes operatoires de la cataracte; paralete et critique. Ann. d'Oc., LIX. Mars et Avril. Paris, in 8o, p. 49.

1139. Graefe, A. v., Ueber das verfahren des peripheren linearschnittes. A. f. O., XIV. 3, p. 106. 1868.

1140. Heymann, Ueber linearextraction. Klin. Monatsbl., VI. 326.

1141. Hoering. Ueber linearextraction. Ibid, 331.

1142. Mannhardt, Cataract operation. A. f. O., XIV, 3, p. 26.

1143. Milliot, Ueber regeneration der linse. Journ. de Brux., XLVII. Dec.

1868. 1144. Sichel, Histor. notiz uber die operation des grauen staars durch die methode des aussaugens od. adspiration. A. f. O., XIV, 3, p. 1.

1145. Tavignot, Ueber die behandlung der cataracte ohne operation. Journ. de Brux., XLVII. Dec.

1146. Taylor, Ch., Ueber cataract extraction. Brit. Med. Journ., Nov. et Dec.

1869. 1147. Blessig, Bericht uber die in den Jahren, 1864-68, ausgefuhrten staar operationen. Petersb. Med. Zeitschr., XV, 3, p. 145.

1148. Tavignot, Phosphorirtes oel gegen cataract. Presse Med., XXI, 8, p. 26.

1149. Turner, Cataract mit complicationen bei der operation. Philadelph. Med. and Surgic. Reporter, XX, 4, p. 61.

1150. Ullersperger, Spontane eilung einer cataract. Wien. Med. Presse, IX, 48.

1151. Wagner, Fremdkorper in der linse. Klin. Monatsbl., VI, p. 15.

1152. Collmann, Beiderseitige linsenverschiebung durch aussere Gewalt. Ibid, VII, p. 48.

1153. Davis, Dislocation der krystallinse. St. Louis Med. et Surg. Journ., VI, p. 38.

1154. Noyes, Henry, Operation bei verschliessung der pupille nach cataractoperation. O. H. R., VI, p. 209.

1155. Taylor, Further observations upon an improved method of e xtract ing in cases of cataract. O. H. R., VI, p. 197.

1156. Dantone, Beitrage zur extraction des grauen staars. Erlangen, Enke.

1157. Galezowski, Ueber die operation der cataract. Gaz. des Hop., p. 86.

1157a. Noyes, Ueber die modificirte lienarextraction. Transact. of the Americ. Opthalm. Society, p. 28.

1158. Iwanoff, Befund eines extrahirten auges. In: Sympathische Gesichtsstorungen v. Mooren. Berlin, p. 168.

1159. ———, Anatomische befunde an reclinirten und extrahirten augen. In: Beitrage zur ablosung des glaskorpers. A. f. O., XV, 2, pp. 35, 38, 39, 41, 45.

1160. Gouvea, Ueber entstehung der glaskorperlosung nach glaskorperverlust. A. f. O., XV, 1, p. 244.

1160a. Horing, Reponirte luxation der linse. Zehender's Monatsblatter. 1869.

1160b. Meyer, Eduard, Ueber luxatio lentis. Ibidem.

1161. Stricker, W., Zur geschichte der augenheilkunde. Virchow's Arch., XLVII, p. 519.

1162. Williams, Ueber cataractoperation bei erwachsenen. Transact. of the Amer. Opth. Soc., p. 30.

1163. Barbour, Cataracte. Philade'ph. Med. and Surg. Reporter, XXI, 231.

1164. Hirsch, Ein wort zur geschichte der cataractoperationen im alterthum. Klin. Monatsbl., VII, p. 282.

1869. 1165. Knapp, Staaroperationen nach der peripherlinearen extraction. A. f. A., u. O., I, 1, p. 44.

1166. Noyes, Linsenluxation in den glaskorper und darauf in die vordere Kammer. Ibid, p. 154.

1167. Reuss u. Wolnow, Ueber corneal-astigmatismus nach staaropera-tionen. Wien., Braumuller.

1168. Williams, Ueber staarextraction. A. f. A. u. O., I, 1, p. 91.

1169. Stephan, Weitere erfahrungen und Studien der Jahre, 1867-69.

1170. Wolfe, Ueber cataractextraction. Glasgow Med. Journ., S. II, 1, p. 82.

1171. Monte, Michele del., Ueber operation des harten staars durch ex-traction. Morgagni, XI, p. 824.

1172. Noyes, Cataractmesser. Transact. of the Amer. Opth. Soc., p. 51.

1173. Oglesby, Entfernung der ganzen iris bei einer staaroperation. O. H. R., VI, p. 269.

1174. Williams, Remarks on the use of the suture to close the corneal wound after removal of the cataract by flap extraction. O. H. R., VI, p. 28.

1174a. Hutchinson, Clinical notes on pyramidal cataracts, with specula-tions as to their cause. O. H. R., VI, p. 136.

1870. 1175. Perrin, Falle von cataract bei diabetikern. Gaz. des Hop., p. 63 u. 70.

1176. Walton, Haynes, Vorlesungen uber cataract. Med. Times e t Gaz., p. 15 u. 26.

1177. Charteris, Falle von staaroperationen. Glasgow Med. Journ., II, 3, p. 481.

1178. Coppee, Doppelseitige cataract operirt mittelst der modificirten lin-earextraction. Presse Medic., XXII, 14.

1179. Giraud-Teulon, Ueber staaroperationen. Gaz. des Hop., p. 159.

1180. Graefe, A. v., Ueber den peripheren linearschnitt. Klin. Monatsbl., VIII, p. 1.

1181. Mourton, Ueber luxation der linse unter die conjunctiva. Recueil de Mem. de Med. Milit., 3 Serie, XXIV, p. 414.

1182. Zereissung des augapfels; verlust der linse und iris; erhaltung des sehvermogens. Brit. Med. Journ., p. 40.

1183. Stilling, Aphorismus uber den erfolg der neueren staaroperations methoden. Klin. Monatsbl., VIII, p. 97.

1184. Taylor, Ueber staaroperation. Lancet. April. Brit. Med. Journal, March.

1185. Wilson, Henry, Ueber extraction des staars durch Graefe's peri-pheren linearschnitt. Dubl. Journ., XLIX, May.

1186. Coccius, und Wilhelmi, Die Heilanstalt fur arme augenkranke zu Leipzig zur zeit ihres 50 jahrigen bestehens.

1187. Blodig, Karl. Ueber die dislocation der linse. Wien. Med. Presse, XI, 44.

1870. 1188. Thiry, Ueber die modificirte linearextration des staars. Presse Med., XXII, 4.

1189. Delagarde, Philip Chilwell, ueber cataractextractionen. St. Barth. Hosp. Rep., VI, p. 56.

1190. Forster, Ueber den peripheren linearschnitt bei staaroperation. 27. Jahresbericht der schles. Gesellsch. fur Vaterl. Cultur., p. 220.

1191. Ritter, Fall von acuter cataractbildung. Klin. Monatsbl.,VIII, p. 256.

1192. Stellwag. von Carion, Lehrbuch der prakt. Augenheilkunde. 4. Aufl.

1871. 1193. Knapp, Ueber staarextraction. Transactions of the American Opthalmological Society. Seventh Annual Meeting, July, 1870.

1194. Hasner, Ueber die staarextraction. Prag. Vierteljahrschr. C. X, p. 73.

1195. Knapp, Ueber knochenbildung im auge. A. f. A., u. O., II, p. 133.

1196. Lindner, Luxation de linse zwischen sclera und bindehautsack. Oesterr. Zeitschr. f. Prakt. Heilk.. XXIV, 2.

1197. Aub, Beitrage zur kenntniss der vorletzungen des auges und seiner umgebungen. A. f. A. u. O., II, 1, p. 252.

1198. Berthold, Cataracta congenita capsularis posterior. A. f. O., XVII, 1, p. 169.

1199. Canstatt, v., Zur operativen heilung des grauen staars, nebst Nach-schrift von Zehender. Klin. Monatsbl., IX, p. 131.

1200. Galezowski, Ueber ein neues verfahren zur cataractextraction. Gaz. des Hop., 36.

1201. Naquard, Etude sur les luxations du cristallin. These. de Paris.

1202. Iwanoff, Glaskorper. Stricker's Gewebelehre. p. 1071.

1203. Babuchin, Linse. Ibid. p. 1030.

1204. Gussenbauer, Ueber die heilung per primam intentionem. Arch. f. Chirurgie, XII. p. 791.

1204a. Guberboch,Studien uber die feineren vorgange bei der wundheil-ung per primam intentionem an der cornea. O. Q. L. Hft., 4.

1204b. Westhoff. De operatie de senile cataract. Utrecht.

1205. Schiess-Gemuseus. Angeborener linsendefect. Klin. Monatsbl., IX. p. 99.

1206. Jeaffreson. Ueber behandlung der cataracte. Lancet, II, 12.

1207. ——, Case of congenital malposition of the lens in each eye. O. H. R., VII, p. 186.

1208. Keller, Karl, 1. Fall von dislocation der linse am rechten auge. 2. Ueber v. Graefe's methode der staaroperation. Wien. Med. Presse. XII. 46.

1209. Oettingen, G. v.. Die opthalmologische Klinik Dorpats in den ersten 3 Jahren ihres Bestehens. Dorpat.

1210. Pagenstecher. Hermann. Ueber cataract operation ohne eroffnung der kapsel. Ann. d'Oc., LXVI. p. 126.

1871. 1211. Perrin. Verfahren zur zerstorung der kapsel bei der cataractoperation. Gaz. des Hop., p. 543

1212. Taylor, Ueber cataractoperation mittelst eines schnittes an der
peripherie der iris ohne verletzung der pupille. Lancet, II, 19.

1213. Tweedy, Ueber eine sichtbare streifung der normalen krystallinse.
Lancet, II, 19.

1214. Critchett, G., Ueber behandlung der cataracte. Presse Med., XXIV,
p. 60.

1872. 1215. Muller, Heinrich, Gesamelte und hinterlassene schriften zur anatomie und Physiologie des Auges. Bd.

1216. Berthold, Ueber verknocherung der krystallinse des menschlichen
auges. A. f. O., XVIII, p. 104.

1217. Salomon. Max, Dir krankheiten des linsensystems. Braunschweig.

1218. Loring, Eduard G., Astigmat. Glas fur starrkranke, nebst bemerkungen uber die statistik des sehvermogens nach cataractoperationen. Transactions of the American Opth. Society. Eighth Annual Meeting, July, 1872.

1219. Liebreich, Eine neue methode der cataractextraction. Berlin, 1872.
St. Thomas Hosp. Rep., II, p. 259.

1220. Milliot, Benjamin, Ueber regeneration der krystallinse bei einigen
saugetheiren. Journ. de l'Anatomie et de la Phys., VIII, 1, p. 1.

1221. Rothmund, A., Die neueren methoden der staaroperation, mitgetheilt von Berger. Blatter fur Heilwissenschaft, III, 1 u. 2.

1222. Wolfe. J. P., Ueber traumat. cataracte und deren operation. Brit.
Med. Journ., Jan. u. March.

1223. Coates, Traumat. cataracte. Operation. Lancet, I, 28.

1224. Forster, Accommodationsvermogen bei aphakie. Klin. Monatsbl.,
X, p. 39.

1225. Jeaffreson, Schichtstaar. Iridectomie. Brit. Med. Journ., p. 612.

1226. Panus. Ueber cataractoperation. Gaz. des Hop., p. 452.

1227. Taylor. Bribosia, Hansen. Discussion uber staaroperation. Klin.
Monatsbl., X, Sept.

1228. Wolfe, Traumat. cataract. Ibidem.

1229. Cowell. George. Entzundung des uvealtractus bei vater und 3
Sohnen; anfangliche affection des rechten auges bei allen, darauf
folgende affection des linken auges bei 2; cataractose linse in 4
augen; congenitale cataract bei der Mutter. Opth. Hosp. Rep.,
VII, 3, p. 333.

1230. Harlan George C., Nuclearcataracte. Phila. Med. Times, II, 43, 47.

1231. Jacobson, Widerlegung der neuesten angriffe gegen v. Graefe's
linearextraction. A. f. O., XVIII, 1, p. 297.

1232. Streatfeild, Ueber die vortheile der anwendung scharfer haken bei
der cataractoperation. Lancet, II, 2.

1233. Driver, Bericht uber 50 staarextractionen nach der A. Weber'schen
methode. A. f. O., XVIII, 2, p. 200.

1872. 1234. Fano, Ueber ein wenig bekanntes vorkommiss bei der cataractoperation nach der "preussischen" methode. L'Union, p. 146.

1235. Goodmann, Cataract operation nach Liebbreich's neuer methode.
Phil. Med. Times, III, 50.

1236. Jeaffrson, Ueber cataractextraction. Lancet, I₁, December.

1237. Lawson, George, Einheilung eines eisensplitters in die linse, extraction derselben mit dem fremden korper. Hilung. Med. Times
and Gaz., p. 569.

1238. Watson, W. Spencer, Ueber lappenextraction der cataracte. Lancet, II, p. 866.

1239. Anagnostakis, Zur geschichte der opthalmiatrischen chirurgie im
Alterthum. Gaz. Hebd., No. 9.

1240. ——. Annual report of the Massachusetts charitable eye and ear
infirmary, 1873. Boston. (Report on 64 cataract extractions according to the method of von Graefe, by Dr. Hasket-Derby.)

1241. Baudry, S., Des principaux procedes d'extraction de la cataracte.
Parallele et critique. 52 pp. Paris. A. Parent. Ann. d'Oc., 70,
p. 107.

1242. Boniver, Use of phosphorous in cases of cataract. Lancet, II, p. 735.

1243. Braun, Gustav (Moskau), Ein beitrag zur nachstaaroperation. Klin.
Monatshefte f. Augenh., p. 142.

1244. Brettauer, Dimonstrazione d'un caso di cataratta corticale posteriore. Indettorina, II. Morgagni

1245. Bibrosia, Modifications a apporter, en certains circonstances, a l'operation de la cataracte par extraction lineaire. Discussion Congres de Londres. Compterendu, p. 41-46.

1246. Chassaignac, Sur les divers modes d'extraction de la cataracte.
Societe de Chirurg., 21 Mai. Gaz. des Hop., p. 667.

1247. Coert, J., De schijabare accommodatie bij aphakie. Dissert. Inaug.
Utrecht. Bijbladen, 14 de Verslag, Nederl. Gasthuis voor oglij-
ders, p. 33-84.

1248. Critchett, G., Einige winke fur die behandlung noch nicht opera-
tionsreifer staare. Opth. Ges. Klin. Monatsbl. f. Augenh., p.
458-467.

1249. ——, Traitement des cataractes en attendant l'operation. Ann.
d'Ocul., 70, p. 161-168. Discussion uber mit beginnender cataract
sich entwickelunde myopie.

1250. Derby, Hasket, Bericht uber 64 staaroperationen nach der methode
von Graefe. ausgefuhrt im Massachusetts Hospital. Arch. f.
Augen-und Ohrenhlk., III, 1, p. 193-198.

1251. Derby, On the importance of an accurate record of all operations
for cataract, and the results of the same, with practical suggestions. Transact. Americ. Opth. Soc., p. 58-64.

1252. Desmarres, Alphonse, Lecons cliniques sur la chirurgie oculaire,
492 pp., avec 27 figures. Paris. Asselin.

1872.   1253. Depres, L'enucleation du cristallin dans l'operation de la cataracte par deplacement. Soc. de Chirurg., 7 Mai. Gaz. des Hop., p. 596.

1254. Dhanens, B., Cataracte senile double. Ann. de la Soc. de Med. d'Anvers, p. 225.

1255. Dolbeau, Sur la valeur des differents procedes d'extraction de la cataracte. Soc. de Chir., 7 Mai. Gaz. des Hop., p. 597.

1256. Donders, F. C., Ueber scheinbare accommodation bei aphakie. Arch. f. Opth., XIX, 1, p. 56-77.

1257. Duplay, Sur la valeur des differentes methodes d'extraction de la cataracte. Discussion. Soc. de Chir., 9 Avril. Gaz. des Hop., p. 429, 451.

1258. Dutrieux, P., Quelques mots a propos de l'operation par l'extraction lineaire peripherique. Presse Med. Belge., No. 12.

1259. Fano, Lettre au redacteur de l'Union Medicale, No. 25, p. 303.

1260. ———, Memoire sur l'operation de la cataracte pendant les 13 dernieres annees (1860-73). Journal d'Oculistique et de Chirurgie de M. Fano, No. 1 u. 2, 1873.

1261. ———, Observations cliniques. 2. Luxation traumatique sous-conjonctivale du cristallin. 3. Cataracte capsulo lenticulaire adherente par la peripherie. Keratotomie superieure a lambeau. Persistance apres l'operation de la presque totalite de l'opacite capsulaire. Resorption complete au bout de deux mois. 10. Opacite capsulaire centrale. Iridectomie en haut. Amelioration considerable de la vision. 15. Cataracte traumatique avec remollissement du corps vitre. Broiement du cristallin. Resorption de la lentille et persistance d'une opicite capsulaire. Extraction consecutive de la capsule opaque par keratotomie lineaire. Retour de la vision. 25. Luxation traumatique en bas, en avant et en dedans du cristallin.

1873.   1262. Fano, Ce qu'etait le diagnostic de la cataracte il y a vingt ans, ce qu'il est aujourd'hui.

1263. Flarer, Giulio. Semplificazione al metodo di de Graefe della estrazione lineare della cataratta. Gaz. Med. Ital., Lombarda, Serie VI, Tomo VI. Annali di Ottalm., III. p. 109.

1264. Fornier, A., Ueber die narbenbildung nach der v. Graefe'schen cataractoperation. L'Union Med., No. 14.

1265. Fubini, S., Beitrage zum studium der krystallinse. Moleschott's Unters zur Naturlehre.

1266. Fumagilli, Un caso di rottura della teoria sul mecanismo dell' accommodatura. Ann. Univers., p. 355. November.

1267. Gayat, J., Experimentalstudien uber linsenregeneration. Opth. Ges. Klin. Monatsbl. f. Augenh., p. 454-458.

1268. ———, Sur la regeneration du cristallin. Congres Med. de Lyon. Seance 22, Aout. Gaz. des Hop., p. 1172. Gaz. Hebd., No. 35, p. 563.

474

1878. 1269. ——, L'operation des cataractes et la regeneration du cristallin. Lyon Med., No. 22.

1270. ——, Disposition des lambeaux de la capsule cristallinienne apres son ouverture. Lyon Med., No. 17.

1271. ——, Modification legere dans un temps de l'operation de la cataracte. Gaz. Hebd., No. 35.

1272. ——, Resultats de l'extraction lineaire dans un service de l'Hotel Dieu de Lyon pendant l'annee, 1872. Lyon Med., 16 Fevr. et 2 Mars. Ann. d'Oc., 69, p. 182-184.

1273. Remarks on cataract extraction. Suggestions for securing greater precision in reporting operations and results. Form of the corneal section. Transact. Amer. Opth. Soc., p. 65-68.

1274. Grossmann, L., Opthalmologisch-casuistische falle in der augenabtheilung des Buda-Pester allgg. Krankenhauses beobachtet. Berl. Klin. Wochenschr., pp. 351, 365. 375. 2. Cataracta calcarea s. gypsea. Entfernung derselben. 3. Cataracta calcarea, welche hinter der iris in schalenform edschien.

1275. Haltenhof, G., Cataracte traumatique luxee, resorption spontanee. Bulletin de la Soc. Med. de la Suisse Romande, No. 12. Lusanne.

1276. Hansen, Edmund, Die Liebreich'sche staaroperation. Hosp. Tidende, No. 3 u. 4.

1277. ——, Observations sur le procede d'extraction de Liebreich. Discussion. Congres de Londres. Compte-Rendu, p. 52-58.

1278. Hasner, v., Die subconjunctival extraction. Vorlaufige Mittheilung. Wien. Med. Wochenschr., p. 829-830.

1279. Haddaeus, Idar, Ueber eine modification der peripheren linearextraction v. Graefe's Klin. Monatsbl. f. Augenh., p. 350-354.

1280. Hersing, Compendium der Augenheilkunde. Erlangen.

1281. Higgens, Charles, Notes on eleven cases of operation for cataract. Med. Times and Gazette, 46, p. 412.

1282. Hogg, Jabez, Indian operation for cataract. Med. Times and Gaz., 46, p. 430.

1283. Jacob, H., The removal of cataract by solution, especially with regard to the soft cataract. The Med. Press and Circular, Febr. 5.

1284. ——, Accidents in flap extraction of cataract and the methods of avoiding them. The Med. Press and Circular, Febr. 19, March 12. Brit. Med. Journ., May 10.

1285. Jager, Eduard v., Der Hohlschnitt. Eine neue staarextractionsmethode. Mit 6 Holzschnitten. 23 pp. Wien. L. W. Seidel u. Sohn.

1286. Jaffreson, Christopher, Flap operation in cataract. Lancet, I, Jan. 11, p. 74.

1287. Jones, H. Macnaughton, Cases of cataract extraction. Cork Med. Chir. Society. Dublin Journ. of Med. Sc., Vol. LVI, p. 85-87.

1873. 1288. Knapp, H., Report of one hundred and fourteen extractions of cataract. Transact. Amer. Opth. Soc., p. 50-54.

1289. Kostecki, Z., Ueber v. Graefe's lineaire methode und deren erfolge. Gazeta Lekarska, No. 26.

1290. Leber, Studien uber den Flussigkeitswecksel im Auge. A. f. O., XIX, 2, p. 87.

1291. Lebrun, Nouvelle methode d'extraction de la cataracte par un procede a lambeau median sphero-cylindrique. Congres de Londres. Compte-Rendu, 215-227.

1292. Lefort, Leon. Sur la valeur des differentes methodes d'extraction de la cataracte. Soc. de Chir., 30 Avril. Gaz. des Hop., p. 565-581.

1293. Lindner, Sigmund, Ein fall von linsendislocation mit vollstandiger resorption der linse. Allg. Wien. Med. Z'g., No. 15, p. 237.

1294. Little, David, Tabular report and remarks on 200 cases of extraction of cataract by Graefe's modified linear section. Med. Chir. Review, January, p. 196.

1295. Logetschnikoff, Ueber die von ihm im Jahre, 1872 und 1873, nach der Graefe'schen methode gemachten linearextractionen. Opth. Ges. Klin. Monatsbl. f. Augenh., p. 483-486.

1296. Mannhardt, Franz, Accommodationsvermogen bei aphakie. Inaug. Diss. Kiel.

1297. Martin, George, Releve statistique des operations pratiquees pendant l'annee, 1872, dans le clinique opthalmologique du Dr. Wecker. Paris. A. Delahaye. 36 pp.

1298. Meyer, Traite pratique des maladies des yeux. Paris.

1299. Michel, J. (Nancy), Quelques faits pour servir a l'histoire de l'extraction de la cataracte par incision dite lineaire ou a petit lambeau de la cornee sans iridectomie. Soc. de Chir. Gaz. des Hop., p. 515-518. Gaz. Hebd., 35, p. 557.

1300. Monoyer, Ueber cataractoperation. Soc. de Chir. Gaz. Hebd., p. 157.

1301. Montmeja, de, Du diagnostic de cataractes. Fausses cataractes. Complications des cataractes. Revue medico-photographique des des Hopitaux de Peris, pp. 10, 39, 61, 104, 144.

1302. Notta, Notes sur un nouveau procede d'extraction lineaire par la cornee sans excision de l'iris. Discussion. Soc. de Chir. Gaz. des Hop., p. 124. L'Union Med., No. 20 et 28.

1303. Pagenstecher, H. u. Genth, Carl. Atlas der pathologischen anatomie des auges. Erste Lieferung. Taf., I-V, mit Text. Wiesbaden C. W. Kreidel's Verlag.

1304. Pagenstecher, 17. Jahresbericht (1872) der Augenheilanstalt fur Arme zu Wiesbaden. 30 pp.

1305. Perrin. Maurice, Des divers procedes d'operation de la cataracte. Soc. de Chir., 2 April. Gaz. de Hop., p. 408.

1306. Robinski, Recherches sur le cristallin. Congres de Londres. Compte Rendu, p. 241.

1873. 1307. Roosa, John, Liebreich's extraction of cataract. Dislocation of lens and failure to escape. Reopening of wound nine days after. Extraction of lens. Good result. Trans. Amer, Opth., p. 69, 70.

1308. Samelson, J., Cas d'aniridie traumatique avec aphakie. Congres de Londres. Compte Rendu, p. 145, 146.

1309. Savary, Sur un nouveau moyen de fixation de l'oeil dans les extractions lineaires combinees et les iridectomies. Ann. d'Oc., 69, p. 116-118.

1309a. Schweiggger, Handbuch der speciellen Augenheilkunde. 2. Aufl.

1310. Secondi, Ricardo, Sulla lussazione spontanea della lente cristallina. La nuova Liguria Med. No. 5, Annali di Ottalm., III, p. 94-97.

1311. Seely, Behandlung der cataract. The Clinic, p. 65.

1312. Stowers, J. H., Cases from the opthalmic wards. St. Barthol. Hosp. Rep., p. 140. (Luxatio lentis.)

1313. Streatfeild, J. F., Section de la cornee comme operation preliminaire. Discussion. Congres de Londres. Compte Rendu, p. 154-159.

1314. Taylor, Ch. Bell, Methode propre a empecher le prolapsus de l'iris apres l'extraction de la cataracte, au moyen de la separation de l'iris de son insertion peripherique, au lieu de l'ablation d'un segment de son limbe. Discussion. Congres de Londres. Compte Rendu, p. 38-40.

1315. ———, On the new method of extracting cataract by peripheral section of the iris without invading the pupil. Med. Press and Circular, 2.

1316. ———, Operations of cataract. Lancet, I, January 4, p. 31.

1317. Terson, Ueber linearextraction der cataract, mit oder ohne iridectomie. L'Union Med., 55.

1318. Tillaux, De l'extraction de la cataracte. Bull. Gen. de Therap., p. 541. Juin 30.

1319. Trelat, L'extraction de la cataracte. Soc. de Chir., 30 Avril. Gaz. des Hop., p. 589.

1320. Worlomont, Ueber die methoden der staarextraction und besonders uber die sog. mediane extraction. Opthal. Ges. Klin. Monatsbl. f. Augenh., p. 368-370.

1321. ———, Quelques considerations sur les procedes de l'extraction de la cataracte, et une nouvelle methode de pratiquer cette operation. Discussion Congres de Londres. Compte Rendu, p. 16-31.

1322. ———, Des procedes d'extraction de la cataracte et specialement d'extraction mediane. Gas., Hebd., No. 50.

1323. ———, Instruments nouveaux; kystotome a dard cache. Crochet cache pour l'iridodialyse. Aiguille-crochet pour la dechirure des fausses membranes, etc. Ann. d'Oc., 70, p. 219-225.

1324. Watson, W. Spencer, Flap operation for cataract. Lancet, I, Jan. 4, p. 31.

1874. 1325. Wecker, L. v., De l'extraction des cataractes adherentes. Ann. d'Oc., 69, p. 256-261.

1326. Welz, v., Ueber linearextraction. Opth. Ges. Klin. Monatsbl. f. Augenheilk., p. 370-376.

1327. ——, Die iridectomie der peripherischen linearextraction vorausgeschicht. 8 pp. Wurzburg. Fleischmann.

1328. Stein, Eine neue modification der v. Graefe'schen linear staarextraction. Med. Centrl. Bl., XII, 2.

1328. Williams (Cincinnati), Communication touchant differents sujets. (Ulcere, serpigineux de la cornee, iritis, granulations palpebrales, conjonctivite neuro-paralitique, atropine, extraction de Graefe, anomalies de refraction.) Discussion. Congres de Londres. Compte Rendu, p. 111-120.

1329. ——, Wilson, H., Des aiguilles pour pratiquer la suture apres l'extraction de la cataracte. Congres de Londres. Compte Rendu, p. 263-265.

1330. Wilson, H., Das Braun'sche verfahren zur operation des nachstaars. Klin. Monatsbl. f. Augenhlk., p. 267.

1331. Wolnow, M., Das accommodationsvermogen bei aphakie. A. f. O., XIX, 3, p. 107-118.

1332. Wolfe, Sur la cataracte traumatique. Discussion. Congres de Londres. Compte Rendu, p. 81-91.

1333. Zehender, W., Kurzer bericht uber die neuesten vervollkommnungsversuche auf dem gebiete der staaroperation. Klin. Monatsbl. f. Augenhlk., p. 313-321.

1874. 1334. Hosch, Das epithel der vordern linsenkapsel. A. f. O., XX, 1, p. 88.

1335. Arlt, Ueber verletzungen des auges in gerichtsarztlicher beziehung. Wien. Med. Wochenschr., XXIV, p. 10-14.

1336. Camuset, Georges, Ueber cataractextraction nacht der "franzosischen methode." Gaz. des Hop., 17.

1337. Del Monte, Michele, Graefe's linearextraction. Riv. Clin., 2, IV, p. 45.

1338. Stein, Eine neue modification der v. Graefe'schen lin-   ? ? ? ??

1339. Affre, Cataracte liquide a noyau flottant. Recueil d'Opth., p. 458-461.

1340. Ayres, C. S., Case of pyramidal cataract not following opthalmia neonatorum. Double iridectomie inward. Excellent visual results. The Cincinnati Lancet and Observer, p. 716-719.

1341. Agnew, C. R., A contribution to the statistics of cataract extraction of 1118 recent cases. P. 192.

1342. Adamink, E., Zur frage uber die gultigkeit der cataract-extractionsmethoden. P. 186.

1343. Becker, Otto, Atlas der patholog. Topographie des Auges, p. 241.

1344. Bresgen, H., Ein fall von angeborenem defect der linse, symmetrisch in beiden Augen. Arch. f. Augen. u. Ohrenh., IV, 1, p. 119.

478

1874. 1345. ———, Ein seltener fall von schichtstaar, Klin. Monatsbl. f. Augenh., p. 194.

Bader, C., A new cataract knife. Lancet, II, p. 760. (V. Graefe's messer unter einem stumpfen winkelgeknicht. wie es schon mehrfach von Anderen namentlich fur Iridectomieen, gebraucht worden ist.)

1347. ———, On extraction of cataract. Guy's Hosp. Rep., XIX, p. 507-516.

1348. Andre, Luxation sous-conjunctivale du cristallin sens traumatisme. Ann. d'Ocul., 72. p. 111-115.

1349. Chauvel, J., Note pour servir a l'histoire de la cataracte centrale et acquise. Arch. Gen. de Med., p. 415-433.

1350. Classen, A., Ueber die beste methode der cataractextraction. S. Oben, p. 190.

1351. Calhoun, A. W., Report of 77 operations for cataract. Atlanta Medical and Surgical Journal, September, p. 330.

1352. Cywinski, Kritik der Liebreich'schen staaroperations-methode. Medycyna Nr., 47.

1353. Coste, Un mot sur les derniers procedes d'extraction lineaire de cataracte. Marseilles Medical, Avril, 1873.

1354. Camuset, Georges, Operation de la cataracte par le procede francais. Gaz. des Hop., p. 131; p. 278.

1355. Coppez, Clinique opthalmologique de l'operation de cataracte. Journ. de Med. de Buxelles, Avril, p. 293-302, 408-422.

1356. Castorani, Raphael, Memoire sur l'extraction lineaire externe, simple et combinee de la cataracte. 106 pp. Paris. Germer-Baillliere. Gaz. des Hop., p. 1026.

1357. Carter, R., Brudenell, Mr. Bader's "new cataract knife. Lancet, II, p. 819.

1358. Chisolm, Julian J., Opthalmic and aural surgery reports. Richmond and Louisville Medical Journal, January, 1873. Ann. d'Ocul., 71, p. 94-101.

1359. Durand, Alphonse, Essai sur les cataractes lenticulaires spontanees de l'enfance. These. de Paris.

1360. Demazure, Essai sur la cataracte. These. de Paris. Nr., 289.

1361. Derby, Hasket, Report on 66 cataract extractions, being those done by the methods of von Graefe and Liebreich. S. Oben., p. 192.

1362. Del Toro, Comparison entre la keratotomie lineaire. Cron. Opthalm. Ann. d'Ocul., 73, p. 184.

1363. Saint-Germain, de, Operation de la cataracte par le procede francais. Gaz. des Hop., p. 278.

1364. Duval, Ferdinand, Quelques considerations sur les luxations spontanees et les luxations congenitales du cristallin. These. de Paris.

1365. Eberhardt, Beitrag zur pathologischen anatomie der cataracta. Sitzungsber. der Krakauer Akad. d. Wiss.

1366. Ewart, Notes on the minute structure of t he retina and vitreous humour. P. 62.

1874. 1367. Merkel, Fr., Macroscopische anatomie des auges in Graefe's und Saemisch's Handbuch der Ges. Augenheilkunde, I.

1368. Fubini, Contributo allo studio della lente cristallina. Riv. Clin. di Bologna, Vol. VIII, 2. Febbrajo und Atti della Reale Accademia delle Scienze di Torino. Vol. VIII, s. d. vorjahr. Ber., p. 57.

1369. Giraud-Teulon, L'operation de la cataracte par l'extraction lineaire. Soc. de Chirurgie. Gaz. des Hop., p. 1197.

1370. Galezowski, Nouvelle modification du procede d'extraction de la cataracte. Recueil d'Opth., p. 357-363.

1371. Gely-Guinard, Considerations sur le traitement de la cataracte par les procedes a petit lambeau median. These de Paris.

1372. Garvens, Ueber die iridotomie. Inaug. Diss. Munchen.

1373. Goldzieher, W., Beitrage zur pathologischen anatomie des auges. Pester Med. Chirurg. Presse. Nr., 28, 29.

1374. Hirschberg, Klinische beobachtungen, p. 38-44; p. 98, 100, 101.

1375. Hirschberg, J., Zur aetiologie und Therapie der cataract. Dt. Zeitschr. f. Prakt. Med., 31.

1376. Horner, Ueber den anatomischen befund bei entzundlicher kapselkatarakt. Mit ein Tafel, Opth. Ges. Klin. Monatsbl. f. Augenh., p. 462-468.

1377. Hogg, Jabez, A modified cataract knife. Med. Press and Circular, April 29, p. 351. (Mittelding zwischen v. Graefe's und Wenzel's messer. Manz.)

1378. Higgens, Ch., A new forceps for tearing through opaque capsule. p. 271.

1379. Arnold, J., Microscopische anatomie der linse und des strahlenplattchens. Mit 20 Holschn. Graefe's und Saemisch's Handbuch d. Ges. Augenheilkund, I, 1, p. 288-320.

1380. Robinski, Severin, Zur pathologie und therapie der cataract. Vorlaufige Mittheilung. Dt. Ztschr. f. Prakt. Medicin,, Nr. 6.

1381. Rydel, L., Cataracta zonularis. Przeglad Lekarski, Nr., 51.

1382. Rothmund, Ueber die contraindicationen der v. Graefe'schen linearextraction. Klin. Monatsbl. f. Augenh., p. 544-352.

1383. Schiess, Zehnder Jahresbericht, pp. 26, 34, 37.

1384. Seely, W. W., Rapid formation of a cataract. The Clinic, December 12, p. 284.

1385. Schlesinger, Adolf, Ueber beiderseitigen schichtstaar. Pester Med. Chir. Presse. p. 292.

1386. Stein, W., Eine neue modification der v. Graefe'schen linearen staarextraction. Centralbl. f. d. Medic. Wiss., p. 17.

1387. Tweedy, John, On a visible stellation of the normal and of the cataractous crystalline lens of the human eye. Opth. Hosp. Rep., VIII, p. 24-38.

1388. Terson, Double pupille artificielle dans un cas de cataracte zonulaire. Revue Med. de Toulouse, No. 10.

1871. 1389. Thompson, J., Operation for artificial pupil and subsequent extraction of a lens which had been couched sixteen years before. Amer. Journ. of Med. Sciences, Vol. LXVII, p, 378, 379.

1390. Arlt, v., Ueber die verletzzungen des auges in gerichtsarztlicher beziehung. Wiener Medic. Wochenschrift. Sept. Abdr. 100 pp. Augenoperationslehre in Graefe's und Saemisch's Handbuch, Bd. III, 1.

1391. Vidor, Sigm., Bericht uber staarextractionen. Szemeszet, Beilagen zum Orvosi Hetilap Nr., 4, 5, 6.

1392. Hippel, A. v., Fall von doppelseitiger spontaner luxation der ungetrubten linsen. Arch. f. Opth., XX, 1, p. 195-203.

1393. Watson, W. Spencer, On the advantage of opening the capsule before making the corneal section in the operation for senile cataract. Med. Times and Gaz., May 9.

1394. Warlomont, Des procedes d'extraction de la cataracte et specialement de l'extraction mediane. Ann. d'Ocul., 71, p. 5-26.

1395. Woinow, M., Seltener fall von linsenluxation. Medic. Bot. Nr., 42.

1396. Zacher, J., Blind. Staar. Eine sprachwissenschaftliche studie. Klin. Monatsbl. f. Augenh., p. 277-303.

1397. Zehender, W., Zur ernahrung der linse, nach versuchen von Bence Jones. Klin. Monatsbl. f. Augenheilk, XII. Jahrg., 1874, p. 152, 153.

1398. Hosch, Fr., Das epithel der vorderen linsenkapsel. Mit 1, Tafel. Arch. f. Opthalmology, Bd. XX, 1, p. 83-88.

1399. Friedenwald, Traumatic cataract. Philadelphia Med. and Surg. Reporter, p. 265.

1400. Assmuth, J., Subcutane injectionen von schwefelsaurem strychnin bei beginnendem staar. Dorpater Medic. Zeitschr., p. 145.

1401. Hirschberg, J., Zur statistik der cataractextraction. P. 191.

1402. Del Monte, Michele, Una mia aggiunta all' estrazione lineare modificata di Graefe. Rivist. Clin. di Bologna, Febbr., p. 45. (Die Bildung des Conjunctival lappens betreffend.)

1875. 1403. Azam, Cataracte double. Extraction des deux cristallin dans la meme seance. Accidents inflammatoires (iritis) du cote droit. Succes complet a gauche. Fausse membrane mobile dans le champ pupillaire droit. Bordeaux Med. Nr., 44.

1404. Becker, Otto, Pathologie und Therapie des linsensystems, im Handbuch der Ges. Augenheilkunde von Graefe und Saemisch, Bd. V, Cap. VII, p. 157-520.

1405. ——, Atlas der Pathologischen Topographie des Auges.

1406. ——, Krystallwulst. Opth. Ges. Klin. Monatsbl. f. Augenheilk, p. 445-449.

1407. ——, Verkalkende linse. Opth. Ges. Klin. Monatsbl. f. Augenheilk, p. 449, 450.

1875. 1408. Bresgen, H., Ein fall von partiellem schichtstaar nach verletzung der linse. Wiener Med. Wochenschr., No. 33.

1409. Briere, Guerison spontanee et rapide d'une cataracte traumatique. Gaz. des Hop., No. 84, p. 668.

1410. Barkan, 'A., Ein durch die hornhaut und pupille in die linse eingedrungenes eisenstuckchen 5 Monate spater mit der cataract erfolgreich extrahirt. Arch. f. Augen. u. Ohrenheilk, IV, 2, p. 264-268.

1411. Bjorken, J., Nyare staaroperationsmethoder. Upsala Lakarefor. Forh., Bd. XI, p. 58.

1412. Bounel, Des accidents inflammatoires consecutifs a l'operation de la cataracte. These. de Paris.

1413. Blessig, Dr., Bericht uber die in den Jahren, 1869, bis 1875, in der St. Petersburger Augenheilanstalt Ausgefuhrten Staarextractionen. Petersburger Med. Zeitschr., No. 3, p. 225-241.

1414. Becker, O., Kapseleroffnung. Opth. Ges, Klin. Monatsbl. f. Augenheilk, p. 440-442.

1415. Brute, Fils, Luxation spontanee du cristallin cataracte dans la chambre anterieure. Extraction; irido-choroldite purulente. Recueil d'Opth., p. 370-372.

1416. Brunhuber, A., Ein fall von traumatischer luxation der krystallinse in den glaskorper. Berliner Klin. Wochenschr., p. 569-585.

1417. Critchett, G., Remarques pratiques sur la cataracte congenitale. Ann. d'Ocul., T. 74, p. 220-223.

1418. Cahnheim, Ein fall von congenitaler cataract. S. Oben., p. 184.

1419. Cuignet, Remarques pratiques sur la keratotomie sclerale (procede de Graefe). Recueil d'Opth., p. 101-126.

1420. Chiralt, V., La cherotomie mediane. Annali di Ottalm., IV, p. 397.

1421. Cywinski, Luxation lentis. Medycyna, No. 13.

Demazure, Essai sur la cataracte traumatique. These. de Paris, 1874.

1423. Derby, Richard H., Report on 38 cataract extractions, performed at the New York Eye and Ear Infirmary, in the year 1874, by the surgeons of the infirmary. Fifty-fourth Annual Report of the Infirmary, p. 43-54.

1424. Toro, Del, La keratotomie mediane. Cron. Oftalm., 2. April.

1425. Dezanneau, De l'iridectomie dans l'operation de la cataracte par extraction. Bull. Gen. de Therap., T. 88, p. 390-398; p. 445-451.

1426. DeWecker, L., Sur un nouveau procede operatoire de la cataracte. Comptes Rendu de l'Acad. des Sciences, Vol. LXXX, p. 1294. Ann. d'Ocul., T. 73, p. 264-268.

1427. Dufour, Rupture du ligament suspenseur du cristallin et mecanisme de l'accommodation. Bull. de la Soc. Med. de la Suisse Romande. 18 pp.

1428. Fleuzal, Observation de cataractes noires nucleaires. Tribune Med., p. 680.

1875. 1429. Fernandez Santos. De l'eserine dans l'operation de la cataracte. La Cronica oftalm., Juin, p. 54. De l'operation de la cataracte chez les oiseaux. Cron. Oftalm., p. 181-184.

1430. Gayat, De la non-regeneration du cristallin chez l'homme et le lapin. Comptes Rendus de l'Acad. des Sciences, 20 Sept.

1431. Gorecki, Xavier, Opacites de la partie posterieure de la capsule du cristallin compliquant la cataracte senile ordinaire. Recueil d'Opth., p. 33-37.

1432. Gayet, De l'etiologie probable des cataractes zonulaires ou stratifiees. Ann. d'Ocul., T. 74, p. 55-61.

1433. Gorecki, X., Myopie progressive; guerison spontanee par absorption du cristallin. Recueil d'Opth., p. 37-41.

1434. Green, John, Notes on the examination of the eyes of a criminal executed by hanging. Transact. Amer. Opth. Soc., p. 354.

1435. Grand, S., Note sur pupille en trou de serrure. Lyon Med., p. 474.

1436. Hutchinson, Jonathan, Imperfect teeth and lamellar cataract. Trans. of the Pathol. Soc., Vol. XXVI, p. 235-244. Lancet, March 6, p. 336.

1437. Humblot, Du choix de la methode dans l'operation de la cataracte. These. de Paris.

1438. Heyl, A. G., Hyphaema following the operation of discission. Phila. Med. Times. January 2, p. 213, 214.

1439. Gayat, J., De la non-regeneration du cristallin chez l'homme et chez les lapins. Compte Rendu, p. 483. T. 81, p. 483, 484.

1440. J. Henle, Ueber die linsenfasern. Nachrichten d. Kgl. Gesellsch. d. Wissensch. zu Gottingen, No. 21, 1 Sept.

1441. Jeffries, Joy, Reports of sixteen cases of cataract operations. Boston Med. and Surg. Journal, No. 4, p. 517-520.

1442. Jacob, A. H., Case illustrative of the pathogeny and treatment of cataract. The Med. Press and Circular. No. 24, p. 421, 422.

1443. Keyser, P. D., Supplemental report of cataract extractions.

1444. Kleingunther, G., Ueber die erfolge, welche durch die Jacobson'sche extractionsmethode in der Greifswalder Klinik in den Jahren, 1873 und 1874, erzizelt wurden. Inaug. Diss. Greifswald.

1445. Lindner, Cataracta perinucleris mit micropthalmos. S. Oben, p. 187.

1446. Leber, Ueber die erkrankungen der augen bei diabetes mellitus. Arch. f. Opth., XXI, 3, p. 206-337.

1447. Lauri, Carlo, Discissione, e reclinazione ad un tempo di una cataratta traumatica, seguita da buon esito. Je Raccoglitore Medico, 20 October, p. 369-371.

1448. Lederle, J., Luxation lentis subconjunctivalis incompleta. Klin. Monatsbl. f. Augenheilk., XIII, p. 30-35.

1449. Massie, F., Des deplacements du cristallin sous la conjonctive. Paris. Delahaye.

483

1875. 1450. Pufahl, Discisio zonulae. Dt. Ztschr. f. Prakt. Medicin.

1451. Poncet, Communication sur les consequences de l'issue du corps vitre dans l'operation de la cataracte. Gaz. Med. de Paris, No. 14.

1452. Pean, Aiguille et couteaux a cataracte. Gaz. des Hop., p. 437.

1453. Pfluger, Zwei falle von plotzlich entstandener myopie in folge traumatischer linsenluxation. Klin. Monatsbl. f. Augenh., XIII, p. 109-111.

1454. Rusconi, Ulr., Caso di completa ossificazione della lente cristallina. Gaz. Med. Ital. Lomb., 17 Luglio. Annali di Ottalm., IV, p. 434. (Verf. fand in einem vor langen Jahren an Blennorrhoe erblindeten auge eine verknocherte linse, deren verknocherung, wie er vermuthet, vom kern ausging manz.)

1455. Rydel, Cataracta. Przeglad Lekarska, No. 10.

1456. Reid, Cataracta diabetica. Glasgow Med. Journ., p. 424. July.

1457. Roder, Ueber kapseldurchschneidung und dadurch bewirkte veranderung der hornhautkrummung. Opth. Ges. Klin. Monatsbl. fur Augenheilkunde, p. 362-366.

1458. Raab, Fritz, Ueber spontane dislocation der linse und ihre folgen. S. Oben., p. 56.

1459. Stoddard, Charles L., Cataract. Transactions of the Wisconsin State Medical Society, p. 56.

1460. Wengler, R., Ueber die heilungsvorgange nach verletzung der vodern linsenkapsel. Gottingen, 1874, 36 S.

1461. Schiess-Gemuseus, Kurzer bericht uber zweihundert scleralextractionen. S. Oben., p. 157.

1462. Solomon, J. V., An improved method of treating certain cases of cataract requiring e xtraction. Lancet, July 31, p. 167.

1463. Santisson, Corectopie mit linsenverschiebung. Petersburger. Med. Ztschr., p. 262.

11464. Talko, Cataractt traumatique. Resorptie lentis. Medycyna, No. 26, 36. (Referat in Virchow-Hirsch's Jahresbericht, p. 492.)

1465. Tesnier, Joseph, De la phosphaturie a forme diabetique et de son influence sur le resultat de quelques operations de cataracte. These. de Lyon.

1466. Taylor, Ch. B., Clinical lecture on a case of cataract extraction. The Practitioner, p. 340-44 and 404-411.

1467. Talko, Luxation lentis. Ibidem, No. 26.

1468. Wecker, L. v., Die periphere lappenextraction. Opth. Ges. Klin. Monatsbl. f. Augenheilk., p. 366-389.

1469. Millingen, E. van, Sur la rehabilitation de la reclinaison dans l'operation de la cataracte. Gaz. Med. d'Orient, No. 5 et 6, p. 76.

1470. Hippel, v., Beobachtungen an einem mit doppelseitiger cataract geborenen. erfolgreich operirten kinde. Arch. f. Opth., XXI, 1, p. 101-131.

484

1875. 1471. Webster, D., Ein fall von lenticonus. S. Oben., p. 185.

1472. Wengler, Rich., Ueber die heilungsvorgange nach verletzung der vordern linsenkapsel. Inaug. Diss. Gottingen, 1874.

1473. Weiss, Ueber den nach dem Weber'schen Hohlschnitt entstehenden cornealastigmatismus. Opth. Ges. Klin. Monatsbl. f. Augenhellk, p. 513-515.

1474. Williams, E., Spontaneous luxation of t he lens. Transact. Amer. Opth. Soc., p. 291-293.

1475. Zehender, Spontane luxation der linse unter die conjunctiva. Klin. Monatsbl. f. Augenh., XIII, p. 84, 85.

1476. Power, Cases of cataract. Lancet, March 27, p. 438; April 3, p. 472; May 1, p. 610.

1477. Elias, Sur la rehabilitation de la reclinaison dans l'operation de la cataracte. Gaz. Med. d'Orient, Avril.

1876. 1478. Ritter. K., Zur Histologie der Linse. I. Ueber den Bau des Centrums der Kalbslinse. V. Graefe's Archiv. f. Opthalmologie, Bd. XXII, Abth. 2, p. 255-270. (Hierzu Taf., III und IV.)

1479. ———, Ueber das centrum der linse bei der neugebornen katze. Ebendaselbst. Abth. 4, p. 26-30.

1480. O. Cadiat, Du cristallin, anatomie et developpement; usages et regeneration. These. de Paris.

1481. Thin, G., and Ewart, J. C., A contribution to the anatomy of the lens. Journ. of Anatomy and physiology, Vol. X, p. 223-231. (Plate IX.)

1482. Hofmann, Fr., und Schwalbe, G., Jahresber. uber die Fortschritte der Anatomie und Physiologie. Jahrg., 1876, p. 397.

1483. Laptschinsky, M., Ein beitrag zur chemie des linsengewebes. Arch. f. die Ges. Physiologie, Bd. XIII, p. 631.

1484. Ritter, C., Ueber den bau des cestrums der kalbslinse. Arch. f. Opthalmol., XXII, 2 Abth., S. 255.

1485. Ritter, C., Ueber das centrum der linse der neugebornen katze. Arch. f. Opthalmol., XXII, 4 Abth., S. 26.

1486. Abadie, Ch., Traite des maladies des yeux. Vol. I. Paris. Octave Doin. 501 pp.

1487. Albert, Jules, Recherches sur l'acuite visuelle mesuree plusieurs annees apres les operations de cataracte et sur la cause la plus ordinaire de sa frequente diminution. These. de Paris.

1488. Bjorken, John, Nyar staroperationsmethoder. Upsala Lakaref. Forh., II, p. 158.

1489. Baudon, Luxation spontanee du cristallin pierreux; ramollissement du corps vitre; extraction avec conservation de l'organe. Recueil d'Opthalm., p. 49-51.

1490. Cadiat, O., Du cristallin; anatomie et developpement; usages et regeneration. S., p. 76.

1876. 1491. Brailey. A., Curator's pathological report. Opth. Hosp. Reports, Vol. IX. (a) Excision of the globe containing cyst of iris following extraction of cataract, p. 55. (b) Cataract extraction followed after six weeks by sympathetic irritation (? iritis) of the other eye, p. 60. (c) Double cataract extraction, with an interval of ten days between the operations; iritis of the second eye, followed by failure of the other, p. 62. (d) Examination of an eye lost after extraction of cataract, p. 82. (e) Glaucoma in an eye which has been previously operated on for cataract, p. 84.

1492. Critchett, G., Practical remarks on congenital cataract. Brit. Med. Med. Journ., March 4, 11, p. 279, 313. Bericht f., 1875, p. 400.

1493. Dufour, M., Guerison d'un aveugle-ne. Observation pour dervir a l'etude des theories de la vision. 20 pp. Lausanne. (Linearextraction mit Erfolg. S. Oben., p. 142.

1494. Driver, Notizz uber die A. Weber'sche Hohllanzenoperation. Klin. Monasbl. f. Augenh., p. 135-137.

1495. Finlay, Ch., Excision ou enclavement d'un lambeau etroit d'iris, par une plaie peripherique independante pendant l'operation de la cataracte. Ann. d'Ocul., T. 75, p. 64-71.

1496. ——, Resultat de deux extractions de cataracte par la nouvelle methode, e tc. Ann. d'Ocul., T. 75, p. 299-301.

1497. Higgins, Ch., Clinical lecture on cataract. Med. Times and Gaz., V. 52, p. 570.

1498. Hay, Thomas., A case of senile cataract of ten years duration in a lady 86 years of age. Philadelphia Med. and Surg. Reporter, Aug. 19, p. 147. (Bei der operation dislocation der linse u. starker glaskorperverlust, ehe der kern herausgebracht wurde. Gute Heilung.)

1499. Hirschberg, J., Ueber die peripher-lineare staar-extraction. Berliner Klin. Wochenschr., No. 1, 2.

1500. Horner, Ueber nasse salicylverbande. Mittheil. aus d. Opth. Klinik. im amt.) Bericht uber die verwaltung des medicinalwesens im Canton Zurich.

1501. Hogg, J., Congenital luxation of the cristalline lens. Lancet, May 27, p. 773.

1502. Hirschberg, J., Zur anatomie der spontanen linsenluxation. Mit 1 Tafel. Archiv. f. Opthalm., XXII, 1, p. 65-72.

1503. Imre, J., Ein beitrag zur kenntniss vom zu sammenhang der linsenkapsel mit der hyaloidea. Klin. Monatsblatt f, Augenh., p. 184-187.

1504. Heyl, Albert G., Coloboma lentis. Report of the Fifth International Opth. Congress, p. 16-28.

1505. Jacob, A. H., Considerations upon soft cataract occurring in middle life, its pathology and treatment. Med. Press and Circular, May 12.

1506. Knies, Zur chemie der altersveranderung der linse. Unters. des Physiol. Instituts in Heidelberg, I, 2.

1876. 1507. Klein, S., Beiderseitige angeborene katarakt erfolgreich operirt. Klin. Monatsbl. f. Augenh., p. 370-377.

1508. Keyser, P. D., On bony formation in the place of t he lens. Report of the Fifth Internat. Opth. Congress, p. 131-134.

1509. Laptschinsky, M., Ein beitrag zur chemie des linsengewebes. S.. p. 78.

1510. Lasvenes, Fracture de la cornee, cataracte traumatique; phenomenes d'irido-choroidite. Iridectomie. Guerison. Gaz. des Hop., p. 979. (N'chts zu referiren. R.)

1511. Magnus, H., Geschichte des grauen staars. 315 pp. Mit einer Tafel. Leipzig.

1512. ———,Die staarausziehung bei den Greichen und Romern. Arch. f. Opth., XXII, 2, p. 141-184.

1513. ———, Die augenoperationen der fruheren Johrhunderte. Ein bild aus der culturgeschichte des arztlichen standes. Dt. Ztschr. f. Prakt. Medicin., No. 34, 35.

1514. Moore, Oliver, Statistical report of 40 cataract extractions. Fifty-fifth Annual Report of t he New York Eye and Ear Infirmary. p. 31-40.

1515. Martin. E., Des pansements de l'oeil apres l'operation de la cataracte par extraction. Lecon de Clinique Opthalmologique, 8. Paris. 16 pp.

1516. Panas, M., Considerations pratiques sur les cataractes. Bulletin Gen. de Therap., pp. 207, 253. 309.

1517. Peszkowski, Ein fall von cataracta traumatica mit schneller und vollstandiger heilung. Wiener Medic. Presse, S. 1260-1261.

1518. Quaglino, A., Sul valore relatico dell' estrazione lineare modificata in confronto cogli altri metodi operativi per la cataratta e sugli accidenti e complicazioni che possono compremetterne l'esito felice. Annali. di Ottalm., V, p. 263.

1519. Rothmund, Ueber den staar. Ein vortrag im Munschener Volksbildungsverein. 12 pp. Munchen. (Popular.)

1520. Schmidt-Rimpler, Ueber zuckergehalt bei cataracta diabetica. Sitzung des arztl. 'Vereins zu Marburg, 5 Jan. Berliner Klinische Wochenschrift.

1521. Sinclair, Julie, Experimentelle untersuchungen zur genese der erworbenen kapsel-katarakt. Inaug.-Diss. Zurich.

1522. Strawbridge, G., Report of forty recent cases of cataract extractions. Philadelphia Med. Times, February 19, p. 245.

1523. Snell, Simeon, On the suction operation for cataract. Brit. Med. Journ., May 13.

1524. Schiess, Ueber antiseptisches verfahren bei extractionen. 12 Jahresbericht, p. 40-45.

1525. Streatfeild, J. F., Congenital malposition of lenses; iridectomies: improvement of vision. Opth. Hosp. Rep., VIII, p. 393.

1876. 1526. Sous, G., Luxation d'un cristallin transparent dans la chambre anterieure. Ann. d'Ocul., T. 75, p. 120-123. Bordeaux Medical, p. 178, 179.

1527. Teillais, Cataracte diabetique. Glaucose dans le cristallin. Ann. d'Ocul., T. 76, p. 238-242.

1528. Taylor, Bell, A met hod of operating for cataract by which the pupil is preserved. Lancet, 5 February. Med. Times and Gaz., 52, p. 183.

1529. Hasner, v., Langbau und katarakt. Klin. Monatsbl. f. Augenh., p. 251-256.

1530. Vidor, S., Die entfernung des grauen staars nach v. Graefe's peripherum linearschnitte. Wiener Med. Wochenschrift, Nos. 45, 46, 49, 51.

1531. Weiss, Schichtstaar und Mangelhafte Entwickelung der Zahne. Memorabilien, p. 308.

1532. Williams, A. D., A brief statement of the present status of cataract extraction, with statistics and individual work. The Cincinnati Lancet and Observer, September, p. 780. (Unter 50 Fallen v. Graefe'scher extraction gingen dem verfasser 2 Augen verloren. R. H. Derby.)

1533. Ware, L., Jaeger's operation for cataract. The Chicago Medical Journal and Examiner, June, p. 496.

1534. Wolfe, Lettre sur l'extraction a lambeau peripherique. Ann. d'Oc., 75, p. 305.

1535. Williams, E., Luxatio lentis. S. Oben., p. 214.

1536. Gayet, J., De l'inutilite des pansements occlusifs apres les keratotomies et les sclerotomies. Lyon Medical. Ann. d'Ocul., T. 75, p. 252-258.

1877. 1537. Brailey, Ein cyste nach staaroperation. Centralblatt fur A. H., Vol. I, p. 2.

1538. Deutschman, Untersuchung zur pathogenese der cataract. Graefe Arch., XXIII, S. 114.

1539. DeWecker, De l'extraction de la cataract senile. Centralblatt fur A. H., Vol. I, p. 113.

1540. Dr. Leopold Weiss, Ueber den nach den Weber'schen Hohlschnitt enstehenden corneal astygmatismus und die ursache des nach extractionen enstehenden astygmatismus uberhaupt. Knapp's Arch., VI.

1541. Galezowski, De la Hermometrie en Opthalmolojie Recueil d'Opth., p. 275-307.

1542. Haskel, Derby, Practical remarks on cataract extraction. Boston Medical and Surgical Journal, November.

1543. Hirschberg, J., Ueber den lanzenschnitt zur kernstaar extraction. Centralblatt fur A. II., Vol. I, p. 2.

1877. 1544. Heyl, Coloboma lentis. Fifth Opth. Congress, held in New York.

1545. Kessler, Zur entwickelung des Auges der Wirbelthiere. Leipzig, S. 49.

1546. Knies, Uber spindelstaar und die accommodation bei denselben. Arch. fur Opth., XXIII, S. 217.

1547. Kruckow, Ein altener fall der traumatischen katarache yahresbericht. Opth. Lit. Russland Db., p. 66.

1548. Ritter K., Zur histologie der linse. Graefe Arch., Vol. XXIII, p. 156-164.

1549. Knapp, Uber capsulitis. Heidelberger Opth. Congress.

1550. Mathiessen, J., and Jacobson, Uber die brechungs coefficienten kataraktoser linsensulstanz. Zehenden Monatsbl.

1551. Lunkiewitz, M., Manie nach der kataract operation.

1552. Pagenstecher, H., Operation des grauen staars in der capsul. Graefe Arch., XXIII, p. 35.

1553. Rumschewitz, Uber die entwickelung der linse und der glaskorpers. Die Schriften der Natur Forscher zu Kiend, Vol. II, 77.

1554. Robinski, Die augen linsensterne des Menschen und der Wirbelthiere.

1555. Sammelson, Über luxation der linse. Heidelberger Opth. Congress.

1556. Teillais, Cataracta diabetica. Zuker in der Linse. (Nante Cen.)

1557. Zehender, Zur chemie der cataract. Heidelberger Opth. Congress.

1558. Diaz Rocafull, Cholesterin der linse. Yahresbericht fur 1877, uber die Opth. Literature Spanien Centralblatt.

1878. 1559. Alfred von Graefe, Die antiseplische wund behandlung bei staar extraction. Graefe Arch., XXIV, B. 1.

1560. Anagnostakis, Über die staar extraction bei alten leuten. Centralblatt fur Prakt A., p. 219.

1561. Bauerlein, 100 staar extractionen nach Graefe. Aertz. Intelligensblatt, No. 9.

1562. Coursserant, Cataracte diabetique. Paris. Centralbl. fur Prakt. A.

1563. Dr. Wodsworth, Six members of one family with congenital dislocation of the lens. Lancet, January 19.

1564. Dr. Ischmursin, Die kunstliche katarakten. Centralblatt fur Prakt A., p. 14.

1565. Del Toro, Staar extraction. Centralblatt fur Prakt. A., p. 16. De la cataracte chezles diathesiques mensuelle, p. 322.

1566. Forestier, J., Operation de cataracti. Bull. Soc. Med. de la Tonne.

1567. Fieandt, K. v., Zwei falle om extraction cataracta cum capsula. Fur Prakt. A.

1568. Martin, Geo., Über die gewonliche ursachen des misserfolgs bei der extraction der Morgagnischen staare und uber die mittel, sie zu besiege. Annales d'Oculistique, January, February.

1569. Guaita, D. L., Subconjunctionate luxation der linse nach consec sympath cyclitis am d'Ottol. Fasc. II and III.

1878. 1570. Haab, O., Beitrag zu den angeboren fehlen des auges. Ach. for Opthal., XXIV, 2, p. 276.

1571. Hassner, Aphakie. Prag. Med. Wochenschrift, No. 1.

1572. Kadyi, Das Maulwurf's Auge. Krakan.

1573. Knapp, Bericht uber ein viertes und funftes Hundert staar operation. Knapp's Arch., VI, 2, p. 314-408.

1574. Leber, Periphere kapsel spaltung. Elfte Heidelberger Congress im Pathologie der Linse Berichte uber das elfte Heidelberger Congress.

1575. L. Rydel, Beobachtungen uber den staar un staaroperationen, p.240.

1576. Mandelstramm, Angeborene luxatio lentis. Zehenten Monatsheft. Marz.

1577. Rampoli, Uber den comparativen Werth d. v. Graefe'schen modific. linear extraction.

1578. Steinheim, Eine nachblutung nach der linear staarextraction. Marz. Centralbl. fur P. A., p. 51.

1579. Tchuchardt, R., Em Pathologische Anat. der Discissionen Mang. Disst. Goettingen.

1580. Reports Gazette des Hopiteaux.

1581. Schmidt, H., Beitrag zur statistik der modificirten linear extraction.

1879. 1582. Briobat, Luxation sous-conjonctirate de cristallin. Gazette de Opth. Par., 1879, 50, p. 40.

1583. Blitz, R., Operations for cataract. Am. Med. Apos., Philad., XXX, 455-458.

1584. Belsone, G., Du operazioni di cateratta per estrazione a grande lembo. Indipendente Torino, XXX, 854-857.

1585. Bresgen, H., Zur heridatat der linsen anomaliven. Centralblatt fur A. H., April.

1586. Colsman, A., Uber die entfernung eines zus ammenhangenden moglich grossen stucke aus der vodern linsenkapsel bei der iridectomie verbundenen staaroperationen. June Centralblatt fur Prak. Augen, p. 215.

1587. Calhoun, 185 cataract extractions. Amer. Med. Apos., Philad., XXX, 455-442.

1588. Caspar, R., Uber die extraction des cataractosen linsen in Geschlosener Kapsel fur Auge., p. 195.

1589. Fitzgerald, O. G., Uber Knapps periphere kapselspaltung. Opth. Sect. of the 47th Meeting Brit. Med. Ap., Cork. August.

1590. Dr. Wecker, Chirurgie Oculare. Paris. Die combinirte periphere lappen extraction. Centralblatt f. Augen, p. 144.

1591. ——,Linear und lappens schnitt. Zehender's Monatsblatt. Oct.

1592. Deutschman, Fortgesetze untersuchungen zur pathogenese der cataract. Graefe Arch., XXV, B. 2.

1879. 1593. ——, Pathogenese der cataracte nephritica.

1594. D'Oench, Beitrag zur kentniss der e ctopia lentis congenita. (St. Louis.) Arch. f. A. H. Kunde, IX.

1595. Fajarnes, R., Cataractas negras. Cron. Optal, Cadiz, IX, 37-39.

1596. Frotingham, Cases of hard cataract operation by the modified linear method. Ann Arbor. P. 346-349.

1597. Froyana de Quintana, Que proceder es preferible para la operation de cataract? Cron. Optal. Cadiz, 159-164.

1598. Graefe, A., Uber congenitalen harten kernstaar. Bericht der Heidelberger Opth. Congress.

1599. Guerinean, Modification des procede par discission. Gaz. des Hosp. Pirs., III, 677.

1600. Caspar, R., Uber die extraction der cataractosen linsen in geschlossener kapsel. Centralblatt fur Auge, p. 195.

1601. Galezowski, Uber das rothsehen der staaroperirten. Recueil d'Opth. September.

1602. Galezowski, Einge worte uber den nachstaar und ceim operationem. Centralblatt fur Auge, p. 182.

1603. Heubel, Uber die wurkung wasser entziehender Stoffe unsbesondere auf die krystal linse. Arch. fur Gesammte Physiologie des Menschen und Thiere. Bonn. S. 24.

1604. Hassner, Uber die staar extraction. Prager Med. Mechanschrift, V. No. 8 and 9, p. 74-82.

1605. Haltenhoff, Congenitalstaar operirt an ein 7-1-2 Yahr Madchen Soc. Med. St. Geneve, Report. Centralblatt fur A. H. K., April 6.

1606. Heubel, Wirkung wasser entziehenden stoffe auf die krystallinse. Pflugger5s Arch. fur die Gesammten Physiologie, S. 21.

1607. Henbe, Zur anatomie der krystallinse. Des 23 Bericht der Kgl. Ges. der Wissenschaft.

1608. Mathiessen und Jacobson, Uber die brechungs coefficient und die chemische beschaffenheit cataractoser linse substans. Zehender's Monatsblatt. f. Augenheilkunde, August.

1609. Jany, Zan falle von beider seitige cataracta diabetica. Arch. fur Augenheilkunde, Vol. VIII. Zwei falle von beider seitigen cataracta diabetica operirt durch suction, nebst einigen bemerkungen uber dieses operations verfahren unf die Genese der diabetische cataracte. Arch. fur Augen., July.

1610. Woef, J. R., Uber die veringerung der ublen ausgange nach staar extraction. Opth. Sect. of the 47th Meeting Brit. Med. Ap., Cork. August.

1611. Knapp, Operations in several forms of complicated cataracts. Transaction of the American Opth. Society, p. 516-609.

1612. ——, Bericht uber ein 6th hundert staar operation. Centralblatt fur Augen., p. 246. December 6.

1879. 1613. Schuchardt, Karl, Zur Path. Anatomie der Discisionen. Goettingen.

1614. Michel, Nagel's Yahres Bericht.

1615. Morton, Operation for senile cataract at Moorfield Hospital during eleven months. Ropal Opth. Hospital Reports, Vol. IX, Part 3. December.

1616. Morano, Intorno agli stomi dell en sotellio della capsula del cristllins Atti del Associaz Ottalmi Ital, Riunione di Napole, Settembre, p. 61.

1617. Morton, Congenital double dislocation of the lenses in various members of one family. Royal Hospital Reports, Vol. IX, Part 8. December.

1618. Minor, Dislocation of the crystalline lens. Transaction Youngstown, Ohio, 80, p. 78.

1619. Monte, Moel, Sibenzig cataract extractionen nach v. Graefe. Ann. di Ottol. Fas., 283.

1620. Nicati, Cataracts at lesions dentaires des rhachitique. Centralblatt fur Auge, p. 159.

1621. Pagenstecher, H., Vodere glaskorper ablosung in beziehung zur bildung der cataracte und operation der cataract. Berichte der 19th Opth. Congress. Heidelberg.

1622. Paoli, C., Cateratte congenita operati dell' eta di 15 anni Sperimentate Firenze, Vol. IV, p. 47-53.

1623. Pedebidon, Deplacement traumatiques du cristallin. Gazette de Opth., Par. 78, p. 40.

1624. Pope, B. A., Extraction of hard cataract. Am. Med. Assoc., Phila., XXX, 417-430.

1625. Rydell, Klin. beobacht der kataract under ubersicht der operation fur 1869-77. April. P. 112.

1626. Sasse, H. F., Chemistry der descemetische membran untersuchung des Phys. Inst. der University Heidelberg, B. 2, Heft. 4.

1627. Sarrazin, Cataracti traumatique du cristallin. Gazette de Opth., Par. 40, p. 40.

1628. Vidor, Staar extraction szemeszet. Budapest, 49-53.

1629. Wolfe, In what manner can we avoid the danger of failure in cataract extractions. The Lancet Reference. Centralblatt f. Augen., p. 144.

1630. ——, Traumatic cataracte. British Medical Journal, February 14.

1631. Landolt, Staar extraction. Centralblatt fur Augenh., p. 282.

1632. Zehender, Brechungs coefficient und chemische bechaffenheit cataractose linsen. Berichte der 19th Opth. Heidelberger Congress.

1880. 1633. Armaignac, H., Note sur la cataracte noire f. de medicale Bordeaux, 1879-80. Vol. IX. 357-359.

1634. Borysiekiewicz, Beitrage zur extraction des grauen staars der erwachsenen. Klin. Monatsbl. f. Augen. Juni, heft.

1880. 1635. Bracchini, Luxation beiden linsen in die voderkammer.

1636. Badal, Deux cas d'ectopia du cristallin observes dans la mene famille. Journ. de Med., Bordeaux, IX, 461.

1637. ———, Coloboma des membrane de l'oed et du cristallin; cataracte noire. Gaz. des Hop., Paris, III, 489.

1638. Berthelemy, Ed., Du diagnostic de la cataracte. Paris. P. 43.

1639. Chittenden, R. H., Histo chemische untersuchung des phys. Ma. der University Heidelberg, B. 3, Heft 1.

1640. Chodin, Uber die anwendung von massage bei discissio cataractae Yahres Bericht der Opth. Literature Russland fur 1880.

1641. Kipp, Chas. H., Concerning a series of cataract e xtractions, etc. Arch. fur Augenheilk., XI.

1642. Culbertson, H., Several cases of cataract, etc. Cincinnati Lancet and Clinic, p. 255-258.

1643. Compton, J. Burnett, Curability of cataract with medicine.

1644. Cheatham, W., Can the process of cataract be stayed. Louisville Med. News, IX, 112.

1645. Chisholm, J. J., A needle operation to mature a senile cataract. Baltimore Med., VII, 19.

1646. Camuset, G., Cataracti d'origin sympathique. Gaz. des Hop., Paris, III, 483.

1647. Deutschman, Die veranderung der linse bei eiter processen im auge. Graefe, B. XXVI, B. 1.

1648. ———, Zusatz zu dem aufsalt von Ulrich. Anat. and Physiology des Canals Petit.

1649. Dr. Luca, Fall secunderehintere kapsel cataract. Inter. Opth. Congress zr. Mailand, Sept. (with discussion).

1650. ———, Healing of cataract by electricity. Medical Journal, New York.

1651. Frank, E., Beitrag zur staar extraction. Arch. f. Augenhelk., XI.

1652. Fand, Subconjunctival luxation der linse. Annali di Opth. Far., III.

1653. ———, Cataracti capsulo. Lenticulaire developpee chez me femme, etc. Journ. d'Oculaire et Chir., Par. VIII, 205-207.

1654. Fernandez Osuma, (G. F.), Bosquejo critico sobre la operation de la cataracta. Prensa. Med. de Granada, 1879-80, II, 476.

1655. Gerbach, Beitrag zur normalen anatomie des auges. Leipsig.

1656. Galezowski, Etude sur les cataractes et sur lens traitement. Recueil d'Opthal., Mars. et April, Mai, June, Juli, Aout.

1657. ———, Cataract dez les syphilitiques. Recueil d'Opth., Oct.

1658. ———, Cataract congenitaales. Ibid., Oct., Nov.

1659. Goldzieher, Die verknocherung im auge. Arch. fur Augenheilk. Knapp-Schwiegger, IX, 3.

1660. Gayet, Communication sur un point s'histologie de la cataracti capsulaire. Lyon Med., XXXIII, 15-17.

1880. 1661. Gastaldo, J., De las cataractas complicadas accident consecutive a la operation aufiteatro. Anat. Med., VIII, 74-83.

1662. Renling, G., On extraction of cataract within the capsule. Tre. N. and Chir. Fac., XXXII. Baltimore, Md.

1663. Heuse, Zwei falle von einseitger zonularer. Cataract mit knochen defecten an derselben korperhalfte. Centralblatt fur Augenheilk. June.

1664. Hirschberg, J., Ist cataract ohne operation heilbar. Virchow Arch., Bd. 80.

1665. Hogg, J., Cure of cataract and the eye aection. London. Ein casuistik der kernstaare im kinder alter. Centralblatt fur Prakt. Augenheilkunde.

1666. Jones, W., Clinical lectures on operations for cataract by discission from behind. Lancet, London, I, 903.

1667. Knies, Pathological anat. mittheilungen. C.) Klin. Monatsheft. f. Augenheilkunde. May.

1668. Leber, Kernstaarartige trubungen der linse nach verletzungen ihrer kapsel. Graefe Arch., XXVI, B. 1.

1669. Levis, R. J., Suction operation for cataract. Med. Bull., Philadelphia, II, 13.

1670. Lundy, O. J., Diabetic cataract. Michigan News, III, 168-170.

1671. Santo Fernandez, Examen de un cataracta en el fondo delojos despues de dos anos operando. Cron. Med.-Quir. de la Habana, VI, 341-344.

1672. Loring, E. G., An improved operation for a new pupil after cataract operation. N. T. Medical Journal, XXXIII, 496-503.

1673. Michelson, Ein fall von cataracta traumatica mit volstandiger resorption der linse. Der Opth. Literature, No. 12.

1674. Mohendra, Senile cataract; extraction of lens by Lawson's method. Md. Med. Gazette, Calcutta, XV. 47.

1675. McIntosh, M., A report of seventeen cases of cataract operation with remarks. Tr. Md. Ap., Atlanta, Ga., XXXI, 193-197.

1676. Marcus, Gunn, Clinical treatment of patients. Royal London Opth. Hospital Report, Vol. X, Part I. August.

1677. Manfredi, Contusionen der kapsel. Intern. Opth. Congress, zn. Mailand, Sept. (with discussion), 14.

1678. Placido, Anomalie der krystallinse. Peno d'Ische Zeitschrift fur Augenheilkunde, Lissabon, I. Mai.

1679. Rosenthal, Die physiologie der thierischen Warme Hermans Handbuch der Physiologie, IV, S. 2, 289.

1680. Rampoli, Stationarer centralstaar. Operation vergrosserung der pupilla. Annali d'Opth., Fasc. II.

1681. Rara, G., Erfolgreiche doppelseitige cataract extraction bei hochgradige hereditare micropthalmen. Annali di Opth., Fas. III.

494

1880. 1682. Reymond, C., Communicazioni sulla medicazini di Lister nel operazioni di cataracta. Gior. de Royal Acad. de Med. di Torno, 3 S.,
XXVLIII, 17-40.

1683. Semper, Die naturlichen existenz bedingungen der Thiere.

1684. St. George's Hospital Reports. Cataracts. 1877-1879, IX, 479-486.

1685. Sinri, A., Cura della cataratta secundaria (casipractisi). Bull. d'Oc.
Fienze, 1878-80, II, 105, 125, 140.

1686. Sincbair, J. G., Traumatic cataract. Trans. Med. Soc., XLVI. Nashville, Tenn.

1687. Teal, T. P., On extraction of cataracts by suction. Lancet. London,
January 29.

1688. Talko, Ein frage uber linsen luxation. Arch. fur Augenheilk., IX, 4.

1689. Ulrich, Richard, Ein anatomie und physiologie des canalis petit und
der anstosaenden den Gewebe Graefe, XXVI, B. 2.

1690. Wicher, Kiewicz, Uber die eis amvendung nach staar extractionen.
Klinische Monatsblatter fur Augenheilkunde. XVIII. January.

1691. Williams, A. D., Traumatic cataract in an old man who has a dislocation of second cervical vertebra. St. Louis Medical Society,
XXXVIII.

1692. ———, Remarkable heredity of congenital cataract in four generations; fifteen cases in one family. St. Louis Medical Journal,
April 5.

———, Bechamp, A., Recherches sur les matieres albuminoides du cristal
lin, an point de non identitate. Compt. Med., XC, No. 22.

1694. Fleury, Luxation sons-conjunctivale du cristallin survenne a la
suite dun tramatisme. Bull. et Mem. Soc. de Chir. de Paris., N.
S., Vol. VI, 135.

1695. Jones, W., Clinical lectures on operations for cataract by discission
from behind. Lancet, I, 903. London.

1696. Lall Madhul Moorje, Notes on lens of vitreo often cataract extraction. Indian Med. Journ. de Calcutta, XV, 91.

1697. Alexander, Zweiter bericht der Augenheilanstalt. Aachen.

1698. Adamuck, Opthal. Beobachtungen. Kasan, 1880.

1699. Barde, Hospital Opthal. a Geneve, Januar, 1879, bis Dec. 1880.
Geneve, 1881.

1700. Durr, Berichte uber die Opth. thatigkeit in dem Yahren, 1877-80.
Hannover, 1881.

1701. Haltenhoff, Dieuxieme rapport de la clinique pour la maladies des
yeux. Geneva.

1702. Hippel, Bericht uber die Opth. Universitats Klinik zu Giesse, 1879-
1881.

1703. Hirschberg, Yahresbericht der Augenklinik, 1881.

1704. Haas, Bericht der Augenheilanstalt zu Rotterdam, 1880.

1705. Jany, 16th Yahresbericht. Breslau, 1881.

1880. 1706. Kipp, First report of Newark Eye and Ear Infirmary.

1707. Knapp, Eleventh report of New York Eye and Ear Clinic.

1708. Kerschbaumer, Rosa, und F., Bericht uber das Yahr. 1879. Salzburg, 1881.

1709. Geppner, 10 Yahresbericht der Augenklinik in Warschau, 1880.

1710. Manhattan Eye and Ear Clinic, 1879-1880.

1711. Maier, Seventh report. Carlsruhe, 1881.

1712. Males, Extraction de cataract. Brit. Med. Journal, July, 1881.

1713. Pagenstecher, Yahresbericht, 1880. Wiesbaden.

1714. Passiatore, Bericht von Prof. Magni und Gatti. Riv. Clin., S. 2, Bd. X.

1715. Presbyterian Eye and Ear Hospital, Baltimore. 1881.

1716. Rosmini, Rendiconto clinico dell instituto opthalmico di Milano, 1874-1878. Gaz. Medital Lombard, No. 8, 9.

1717. Raehlmann, Bericht der Augenklinik. Dorpat. Oct., 1879, to April, 1881.

1718. Reymond, Alcune annotazioni sulla medicazioni di Lister, etc. I Genuaio, 1880.

1719. Rudolph, Stiftung, Bericht du K. K. Krankenstalt, in Mei, 1881.

1720. Sammelsohn, Six Yahresbericht der Colner Augen Klinik.

1721. Scholer, Yahresbericht uber die Wirksamkeit seiner Klinik im Yahre, 1880.

1722. Scellnigo, Ambulatorio clinico oculistic. Rapport per l'Anno, 1880. Roma, 81.

1723. Schiess-Gemuseus, 17 Yahresbericht der Augenheilanstalt zu Besel. 1881.

1724. Steffan, 19 Yahresbericht der Augenklinik in Frankfort. 1881.

1725. Wicheikiewicz, 3 Yahresbericht der Augenklinik fur Annen Posen.

1881. 1726. Arlt, Spontane berstung der vodern kapsel einer cataractoser linse. Bericht uber den XIII Versammullung des. Opth. Ges.

1727. Abey, Der canalis Petit und die zonuba Zinii beim Menschen und Wirbelthieren Graefe Arch., XXXVIII, B. 1.

1728. Aret, Opth. Congress Heidelberg. Klinisches Monatsblatt fur Aug., XX, B. S. 230. Marz.

1729. Belloward, V., Bemerkungen uber ein fall von spontaner linsenluxation in die vorder kammer. Arch. S. Opthal., January, February.

1730. Bresgen, Zur kentniss der linsenkapsel verletungen. Arch. fur Augenh., April.

1731. Baudon, Luxation congenitale double du cristallin en haut et en ded ans. Recueil d'Opth., April.

1732. Becker, Falle von Cataracta Axialis Finska Lakar Handb., Bd. XXXIII, 1, p. 45.

1733. Brudenell, Carter, Two cases of cataract. Lancet, No. 23.

1881. 1734. Bache, Etude sur la cataracte secondaire et sur son traitement en particulier. These. de Paris.

1735. Carreras Arago, Zundhutchen in der linse. Extraction des Fremd Korpers aus der linse. Revista di Cencias Medicas de Barcelona.

1736. ———. Arteria hyaloidea persistens in nur ein auge ablosung ihres voderes endes welches im glaskorper flottirt; cataracta corticalis posterior. Centralblatt, February, p. 44.

1737. Crittchett, George. Practical remarks on cataract. Opth. Review, Vol. 1. December.

1738. Cahn, Zur physiol. und patholog. chemie des auges. Zeitschrift f. Physio Chemie, Heft., 4.

1739. Casablanca. De l'iridectomie principal element dans les applications a l'extraction de la cataract. These. de Montpellier.

1740. Deutschmann, R., Zur physiologischen chemie der augenflussigkeit. Graefe Arch., Vol. XXVII. B. 2.

1741. Derby, Anaesthesia and non anesthesia in extraction of senile cataract. Am. Opth. Soc. of Newport.

1742. Feuer, Die operation des weichen staars. Wiener Med. Presse, No. 14-17.

1743. Fort, Uber die verbesserung bei staar operation. Gaz. des Hop., No. 4 and 5.

1744. Foerster, Uber kunstliche reifung der staare. Bericht der 13 Versammulung der Opthal. Gesellschaft, S. 133.

1745. Grandenigo, La thermometria dell ochio. Annales di Ottal., VI, 2, p. 177.

1746. Foerster, Uber kunstliche refung des staars. Arch. fur Augen., B. XII. Also, discussion. Zehender's Monatschaft. Beilagheft, p. 133.

1747. Galeszowski, De ane'gues formes particulieres des cataractes congenitales. Recivel d'Opth., No. 3. Les cataractes traumatique. Arch. d'Opth. December.

1748. Gayet, Procede d'iridectomie dans be cas de cataractes secondaires. Congress de Reines.

1749. Gaillet, Operation da la cataracte per extraction au moyen l'iridectomie simple. Gaz. Held. de Med., No. 9.

1750. Girard, La cataracte secondaire. Rev. Trimestielle d'Opthal. Praeb. October.

1751. Horner, Die antiseptische. Chirurgie Augenkrankheiten Interh. Med. Congress, London.

1752. Jany, Zur behere von der diabetischen cataract und operation derselben. Deutsch. Med. Wochenschr., No. 49.

1753. Ein frage der antisepsis bei augenoperationen. Centralblatt fur Prakt. Augenheilkunde, p. 171.

1754. Knapp, H., Bericht uber ein siebentes Hundert staar extractionen, mit historischen undkritischen bemerkungen besonders uber die periphere kapsel offnung. Arch. f. Augenheilkunde, XI, 1.

1881 1755. Landesberg, Beiderseitige spontane linsen luxation. Klin. Monatsblatt, Bd. XIX, p. 251.

1756. Laurent, Contribution a l'etude des deplacements traumatiques du
cristallin. These. de Paris.

1757. Levis, Uber aussaugung der cataract. Phila. Med. and Surg. Reporter, XVIII, 22, p. 463.

1758. Lloyd, Owen, Extraction of cataract by small angular flap at the
lower section. Birmingham Med. Review, July, p. 254.

1759. Moura, Un nouveau (?) procede pour l'operation de la cataracte;
petit lambeau mixte avec iridectomie. Periodic Dopthal, No. 5.
Lisbon.

1760. Michel, Das verhalten des auges bei storungen in circulations gebiete der carotis. Wiesbaden.

1761. Morano, Francesco, In guali forme di cataratta convenga l'extrazione della capsula in sieme alla leute. Giorn. Della Mallattive
Degli Occhi, Anno, IV.

1762. Manfredi, La profilassi antisettica nella chirurgica oculare. Colle-
zioni Italiana di Letture swiba Medicine. Lettur, 5 Maggio.

1763. Nettleship, A dislocated and opaque lens lying at times between
the sclerotic and the outer surface of the retina. Opth. Soc. of
Newport.

1764. Purtscher, O., Zwei falle Rothsehen by aphakischen. Centralblatt
fur Augenheilkunde. November.

1765. ———, Ein fall von linsen verletzung ohne folgende cataract. Augenheilkunde. June.

1766. Pagenstecher, Uber extraction der cataract in geschlossener kapsel nebst berichti uber weitere 117 Fathe. Arch. fur Augen., January 2.

1767. Placido, Un nuova anomalie de conformeciao du cristallini. Cris-
talocone polar anterior Periodico d'Opth. Practica, No. 5 and 6,
p. 80.

1768. Power, Notes on a case of congenital luxation. Lancet, April 9,
p. 155.

1769. Poloni, Recuperative tardive de la owe apres nue operation de la
cataract. Rev. d'Oculistique, No. 12, p. 273.

1770. Purtscher, Ein fall von erythropsie nach traumatic cataract. Centralblatt fur Prakt., August, p. 333.

1771. Rheindorff, Glaskorpers hexis bi scleral extraction. Leipsig.

1772. Rampoli, R., Die der cataract extraction vorausgeschickte iridectomie als vorbengungmittel. Annali d'Opth.

1773. ———, Della iridectomie considerata come atto premmutoria alla
etrazione. Annali d'Ottal., X, 109.

1774. Reymond, Alcune anauotazioni sulla medicazioni di lister nelle
estrazione della cataracta et quadri statistici delle operazioni
d'estrazione. Mt. Med. Congress zu London Opth. Soc.

498

1881. 1775. Sammelsohn, Zur flussig kelterstrommung in der linse. Klin. Mo
natsblatter fur Augenheilkunde. July.

1776. Sedjaewsky, K. W. Kurzer bericht uber die operationen von extractio cataractae nach v. Graefe. Protocall der 3 Versammulung de
Aerzte de Woroneg'schen Gourvernements.

1777. Schaefer, Ein fall von congenitalen einseitigen schicht staar. Klin.
Monatsblatt f. d'Opth., B. XIX, p. 455.

1778. Schenkl. Uber antisepsio bei augen operationen. Prag. Med. Wochenschrift, Bd. VI, S. 11.

1779. Sichel, De l'opthalmire sympathetique consecutive a l'operation de
la cataract. Rev. d'Ocul. du Sud-Oerest, II, No. 9.

1780. Saltina, Sopra alcuni casi di delirio in sequito all estrazione di cateratta. Spalanzoni.

1781. Ullmann, G., Contribution a l'etude de l'etiologie de la cataracte.
p. 102. Paris.

1782. Vidor, Uber congenitalen harten kernstaar. Wiere Med. Wochenschrift, Nos. 23 and 24, pp. 644, 676. Die Antiseplik in der Augenheilkunde.

1783. Wordsworth, A case of simultaneous dislocation of both lenses,
caused by the kick of a horse. Royal London Opth. Reports, X,
p. 204.

1784. Watson, Spencer. On the advantage of opening the capsule before
making the corneal section for cataract. Med. Times and Gazette,
No. 1610.

1785. Webster, Sympathetic infection, following operation for cataract.
Trans. of American Opth. Soc.

1786. Rymarkiewicz, Fall von angeborener partieller cataract. Medycyna.

1787. Armaignac, Cataracta congenitale double adherent a gauche. Rev.
d'Ocul. du Sud-Onest, II, No. 10.

1788. ———, Cataracte traumatique. Rev. d'Oculistique, II, No. 10, p. 221.

1789. Recuperative tardive de la vue apres une operation de la cataract.
Rev. d'Ocul., September, pp. 241, 246.

1790. Fernandez Santos, Schuss verletzung der beiden augen; resorption
der linken linse. Arch. f. Augen., Bd. X, 3. Die antiseptic bei
catteract extraction. Cronic Opthal., X, p. 81. Cadiz, 1880-81.

1792. Holmes, Ein merkwurdiger fall von verletzung des augapfels. Arch.
f. Augen., Bd. X, 3.

1793. Theobald, S.. Total congenital luxation of the lens. Amer. Opth.
Soc. Reuort.

1794. Haab, Antiseptik und operative. Fortschritte under Augenheilkunde Schweiz Cork, B. 1, Bd. XI, 2, 3 and 4.

1795. Goldzieher, Knochen bildung im umkriese der linse. Bericht der
13 Versam der Opth. Gesellschaft zu Heidelberg.

1882. 1796. Abey, Der canalis Petit und die zonula Zinnii beim memschen und wirhelthiere. Graefe Arch., XXXVIII, B. 1.

1797. Berger, Bemerkungen uber die linsen kapsel. Centralblatt fur Prakt. Augenheilkunde.

1798. Critchett, George, Practical remarks on cataract. Opth. Reviews. February.

1799. Aret, Opth. Congress, Heidelberg. Klinischen Monatsblatt fur Aug., XX, B. S., 230. Marz.

1800. Foerster, Uber die riefe des staars kunstliche reifung desselben korrelyse. Extraction der vodern kapsel. Arch. fur Augenheilkunde, XII.

1801. Galezowski, Des cataractes traumatique. Reciverild Opthal., January, 82.

1802. ———, De la aetiologie des cataract. Recueil d'Opthal. November.

1803. Gastaldo, Luxation traumatique du cristallin. Revue Clinique d'Oculistique du Sud-Ouest. May, 1882.

1804. Hirschberg, Anatomische und praktische bemerkungen zur alter-staar ausziehung, pupillen bildung und hornhaut farbung. Graefe Arch., Vol. XXVIII, 1.

1805. Hasner, Drei falle von ektopie und luxation der linse. Prager Med. Wochenschrift, VII, No. 46.

1806. Hock, Uber die operation des ange-wachsenen staares. Wiener Med. Blatter, 43 and 44.

1807. Kipp, Second Report of Eye and Ear Hospital. Newark, 1882.

1808. Kuhnt and Berger, Beitrage zur anatomie der zonula zinii. Arch. fur Opthal., XXVIII, 28, B. 2.

1809. Lowengren, opver staar extractionen. Nord. Med. Arch., Bd. 14, No. 22.

1810. Leber, Uber cataract und sonstige augen affectionen durch Blitz-schlag. Graefe Arch., Path., Vol. XXVIII, Bd. 3.

1811. Mayerhausen, Ein kentniss der erythopsie. Wiener Med. Presse, No. 42, S. 1320.

1812. Morris, Wm., Use of anesthetics in Bright's disease, and several cases of sudden death after cataract operation. American Opth. Soc., Newport.

1813. Memorsky, Uber die erkennung artificieller cataracte bei. Soldaten Wojenno-Sanit dje'lo, 1882, No. 45.

1814. McHardy, McDonald, Cataracta nigra. Opth. Society Report, January, 1882, Part II.

1815. Nettleship, Diabetic cataract. Opth. Society Report, January, 1882.

1816. Prof. Michel, Uber die naturliche und kunstliche linsentrubungen. Festschrift zur dutten Sacular feier der Alma Julia Maxamilia gewidmet von der Med. Facultate. Wurzburg. P. 53.

1817. Priestly Smith, The growth of the crystalline lens. Opth. Society of the United Kingdom. January 11.

500

1882. 1818. Presbyterian, Fourth Report of Eye and Ear Hospital, Baltimore. Chisholm.

1819. Steiner, Ein kentniss der erythropsie. Mene Med. Presse, No. 44, S. 1887.

1820. Schmeichler, Die staaroperationen an der klinik des Prof. Hofrathes, Dr. v. Arlt. Wiener Med. Wochen. Hosp., 16, 17, 19.

1821. Scholer, Flourescein und seiner bedeutung fur forschung der flussigkeitswechoel im auge. Deutschen Med. Wochenschrift, No. 2.

1822. Swan, M. Burnett, Second report of Eye and Ear Hospital, Washington.

1823. Ulrich, Ein spontane aufsugung einer cataractoser linse. Klinischen Monatsblatt fur Aug., XX, B. S., 230.

1824. ———, Klinische mittheilungen. Klinische Monatsblatter, July, 82.

1825. Wiecherkieiorcz, Fourth report of Eye and Ear Hospital, Posen.

1826. Milles, W. J., Sympathetic inflammation after linear extraction. London Opth. Review, Vol. X, Part III.

1827. Armaignac, Cataracte capsulo lenticulaires, etc. Rev. d'Ocul. du Sudoest Annee, II, 1882.

1828. ———, De l'operation de cataract chez les diathesiques et les cachectiques. Rev. d'Ocul. du Sudoest, No. 12. 1882.

1829. Angelucci, Lussazione del cristallins dell' ochio destro miopia consecutiver, etc. Quadri Statistie fram menti d'Optalmologia. Roma, 1882.

1830. Ayres, W., Gliomatose infiltration der linse. Arch. f. Augen., XI, 3, p. 327.

1831. ———, Knochen bildung in der linsenkapsel. Arch. f. Augen., XI, 3, p. 327.

1832. Abadie, De certain complications consecutives a l'operation de la cataracte et ches moyens d'y remedier. Annal d'Oculistique, LXXXVIII, p. 145.

1833. Ausset, Du traitement de la cataracte molle par le methode de l'aspiration. These de Paris.

1834. Alexander, 3 Bericht der Augenheilanstalt-Aachen. 1882.

1835. Adler, 9 Bericht St. Joseph's Kinderspital. Mel.

1836. Angelucci, Quadro de numero totale der malatti, etc. Oct., 1880, al Maggio, 1882. Roma, 82.

1837. Briere, Cataracte senile compliquee des synechis totales et d'vitis sympathetique. Gaz. des Hop., No. 12.

1838. Badal, Lecons sur l'extraction de la cataract. Gaz. Hebd. des Sciences Med. de Bordeaux, Nos. 9, 12, 15 and 18.

1839. Cohite. First Yahresbericht des Richmonder A. Klinik, 1881.

1840. Critchett, Zonular cataract. Fransc. Opth. Society, London. Vol. II, 82.

1841. ———, Practical remarks on cataract. Opth. Revue, I, 82, No. 4. February.

1882. 1842. Davidson and Lawford, Statistics Eye Department of St. Thomas' Hospital Report, IX. 1882.

1843. Donders, Twenty-third report. Utrecht, 82.

1844. Dor, Fifth report. Lyons.

1845. Dickenson, Congenital cataract. St. Louis Med. and Surg. Journ., Vol. XIII, No. 1, p. 53.

1846. Derby-Haskett, Anaesthesia and non-anaesthesia in extraction of cataract. Cambridge, 82.

1847. Galezowski, De l'influence des irites et chez choroidites sur le developpement des cataractes. Rec. d'Opth., p. 74.

1848. ———, De le valeur semi ologique des phenomens visuels chez les cataractes. Rec. d'Opth., p. 653.

1849. Gayet, Distribution de la cataract dens la region Lyonaise. Ass. Franc. pour l'Avanc. des Sciences, Sess. de 1882, al Rochelle. Prog. Med., 1882. Gaz. Opth., X, 1882. Rev. d'Ocul., III, 9, p. 208.

1850. Hodges, Preliminary iridectomie; extraction. British Med. Journal, September 2, p. 424.

1851. Henle, Zur entwickelung der krystallins und zur theilung des zellkerns. Arch. f. Mikr. Anat., 1882, p. 413.

1852. Harlan, Two cases of irideremia with lamellar cataract, etc. Med. News, April, 82.

1853. Hemeway, Soft cataract, its cause and pathology. Chicago Review. p. 88-90.

1854. Galezowski, Du spray phenique, etc. Rec. d'Opthal., III, No. 5, p. 290.

1855. Jany, Seventeenth report. Breslau, 82. Thirtieth report of Schlesischen Verein, 81.

1856. Jeffries, B. T., Eighty-six cases of cataract operation. Boston Medical and Surgical Journal; June, p. 660.

1857. Kipp, Yahresbericht Newark Eye and Ear Infirmary.

1858. Knapp, H., On extraction of cataract: clinical remarks. Medical Review, Vol. XXI, No. 7, p. 169.

1859. ———, Ein seventh hundert staar extraction. Arch. f. A., X, p. 49.

1860. Moyne, Guarigione della cataracta incipiens. Bolletino d'Oculist, IV, No. 7, p. 77.

1861. Moreal, Ricardo, La iridectomia antes de la operacione de la catarata. Opthalm. Prat. Amor., No. 2, p. 185.

1862. Massachusetts, Fifty-sixth report of Eye and Ear Infirmary. 81; Boston, 82.

1863. Mazza, Pietrification, degenerazione calcarea della lente cristallina. Genoa, 82.

1864. Muralt, Die staar extraction. Opth. Klin. in Zurich, 1870-1880. Inaug. Dis., Zurich, 82.

1865. Moyne, l'Operacione della cataracta nel grand ospedale di venezia.

1882. 1866. ———, Bolletino d'Oculo, Anno., V. No. 3, p. 91.

1867. Moura, Noro processo para a extraccao da cataracta, etc. Rio Janeiro, 1882.

1868. Nagel, Statistiche Notizen.

1869. Pena, A., De la tratamento consecutivio a extracio de la cataratta. Optalm. Prat. Anno., 1, No. 2, p. 25.

1870. Pfluger, Report of Universitatn Bern.

1871. Pagenstecher, Yahresbericht Augenheilanstalt. Wiesbaden.

1872. Presbyterian, Eye and Ear Hospital. Baltimore, 82.

1873. Pannas, Sur la cataracte nucleaire de l'enfance simulant la cataracte stratifiee on zonulaire deductions operatoires qui en deconlent. Arch. d'Opth., II. 6; p. 461.

1874. Proust, Trois observations de cataracte zonulaire. Rev. d'Ocul. de Sudouest, No. 8, p. 172.

1875. Kerschbaumer, Rosa, Fourth report of A. Salzburger.

1876. Reynold, Cataract Ext. Medical Herald. Feby., 82.

1877. Robinski, Untersuchungen zur Kenntniss der Lange und Anordung der Augenlinsen f. asern, No. 21.

1878. ———, Die structure der augenlinsenrohren. Centralblatt f. d'Med. W., No. 28.

1879. Untersuchungen uber die sogen augenlinsen fasern. Arch. f. Augenheilkunde, XI, S. 477.

1880. Robert, Essai sur le pathogenie des cataractes spontanees. These, Paris, 82.

1881. Roosa, Ll. J., Cataract Rep. Opth., Manhattan Eye and Ear Infirmary, 82.

1882. Reynolds, Dudley, Cataract extraction. Med. Herald; Feby., 82.

1883. Scholer, Yahresbericht. Berlin, 82.

1884. Samuelsohn, Kolner Yahresbericht.

1885. Scellingo, Ambulatorio clinique. Gaz. Med. di Roma.

1886. Smith, Eye and Ear Department of St. Mary's Hospital, Detroit, Mich.

1887. Struwe, First Yahresbericht. Gleiwitz.

1888. Sundy, First Report Eye and Ear Hospital of State of Michigan.

1889. Steffan, Twentieth Report, Frankfort.

1890. Stor, Ubersichtliche Zusammen stellung. Regensburg, 82.

1891. Smith, Priestly, Spontaneous dislocation of the lens into the anterior chamber, with secondary glaucoma. Opth. Rev., 1, No. 8, p. 209.

1892. Schroder, Uber eine neue Methode der Kapselspaltung. Berlin Med. W., Nos. 2 and 3.

1893. Ulrich, Rupture der Linsenkapsel. Klin. Monatsblatt, f. A., XX, p. 181.

1894. Uthoff, Uber congenitale linsenkrankungen. Scholer's Yahresbericht.

1895. Verbardi, Cataracta a forma congenita, verificata in trepatelli. Bolletino d'Oculo, Anno. V, No. 3, p. 91.

1882. 1896. DeWecker, Quelques perfestionments apportee a l'extraction de la cataract. Annal d'Oculistique, XXXVIII, p. 215.

1897. Wicherkiewicz, Ein seltener Heilungs verlauf nach ein glaucoma iridectomie nebst ein beobachtung uber traumatische linsentrubungen. Klin. M. Bl. f. A., XX, p. 181.

1898. Zestieden. Verslag van bet bestur der vereenigung; tot let verleenen van hup nind vermogenden oogliders voor. Zuid Holland-Rotterdam.

1899. Zehender, Ein Fall einseitiger congenitaler zonular cataract. Klin. Monatsblatt, XX, p. 53.

1900. Rampoldi, Sublussazione traumatica della lente cristallina. Ottalm. Ann. Univ. di Med., No. 261.

1901. Just, Tenth report. Zitau.

1883. 1902. Aix, Inaug. Dissert. Olten.

1903. Andrero, E., Extraction in the capsule.

1904. Abadie, Uber die unmittelbare Zufalle nach cataract extractionen. Societe Francaise, d'Opth., Jany., 83.

1905. Albert, Muller, Beitrag zur Lehre von der traumatischen cataract Inaug. Dissert. sub ausp. Prof. Schies Basel.

1906. Anagnostakis, At Congress of Greek Physicians. Results of 52 cataract extractions. Gaz. Med. Orient, (Min-Med-chir).

1907. Abadie, Moyens de combattre les accidents de suppuratiar consecutifs a l'operation de la cataract. Annales d'Oculistigue, Sept. and Oct.

1908. Alexander, Vierter Bericht der Augenheilanstalt fur den Regierungs Bezirk Aachen.

1909. Annual Report of Presbyterian Eye and Ear Hospital; Dec. 1, 1881, to Jany. 1, 1883.

1910. Becker, O. Wo., Uber die Wirbel und der Kernbogen in der menschlichen linse. Arch. f. Augenheilkunde, XII, 2.

1911. Breton, Cataracte Liquide d'une jaunatre, XI, Recueil d'Opth. Nov.

1912. Benson, On erythropsia in aphakia. Opthalmic Review, No. 26; Dec.

1913. Berger, Anatomische Untersuchung eines Falles Cataracts. Bsea· Braef, Arch., XXIX, 4.

1914. Badal, Lecons sur la operation de la cataracta. Paris, 83.

1915. Borthen, Lyder, Ainridin et Aphakia Traumatica, Klin. Monatsblatt fur Augenheilkunde, XXI, p. 62.

1916. Brignone, Un caso di catterata diabetica. Bolletino d'Ocul., VI, 1., p. 9.

1917. Chavernac, Extraction de la Cataracte. Retour a la Methode de Dairel Annales de Oculistique. Tomo, LXXXIX; Jan., Fevrier.

1918. Carreras-Arago, Einige Ermwagungen die bei der operativen Behandlung des Staars zu beachten sind. Reirsta de Ciencias medicas, Barcelona. Marz, 1883.

504

1883. 1919. Chardomet, Communic a l'Acad. des Sciences. Feby. 19.

1920. Carre, Cataracte Senile Manuel operation de la extraction. Gaz. d'Opth., No. 1, 2.

1921. Cano. Die Disinfection in der Augenheilkunde. La Cronica Optalmologica, April.

1922. Chisholm, J. J., Fifth annual report of the Presbyterian Eye and Ear Charity Hospital.

1923. ———, Zweiter bericht des Vorstandes des Verinnes zur Unterhaltung der Augen-med ohren heilaustalt in Gleiwirtz; Oct. 8, 15; Sept. 31, 82.

1924. Dessaner, Klinische Monatsblatter fur Augenheilkunde, XXI, p. 89. (Report. Czermak). Zur Zonula Frage.

1925. Dimmer. Zur Erythropsie, v. Wiener Med. Wochenschrift: No. 15, S. 436.

1926. Deutschman, R., Uber nephritische cataract. Graef, Arch. XXIX, B, 3.

1927. DeLaperonne, Etude clinique sur la maturation artificielle de la cataracte. These de Paris.

1928. Dor, Sixieme rapport, annuel de la clinique opthalmologime de M. le Prof. Dor a Lyon.

1929. DeHaas, Vereenigen tot het verleenen von hulp oon minvermogende ooglider voor Zind-Holland. Zeventiende Verlags Ioohende over hat jaar. 1882.

1930. Donders, Vier-en-twintiquste jaarlijksch verslag betrekklelijk de verplegnig en hot onderwijs in het Nederlandsch Gasthuis voor ooglyders. Utrecht.

1931. Dritter Yahresbericht des Vorstandes des ver eins zur Unterhaltung der Augen und Ohren heilanstael fur oberschlesein in Gleewitz. Oct., 82; Oct., 83.

1932. Eales, Three cases of traumatic dislocation of the lens. British Med. Journal, Feby.

1933. Falchi, Ld produzione dell Episthelio della cristallirde anteriore negle animali adulti allo stato sano e pathologico. Arch., p. 1, Med., VII, No. 14.

1934. Ferge, Bericht uber 100 staar extractionen nebst einigen Mitthelungen aus der Praxis Braunschivey.

1935. Fienzal, Bulletin de la clinique naturial opthalmologique de Hspice de Quinze-Vingts, Tom. 1, Fasc.

1936. George Cowell, Certaire modifications of Graefe's Linear Extraction. British Med. Journal, Jany.

1937. Galezowski, Uber die staar extraction mit und ohne Iris auschneidung. Societe Francaise. d'Opth., Jany., 83.

1938. ———, Aetiologie de Cataract. Recuell d'Opthalmologie, Janwier.

1939. ———, Extraction ohne Iridectomie Recuell d'Opthalmologie, Feb.

1888. 1940. ———, Diagnostic des Cataractes. Recueil d'Opthalmologie, Juillet, No. 7.

1941. Gallenga, Die methode per accelerare la maturzione della cateratta ecrevi cenni sulla corelisi dee torster. Giornale della R. cucademia de Medici di Torino. Aug., Fas. 8.

1942. G. Vassaux, Persistance de l'artere hyaloidienue et de la membrane pupillaire ayant determine des alterations intra ocula:res, sini ulant cliniquement un neoplasme. Arch., d'Opth., III, No. 6; Nov.-Dec.

1943. Grandenigo, Antisepsis in oculistica, Ann. d'Opth., XII, I.

1944. Holtske, Micropthalmus and Coloboma, von Kaninchen. Arch. fur Augenheilkunde, XII.

1945. Hirschler, J., Zum Rothsehen der Aphakischen. Wiener Med. Wochenschrift, 4-6.

1946. Heuse, Ein Dritter Fall von einseitiger cataract mit Knochenanomolie derselben Seite, auch fur prak Augenheilkunde; Dec., p. 367.

1947. Heitzman, C., Uber den feineren bau der linse und des Glaskorpers Ber. d'Opth. Heidelberg, XV.

1948. Hocquard el Masson, Etude sur les rapports, la forme et le mode de suspension du cristallin e l'etat physiologique. Arch. f. Opth., III, No. 2.

1949. Hirschberg, J., Anatomische und praktische Bemerkungen zur staarextraction. Berlin Med. Woch., No. 3.

1950. Holstein, Die Antisepsis in der Augenheilkunde. In Dis Berlin, 83.

1951. Haltenhoff, Troisieme rapport de la opthalmique du Mqlard. Geneva.

1952. Hirschberg, Yahresbericht seiner Augenklinik.

1953. Jnhasz, L., Zur operation des grauen staars. Yahresbericht Opth. Literature Ungarns. Szemeszet.

1954. Jefferson, A New Cataract Operation. Lancet, Jany. 27.

1955. Jany, Achzehnter Yahresbericht, 1882, uber die Wirksamkeit der Janjochen Klinik in Breslau.

1956. Karwat, Beitrag zur Erkrankung der Auge bei Carotis Atherom, Inaug. Dis. Wurzburg.

1957. Knapp, H., Farbung des Licht reflexes am Rande von in die vodere Kammer dislocirte Linsen. Ein einfaches Klinischen Exper'ment. Arch. fur Augenheilkunde, XII, 3.

1958. ———, Annual report of New York Opthalmic and Aural Institute.

1959. ———, Manchester Royal Eye Hospital, the sixty-seventh annual report.

1960. Kerschbaumer, Funfter Bericht der Augenheilanstalt in Salzburg. Yahresgang, 82.

1961. Karwal, Mariano, Beitrag zur Erkrankung des Auges bei Carotis atherom. Inaug. Dist. Wurzburg.

1962. Max, A. Arx, Ein pathologie des Schicht staars. Inaug. Dissert. Olten; sub ausp. Prof. Horner.

1883. 1964. Mayerhausen. Ungewohnliche langes persistiren der Tunica vasculosa lentis bei Kaninchen. Zeitschrift f. Vergleichende, Augenheilkunde, Thier Med., IX.

1965. Mauthner, Phlebotomie apres l'operation de la cataracte. Fasc. Med.

1966. Mazza, A., Lussazione spontanea della leute cristallino nella camera del vitreo. Annal d'Opth., XII, p. 320. Mules' Hereditary Transmission of Ectopia Lentis. Opth. Rev., 1883, Vol. 2.

1967. Massachusetts Charitable Eye and Ear Infirmary, fifty-seventh annual report, for, the year 1882.

1968. Manhardt, Poliklinik der vaterlandischen Frauen hilf verein fur 1882.

1969. Nikolsky, D., Mangel der Linse Matschebnija Wjedomoski, No. 36. Yahresbericht der Opth. Literature. Russland.

1970. Noyes, H. D., Foerster's operation for ripening of cataract. Med. Record, 4, Aug.

1971. Purtscher, O., Ein Frage der Erythropsie Aphakischer. Centralblatt fur Augenheilkunde. Juni, 83.

1972. Ph. Steffan, Der periphere flache Lappenschnitt nebst einem Referat uber 300 weitere cataract extraction. Graef Arch., Vol. XXIX, 2.

1973. Smith, Priestley, Growth of crystalline lens. Opth. Soc. of United Kingdom, Jan. 11, 1883.

1974. Prouff. J. M., Procede simple, facile sur de la cataracte Morgagnie nue a noyau flottant. Revue Clin. d'Oculistique, No. 5, 80.

1975. Pflugger, Hemorrhage in dem Canalis Petit. Berlin Méd. Wochenschrift, No. 42.

1976. Panas, Cataracte Traumatique Jour de Med. et de Chirr Feovier.

1977. Pfluger. Yahresbericht der Universitats Augenklinik in Bern uber Yahr, 81.

1978. Pagenstecher. Yahresbericht pro 1882 der Augenheilaustell fur Arme in Wiesbaden.

1979. Quaglino. Intorno alla hissaziono del cristallino. Annal di Ottalm.. XII, p. 522.

1980. Rodero, F., Uber die staar operation. Revista Estramena de Medicina Cirujia of Farmacia Mai el Juni.

1981. Rossander, Carl J., Om Kapsel in di Klamming vid starextractioner och om iridotomien, (Hygiea, S. 209). Yahresbericht der Scandinavischen Opth., Sit., 83

1982. Rheindorf. Discission einer angeborenen cataract bei einem 5 monat, 1 kinde. Tod. 15, Stunden nach der operation. Klinische Monatsblatter fur Augenheilkunde; Dec.

1983. Rampoldi, Cateratta nucleo-corticale in quattro indiudin della is tessa faringlia. Annal d'Ottal.

1984. Rosmini, G.. Sull estrazione lineare simplificata della cataracta molle. Annal d'Ottal. XII, 2. p. 189.

1883. 1985. Rossander, Om Kapsel, im Klamming vid starextraktionen och om iridotomien, Hyglea, p. 309.

1986. Schwalbe, Lehrbuch der Anatomie des Eirnes organ, p. 141.

1987. Snell, Simeon, Extraction of cataract through a flat, lower flap incision. British Med. Journal; Jany.

1988. Schmidt, Rimpler, Ein Aetiology der Kataract Entwickelung im mittleren Lebensalter. Klin. Monatsblatter, Mai.

1989. Scherk, Iridotomie und Discision. Klinische Monatsblatter für Augenheilkunde. August.

1990. Schmitz, George, Notizen zur staar operation. Klinischen Monatsblatter fur Augenheilkunde; Dec.

1991. Sarwage, A., De l'extraction de la cataracte method a lambeau peripherique sans iridectomie. These de Paris.

1992. Saint, Martin, Aphacie traumatique de l'oeil droit avec ectasie de l'iris. Bulletin de la Clinique de Quinqe Nigts, I, No. 2.

1993. Secondi, S., Sulla medicazozne antisettica nelle operazioni di cateratta. Annal d'Ottal, XII, p. 512.

1994. Sedan, De Hemorrhagie Consecutive a l'extraction de la cataracte. Rev. Clin. Ocul., No. 9, p. 177.

1995. Scherk, Iridotomie und Discission. Klin. Monatsblatter, XXI, p. 315.

1996. St. Mary's Hospital Annual Report. Detroit.

1997. Schies-Gemuseus, Neunzehnter Yahresbericht von Jan. 1, 1882, to Jany., 1883.

1998. Steffan, Ein und zwanziste Yahresbericht, Frankfort on M.

1999. Tepliaschin, A., Ein Casuistick des Einflusses des Ergotismus auf die Enstehung von Cataracten. Medic Wjestnik, No. 45. Yahresbericht der Opth. Literature; Russland.

2000. Terson, Des moyens d'evitur la suppuration de la plaie d'aus l'extraction de la cataracte dans le cas de catarrhe au sac lachryval. Soc. Franc., d'Opth.

2001. V. Candron, La maturation artificielle de la cataracte. Revue Gen. d'Opthal., No. 6.

2002. Van Milligan, Augenheilaustalt in Constantinople, Bericht uber Yahre, 81-82.

2003. Warlamont, De hemorrhage consecutive a l'extraction de l'cataracte.

2004. G. Bono, Astygmatie negli operati di catteratta.

2005. Robinski, S., Zur Kenntniss der Augen linse und deren Untersuchungs methoden. Berlin.

2006. Alvarado-Gomez, Juan, Consideraciones generdles practicas acerca de la operation de la cataracta. Salamanca, 1883.

2007. Armaignac, De l'operation de la cataracta chez les diathesique et cachectiques. Rev. Clin. d'Ocul. du sud ouest, Dec., 82.

2008. Hock, Bericht der Privataugen heilanstalt, von 1 Marz, 1882, to May, 1883; Merier Med. Blatter, No. 12-16.

1884. 2009. Alfred Graefe, Wund behandlung bei Augen-operationen mit besondere Berichsichtigung der Staar Extraction; operation unreife staars.

2010. Appenzeller, Ein Beitrag zur Lehre von der Erblichkeit des grauen staars. Mittheilungen an as Opth. Klinik in Tubingen. Dr. Nagel Bd., II, Heft. I. Lutingen.

2011. Aleksejew, A., Uber artificielle traumatische cataracten. Prof. der Kankas Med. Gaz., 1883, No. 12.

2012. Alexander, Funfter Bericht der Augenheil anstalt fur die Regierungs bezirk Aachen. Aachen.

2013. Adler, Zehnter Bericht uber die Augen kranken abtheilung am K. K. Krankenhause Wieden und im St. Joseph's spitale fur 1882.

2014. Birnbacher, Uber Phakokele. Graefe Arch., XXX, B., 4.

2015. Burnett, J. C., Die Heilung des Auges auf Arzneilichen Wege. Leipsig.

2016. Bull, Ch., Forster's operation for the rapid artificial ripening of cataract, with an analysis of thirty cases. New York Med. Journal, XXXIX, No. 21, p. 572.

2017. Baudin, Die Hemorrhagies intra-oculaires apres l'operation de la cataracte. Rec. d'Opth., No. 8, p. 454.

2018. Baas, J. H., Allegemeins storungen im Folge des Fragens von staarbrillen.

2019. Bull, St., The hydrochlovate of cocaine as a local anaesthetic in opthalmic surgery. New York Medical Journal, XII, 22, p. 609.

2020. Brauerlein, Augenklinik zu Wurzburg; 400 staar operationen. Wurzburg.

2021. Berger, A. M., Bericht uber die Augenheilanstalt in Munchen fur Yahr 1882.

2022. Ciaccio, Memoire della Accademie delle Scienze dell Institutio di Bologna; Sec. III, IV.

2023. ———, D'Osseraziona anatomico comparte intorno agli occhi; della Talpa illumimata equelli della Talpa cieca. Men dell Instituto di Brogna.

2024. Critchet und Juler, Case of zonular cataract. Opth. Society of United Kingdom, June, 1884.

2025. Chodin, Bericht uber die Wirksamkeit der Augenklinik an der St. Waldamar-Universitat warend Ihres, 12, Yahrigen Bestehen om Kassich Zelschrift fur Opth. July-Oct.

2026. Carreras, Y. Arago, Von den erblichen cataracten und ihrer Ubertragung auf Individwen des gleichen Geschlescts. Referal in Centralblatt fur prakt Augenheilkunde; p. 466.

2027. Carter, B., Modern operations for cataract. Lect. I, II, III, Med. Times and Gaz., No. 1750, 1752, 1754.

1884. 2028. Castorani, Memoria sull estrazione lineare inferiore della cateratta con la capsula Resoconto della. R. Acc. Med. chir. di Napoli. 1884. Tom. 38.

2029. Dehenne, Vereiterung nach staarextraction bei einem Leberkranken. Bull. de la Clinique Nat.

2030. Drake-Brockman, A statistical review of 1,767 cases of cataract extraction. Opth. Review, Vol. III; August, No. 34.

2031. DeWecker, Le Extraction Simple. Annales de Oculistique, Tom. XCI, Oct., Nov., Dec.

2032. Dubruell, De l'operation de la cataract clinique faite a l'Hospital St. Elvi de Monpellier Gaz., Med. de Par's; Juni 21, No. 25, p. 289.

2033. De Haas, J. H., Een geval van Genezing von Cataract door Reclinatio Nederl Tijdschrift voor Geneeskonde, XX, 2.

2034. Danesi, G., Sulla cataratta traumatica. Bollextino, VI, No. 6, p. 101.

2035. Dr. Jardin, Luxation traumatique du cristallin; extraction Jour des Sciences, Med. de Lille, No. 23.

2036. Duyse, van, Panopthalmie tardive apresinne operation de cataracte avec enclavement irien. Annal d'Ocul., XLII, p. 44.

2037. Dor, Septieme rapport annual de la clinique opthal. Lyon, 1884.

2038. Donders, Heft. 24, Bessaan van het Nederlandsch Gasthuis voor ooglijders Utrecht, 84.

2039. Everbusch and Pemerl, Bericht fur 1420 in der Munchener Augenklinik, Augefuhrte Staar entbindungen Arch. fur Augenheilkunde, Knapp, Schweigger, XII, 4.

2040. Fryer, B. E., Two cases of double congenital symmetrical ectopia lentis in sisters. Amer. Jour. of Opth., l., 2, p. 54.

2041. Fryer, B. C., Double congenital zonular cataract in an infant four months' old, in which atropia and duloisine produced but slight pupillary dilatation. Zeitschrift f. Ethmologie, S. 55.

2042. Fano, Des resultats fournis par les operations dans les cataracte traumatique. Journal d'Oculist, April-May.

2043. Fryer, B. C., Traumatic luxation of lens, inward, downward and backward; restoration of the normal position with fair vision. American Journal of Opth., l., 6, p. 183.

2044. Gayet, Absorption der Ultra violetten Strahlen durch Die Linse. Bull. de la Clinique Nat.

2044. Gayet, Absorption der Ultra violetten Strahlen durch Die Linse. Rec. d'Opth., No. 12, p. 703.

2046. ——, Lecon clinique sur l'operation de la cataracti. Rec. d'Opth. No. 12, p. 703.

2047. Girard, Cataractes spontanes et privitions operatoires. Rev. Trimestr, d'Opth., prak Roril, l. No. 6.

2048. Green, John, A case of rupture of zonula. Am. Jour. of Opth., l. 2. p. 43.

1884. 2049. Grandelement, Observations de luxation du cristallin. Rev. d'Ocul-istique. April, p. 101.

2050. Gieleu, Borsame in der Augenheilk der Augenheilkunde. Deutsch Med. Woch., No. 10.

2051. H. Fieunzal, Cataracte Hemorrhague. Societe Francaise d'Opth.; Jany., 31.

2052. ——, Atresis progressive du colobom artificial a la suite de certain operation de cataracte. Bull. de la Clinique Nat. Opth. de Trospice de quinzi-vingts, II., I., p. 29.

2053. Holbert, Uber eine Augen thumliche Ermudungs erscheinung des nervosen Schapparante und seine beziehung zur Erythropsia. Zehenders Klin. Monatschrift, Vol. 22, No. 7.

2054. Hirschberg, J., Cataracta diabetica. Centralblatt, S. 186. Cataracta gypsea, procidna, Centralblatt fur Augenheilkunde, S. 321.

2055. Uber die Anaestheire bei Augen operationen. Berl. Clin. Wochen-schrift, No. 50 and 51.

2056. Higgens, Extraction of Cataract. The Lancet, No. 20. Five cases of extraction of cataract in which the eye operated on successfully, was subsequently lost by sympathetic opthal., following an un-successful extraction of the second eye. Lancet, II, p. 13.

2057. Hartridge, The action of hydrochlovate of cocaine in the eye. Med. Times and Gazette. No. 1705.

2058. Horstman, Uber cocain muriaticura. Deutsche Med. Wochenschrift. No. 49.

2059. Hirschberg, Yahresbericht der Augenklinik fur 1883. Notz. Central-blatt.

2060. Hellferich, Uber Kunstliche Reifung des Staares Sitzungs bericht der Wurzburger Phys. Med. Gesellschaft, p. 115.

2061. Inonye, Privat augenklinik zu Tokio, in Japan. Report, 83; Tokio, 84.

2062. Jegorow, Bericht uber 152 staar operationen. Russiche Zeitschrift fur Opth. May.

2063. Jany, Nineteen Yahresbericht der Jany. Augenklinik in Breslau.

2064. Knapp, H., Berichti uber an achter Hundert staarextractionen nebst Bemerkungen. Arch. fur Augenheilkunde, XIII, 243.

2065. Katzaurow, J., Zur Frage der Erythropsia in folge von aphakia. Wratsch, No. 15.

2066. ——, Bericht uber das Erste Hundert von Cataract extractionen.

2067. ——, Zur Frage der Erythropsia in folge von Aphakie. Wratsch. 1884, No. 15.

2068. ——, Blutung aus dem Auge gleich nach Extraction einer Cataract, 1884, No. 36.

2069. Knapp, Hydrochlorate of Cocaine. Experiments and applications. Med. Record, Vol. XXIX, No. 17, p. 461.

.1884. 2070. Kazaurow, Ein vereinfachtes der cataract extraction. Centralblatt, f. p. A. S., 372.

2071. Klein, Erster Yahresbericht der Augenklinik im Neisse, 1884.

2072. Kolner, Augenheilanstalt fur Arme. Ninth Yahresbericht; 1883-1884.

2073. Landesberg. M., Uber das auftreten von myopie wahrend der senilen Staarbildung Centralblatt fur Augenh., April. Cataracta Diabetica Beiderseits, Philadelphia.

2074. ———, Zur Nephritioche Cataract. Graefe Arch., XXX, B., 4.

2075. Lange, O., Ein Antiseptik bei Staaroperationen. Zehenders Klinische Monatsblatter, XII, Nov.

2076. ———, Zur Frage uber die spontane resorption cataractoser. Linsentrubungen, Graefe Arch., Vol. XXX, B., 3.

2077. Landolt, La Cocain. Arch. d'Opth., No. 6, p. 535.

2078. Mengin, Iridectomie dans la operation de la cataract. Recueil d'Opth., Feby., p. 103.

2079. McKeonn, Treatment of unripe cataracts by means of injections of water. British Med. Ap., Belfast. July 92-Aug. 1.

2080. Meyer, (of Paris), Kunstliche Reifung des Staars. Eighth Internat. Med. Congress, Copenhagen. Opth., Dec.

2081. Michel, Die chemische zusammensetzung der iinsensubstanz, Copenhagen, Opth., Dec.

2082. Maklakoff, Un procede operatoire de la cataracte. Arch. d'Opthalmologie. Mai-Juni.

2083. Machek, E., Yahresbericht aus der Prof. Rydelschen Universitats Klinik-Krakau.

2084. Maufredi, Nicolo, La Lussazione spontanea del cristallino da sctopia lentis congenita et il glaucoma secundaria consecutive; Studio clinico critico. Arch. per le Scienze Med., VIII, No. 9.

2085. Matthewson, A., The natural history of the cataract. New York Med. Journal, Vol. XL, No. 5, p. 132.

2086. Meyhofer, Iodoform nach Staarextraction. Beh. Klin. Monatsblatter f. Augenh., XXII, S. 166.

2087. Martin, G., Hygiene des Instruments, gui servent a l'extraction de la cataracte. Gaz. Opth. April.

2088. Meyer. E., Anaesthesie locale de l'oeil par la cocain. Aev. Geuer d'Opthal. III, No. 10, p. 433.

2089. Manchester, Royal Eye and Ear Infirmary. Sixty-eighth Annual Report, 83-84.

2090. Massachusetts Charitable Eye and Ear Infirmary. Fifty-eighth Annual Report; 83.

2091. Meyhofer, Bericht uber die Wirksamkeit der Augenklinik in Gorlitz; 1874-1883.

1884. 2092. Mitau, Augenheilanstalt, in St. Petersburger Med. Wochenschrift, No. 1.

2093. Maier, Nermter Bericht der Augen abtheilung des Vereinsklinik Karlsruhe, 1884.

2094. Noyes, Luxation der Linse in das Corpus Vilrium, Sixteenth Opth. Congress; Heidelberg, 84.

2095. Namias, M., l'Antiseptic nella chirurgia ocular. Tese di Laurea Giornale la Revista Clinica, 1884. Marzo.

2096. New York, Opthalmic d'Annal Institute; Fourteenth Annual Report.

2097. Ottava, I., Steinplitter in der Linse. Centralblatt fur Augen, p. 420.

2098. Pagenstecher, H., Augen affectionen nach Blitzschlag. Arch. fur Augenh., XIII, p. 146.

2099. Pegrot, Retreation d'urine consecutive a une operation de cataracte. Gaz. d'Hosp., No. 134.

2100. Pflugger, Universitats-Augenklinik in Bern. Bericht uber das Yahr 1882; Bern., 1884.

2101. ——, Zur Frage der Erythropsie. Yahresbericht d'Universitate Augenklinik in Bern., 1883, S. 49.

2102. Panas, Anaesthesie locale de l'oeil par instillation de chlorhydrate de cocain. Bull. de l'Acad. de Med., No. 47.

2103. Quaglino, A., Degli antisetti nella cura consecutiva all estrazione della cateratta. Milano, 1884. Gaz. d'Hospital, No. 17.

2104. Reich, M., Die oculistik inr Kaukasus im Yahre, 1883. Wojenno. Medicinsky Journal, Oct. to Dec., 1884.

2105. Rossander, Fall af dubbelsidig linsen luxation. Hygeia, 1884. S. R. Lakeresalesk Forh., p. 30.

2106. Prof. Rydel, Eine neue methode der eroffnung der linsenkapsel bei staar operationen. Bericht uber die Augenartliche Section der IV Polnichen Natur Fovscher und Aerzte Versammelung. (Posen, Juni, 1884.)

2107. Rampoli, R., Opthal. Beitrage. Annali d'Opth., Fasc. 304.

2108. Rohmer, Cataractes congenitales completes. Soc. de Med. de Nancy Compte Rend. Gen. des Acad., Avril, No. 14.

2109. Szill, Adolp., Spontane aufsaugung einer cataractosen lins. Centralblatt fur Prakt. Augenheilkunde. January.

2110. Steinheim, B., Zur casuistik der erythropsie. Centralblatt fur Prakt. Augenheilkunde. February.

2111. Schofer, Dr. H., Der graue staar und seine behandlung. Heidelberg.

2112. Schenkl, Berichti uber die im Yahre, 1883, im Poliklinischen Institute der Deutschen Med. Facult. Prag. in Centralblatt fur Augenheilkunde, 1884, Yahresbericht der Opth. Literatur Russland Russiche Zeitschrift fur Opth. January.

2113. Sauvage, Etude historique et critique de l'extraction de la cataracte et de ses differents procedes, VIII. Recueil d'Opth., No. 3. Maro.

1884. 2114. Steinheim, Contributions a l'etude de la erythropsia. Recueil d'Opth. No. 3. Avril.

2115. Secondi, Uber die antiseptische medication bei cataract extraction-en. Annali d'Opth., Fas. 6.

2116. Schafer, Der graue staar und seine behandlung. Deutsche Med. Zeitung, No. 31.

2117. Simi, A., Intorno al secondo tempo della estrazione della cataracte capsulo lenticulari e di quelle lenticulo mature ed immature e della maturazione artificiale di quste ultime. Bollento, VII, No. 1, p. 14; No. 2, p. 47.

2118. Snell, Thermometry in cataract extraction. The Opth. Review, III, No. 10, p. 105.

2119. Salame, J., Dis hemorrhages consecutive a l'operations portant sur le globe de l'oeil. Rec. d'Opth., No. 4, p. 233.

2120. Schenkel, Das cocain ein mittel zur locale anaesthesie des auges. Prag. Med. Wochenschrift, No. 45.

2121. Schreiber, Yahresbericht der Augenheilanstalt in Madgeburg von Oct., 1882; Dec., 1883. Madgeburg.

2122. Schiess-Gemuseus, Augenheilanstalt in Basel. Zwanziqster Yahres-bericht von Jan. 1, 1883-84.

2123. Scholer und Uthoff, Beitrag zur pathologie des schuewln und netz-haut bei allgemein erkrankungen nebst ein operation. Statistik. 1882-83. Berlin, 1884.

2124. Steffan, Zwei und Zwanzigster Yahresbericht der Steffanischer Augenheilanstalt, Frankfort. Frankfort, 1884.

2125. Struve, Three Yahresbericht der Augenklinik in Gleiwitz fur 1883.

2126. Tzihi, Centralblatt fur Augenheilkunde. Eighth Year.

2127. Theobald, S., Zwei falle von maturatio corticis durch iridectomie zur beschleunigen der langsamen cataract bildung. Trans. of the Opth. Soc.

2128. Van Duyse, Aniridie double congenitale avec deplacement des cris-tallins. Annal. de la Societe de Medicine de Gand.

2129. Waldhauer, C., Vier falle von diabetischer cataract. St. Peters-burg Med. Wochenschrift, Nos. 51, 52.

2130. Wolf, J. R., An operation for cataract. Med. Times and Gazette, No. 1781.

2131. West, S., Posterior dislocation of the lens of twelve years standing, following a blow. Trans. of Opth. Eoc. of United Kingdom, III, p. 100.

2132. Weber, A., Uber die locale andwendung des cocains am auge. Zeh. Klin. Monatsbl. f. Aug., XXII, S. 443.

2133. Walker, F. P., Statischer bericht uber 63 cataract extractionen. New York Eye and Ear Inf. Trans. Am. Opth. Soc. 1883.

2134. Webster, Bericht uber 35 cataract extractionen. Trans. of the Amer. Opth. Soc.

514

1884. 2135. Wickerkiewicz, Sechster Yahresbericht uber die Wirksamkeit der Augenheilanstalt fur Arme. Posen 1884.

2136. Just, Elfter Yahresbericht uber die Augenheilanstalt zu Zittau, 1882-83. Zittau, 1884.

2137. Jacobson, Sen., Prepatorische iridectomie und antiseptische behandlung. Graefe Arch., Vol. XXX, B. 2.

2138. Creniceanu, George, Klinische erfahrung uber den zustand der zonular zinii bei gewissen staar formen bericht uber die Opth. Lit. Ungsans, 1883-84, by Dr. Szili. Centralblatt fur Augen., p. 420.

2139. ———, Cataracti traumatica partialis. By Dr. Szili, p. 23.

2140. Dr. Chilret, Technique de la operation de la Mai, June.

2141. Berger, E., Membrana pupillairs perseverans eines auges. Schichtstaar beider augen. Zeh. Klin. Monatsblatt fur Augenheilkunde, XII, S. 281.

2142. Pinto de Gama, Des hemorrhages consecutives a l'extraction de la cataract. Rev. Gener. d'Opth., No. 3, p. 97.

2143. Armaignac, A., De la hemorrhagie intra-oculaire a la suite de l'operation de la cataracte.

2144. ———, Operations de zuerison avec conservation de la vue. Rev. Clinique d'Ocul., No. 7, p. 154. Observations d'hemorrhagie operatoire a repetition chez une operee de cataracte par extraction. Paracentese tardive. Guerison. Rev. Clin. d'Ocul., No. 7, p. 163.

2145. Cuignet, Hemorrhagieo anterienres de l'ail operatoires et post operatoires. Rec. d'Opth., No. 9, p. 523.

2146. Gotti, Del emorragia consecitiva all estrazione del cataratta. Rev. Clin., No. 6.

2147. Koller, Uber die verwendung des cocaino zur anaesthesirung des Auges. Wiener Med. Wochenschrift, Nos. 43, 44.

2148. Koenigstein, Uber das cocain mevriaticun in seiner anwendung in der Okulistic Wiener Med. Presse, Nos. 42 and 43.

1885. 2149. Arlt, Winke zur staar operation. Graefe Arch., Vol. XXXI, p. 3.

2150. Aret, Verwendung der reisen gerische pincette bei der cataract extractionen. Graefe, XXXI, B. IV.

2151. Hagen, Dr. O., Torn. ein fall von entfernung des luxirten linsen kernes durch eine von den ublichen methoden. Casiustick Centralblatt fur Augenheilkunde. June.

2152. Rogman, A., Un cas de cataracte traumatique opere l'asperation. Sept., Oct.

2153. Alt, A cataract extraction followed by death. Amer. Journ. of Opth., 1885, No. 2.

2154. Agneu, A new operation for the removal of dislocated cristallin lens. Opth. Soc.

2155. Armaignac, La defaut de usage d'un oeil. Rec. d'Opth., No. 9, p. 209.

2156. Berger, E., Zur zonula frage. Graefe Arch., Vol. XXXI, B. 3.

1885. 2157. Brettauer, Spontane aufhellung cataracte linse. Heidelberger Congress, 17th.

2158. Birnbacher, Uber Phakokell. Graefe, XXXI, B. 4.

2159. Berger, E., Ein fall von erythropsie. May, 1885.

2160. St. John Rooosa, D. B., Extraction of the lens in its capsule. Med. Record, February 7, 1885.

2161. Brettremieux, Paul, Etude sur l'extraction de la cataracte. Arch. d'Opth., Tom. 5. November and December.

2162. Beiro, A l'etude de l'embryologie de c'oeil du developpement du corp vitre et de la capsule vascularise du cristallin. Rec. d'Opth., IV, 6, 7, 8.

2163. Boe, E., De cataracte syphilitique. These. de Bordeaux.

2164. Brignone, Lecado csao di cateratto diabetica. Boll. d'Ocul. Sept. 1.

2165. Baker, 27 cases of senile cataract operated by Graefe. Linear extraction. Amer. Journal of Opth.

2166. Bonagente, Operazizone di cateratta dura lenti colare el capsulo. Lenticulare per expulsione o extrazione.

2167. Bacchi, Sur l'extraction lineare inferieure de la cataracte avec la capsule. Bull. de la Clinic d'Opth., I, p. 70.

2168. Blanc, La contribution e l'etude sur la extraction du cristallin dans la capsule. Geneve, 1885.

2169. Berry, Note on the after treatment of cases of cataract extraction. Opth. Rev., IV, No. 47, p. 257.

2170. Begue, Corps etrangers du cristallin. Bull. de la Clin. Nat. Opth., No. 1, p. 69.

2171. Cozermak, Wilhelm, Zur zonula frage. Graefe Arch., Vol. XXXI, B. 1.

2172. Cross, J. F., Symmetrical dislocation of lenses upward. Congenital. Trans. of Opth. Soc.

2173. Chauvet, De la extraction de la cataracte a la clinique. Opthal. de la Facultie de Bordeaux. These. de Bordeaux.

2174. Coppez, De la extraction de la cataracte molle et particulier de la catracta traumatique par aspiration. Trans. d'Opth.

2175. DeHaas, Dr. Yahresbericht de Augenklinik zu Rotterdam f. 1884.

2176. Hock, Dr., Yahresbericht der Augenklinik Wien Privart.

2177. Sammelsohn, Dr., Yahresbericht der Kolner Wien.

2178. Huschberg, Dr., Yahresbericht der Hirschberger Wien. Berlin.

2179. Donders, Yahresbericht der Nederlandsch Gasthuis voor Coglijders. (Utrecht.)

2180. Jany, Dr., Yahresbericht der 1884, in Breslau.

2181. McKneown, Dr., Intra-capsular injicIion in cataract extraction. North Ireland Branch of Opth. Society. Hirschberg's Centralblatt fur Augenheilkunde, p. 238.

2182. Blanc, Dr. Louis. Contribution a l'etude sur l'extraction du cristallin dans sa capsule. Recherches sur la developpement du cristallin chez l'homme et quelques.

1885. 2183. Webster, Daniel, Extraction of a lens dislocated into the vitreous, with the aid of Dr. Andrew's bident.

2184. Fieunzal, Dr., Dumeillur procede de l'extraction de la cataracte senile. Bulletin de Clinique Nat. April, June. Sulla lussazione del cristallino sotto la conjunctiva.

2185. LeBlat, De la cataracte congenitale esti des Annal. de la Societe Med. et Chir. Liege.

2186. Dickey, J. L., Ein fall von angeborener ektopia lentis. Amer. Jour. of Medical Sciences. April, 1885.

2187. Dickerton, Traumatic cataract; absolute disappearance of lens and capsule without operation; perfect vision, with power of accommodation. The Lancet, 1885, II, No. 12.

2188. Dehenne, De l'intervention chirurgicale dans la luxation du cristallin. Union Med., No. 92, p. 26.

2189. Eosenko, Uber die ungunstige wirkung des cocaines bei cataract operationen. Wjestnik Opth., 1885, No. 6.

2190. Franzosichen Congress. Sitzung, April. Referat im Centralblatt fur Prakt. Augenheilkunde.

2191. Fieunzal, Compto Rendu de la Clinique pour l'Anee. 1884.

2192. Fano, Condute a suivre dans les cataractes han lantes et eu voie de deplacement. Journal des Sciences, November.

2193. ———, Hemorrhagie intra-oculaire consecutive a l'extraction du cataracte. Journal des Sciences, September.

2194. Galezowski, Staaar operation und nachbehandlung. Societe Francaise d'Opth. January, 1885.

2195. Berry, Geo. A., Note on the after treatment of cases of cataract extraction. Opth. Review, September.

2196. Galezowski, De la marche el du prognostir des cataractes. Recueil d'Opth., No. 5.

2197. ———, Traitement de la cataracte. Recueil d'Opth., No. 6.

2198. Emploi des rondelles de gelatine pour l'occlusion de la plaie. Opth., No. 8. Corneene apres l'extraction de la cataracte. No. 10.

2199. Gualta, A proposito dell 'esame anatomico di due bulbi oculare operati di ablazione della cateratta, etc. Gion. International Scienze Med., VII, 1, p. 4.

2200. Gorecki, Conduite a tenir dans les cas de cataracte incomplete. Le Pract., 1885, p. 599.

2201. Girard, Hemorrhages post. operatoires. Rev. Trimesti d'Opth.

2202. Hirschberg, J., Ein fall von Blausehen. May, 1885.

2203. Schmidt, H. and Rimpler, Zur extraction centraler rudimentarer staare und dicker nachstaare. Centralblatt fur Prakt. Augenheilkunde. June.

2204. Horning, Privart augenheilanstalt zu Ludwigsburg. Stuttgart, 1885.

2205. Hirschberg, Schadelmisbildung neben schichtstaar. Centralblatt fur Prakt. Auge., p. 235.

1885. 2206. Schiotz, Hj., Ein fall von hochgradigen hornhaut astigmatismus nach staar operation. Besserung auf operation. **Wege Central-blatt fur Auge.**, p. 469.

2207. ———, Ein fall von linsen astygmatismus nach iridectomie. Centralblatt fur Augen., p. 470.

2208. Higgens, Cataract extractions. Trans. of the Opth. Soc. of the United Kingdom, V, 116.

2209. Harlan, Two cases of subconjunctual dislocation of crystalline lens. Amer. Opth. Soc., 1885.

2210. Knapp, H., Yahresbericht der 1884. New York Augen. and Ohren. Klinik.

2211. Kasaurou, Fall von extract eines staares der 40 yahre estanden hat. Wratsch., 1885.

2212. Landesberg, Zur kentniss der transitorischen psychosen nach staar operationen. Centralblatt fur Prakt. Augenheilkunde. May, 1885. Ein nephritisch cataract. Graefe Arch., XXX, 3, S. 143.

2213. DeWecker, L., Les indication de l'extraction simple. Annales d'Oculistic, 1885, Tim. XCIV. Juillet-Avat.

2214. ———, Les causes de suppuration et d'inflammation apres l'extraction de la cataracte. Juillet, Avet, Nov., Dec.

2215. Mathiessen, Ludwig, Uber das Gesetz der Zunahme der Brechungs indices unnerhalt der krystallins der sauge thiere. Graefe Arch., Vol. XXXI, B. 2, p. 31.

2216. Magnus, Erster Yahresbericht der Augenklinik in Breslau.

2217. Mathewson, A., A case illustrating the natural history of cataract. Trans. of Amer. Journ. Opth. Soc., 1884.

2218. Nordman, Arch. fur Augenheilkunde, Vol. XIV. Fall von cataracta Morgagia mit Wasserklarer cortical flussigkeit.

2219. Nettleship, E., Note en the spontaneous disappearance of diabetic cataract. Trans. of Opth. Soc.

2220. Oettinger, Uber kunstliche reifung des staars. Inaug. Dissert. Breslau.

2221. Purtscher, O., Weitere beitrage zur erythropsie. Vol. IX, February and March.

2222. Pfluger, Universitates Augenklinik in Bern, fur yahr 1883. Bern, 1885.

2223. Panas, F., Sur la cataracte oportuite de la operation Clin. d'Opth. de Hosel Dieu. Journal de Med. et Chir., 1885, 61.

2224. ———, Du choix du meilleur procede d'extraction de la cataracte. Arch. d'Opth., 1885, Tom. V, No. 4. Juillet, Aout.

2225. Prouff, M. J., Capsulotouire simple avec cataracte cystotome et capsulotomie croisee dans cataracte cas de cataracte secondaire prodinte par les depsts vitreux on des opacities sur le capsule. Rev. Clin. Ocul., No. 4, p. 249.

1885. 2226. Rubatel, Recherches sur la developpement du cristallin. Geneve.

2227. Rubbatel, Rod., Animaux superieurs. Inaug. Diss. Geneva. 1885. (Sub. ausp. Prof. Bugnion.)

2228. Rossander, C., Om artificial staar mognad. Yahresbericht der Scandinavischen Opth. Literatur fur 1885. Referet Hirschberg's Centralblatt, p. 385.

2229. Royal Manchester Eye and Ear Hospital. Report for 1884.

2230. Redard, Note sur les procedes operatione pour la cataracte molle chez le eufante. Rev. Clin. d'Ocul.

2231. Schiess-Gemuseus, Ein beitrag zur Lehre von den angeborener linsen anomalien. Graefe, XXXI, B. 4.

2232. Schweigger, Uber cocain. Centralblatt fur Augenheilkunde, Vol. IX, January.

2233. Szili, A. Solp., Uber erythropsie. Centralblatt fur Augenheilkunde, Vol. IX, February.

2234. Schreiber's Augenheilanstalt in Madgeburg. Yahresbericht fur 1884.

2235. Schies-Gemus, Augenheilanstalt in Basel. Yahresbericht, 1884.

2236. Schenkel, Uber 100 frontal extractionen. Prag. Med. Wochenschr., 33, 34, 35.

2237. Solomon, J., Clinical lectures on congenital cataracts. Lancet, 1885, No. 9.

2238. Streatfield, Cataract extractions. Trans. of the Opth. Soc. of the United Kingdom, V, p. 116, 269.

2239. Schenkel, Uber 100 frontal extractionen. Prag. Med. Wochenschr., 1885, No. 32.

2240. Story, Cystoid cicatrix. Trans. of the American Opth. Soc. of the United Kingdom, V, p. 126.

2241. Sedan, Noe sur an corps etranger du cristallin. Rec. d'Opth., No. 12, p. 734.

2242. Schiotz, Ein fall on hochgradigen hornhaut astigmatismus nach staar extraction. Rec. d'Opth., No. 12, p. 283.

2243. Inoye, T., Yahresbericht der 1884. Privart Klinik in Tokio.

2244. Tom, Ein fall entfernung des luxirten linsenkerns durch eine von der ublichen abweichen methode. Centralblatt f. Augen., 1885, S. 176.

2245. Teillais, De la luxation spontanee des cristallin. Soc. Franc. d'Opth.

2246. Vachez, Astygmatismus et cataracte. Soc. Franc. d'Opth., 1885.

2247. Waldhauer, Dr. Sen., Zwei falle von cataracta punctata. Graefe Arch., XXXI, B. 1. Quatre cas de cataractes diabetiques. Revue Generale d'Opthal., III, 1885, Tom. IV, No. 1.

2248. Wicher Kiewicz, Uber ein neues verfahren unreife staare zu oprrieren, nebst beitrag zur augen antiseptic. Zehender's Klin Monatsblatt f. Augenheil.. XXIII, S. 478.

2249. Wadsworth, Luxation of the lens beneath Teuono capsule. Trans. of Amer. Opth. Soc.

1885. 2250. Weeks, Monocular diplopia. Trans. Amer. Med. Apos., 1884.

2251. Cuignet, Cataracte traumatque sans overture de la cristalloide. Recueil d'Opth., No. 4.

2153. Falchi, F., Sulla lussazione del cristallino sotto la conjunctiva. Annals d'Opth., Prof. Quaglino, Fas. 4.

2253. Pooley, Foerster's method of trituration. Med. Recu. S., Dec., 1885.

2254. Robinski, S., Untersuchungen und pathologischen augen linse. Ber liner Klin. Wochenschrift, No. 23.

2255. Power, Case of black cataract. Trans. of Opth. Soc.

2256. Callisti, Ublichen abweichen den methode. Centralblatt fur Augen. 1885, S. 176.

1886. 2257. Agnew, An operation with a double needle or bident for the re-moval of a crystalline lens, dislocated into the vitreous chamber, by C. R. Agnew. Hirschberg's Centralblatt, p. 236.

2259. ——, The after treatment in cataract and iridectomie operations. The Medical Record, 1886.

2259. Abadie, Des procedes actuels d'extraction de la cataracte. Annales d'Oculistique, November.

2260. ——, Des enclavement iriens et capsularis consecutive a l'extrac-tion de la cataracte avec iridectomie. Annales d'Oculistique, p. 128.

2261. Bommel, Beitrag zur aetiologie der cataracte senilis. Inaug. Dissert. Wurzburg.

2262. Bouchard and Charrin, Napthalinstaar. La Semain Medicale, No. 52.

2263. Bertrand, Des variations de forme de cristallin a l'etat patholo-gique. These. de Lyons.

2264. Becker, E., Anatomischer befund einer congenitaler eigenthumlich geformte cataract. Zehender's Klin. Monatsblatt, p. 227.

2265. Boe, F., Recherches experimentales pour servir a l'etude de la cata-racte; traumatique. Arch. d'Opth., VI, No. 4, p. 308.

2266. Brettremieux, Etude sur l'extraction de la cataracte. Arch. d'Opth. VI, No. 3, p. 268.

2267. Bucklin, Report of 200 cataract operations. Med. Record, No. 20, 1886.

2268. Bull, the employment of the thermo cautery in cataract operations. New York Med. Journal, XLIII, No. 13, p. 366.

2269. Bickerton, Cataract extraction performed on an insane patient. Lancet, I, p. 435.

2270. Bevan, Rake, Successful cataract extraction from an insane leper. Lancet. II, 587.

2271. Cuignet, Accidents apres l'operation de la cataracte. IV Recueil d'Opth., No. 5. May.

2272. Chisholm, Julian, The national method of treating cataract patients to the exclusion of compresses, bandages and dark room. The American Journal of Opth.. No. 6. June.

1886. 2273. Culberson, H., Four cases of Galezowski's method of cataract extraction, the last slightly modified. The American Journal of Opth., No. 6. June.

2274. Chibret, Indication de la iridectomie dans la operation de la cataracta. Arch. d'Opth., VI, No. 4.

2275. ——, Lois des deformations astygmatiques consecutives a operation de la cataracte. Bulletin et Memoires de la Societe Francaise d'Opth.

2276. Cuche, Du traitement de la cataracte pendant les guinz demieres annes dans le service opthalmique de Lyon. These. de Lyon, 1886.

2277. Oritchett, Practical remarks on extraction of cataract. Lancet, I. p. 913.

2278. Carter, B., Cataract extractions. Opth. Soc. of United Kingdom.

2279. Deutschman, R., Pathological anat. Untersuchung eines Menschlichen Schichtstaares. Graefe, XXXII, B. 2.

2280. DeWecker, L'avenir del extraction lineaire et de l'extraction a lambeau. Annales d'Oculistique, Tom. XCV. May and June.

2281. ——, Aetiologie de cataract. Rev. Clin. d'Ocul., 1885, Nov. 11, 12. Annales d'Oculistique, Tom. XCV. May and June.

2282. ——, Injections et pausements a l'eserine et antisepsie oculaire. Annales d'Oculistique, p. 121 to 126.

2283. ——, Traite complete. De Opth., Tom. 4, p. 702. 1886.

2284. Deuti, Eigenthumlicher fall von beider seitigen fehlen der netzhaut gefasse, nabst angeborener beider seitige trubung der hinteren linsenschichten. Gazette Medica. Italiana. Lombarda.

2285. Dufour, Sur la cataracte hemorrhagique. Soc. Franc.

2286. Eales, Extraction of cataract. Lancet, I, 977.

2287. Keibel, Fr., Zur entwickelung des glaskorpers. Arch. fur Anatomie und Physiologische Anat., Abth. 5 und 6 Heft.

2288. Fieunzal, Cataractes hemorrhagiques et hemorragies divers consecutives aux operations de cataracte. Bull. de la Clin. Nat. Opth. des Quinze-vingts, No. 4, p. 145.

2289. Faucheron, Luxation spontanee du cristallin dans la chambre anterior. Rev. d'Opth., p. 42.

2290. Frost, A., DeWecker on use of eserine and antisepsis in cataract extraction. London Med. Record, No. 133.

2291. Falchi, S., Sulla lussazioni del cristallino sotto la conjunctiva. Annal. di Ottalm., IV.

2292. Galezowski, Allgemeine indications fur die staar operations.

2293. ——, Recueil d'Opth. May.

2294. Recueil d'Opth. April. Instructions generales pour l'operation de la cataracte.

2295. ——, Soine preliminaires a donner aux malades avant l'operation de la cataracte. Recueil d'Opth. December.

1886. 2296. ——, Corneal wound in cataract extraction. Congress L. Societe Francaise. May, 1886.

2297. ——, La cataract. Progres Med., 1886, Nov. 11, p. 214.

2298. ——, Cataracte capsulaires. Progres Med., 1886, No. 11, p. 214.

2299. ——, Lettre du Dr. Rewillout sur la cataract operation. Gaz. des Hop., No. 1.

2300. ——, Instructions generales sur la operation de cataract. Revue de Sciences Med., 1886, p. 193 and 269.

2301. Gotte. Par la storia del operazione della cataracte. Revist Clin., XXV, 4, p. 286.

2302. Gayet, De la keratocystotome dans l'operation de la cataracte. Unne d'Oculistique, XCV, p. 227.

2203. Gross, Symmetrical dislocation of lenses upward. Cong. Trans. of Opth. Soc. of United Kingdom, V, p. 3.

2304. Gingnabert, Luxation dans la chambre anterieur d'un cristallin cataracte depuis 20 ans extraction. Journal de Science Med. de Lille, p. 615.

2305. Hotz, C. A., The rational treatment of cataract patients. Chicago Society of Opth., No. 11.

2306. Hirschberg, Uber staar operation. Deutsche Med. Wochenschrift, No. 18, and Centralblatt fur Prakt. Augenheilkunde, p. 410.

2307. Hilbert, Zur kentniss der erythropsie. Zehender's Klin. Monatsbl., p. 483.

2308. Jacobson, J., sen, Ein motivirtes uhrteil uber Daviel's lappen extraction und Graefe's linear extraction. Graefe, XXXII.

2309. Jegorow, J., Ein fall von cataracta calcarea accreta. Wjestnik Opth., No. 4.

2310. Jefferson, Cataract. Lancet, 3262.

2311. Kasaurow, Zur prophylaxes der septischen erkrankungen des auges nach staar operationen. Wjestnik, No. 4.

2312. ——, Cataracta hemorrhagica. Wjestnik, No. 1.

2313. Knapp, H., Cataract extraction without iridectomie. Amer. Opth. Society.

2314. Kamocki, Einige bemerkungen uber die gegenwartige cataract extraction. Gaz. le Karska, No. 34.

2315. Kramszty, R., Eine unwilkurliche mit einem holz stab vollbrachte linsen extraction. Gaz. le Karska, No. 39.

2316. Lawrentjeff, A., Eine kleine modification zur staar operation. Arch. f. Augenheilkunde, XVII, p. 125.

2317. ——, Iris. Cataracta stellata.

2318. Landesberg, Riss der voderen kapsel durch contusion. Zehender's Klin. Monatsblatter, XVIV, p. 320.

2319. ——, Aufhelung einer traumatischen cataract. Zehender's Klin. Monatsblatter, XVIV, p. 320. August.

1886. 2320. Lebedow, Zur frage der antisepsis in der Optha Chirurgie. Wjestnik Opth., No. 3, p. 191.

2321. Michel, Prof., Die temperatur topographie des auges. Graefe Arch.,
Vol. XXXII, B. 2.

2322. Michel and Wagner, Physiologisch chemische untersuchungen des
auges. Graefe, XXXII, B. 2.

2323. Meyhofer, Ein weiterer fall von cataract nach blitzschlag. Zehender's Klin. Monatsblatter f. Augen. Felmar.

2325. ——,Bemerkungen zur staar operation. Augenklinik, 1884-85.

2326. Martin, A., Maturation artificielle de la cataracte. Journ. de Med.
de Bordeaux, 1885-86, 19, p. 177-180, 189-192.

2327. Monoyer, F., Extraction de la cataracte par le procede guasi-lineaire
on a section meso cyclique simple on compose. 84 pp. Avec 6 fig.
et 6 pl. 8 Nancy. Impr. Berger-Levranet & Cie.

2328. Bordallo Pinneiro, M., Cataracta lenticulas. Hemorrhagia intra-
ocular secondaria. Gazette Medica Italiana. Lombardia.

2329. Manolescu, Extraction de cataracte molle. Annal. d'Ocul., XCV,
p. 226.

2330. Motais, Observation de cataractes congenitales et traumatiques,
traites par l'aspiration du Dr. Redard. Gaz. Med. Aout.

2331. McKeown, Intraocular injection in the extraction of cataract. Brit.
Med. Journ., I, p. 325.

2332. Martin, Maturation artificielles de la cataracte. Journ. de Med. de
Bordeaux, 1885-86.

2333. Moeller, Causistische mittheilungen uber das vorkommen und die
operative behandlung des grauen staars beim hunde. Zeit. fur
Vergl. Augenheilkunde, p. 138.

2334. Nettleship, Traumatic hemorrhage behind the lens. Opth. Hosp.
Reports, XI, 1, p. 62.

2335. ——, Neuralgia in cataractous eyes. Opth. Hosp. Reports, XI, 1,
p. 57.

2336. ——,Spontanem disappearance of diabetic cataract. Trans. of
Opth. Soc. of United Kingdom, p. 107.

2337. Noyes, Death of a patient under extraction of hard cataract. Opth.
Society.

2338. Mobius, Uber die Foerster'schen iridectomie maturans zur kunstliche reifung immature cataracte. Journ. Diss. Kiel.

2339. Perrin, Operation de la cataracte. Prog. Med.

2340. Panas, Des dernier progres realises dans operation de la cataracte
par extraction.

2341. ——, Bulletin de l'Academie de Medicine. Seance du Jar., 57, 1886.

2342. Power, Case of black cataract.

2343. Randall, B., A case of subluxation of the lens, with double rupture
of the choroid. Trans. of the Amer. Opth. Society.

1886. 2344. ———, A case of multiple rupture of the eyeball, with partial dislocation of the lens. Trans. of the Amer. Opth. Society.

2345. Robinowitch, Ein fall von ectopsie der linse mit luxation derselbe
in die vodere kammer. Wjestnik Opth., No. 1.

2346. Rothziegel, Uber die coincidence von cataract und nephritis allg.
Wiener Med. Zeitung, 1886, No. 30.

2347. Rodzewitch, Bericht uber das erste hundert nach von Graefe methode extrahirte staare. Wjestnik Opth., 1886, No. 4.

2348. Reynolds, Bandage after operation. Med. Record, August.

2349. Rampoli, Lussazizone spontanea della lente cristallina della camera
anteriore. Annal. di Ottalm., XV, 2-3, p. 179.

2350. Rothmund, Uber die gegenwartige nachbehandlung der staar operation. Munchener Med. Woch., 1886, No. 19.

2351. Renton. Note on the value of corrosive sublimate solutions in opth.
operation. British Medical Journal. No. 1340.

2352. Renard. H., De la valeur de l'iridectomie dans l'extraction de la
cataracte au point de vue des resultats de l'operation; contribution
e l'etude comparee des procedes de v. Graefe et de Daviel. These.
Nancy.

2353. Schoen, Uber die Genese der aegnastinellen cataract durch uber-
anstorengung der acc. Graefe Arch., Vol. XXXII, B. 3.

2354. ———,Zonula und grenzhaut des glaskorpers. Graefe Arch., Vol.
XXXII, B. 2, p. 149.

2355. Stellwag, Neue abhandlung aus dem gebiete der praktische Augenheilkunde. Wien.

2356. Staderini, Zwei falle von zehr seltener angeborener affection der
linse und der zonula. Annali di Ottalmologia del Prof. Quaglino,
1885, Fas. 5 and 6.

2357. Schweigger, Staar und nachstaar operationen. Versammelung
Deutscher Natur. Forscher, Sept., 1886. Centralblatt fur Augen.,
p. 282.

2358. Szili, A., Einige bemerkungen zur erythropsie frage. Zehender's
Klin. Monatsblatter. July.

2359. Strawbridge, H. G., Cataract extraction; 263 cases and discussion.
Twenty-second Annual Report of the Amer. Opth. Society, July
21 and 22, 1886.

2360. Starkey, H. M., Three cases of congenital ectopia lentis. Chicago
Society of Opth., December, 1886.

2361. Ayres, S. C., Cataracta pyramidalis. Amer. Journal of Opth., 1886.
No. 1.

2362. Story, Zonular cataract and dental malformations. Opth. Review.
p. 354.

2363. Sulzen, In vivo sichbare sternfigur in der vodern corticales bei zonula zonularis, etc. Zehender's Klin. Monatsblatt, p. 99.

1886.	2364. Staderini, Due casi di rarissima affezzione morbosa della lente cris-
	tallina e del suo legamento. Annual. di Opth., XIV, 5-6.

2365. Spalding, Radical changes in the after treatment of cataract. Brit.
	Med. Journal, November.

2366. Story, Dental malformations and zonula cataracts. The Opthalmia
	Review, October, 1886.

2367. Sprimon, Medycyna, 1886, S. 176.

2368. Telnekinn, De la capsulotomie. Annales d'Oculistique, Tom. XCV,
	1, et livraisons, 1886. Janv., Fevr.

2369. ———, De la capsulotomie. Ann. d'Oculistique, XCV, p. 43.

2370. Tyrman, J., Ein beitrage zur lehre von der erythropsie. Deutsche
	Med. Zeitung, No. 12.

2371. Uhle, Ungewohnliches sehvermogen eines operirtern auges. Ze-
	hender's Klin. Monatsblatt, p. 431.

2372. Vachez, De la operation de la cataracte. Graefe Hebd. de Med. et
	de Chir. Avril.

2373. Reuss, V., Die operation and der Second Wiener Klinik, 1884-85.
	Wiener Med. Presse, No. 49.

2374. Warlomont, Le extraction de la cataracte. Vingt-cingt and de son
	histoire. L'extraction de la cataracte. Vingt-cingt de son histoire.
	Annales de Oculistique, Tom. XCV, 1, et 2 livraisons, 1886. Janv.
	Fevr.

2375. Webster, 50 cases of cataract extraction. New York Med. Monthly.

2376. ———, Removal of a piece of steel from t he crystalline lens. New
	York Medical Monthly.

2377. Wickerkiewicz, Irrigation of anterior chamber in cataract extrac-
	tion. Congress de la Societe Francaise d'Opth. May, 1886.

2378. Lange, O., Nachtrage zu einem falle von spontanea aufhelung
	einer cataractosen linse. Graefe Arch., Vol. XXXII, B. 4.

2379. Green, R. L., Cataract. St. Louis Med. and Surg. Journ., No. 2, p. 81.

2380. Dujardin, eDux cataractes molles opera l'aspiration. Journal de
	Sciences Med. de Lille, 1886. Aout.

2381. Gunning, Sur la maturation de la cataracte. Ann. d'Oc., XCV, p. 226.

1887.	2382. Ayres, S. C., After treatment of cataract patients. The American
	Journal of Opthalmology. January.

2383. Abadie, Ch., Des procedes actuels d'extraction de la cataracte.
	Progres Medical, March 26.

2384. Baker, A. R., A further report of extractions of senile cataract.
	The American Journal of Opthalmology. January.

2385. Berlin, Staar operationen by Thieren. VII Versammelung Opth.
	Gesellschaft, September, 1887.

2386. Bull, C. S., Simple extraction of cataract without iridectomie.
	Twenty-third meeting of American Opth. Society, 1887.

2387. Borthen, Cataract extraction med. Three instrumenten. Norsk
	Mag. Marz.

1887. 2388. ——, Om for beredelserne till katarakt operationer og iridekto-
mier of om efter behandlingen efter disse operationer. **Nork.
Mag. May.**

2389. Burnett, S., Remarks on cataract extraction. **Amer. Med. Apoc.
April.**

2390. Bettman, Boerne, Artificial ripening of cataracts. **Journal of Amer.
Med. Apoc. December 3, 1887.**

2391. Beverini, De l'enclavement de l'iris de la crystalloide apres l'operation de la cataracte par l'extraction lineaire combinee a l'iridectomie. **These. de Paris, 1887.**

2392. Boe, Recherches experimentales pour servir a l'etude de la cataracte traumatique. **Arch. d'Opth., VII, 3, p. 193.**

2393. Besselin, O., Ein fall von extrahirtem und microscopisch untersuchtem schichtstaar eines erwachsenen. **Arch. f. Augenheil.,
XVIII, 1, S. 71.**

2394. Bass, Uber staar erythropsie. **Klin. Monatsblatt, Bd. XXV, S. 453.**

2395. Bogaiewzki, Kurzer bericht uber 173 staar operationen im Land-
krankenhause zu krementschug. **Wjestnik Opth., 1887, IV, 6, S.541.**

2396. Alt, Adolph, Some remarks on congenital cataracts. **Amer. Journal
of Opth., June.**

2397. Chodin, Auswashung der vodern kammer bei staar operationen.
Congress Russicher Aerzte in Moskau. January, 1887.

2398. ——, Uber thermometrie bei Augen operationen. **Congress Russicher Aerzte in Moskau. January, 1887.**

2399. Chisholm, J. J., After treatment of cataract extraction. **The revo-
lution in the after treatment of cataract. Amer. Journ. of Opth.
June.**

2400. Coleman, J. E., Use of galvanic current in the treatment of certain
forms of cataract. **Chicago Society of Opth. and Otology. June.**

2401. Collins, Fuachen, Statistics of cataract operations before and after
the introduction of cocaine. **Opth. Hosp. Reports, XI, 3, p. 338.**

2402. Classen, Uber ein eigenthumliche methode der cataract extraction.
Munchener Med. Wochenschrift, 1887, No. 46, S. 903.

2403. Dor, Napthalin cataract. **Congress Opth. Mai. Bulletin et Memoires de la Societe Francaise d'Opthal., p. 150.**

2404. ——, De la production artificielle de la cataracte par la napthaline.
Rev. General d'Opthal., VI, 1, p. 1.

2405. Deutshman, Pathologisch-anatomische untersuchungen augen von
diabetikern, nebst bemerkungen uber die pathogenese der diabetischen cataract. **Graefe, XXXIII, B. 2.**

2406. ——, Pathogenese der diabetischen cataract. **Graefe, XXXIII, B.2.**

2407. Kasaurow, Dr. Uber ein vereinfachtes methode der staar extraction. **Russicher Congress in Moskau. January, 1887.**

2408. DeWecker, De l'extraction de la capsule anterieure dans l'operation de la cataracte. **Congress Opthal. May, 1887.**

1887. 2409. Dobrowolsky, W., Uber die ursachen der erythropsie. Graefe Arch., XXXIII, B. 2.

2410. Evetsky, Ch. O., L'albuminurie et la cataracte. Arch. d'Opthal. Juillet, Aout.

2411. Smith, Frank Tester, Cataract operations in New York. The Amer. Journal of Opthal. April.

2412. Fontan, J., Sur la cataracte pointille post-typhoidigue. Revue General Opth., No. 4, Avril.

2413. Foerster, Uber luxatio lentis. Eighth Versammelung Opth. Gesell-schaft zu Heidelberg. September, 1887.

2414. Galezowski, Operation de la cataracte. Congress Opthal. Mai. 1887.

2415. ——, Choix de la methode operatoire de la cataracta. Revue General Opth., No. 5. Mai; No. 6, Juin.

2416. ——, Choix de la methode operatoire de la cataracta. Recueil d'Opth. Juillet, Aout.

2417. ——, Du meilleur mode operatoire de la cataracte moyens d'eviter les complications statistique. Recueil d'Opth. Juillet, August.

2418. ——, Aniridie traumatique avec luxation du cristallin; discision; guerison. Recueil d'Opth. July, November.

2419. Gottschau, Uber die entwickelung geschichte der augen linse. Centralblatt Ref., p. 157.

2420. Grandelement, M. E., Indications des lavages intraoculaires apres l'extraction de la cataract. Annales d'Oculistique, XCVII, 1 et 2 livr. January, February.

2421. Gayet, Antisepsis oculaire. Rec. d'Opth., No. 5.

2422. Hess, C., Berichte uber Nineteenth Versammelung der Opthal. Ge-sellschaft. Heidelberg.

2423. ——, Napthalin veranderung im kaninchen auge und uber die massage cataract.

2424. Heule, Entwickelungs geschichte der krystallinse u. s. w. Arch. fur Microscop. Ant., B. XX, p. 418.

2425. ——, Uber albuminurie und cataracte. Russicher Congress in Moskau. January, 1887.

2426. Lawford, J. B., Concussion cataract; two cases. Opth. Review, 1887. Twenty-five cases of luxation of the lens. The Royal London Hospital Report. January, 1887.

2427. Jesop, W., Lamellar cataract. Opth. Soc. of United Kingdom, 1886-87, VII, p. 171.

2428. Knapp, Lenses of 1,000 successive extractions with iridectomie. Twenty-third Meeting of American Opth. Society. 1887.

2429. Kipp, Case of spontaneous absorption of senile cataract without injury to the capsule of the lens; restoration of excellent vision. American Journal of Opth. June.

2430. Lagner, Case of Recklinghausen in Nineteenth Opth. Congress. Heidelberger.

1887. 2431. Lee, On the extraction of soft cataract by injections. Brit. Med. Journal. January.

2432. Magnus, Therepeautischer Monatschrift. October. Uber einfius des napthalin auf dem sehorgan.

2433. Meyer, Paul, Die spontane aufsugung cataracta senilis. Graefe, XXXIII, B. 1.

2434. Moeller, Casuistische mittheilung uber das vorkommen und die operative behandlung des grauen staars beim hunde. Zeitschrift fur Augenheilkunde.

2435. Mules, Cataract extraction. A new method of treating an old complication. British Medical Journal. June 11.

2436. Mathiessen, Ludwig, Beitrag zur dioptrie der krystallinse. Berlin. Everbusch Zeitschr. fur Verg. Augenheilkunde.

2437. Mooren, simple method of extraction. International Med. Congress, Washington, D. C. September, 1887.

2438. Manolesca, Comapres cataract extraction with and without iridectomie. International Med. Congress, Washington, D. C. September, 1887.

2439. Montgomery, W. J., After treatment of cataract extraction. Amer. Med. Apo.

2440. McKeown, Intra-capsular injections in cataract extraction. Brit. Med. Journal, September 3.

2441. Mandelstamm, Ein fall von beiderseitger spontaner linsen luxation. St. Petersburg Med. Wochenschrift, No. 16.

2442. Montagnon, M. P., Luxation lens. Amer. Journal of Opth., IV, 6, p. 157.

2443. McKeown, Intra-capsular injections in the extraction of cataract. British Medical Journal, No. 1412, p. 1589.

2444. Neese, E., Uber das verhalten des epithels bei der heilung von linear und lanzen messer wunden in der hornhaut. Graefe, Vol. XXXIII, B. 1.

2445. Nieden, Cataract bildung bei teleangiectatischer ausdehnung der capillaren der ganzen gesichtshaut. Centralblatt f. Prakt., 1887, S. 353.

2446. Pannas, Etudes sur la mitritiar de l'oeil apres des experiences faites avec la flourescine et la napthalin. Arch. d'Opthal. Mars, Avril.

2447. Purtscher, Neue beitrage zur frage der erythropsie. Arch. f. Augenheilkunde, XVII, p. 260.

2448. Peignon, De l'extraction de la capsule anterieur dans l'operation de la cataracte. Paris, 1887.

2449. Randolph, R. C., Ein beitrag zur nachbehandlung von cataract patienten. Centralblatt fur Prakt. Augen, Mai.

2450. Rohmer, Maturation artificielle de la cataracte. Congress Opthal. Mai, 1887.

528

1887 2451. Rampoli, Maturation artificielle de la cataracte. Congress Opthl. Mai, 87.

2452. E. Ancora indicata in qualche caso la depressione della catteratta. Annal d'Opth., XV, p. 423.

2453. ——, Sulla matura infettiva della panotalmite chetalora conseque alla estrazione della cataratta. Annal d'Ottal., XV, 5-6.

2454. Randolph, Ein Beitrag zur Nachbehandlung von Cataract patienten. Centralb. f. pr. A.

2455. Rheindorf, J., Zur Staaroperation. Arch. f. Augenheilkunde, XVIII, S. 180.

2456. Schlosser, K., Experimentelli Studie uber traumatischer kataract. Munchen, 87.

2457. Schoen, Wm., Die Accommodation und deren folgen Aetiologie des Glaucom und der Alters Cataract. Graefe Arch., XXXVIII, B. I.; also, Arch. fur Augenheilkunde. XVII.

2458. Schirmer, Experimentel Studie in Reine Linsen Contusion. Dissert. Inaug. Greifswald.

2459. Stolting, Glaucom nach Linear Ext. Graefe Arch., Vol. XXXIII, B. 2.

2460. Stein, Stanislaus. Staar durch Tone erzeught. Centralblatt f. Augenheilkunde; 1887, Jan., p. 6.

2461. Saurez, Success immediat et insuccess tardif dans operation de la cataracte. Congress Opthal., Mai, 87.

2462. Suarez de Mendozza, Sur la success immediat et l'insuccess tardif dans operation de la cataracte. Revue General Opth., Mai.

2463. Schweigger, Cataract Extraction. VII, Versammelung Gesellschaft zu Heidelberg; Sept., 87.

2464. Silex, P., Bericht uber 122 Extractionen von Altersstaar mit Eroffnung der Linsenkapsel durch die Kapselpincette. Arch. f. Augenheilkunde, XVII, 4.

2465. Swanzy, Intracapsular injections in cataract extractions. British Med. Journal, Sept. 17.

2466. Tetzer, Compendium der Augenheilkunde, 4, Auflage, S. 282.

2467. Thompson, J. L., Congenital and spontaneous displacement of the crystalline lens. American Med. Apoc.

2468. Vachez, Du lavage de la chambre anterieur. Congress Opthal., Mai, 87.

2469. Valk, Franc, Report of four operations for removal of cataract without an iridectomie, by an entirely new method.

2470. Williams, The latest phases of cataract extraction. St. Louis Med. and Surg. Jour., No. 5, p. 358. The grand effect of cocaine in cataract extractions. St. Louis Med. and Surg. Journal, p. 359.

2471. Zancoval-Terson, Du lavage de la chambre anterieur apres l'operation de la cataract. Anna. d'Ocul., XCVII, p. 302.

1887. 2472. Zehender. W., Cataract Ext. Tod. in folge von Echinococcus der Wilz. Klin. Monatsblatt. XXV, S. 315.

2473. Jacobson. J., Uber cataract extraction. Deutsche Med. Wochenschrift, VIII, No. 78.

2474. Critchett, Dislocation of the lens. British Med. Journal, January.

2475. Kubli, Vier Falle von Erythropsie. Wjestnik Opth., IV, 3, p. 269.

2476. Scholler, Zur Staaroperation. Berliner Klin. Wochenschrift, 87, No. 38.

1888. 2477. Abad'e, De l'antisepsis et l'asepsis dans operation de la cataracte. Arch. d'Opth., Jan.

2478. Armaignac, Nouvelle pince pour extraction dun lam becum de capsule anterieur dans l'operation de la cataract. Rec. d'Opth., No. 3, p. 177.

2479. Beselin, Ein Fall von extrahirten und microscopischen untersuchtem Schichstaar einer erwachsenen. Arch. f. Augenheilkunde, B, XVIII.

2480. Burchardt, Schichstaar mit ungewohnlicher Zeichnung der Voder flache. Indication fur die Art der Operation. Charite Annalen, 1888.

2481. Ball, Case of cataract extraction, with remarks on use of cocaine. Med. Reg., IV, 21, p. 485.

2482. C. Vian, Des progres accomplis dans le traitement; chirurgical de la cataracte et du procede de choix. Recuel d'Opth., Jan.

2483. Chibret, Infection secondaire de l'oeil apres l'operation de la cataracte. Rev. General d'Opth., VII, 1., p. 1.

2484. Cauldron, Traumatismus du critallin un cas de contusion simple. Rev. General d'Opth., No. 12.

2485. Charrin and Roger, Experimentel Cataract. (Menthol). Arch. f. Prakt. Augenheilkunde, Febry., 1888; p. 60.

2486. Dixti, Die Kunstliche Reifung der Cataract. Mailand.

2487. Doyne, A peculiar form of degeneration of the lens. Opth. Society of United Kingdom; Oct., 88.

2488. Drake-Brockman, A statistical review of 1,626 cases of cataract extraction. Madras. Opthalmie Review, Nov.

2489. Dufour, Sur la one rouge ou l'enthropsie. Mai.

2490. Deuot Kin, Uber die Dilatatorectomie bei Cataracta mularis. Wjestnik Opth., Vol. I.

2491. Derby, H., On the dangers of simple extraction of cataract. Boston Med. and Surgical Journal, CXVIII, 8, p. 189.

2492. Doyne, A peculiar degeneration of the lens. Opth. Soc., Dec. 13.

2493. Eoliver, Belt, Bericht uber 100 staaroperation. Knapp Arch., Vol. XIX, B. 2.

2404. Fuchs, Uber traumatische. Klinische Wochenschrift, No. 8 and 4.

2495. Falchi, Micropthalmus Congenita. Annali di Opthalmologi, XIII.

1888. 2496. F. Meyer, Ein Fall von Lenticonus posterior. Arch. fur Prakt.
Augenheilkunde; Febry., 1888.

2497. Fienzal, Discission mit dem Lanzenmesser bei den verschiedenen
Arten von Angeborener Cataract. Societe Francaise d'Opth.,
May 9, 1888.

2498. Freyer, B. E., Excessive hemorrhage of several hours' duration after
cataract extraction (senile). (1 case). American Journal of Opth.,
February.

2499. Fischer, F., Bericht uber ein acht yahriges kind mit angeborener
totaler cataract und dessen verhalten wahrend der Ersten Wochen

2500. G. A. Berry, Note on an instance of marked hereditary in a form of
nach augelangtern Sehen.
cataract developed in early life. The Opthalmic Review, Jany.

2501. Galezowski, Extraction des cataractes luxees. Societe Francaise
d'Opth., Mai 9, 1888.

2502. ———, Traitement de la cataracte luxee. Recueil d'Opth., Mai.

2503. Goldzieher, W., Zwei Falle von beiderseitiger angeborener cataract
nebst Bemerkungen uber das Schenlernen Blindgeborener. Wiener Med. Wochenschrift. No. 3. 1888.

2504. Gayet, Report of cataract extraction. Seventh Internation Opth.
Congress. Heidelberg; August, 88.

2505. Gauita, Proliferazioni degli epiteli corneale sull iride a nella pupilla in seguito od ablazione di cat. Annal d'Opth., 2, p. 145.

2506. Gad, A., Et Tilfaelde af Resorptio cataractae senilis intracapsularis.
Wordisk Opth. Tidsskr, 4, p. 262.

2507. Graefe, A., Ein wort fur Beibehaltung der Iridectomie bei Ext.
harter Cataracte. Graefe Arch., XXXIV, 3, p. 223.

2508. Hess, Zur Pathogenese des Micropthalmus. Arch. f. Opth., XXXIV,
B. 3.

2509. Resopnse a'M. Pr. Panas sur la cataracte napthalinique. Rev. General d'Opth., VII, 6, p. 260.

2510. ———, Experimentelles uber Blitz cataract. Opth. Congress, 1888;
p. 147.

2511. Hirschberg, Geschictliche Bemerkungen Noch einmal die Staraus-
ziehung bei den Griechen. Arch. f. Prak. Augenheilkunde; July.
1888.

2512. ———, Zur Wundbehandlung des Starschnitts. Berliner Med.
Wochenschrift, No. 38.

2513. ———, Tropfen bildung bei beginnenden staar. Centralblatt, p. 321.

2514. Hedeus, Ectopie lentis, atrophischer zonula. Vier fachsehen. Zehender's Klinische Monatsblatter; Mai.

2515. Herman Becker, Ein Fall von Micropthalmus congenitus unilat-
teralis nebst einigen Bemerkungen uber die vermuthliche Aetiologie und Entwickelungs geschicte desselben. Graefe Arch.,
XXXIV, B. 3.

1888. 2516. Hosch. Zur Erblichkeit des grauen staares. Con-Bl. of Schweizer
Aerzte., XVIÏI, No. 19, p. 599.

2517. Jacobson, J., Sr., Von Graefe's Modifirote Linear Extraction und der
Lappenschnitt nach einigen Erfahrung aus der Zeit. 1854-1888.
Graefe Arch., XXXIV, B. 2.

2518. J. Bejerrum, Statistik uber inflammatorische Falle von Cataract
Extraction. Arch. f. Augenheilkunde, p. 381.

2519. Jessop, Symmetrical rings of pigment on the anterior capsule of
lenses, resulting from foetál iritis. Trans. of Opth. Soc., 1887-1888,
p. 126.

2520. Kniess, Grundriss der Augenheilkunde, S. 282.

2521. Knapp, Extraction of cataract without iridectomie. N. Y. Medical
Record, Febry. 11, 1888. (Arch. f. Aug., p. 85). Also, Arch. fur
Augenheilkunde, Vol. XIX, I.

2522. ——, Simple extraction of cataract. Boston Med. and Surgical
Journal, CXVIII, No. 14.

2523. Knox, Shaw, Two cases of dislocation of the crystalline lens. Opth.
Review, No. 83.

2524. Lawford, Pathological Anat. of Lamellar or Zonu'ar Cataract.
Royal Lond. Opth. Hospital Reports, Vol. XII. P. II. p. 184.

2525. Little, David, Operative treatment of zonular cataract. British Med.
Journal.

2526. Landesberg, M., Zur aetiologie der cataract bildung. Arch. fur
Prakt. Augenheilkunde. February, 1888.

2527. Laske, Die sescharfe nach cataracte extraction. In Din. Kiel.

2528. Magnus, Hugo, Linsenernahrung und lens ertrubung. Deutsche
Med. Wochenschrift, No. 40.

2529. ——, Zur Historische Kentniss der Vodere Kammer Auswaschun-
gen, No. 40, B. 2.

2530. ——,Zur Klinische Kentniss der linsen contusionen. Deutsche
Med. Wochenschrift, January 28, No. 3.

2531. McKeown, On one hundred cases of cataract. mature and immature, treated by intraocular injections. Brit. Med. Journal.

2532. ——, Instrument pour les injections intraoculaire dans l'extraction de la cataracte. Annal. d'Oculistique, XCIV, p. 144.

2533. Norris, Gordon, Acutu linsen astygmatismus. Arch. fur Prakt.
Augen., August, p. 234.

2534. Nicati, Spontan heilung der cataracte senilis. Academie der Wis-
senshaft zur Paris. May, 1888.

2535. Becker, Otto, Die Universitats Augenklinik in Heidelberg. Zwanzig
Yahre Klinischer Thatigkeit. Heidelberg.

2536. Motais, Nach staar operation. Societe Francaise d'Opth. May
9, 1888.

2537. Pagenstecher, Herman, Uber staar extractione mit und ohne entfernung der kapsel. Graefe. XXXIV, B. 2.

1888. 2538. Panas, Cataract extraction. Pariser Academie der Medicin. Arch. fur Prakt. Augenheilkunde. February. P. 60.

2539. ———, Des operatione de cataracte par extraction pratiquees a la clinique de l'Hotel. Dien dans les trois dernieres annes avec lavage a la chambre anterieur. Arch. d'Opth., VIII. 1. p. 64.

2540. Proudfood, A., Excessive hemorrhage after cataract extraction (one case). October, March.

2541. Pomeroy, Removal of the dislocated lens with bident. Amer. Jour. of Opth., No. 10.

2542. Carter, R. Brunadel, Introduction to the discussion on the treatment of senile cataract. Brit. Med. Journal, November 24.

2543. Reigel, Zur pathologie der subconjunctivalen linsen luxation. In Dis. Munchen.

2544. Rodsewitch, Bericht uber das zweite hundert von cataracte extractionen. Wjestnik Opth., Vol. III. p. 248.

2545. Schoen, Die ursache des grauen staars. Arch. fur Augenheilkunde, XVII and XIX.

2546. Schirmer, Otto, Experimentelle studie uber die Foerster'sche maturation der cataracte. Graefe, XXXIV, B. 1.

2547. Snell, Simon, On the after treatment of cataract. British Med. Journal.

2548. Schnabel, Die entwickelung der staar operations methoden in den letzen 20 yahren.

2549. Swanzy, Intracapsular injections in the extraction of cataract. Brit. Med. Journal, February 18.

2550. Schweigger, Zur cataract extraction. Erweiderung an Prof. Jacobson. Greaefe Arch., XXXIV, B. 3.

2551. ———,Die Ruckkehr zum lappenschnitt. Knapp Schweigger Arch., B. XVIII.

2552. Steffan, Ch., Ein technik des peripheren flachen lappenschnitt. Zehender's Klinische Monatsheft. June.

2553. Scimeni, Case of zonular cataract. Bolletino d'Oculistica, No. 8-9. Arch. fur Augenheilkunde, p. 308.

2554. Silex, Paul, Zur frage der accommodation die aphakischen auges. Knappach, Vol. XIX, B. 1.

2555. Sulzer, D. E., Over blijfselen van het achterste gedeelte van de vaa thouden de foetale len kapsel bij een volwassene aan een oog met membrana pupillaris perseverans en andere out wikkelings anomalien. Geneeskundin Tydschrift voor Nedeklandsch. Iridie Deel, XXVII, Af. 1.

2556. Tomatola, Luxation of lens under the conjunctiva. Bolletino d'Oculistica. No. 12. Arch. fur Augenheilkunde.

2557. Treacher, Collins. Some of the complications after extraction of cataract. Ropal Opth. Hosp. Reports, January.

1888. 2558. Valude, Erythropsie. Clinique d'Opth. de la Faculte de Bordeaux. Mars, Avril.

2559. Vian, Des progres accomplis dans l'traitement chirurgical de la cataracte et du procede du cholx. Rec. d'Opthal., No. 1. p. 41; No. 2, p. 92.

2560. Valude, L'erythropsie. Arch. f. Opth., VIII, 2, p. 130. St. Louis Med. and Surgical Journal.

2561. Westhoff, Erythropsie bei aphakie. Centralblatt fur d.

2562. Webster, David, Extraction of a partially absorbed calcareous cataract. N. Y. Med. Record, September 29, 1888.

2563. Williams, Hemorrhage long after cataract extraction. St. Louis Med. and Surgical Journal, LIV, 2, p. 106.

2564. ———, Apparent ossification of an old lens. St. Louis Med. and Surgical Journal, No. 3, p. 178.

2565. ———, Cocaine and loss of vitreous in cataract extraction. St. Louis Med. and Surgical Journal, No. 4.

2566. ———, Subluxation of both lenses by separate blows. St. Louis Med. and Surgical Journal, LV, p. 36.

2567. Wickerkiewicz, Einige bemerkungen uber die augenkammer auswaschung. Seventh Int. Congress Opth.

2568. Wickerkiewicz, Bogdan, Beitrag zur kentniss der Paris tirende pupilla membrane. Graefe Arch., XXXIV, 64.

2569. Holtz, F. C., Excessive hemorrhage after cataract extraction; two cases. American Journal of Opth. March.

2570. Little, D., On operative treatment of zonular cataract. British Med. Journal, No. 1413, p. 178.

2571. Arcoleo, L'estrazione della capsula anteriore del cristallino nella operazione della cataratta. Annal d'Ottalm., XVII, 4.

2572. Czermak, Uber extraction der cataract ohne iridectomie mit naht der Wunde. Wiener Klin. Wochenschrift, No. 29 and 30.

2573. Norsa, Un cas de luzzazione spontanea della lenta cristalline nella camera anterior. Bollet della Soc. Lancisiana Roma.

2574. Gunn, Growth of new lens fibres after spontaneous absorption of traumatic cataract. Trans. of Opth. Soc., 1887-88, S. 126.

1889. 2575. A. Wagenmann, Neubildungen von glashautige substanz an der linsen kapsel, etc. Graefe Arch., Vol. XXXV, B. 1.

2576. Alfred v. Graefe, Fortgesetzte bericht uber die mittelst antiseptische wundehandlung erzielte erfolge der staaroperationen. Graefe Arch., Vol. XXXV, B. 3.

2577. Abadie, De certaines complications, qui surviennent quelques jouss apres l'operation de la cataract. Ann. d'Oculistique, Marz, April.

2578. Baker, A. R., A few observations on the etiology, prognosis and cure of incipient cataract without operative interference. Cleveland Med. Gazette, July, 1889.

2579. DaGame, A., Cataract operation without iridectomie. British Med. Journal, No. 1507, p. 1093.

1889. 2580. Brunedell, Carter. Treatment of senile cataract and discussion. British Med. Ap. Opth. Review, September, 1888.

2581. Bribosia, Avant pendant et apres l'extraction de la cataracte. Ann. d'Oculistique, January.

2582. Brettrenieux, P., Une modification du couteau a cataracte. Arch. d'Opthal., January, 1889.

2583. Baudon, Note sur la resultats obtenus dans cent quarente operations de cataract. July, 1871, 1888.

2584. Blanch Aguilar, Quelle est la meilleure methode d'extraction de la cataracte. August, 1871, 1888.

2585. Hess, Carl, Beschreibung des auges von Talpa Europea und von Proteus Auginens. Graefe Arch., Vol. XXXV, B. 3.

2586. Lee, Chas. G., Extraction of soft cataract by intracapsular injection. British Med. Journal, March 30, 1889.

2587. Cereseto, 460 cataract extractionen von Panas ausgefuhrt. Gazette Med. di Torno, 1888, No. 14.

2588. Curatulo, Exeprimente uber die napthalin cataract. Centralblatt fur Augen, p. 352.

2589. Kunn, C. G., Vererbung des schichtstaars in einer familie. Wiener Klin. Wochenschrift, No. 3.

2590. Curatulo, Uber die durch napthalin erzeugte cataract. Lee Morgagni, February, 1889.

2591. Bull, Chas. S., Extraction of cataract without iridectomy. The New York Med. Record, October 5, 1889.

2592. Berry, De l'enclavement de iris consecutive a l'extraction de la cataracte. Paris, 1889.

2593. Little, David, Extraction of senile cataract. Brit. Med. Journal, February 23, 1889.

2594. Deeren, Quelques observations sur les procedes de maturation artificiele de cataract. Recueil d'Opth., May.

2595. Doyne, Peculiar form of lens degeneration. Ibid., p. 113.

2596. Eales, Foreign bodies in the lens. British Med. Journal, October 26.

2597. Martin, Emil, La suture de la cornee dans operation de la cataracte. Recueil d'Opth., May.

2598. Hosch, Fr., Zur casuistic der linsen kapsel verletzung. Arch. fur Augenheilkunde, XX, 1, 2. Zur Erblichkeit des grauen staars. Korresp. Blatter fur Schweizer Aerzte, No. 19.

2599. Fuchs, E., Uber traumatische linsen trubung. Wiener Klin. Wochenschrift, No. 3, S. 53.

2600. Fage, A., Contribution a l'etude des hemorrhagies intraoculaires consecutives a la extraction de la cataracte. Arch. d'Opthal., July.

2601. Grolman, W. von, Uber micropthalmus und cataracta congenita vaculosa. Graefe, Vol. XXXV, B. 3 and 4.

2602. Guerison, Ossification totale de la choroide: glaucoma sympathtique dans un oeil punutivement opere de cataracte; rupture spontanee de la cicatrices: enucleation de l'oeil sympathisant. Recueil d'Op. Jannary.

1890. 2603. Groenon, Zwei falle von aderhaut ablosung nach cataract operation mit spontaner heilung. Arch. f. Augenheilk., XX, 1, 2.

2604. Gunn, M., On the action of the aqueous on lenticular substance. Opth. Review, 1889, No. 94, p. 235.

2605. Galezowski, Extraction de la cataracte et iridectomie. Soc. Opth. Paris, 1889.

2606. Higgins, Charles, On extraction of immature cataract. Lancet, No. 19.

2607. Hirschberg, J., Uber staar operation und diabetischer alterstaar. Centralblatt fur Prakt. Augenheilkunde, p. 264.

2608. Noyes, Henry D., Considerations concerning extraction of hard cataract, with an analysis of 309 cases. Med. Record, March 30, 1889.

2609. Hache, Edmond, Sur la hyaloide et la zone de zinii. Recueil d'Opth. May.

2610. Muttemaier, Herman, Uber das vorkommen von glaucom in cataractosen augen. Ing. Dissert.

2611. Ferrer, H., Report of a series of 106 cases of extraction without iridectomie.

2612. Jacobson, J., Die extraction mit der kapsel. Centralblatt f. Prakt. Augenheilkunde, May.

2613. Chisholm, Julian J., The after treatment of cataract extractions. The Internat. Journal of Surgery. June.

2614. Knapp, H., Cataract extraction and discussion. New York Academy of Medicine. February 18, 1889.

2615. Keyser, P. D., Two cases of removal of spontaneous dislocated lenses from the anterior chamber of the eye. Centralblatt fur Prakt. Augenheilkunde, p. 255.

2616. ———, Discission of cataract. The Times and Register, May 25.

2617. Kazarow, J., Zur frage der suctions methode der cataract extraction. Wjestnik Op., 1889, No. 4, p. 329.

2618. DeWecker, L., Lavenir de l'extraction de la cataracte. Annales d'Oculistique. May and June.

2619. Lawrentiew, Bericht uber das dritte hundert der cataract extraction. Wjestnik Opth., Vol. III. p. 269.

2620. Lippincott, J. A., Irrigation of the anterior chamber. Amer. Opth. Soc. 1889.

2621. Magnus, Hugo, Anatomische studien uber die aufange des alterstaars. Graefe Arch., Vol. XXXV, B. 3.

2622. Martin, E., La suture de la cornee dans operation de la cataracte. Rec. d'Opth., 1889, No. 5.

2623. Pagenstecher, H., Uber cataract extraction in der kapsel. Seventh Opth. Congress. Heidelberg. 1888.

2624. Parisotti, Sur la maturation artificielle de la cataracte. Recueil d'Opth. Marz.

536

1889. 2624a. ———, Sur la maturation artificielle de la cataracte. La Riforma Medic., No. 11 and 12.

2625. Romie, De la panopthalmie chez certains operes de cataracte. Ann. d'Oculistique. January.

2626. Rogman, Considerations relative a la structure et la traitement operatoire de certaines formes de la secondaire. Zehender's Klin. Monatsblatter. May.

2627. Schirmer, Otto. Histologische und chemische untersuchungen uber kapsel narbe und kapsel cataract nebst bemerkungen uber die physiologische wachstum und die structure der vodere linsenkapsel. Graefe Arch., Vol. XXXV, B. 1.

2628. ———, Zur pathologischen anatomie und pathogenese des schichtstaars. Graefe Arch., XXXV, B. 3. Nachtrag. Graefe Arch., Vol. XXXVI, B. 1. 1890.

2629. Steffan, Phil., Weitere erfahrungen und studien uber die cataract extraction. 1887-88. Graefe Arch., Vol. XXXV.

2630. Suarez, Ferdinand, Sur la suture de la cornee dans operation de la racte. Recueil d'Opth. September.

2631. Ayres, S. C., Extraction of cataract without iridectomy or simple extraction. American Journal of Opth. May.

2632. Schlosser, Uber die lymphbahnen der linse. Munchener Med. Wochenschrift, No. 7, 1889.

2633. Saunders, A. R., Traumatic dislocation of the lens, fluminating glaucoma, etc. British Med. Journal, March 2.

2634. Serebreniucowa, E., Bericht uber zwei hundert von cataract extractionen in Land krankenhaus zu Perm. Wjestnik Opth., No. 1, p. 41.

2635. Scimeny, Sull astygmatismus corneale in seguito ad estrazioni di cateratta. Annali di Ottalm., XVIII, 4, 5, p. 299.

2636. Thomas, Chas.. A report of 120 cases of cataract extraction. Journ. of Opthal. Otologie and Laryngologie, Vol. I. January.

2637. Treacher Collins, Hernia of the lens through a corneal perforation. Opth. Hosp. Rep., XII, 4, p. 334.

2638. Wagenman, A., Uber die von operations narben und vernarbten iris vorfallen ausgehenden glass korperertenung. Graefe, XXXV. B. 4.

2639. Collins, W. J., Paralysis of fifth nerve, associated with cataract. Opth. Society of United Kingdom. Brit. Med. Journ., June 28.

2640. Wickerklewicz, R., Uber das geeignetste verfahren der kapseleroffnung behap staar entfernung. Zehender's Klinische Monatsblatter. May.

2641. Wickerklewicz, Bolelas, Cur la cystotomie par rapport, a l'extraction de la cataracte. Recueil d'Opth. May.

2642. Collins, W. J., The composition of the human lens in health and in cataract, and its bearing upon operations for the latter. Opthalmic Review. November.

1889. 2643. Wurdemann, Traumatic cataract with occlusion of the pupil by false membranes and coloboma of the iris. American Journal of Opth. July.

2644. Collins, W. J., Sequel to a case of paralysis of the right fifth nerve with cataract. Trans. of Opth. Soc., Vol. IX, p. 165. 1888-89.

2645. Kuhnt, Uber staar und nachtstaar operationen. Carr. Bl. d. Algem. Aertz Vereins von Thuringen, XVIII, No. 9.

2646. Tepljaschin, Uber cataract in folge chronischer vergiftung mit Mutter Korn, III. Russicher Congress Aerzte zu St. Petersburg. January 4, 1889. St. Petersburg Med. Wochenschrift, No. 3. 1889.

2647. Norsa, Spontane luxation der linse in die vodere kammer. Centralblatt fur Prakt. Augenh., p. 350.

2648. Tatham Thompson, Note on a case of hereditary tendency to cataract in early childhood. Opth. Society of United Kingdom. November, 1889.

2649. Critchett, Anderson, The treatment of immature cataract. British Med. Journal, August 24, 1889.

2650. Haase, C. H., Beitrage zur operation des grauen staars. Festschr. Hamburg Eppendorf. 1889.

2651. Rendon, Results de 140 operations de cataracte. Rec. d'Opth., No. 7, p. 395. 1889.

1890. 2652. Graefe, Alfred v., Fortgesetzte berichte uber die mittelst antiseptischer wundbehandlung erzielten erfolge der staaroperation. A. f. O., 85, 3.

2653. Fager, A., Infection tardive de l'oeil apres operation de la cataracte. Annales d'Oculistique. May, June.

2654. Angello, Leda, Delire chez les operes de cataracte. Recueil d'Opth. July.

2655. Bourgeois, A., De la kystectomie dans operation de cataracte. Recueil d'Opth. August.

2656. Berry, Spontaneous purulent hyalitis nine months after a successful cataract extraction. Opth. Society of the United Kingdom, March, 1890. Arch. fur Augenheilkunde, p. 271.

2657. Brailey, Points in the development of cataract. Opth. Society of United Kingdom. British Med. Journal, No. 9, p. 240.

2658. Dickson, Ban, An early extraction of cataract. New York Med. Journal, No. 9, p. 240.

2659. Blubaugh, The removal of a dislocated lens with the aqueous bident. Times and Register, August 30, 1890, p. 199.

2660. Bull, Simple operation for the extraction of cataract. Amer. Opth. Soc. 1890.

2661. ———. The extraction of dislocated lens from the eye, whether transparent or cataractous. Amer. Opth. Soc.

1890. 2662. ———, The extraction of lens dislocated into vitreous. New York Med. Journal, LII, No. 10, p. 261.

2663. Collins, Treacher, Abnormalities of the zonula of Zinn. Royal London Opth. Hosp. Reports, Vol. XIII, Part I. December.

2664. Cicardi, Uni casi di sublussazione della lenti cristallina. Annal. d'Opth., XVIII, 6, p. 548.

2665. Cisseb, E., Eine seltene angeborene anomalie der linse. Zeheder's Klin. Monatsbl. August.

2666. Dobard, Considerations generales sur l'operation de la cataracte chez les enfants. Recueil d'Opth. September.

2667. Dufour, Des cataractes secondaires au point de vue operatoire. Soc. Franc. d'Opth., May 5.

2668. DeWecker, Un quart de siecle consacre an perfectionnement de l'extraction de la cataracte. Progres Med., 1890, No. 47, p. 416.

2669. Bock, E., Fun falle von cataracta nach menningitis bei jugendliche individuen. Wiener Med. Woch.

2670. Ferri, Complicazioni postume dell operazione di cataratta e loro cause. Annal. d'Opth., XVIII, 6, p. 493.

2671. Fox-Webster, The absorption of immature cataract by manipulation conjoined with installation. Times and Register, 1890, No. 25.

2672. Gefaner, Beitrag zur kentniss der glasshautigen auf der linsenkapsel und die descemetischen. Memlian. Graefe Arch., XXXVI, B. 4.

2673. Norris, Gordon, George Henermant seine deutsche beschriebung der staar ausziehung (1756), etc. Arch. f. Augenheilkunde, XXI, 2, S. 261.

2674. Gifford, Ein neuer staar extractions verband. Arch. f. Augenheilkunde, XXI, 2, S. 181.

2675. Grandelement, Des conditions des success dans l'operation de la cataracte. Lyon Med. Journal, No. 29. 1890

2676. Graefe, R., Uber 450 extractions von cataracta senilis ohne iridectomie. Arch. f. Augenheilkunde, XXII, S. 355.

2677. Hess, Carl, Weitere untersuchungen uber angeborene misbildungen des auges. Graefe Arch., XXXVI, B. 1.

2678. Haskel-Derby, Eight cases of double zonular cataract in ten members of same family. Ann. Opth. Soc. 1890.

2679. Hirschberg, J., Zur geschichte der staar ausziehung. Hirschberg's Centralblatt, p. 198.

2680. J. Accacis da Gama, Cataract operation without iridectomy. Brit. Med. Journal, November 16, 1889.

2681. Lippincott, J. A., On intraocular syringing in cataract extraction, with a report of 53 operations. Opthalmic Review. July.

2682. Kazarow, J. N., Zur frage der cataract operation durch aussaugen. Wjestnik Opthal. July. December.

1890. 2683. Kirkpatrick, Capsulitis purulenta et hemorrhagica. Amer. Journal. April, 1890.

2684. Knapp, H., Ein fall von lenticonus posterior. Arch. f. Augenheilkunde, XXII, B. I.

2685. ———, Uber extraction in der glaskorper dislocirten linsen. Arch. f. Augenheilkunde, XXII, Heft. 2.

2686. ———, Bericht uber ein drittes hundert extractions ohne iridectomie. Arch. f. Augenheilkunde, Heft. 2.

2687. Keyser, Soft cataract. Times and Register, XXI, 20, p. 257.

2688. Iwan M. Burnett, Regular astygmatism following cataract extraction. American Journal Opth. 1889.

2689. Lucanus, Ein fall von monocularem doppelsehen. Klin. Mon. Bl. f. A., XXVIII, S. 282.

2690. Magnus, Hugo, Experimentelle studien der ernahrung der krystallinse und uber cataractbildung. Graefe Arch., Vol. XXXVI, B. 4.

2691. McHardy, Artificial maturation of immature senile cataract by trituration. Opth. Society of United Kingdom. Arch. f. Augenh., p, 274.

2692. Straub, M., Die concavitate des vodern zonula blattes nach vorn. Arch. f. Augenheilkunde, Heft. 2.

2693 McKeown, Cataract operations. Brit. Med. Journal, 1890, No. 1560, p. 1186.

2694. Marlow, J. W., Preliminary capsulotomy in the extraction of cataract. New York Med. Journal, LII, No. 13, p. 357.

2695. Parinaud, Du delire apres l'operation de la cataracte. Societe Francaise d'Opthal. Arch. f. Prakt. Augenheilkunde, p. 334.

2696. Rolland, Mayens tres practiques et asepsis pour la cataract. Recuell d'Opth., March and February, 1890. De la operation de la catracte chez la maladies ambulants et de la responsabilite modicale quelle entraine. Recueil d'Opth., April.

2697. Kerschbaumer, Rosa, Bericht uber 200 cataract extractions. Arch. f. Augenheilkunde, XXII, Heft. 2.

2698. Kalisch, Richard, The arrest and partial resorption of immature cataract, with restoration of reading power. Medical Record, March 29.

2699. Schoen, Bericht zu Prof. Magnus Aufsatz. Graefe Arch., XXXVI, B. 1.

2700. Schweiggger, Uber die operation unrifer stare. Berliner Med. Gesellschaft. Hirschberg's C. Blat., 206.

2701. Schnabel, Uber cataract operationen. Wiener Med. Presse, No. 19.

2702. Schirmer, R., Uber indirecte verletzung der voderen linsenkapsel und des sphincter iridis. Zehender's Klin. Monatsch. May, 1890.

2703. Scimeni, Sull modificazione della curvatura della cornea in seguita ad estrazione di cataratta. Annal. d'Opth., XIX, 3, 4, p. 209.

540

1890. 2704. Shields, Chas., When shall we operate cataract and strabismus in children? New York Med. Journal, LII, p. 384.

2705. Swanzy, Series of 100 cataract extractions. New York Medical Journal, LII, p. 146. Remarks on cataract extraction. British Medical Journal, No. 1523. 1890.

2706. Treacher Collins, Glauoma after cataract extraction. Opth. Soc. of the United Kingdom. British Med. Journal, February 8, 1890.

2707. Trousseau, Les maladies generales et l'operation de la cataracte. Recueil d'Opth. March.

2708. Tyner. T. J.. Preliminary capsulotomy in the extraction of cataract. Opth. Review, IX, 108, p. 320.

2709. Vetrch. Uber das Rothsehen (3 cases). Corresp. Bl. f. Schweizer Aerzte. 1889.

2710. Valk. Francis, Operation of cataract without iridectomy. N. Y. Med. Journal, LI, 16, p. 481.

2711. Valude, Accidents centraux consecutive a l'operation de la cataract. Soc. Franc. Opth. 1890.

2712. Wood, Hiram, Intraocular hemorrhage, consecutive to cataract extraction. Med. Record, May 31.

2713. Webster, Traumatic dislocation of the lens. N. Y. Med. Record, LII, p. 11 and 295.

2714. ——, Fatal meningitis subsequent to panopthalmitis after extraction. Arch. f. Augenheilkunde, XXI, 2, S. 191.

2715. Grosz, Emil, Cataracta partiales traumatica. (Szemeszet, No. 1.) Arch. f. Prakt. Aug., p. 316.

2716. Ieweski, F. O., Cataract and xerosis conjunctivae bei den arbeitern der Glasfabriken Wjestnik Opth. May and June.

2717. Guaita, Panopthalmitis six monat nach staar operation. Italienisches Congress. Piss., 189. Hirschberg's Centralblatt, p. 558.

2718. ——, Experimentell reifung des staares.

1891. 2719. Berry, Unusual results of cataract extraction. Opth. Society of United Kingdom, January, 1891. British Med. Journ., Feb. 7, 1891.

2720. Czermak, W., Drei falle von intracapsularer aufsaugung des alterstaars. Zehender's Klin. Monatsblatter, April, 1891.

2721. Chibret, A prospus du mechanisme de l'infection apres l'operation de cataract. Revue General d'Opth.. January. 1891.

2722. Bernhard, Dub., Beitrag zur kentniss der cataract zonularis. Graefe Arch., Vol. XXXVII, B. 4.

2723. Dimmer, F., Zur glaser correction bei aphakie. Zehender's Klin. Monatsblatter, February, 1891.

2724. Fischer, Rich., Stich verletzung eines auges. Wahrscheinlich ungedehnte zerreissung der voderen linsenkapsel—volkommene wiederstellung. Zehender's Klin. Monatsblatter, February, 1891.

1891. 2725. Fuchs, E., Uber linsen praecipitate. Beitrage zur Augenheilkunde, Heft. III.

2726. Haab, O., Bemerkungen zur staaroperation. Hirschberg's Centralblatt, p. 339. 1891.

2727. Thompson, J. Tatham, Note on Foerster's artificial ripening of cataract. Royal London Opth. Hospital Reports, Vol. XIII, Part I.

2728. Mellinger, Carl, Experimentelli Untersuchungen uber die enstehung der in letzere zeit bekannt gwordene trubung der hornhaut nach staarextraction.

2729. Mules, The formation and pathology of pyramidal and central anterior capsular cataracts. Opth. Society of the United Kingdom, October 16, 1890. Hirschberg's Centralblatt, p. 339. 1891.

2730. Natanson, Spontane aufsaugung cataracte linse. Zehender's Klin. Monatsbl. f. A., XXIX, Bd., S. 423, December, 1891.

2731. Risley, S. D., Incipient cataract; aetiology, treatment and prognosis. Opthal. Review, August, 1891.

2732. Schirmer, Otto, Zur pathologischer anatomie und pathogenese des centralstaars. S. Arch., XXXVII, B. 4.

2733. Seabrook, The natural course of cataract. Med. Record, September 12, 1891.

2734. Topolanski, Dr. A., Uber den bau der zonula und umgebung nebst bemerkungen uber das albinotische auge. Graefe Arch., Vol. XXXVII, B. 1.

2735. Treacher, Collins, On the development and abnormalities of the zonula of Zinn. Royal London Opth. Hospital Reports, Vol. XIII, Part I.

2736. Wagenman, A., Zur anatomie des dunnhautigen nachstaars, etc. Graefe Arch., XXXVIII, B. 2.

2737. Webster, Note on a case of diabetic cataract.

2738. Wray, Chas., Points on the treatment of lamellar cataract. Opthal. Review, September, 1891.

2739. Alexejew, Angeborener staar auf beiden augen. Wroschdjonnaja katarakta na oboich glasach. Russkaja Medizina, No. 45, p. 716.

2740. British Medical Association, Section of Opthalmology. July. The treatment of infantile cataract. Opth. Review, p. 315.

2741. ——, Some points in the treatment of lamellar cataract. Ibid.

2742. Burnham, A few remarks on the treatment of lamellar and senile cataract. New York Med. Record, August 22.

2743. D'Oench, A case of muscular zonular cataract. Arch. Opth., XX, p. 258.

2744. Kessler, Ein bijzonders vorm van angeborener cataracta zonularis. Graefe's Arch. f. Opth. voor Geneesk, II, No. 21.

2745. Philipsen, H., Einige notizen von opthalmologisch diagnostischem inhalt. (1) Die diagnose des schichtstaars durch die form der pupille bei schrag einfallendem licht. Hosp. Tid., p. 783 u. S. 868.

1891. 2746. Schnabel, Ueber cataracta der kinder. Wiener Med. Wochenschr., No. 4.

2747. ——, Bemerkungen uber die katarakte der kinder. Mitteil. der Ver. d. Aerzte in Denmark. 1890. Craz., XXVII, S. 65.

2748. Wray, C., Points in the treatment of lamellar cataract. Opth. Review, p. 263.

2749. Wilson, Harold, Hereditarer kongenitaler staar. Journ. d'Opth. Otol. and Laryng., Oktober. (Von 31 nachkommen bis zur 4. Generation waren 16 mit kongenitalem staar behaftet.)

2750. Collins, Extensive rupture of the posterior capsule of the lens following a blow on the eye from a stone. Trans. of the Opth. Soc. of the United Kingdom, XI, p. 126.

2751. Wood. Rupture of the capsule of both lenses, with other damage to the eye; from pleuro-pneumonia, cough (?). Montreal Med. Journal, XX, p. 87. 1891-92.

2752. Achun, A., Ein fall von luxation der linse und abreissung der regenbogenhaut mit ciliarkorper bei integritat der ausseren augenhaute. (Slutschaj wiwicha chrustalika i otriwa, radus schnoj obolotschki s ciliarnimtjelom prizelosti naruschnich obolotschek glaza.) Wjestnik Opth., VIII, 3, p. 222.

2753. Bettmann, Boerne, Dislocation of the lens into the anterior chamber. American Journ. of Opth., p. 159, und Chicago Med. Record, p. 317.

2754. Deschamps, A., Deux observations de luxation traumatique des cristallins. Dauphine Med. Grenoble, XV, p. 57.

2755. Mercanti, Un raro caso di lusazione incompletamente sottocongiuntivale del cristallino. Annali di Ottalm., XX, p. 365.

2756. Rossigneux, Luxation du cristallin et decollement du corps ciliaire. Province Med., 21. Fevrier et France Med., No. 10, p. 152.

2757. Sureau, H., Contribution a l'etude des luxations spontanees du cristallin. These. de Paris.

2758. Theobald. Dislocated lens. (Amer. Opth. Soc.) Amer. Journ. of Opth., p. 231, und Med. Record, October 3.

2759. Trousseau. L'intervention dans les luxations du cristallin. La Pratique Medic. de Baratoux, January 13.

2760. Wood, White, Subconjunctival dislocations of the lens. Lancet, No. 3522. February 28.

2761. American Opthalmological Society, Annual Meeting September, 1891. Dislocated lens. Amer. Journ. of Opth., p. 231.

2762. Puschkin, Ectopia lentis utriusque oculi. Wjestnik Opth., VIII, 3, p. 224.

2763. Neve, C. F., Remarks on diabetic cataract. Indian. Med. Record, p. 373.

2764. Williot, M., De la cataracte hemorrhagique. These. de Paris.

1891. 2765. American Opthalmological Society, Annual Meeting September, 1891. Glaucoma after extraction of cataract. Amer. Journ. of Opth., p. 281, and Opth. Review, p. 376.

2766. Antonelli, Studio critico ed osservazioni cliniche intorno alla naturazione artificiale della cataratta. Napoli.

2767. Archangelskaja, A., Bericht uber 100 staarextractionen in der land. (Sems two.) Praxis. (Ottschjoz o sotne extraktij katarakt w skemskoj praktika.) Medizinlskoje Obozrenje, XXXI, Nr.15, p.198.

2768. Barr, S., Die extraktion des beginnenden staares. New York Med. Record, December 12.

2769. Bono, Ueber staarextraction. Verh. d. X. Internat. Med. Kongr., 1890, IV, 10, p. 154.

2770. Brockmann, Drake, Preliminary capsulotomy in the extraction of cataract. Amer. Journ. of Opth., p. 90.

2771. British Medical Association, Section of Opthalmology, July, 1891. Iridectomy or non in cataract extraction. Opth. Review, p. 315.

2772. Buller, F., Glaucoma after extraction of cataract. Trans. of the Amer. Opth. Soc., 27th Meeting, p. 120, and Amer. Journ. of Opth., VIII, p. 313.

2773. Carrow, F., A review of a year's work in the treatment of cataract. Trans. Michigan Med. Soci., XV, p. 214. Detroit, 1891.

2774. Chisholm, J. J., How should cataract operation be performed? Journ. Amer. Med. Assoc., XVII, p. 329. Chicago, 1891.

2775. ———, The after treatment of cataract operations. Verh. d. X. Internat. Med. Kongr., IV, p. 13. 1890.

2776. Critchett, A., Capsulotomy knife. Trans. of the Opth. Soc.

2777. Aguilar, Blanche, Cataracte hereditaire. (Compt. rendu de la section opthalmologique du Congres Medic. de Valence.) Revue Generale d'Opth., p. 352.

2778. Bleibaugh, C. B., Report of six recent cases of cataract. Trans. Med. Soc. of West Virginia, p. 865. Wheeling.

2779. Brailey, On some points in the development of cataract. Trans. of the Opth. Soc. of the United Kingdom, XI. p. 66.

2780. Dubief, Note sur quelques recherches bacteriologiques dans les cataractes. Annal. d'Oculist, T. CVI, p. 182.

2781. Green, J., Notes of twenty-one cases of cataract occurring in a single family. Trans. of Amer. Opth. Soc., Twenty-sixth Meeting. p. 690. (Bei 70 bekannten nachkommen einer familie 21 staarfalle.)

2782. Hall, G. C., Cases of hereditary cataract. Indian Med. Record, p. 194. Calcutta.

2783. Knaggs, L., On lenticonus. Lancet, II, p. 657.

2784. Magnus, H., Die grundelemente der staarbildung in der senilen linse. Arch. f. Augenheilkunde, XXIV, S. 1.

544

1891. 2785. ——, Ueber blasenbildung am linsenaquator. Klin. Monatsbl. f. Augenheilk., S. 291.

2786. Natanson, A., Spontane resorption des alterstaares. (Samordnoje wsariwanje startscheskoj.) Wratsch., No. 45, p. 996.

2787. ——, Spontane intracapsulaire recorption eines alterstaares. Klin. Monatsbl. f. Augenheilk., S. 423.

2788. Norris, G., Die katarakt depressionen in Skandinavien in der letzten Halfte des 18. Jahrhunderts, Nord. Opth. Tidskr., IV, 1.

2789. Panas, Cataratte mature ed impermature. Boll. d'Ocul., XIII, p 23.

2790. Venneman, E., Un cas de lenticone double anterieur. Annal. d'Oculist, T. CV, p. 158.

2791. Weeks, A case of lenticonus posterior, with remarks. Arch. Opth., XX, p. 260.

2792. Collins, W. J., On some exceptional cases of operation for cataract. Lancet, II, p. 479.

2793. Cross, F. R., Iridectomy or no in cataract extraction. Brit. Med. Journ., II, p. 472.

2794. Dimissas, Sur la simplification de l'extraction de la cataracte. Recueil d'Opth., p. 136.

2795. Finck, L., Method of operation for cataract in Bijnor Dispensary, with the result of 100 cases during 1890. Indian Med. Gaz., XXV, p. 358. Calcutta, 1890.

2796. Fox, L. W., Improved eye-pairs for the after dressing in cataract operation. Med. News, Philadelphia, p. 851.

2797. Frothingham, C. E., Remarks on the need of more efficient protection of the eye after cataract extraction, and an improved apparatus for the purpose. Journ. Amer. Med. Assoc., Chicago, p. 385. (Eine Augenmaske statt des Occlusiv-Verbandes.)

2798. Fulton, J. F., Treatment of immature cataract. Amer. Journ. of Opth., p. 165.

2799. Gaupillat, Pansement apres l'operation de la cataracte a grand lambeau superieur. Revue Generale d'Opth., p. 339.

2800. Gayet, Essai sur la recherche de l'acuite visuelle apres l'operation de la cataracte. Necessite d'employer partout une methode uniforme. V. Helmholtz'sche. Festschr., S. 62.

2801. Gualta, Cenno preventivo di uno studio sperimentale e clinico nella maturazione artificiale della cataratta. Annali di Ottalm., XIX, 5, 6, p. 517.

2802. ——, Panoftalmite tardiva siluppatata sei mesi dopo un ablazione di cataratta. Ibid., p. 515.

2803. Graefe, A., Zur wundbehandlung der katarakt extractionen. Deutsche Med. Wochenschr., No. 43.

2804. Graves, A. C., Cataract extraction. West. Med. and Surg. Reporter. St. Joseph, 1891-92, I, 27.

1891. 2805. Greef, R., Report of 450 simple extractions of senile cataract. Translated by Dr. A. J. Spahling. Arch. Opth., XX, p. 303.

2806. Deutschmann's Beitrage zur Augenheilk., III, S. 52.

2807. Hansen, C. M., Extraktion der linsekapsel. Hosp. Tid., S. 685.

2808. Harlan, H., Successful cataract extraction in a case of adavanced retinitis pigmentosa. Maryland Med. Journ., XXIV, p. 265. Baltimore, 1891-91.

2809. ——, Ein fall von iris prolaps am 3. Tage nach einer katarakt extraktion ohne iridektomie. Prolaps reponiert; Heilung. Arch. f. Augenheilk., XXIV, S. 50.

2810. ——, Case of hernia of iris occurring on third day after cataract extraction without iridectomy; hernia replaced; recovery. Arch. Opth., XX, p. 81.

2811. Hjort, Ueber katarakt extraktion ohne iridektomie. Norsk. Magaz., p. 648.

2812. Holmes, Spicer, Hemorrhage following extraction of a black cataract in a highly myopic eye, probably associated with choroidal changes; enucleation. Journ. Amer. Med. Assoc, XVI, p. 83. Chicago.

2813. Jacquin, Pressure on the globe after cataract extraction. Ibid, XVI, p. 331.

2814. ——, The simple extraction of cataract. Maryland Med. Journ., XVI, p. 67. Baltimore, 1891-92.

2815. Johannson, E., Katarakt operationen in ausserklinischer behandlung. (Livlandischer Aerztetag.) Walk, September, 1891. (St. Petersburger Med. Wochenschr.)

2816. Kerschbaumer, Rosa, Report of two hundred cataract extractions. Translated by Dr. C. A. Wood. Arch. Opth., XX, p. 349.

2817. Knapp, H., Ein fall von glaskorperblutung nach einer staar extractraktion. Arch. f. Augenheilk., XXIII, S. 272.

2818. ——, The occurrence, prevention and management of prolapse of the iris in simple extraction of cataract. Trans. of the Amer. Opth. Soc., 27th Meeting, p. 80.

2819. ——, Die behandlung der kapsel wahrend und nach der staar extraktion. Verh. des X. Internat. Med. Congresses, Bd. IV, 4, S. 1.

2820. Kollock, C. N., Report of cataract cases. Trans. South Carolina Med. Assoc., p. 107. Charleston.

2821. Lacqueur, Ueber den gegenwartigen stand der lehre von der staar operation. Deutsche Med. Wochenschr., No. 5. (Naturwissensch. Med. Verein in Strassburg. Sitzung vom 29. November, 1890.)

2822. Landolt, Presentation; de quelques instruments ayant trait a l'operation de cataracte. (Societe Francaise d'Opthalmologie.) Arch. d'Opth., XI. p. 463, 545, et XII. p. 323, et Annal. d'Oculist, T. CV, p. 227.

1891. 2823. Lerebzenicowa, E., Bericht uber 300 katarakt operationen. Wjestnik Opth., VIII, 1, p. 32.

2824. Lippincott, J. A., Routine syringing out of cortical matter in cataract extraction, as illustrated by 100 cases. Trans. of the Amer.
Opth. Soc., 27th Meeting, p. 85.

2825. Logetschnikow, S., Eine staar extraktion bei morbus basedowii.
Klin. Monatsbl. f. Augenheilk., S. 277.

2826. ———, Staarextraction bei einer kranken mit morbus basedowii.
(Slutschij i swletschenja katakakti, osloschnjonnoj bolesnju base-
dowa.) Westnik Opth., III, p. 219.

2827. Martin, G., Une complication post-operatoire de la cataracte de
Morgagni. Societe d'Opth. de Paris, November 3.

2828. Mellinger, C., Experimentelle untersuchungen uber die entstehung
der in letzter zeit bekannt gewordenen trubungen der hornhaut
nach staar extraktion. V. Graefe's Arch. f. Opth., XXXVII, 4,
S. 159.

2829. Millee, E., Extraction du cristallin a la curette. Nouvelle anse
fenetree. Annal. d'Oculist, T. CVI, p. 2. (Durch einen in der
Mitte verlaufenden Langsleistep gefenstert.)

2830. Minor, J. L., A report of twenty-five cataract extractions. Arch.
Opth., XX, p. 69

2831. Murrell, T. E., To what extent are personal restraints essential
during healing of corneal wounds? Journ. Amer. Med. Assoc.,
XVII, p. 333.

2832. Neuschuler, De l'astigmatisme post-operatoire. Recueil d'Opth.,
p. 515.

2833. Nikoljukin, J., Bericht uber 97 staar operationen in der Land (Sems-
two) Praxis. (Ottschjot o 97 operatijach katarakti w semskoj
praktike.) Wjestnik Opth., VIII, 3, p. 226.

2834. Nuel, Sur la prophylaxie de la suppuration apres l'operation de la
cataracte. (Societe Francaise d'Opthalmologie.) Arch. d'Opth.,
XI, p. 463, 545, et Annal. d'Oculist, T. CV, p. 227.

2835. Norrie, G., Die katarakt operation in Skandinavian in der letzten
Halfte des Jahrhunderts. Nord. Opth. Tidsskr., IV, p. 1.

2836. Ostwalt, F., Einige Worte uber glaserkorrektion bei aphakie. Klin.
Monatsbl. f. Augenheilk., S. 283.

2837. Parinaud, H., Le prolapsus de l'iris dans l'extraction simple de la
cataracte. Recueil d'Opth., p. 321.

2838. ———, L'enclavement de l'iris dans l'extraction de la cataracte.
(Societe Francaise d'Opthalmologie.) Arch. d' Opth., XI, p. 463,
545, et XII, p. 323, et Annal. d'Oculist, T. CV, p. 227.

2839. ———, Il prolasso dell'iride nella estrazione della cateratta. Boll.
d'Ocul., XIII, 10.

1891. 2840. Pitts, B., Cataract extraction. Trans. Medical Assoc., XXXIII, p. 64.

2841. Pooley, T. R., Operation for secondary cataract, followed by irido-cyclitis and consecutive glaucoma. Amer. Journal of Opth., p. 377.

2842. Rider, W., Report of a case of fatal meningitis following suppuration of the cornea after cataract operation. Trans. Med. Society New York, p .402. Philadelphia.

2843. Roosa, The results of various methods of extraction of cataract, illustrated by 206 cases. Arch. of Opth., XX, No. 2, p. 207.

2844. Santos, Fernandez, Extraction du cristallin dans myopie. Compte rendu de la section opthalmologique du Congress Medic. de Valence. Revue Generale d'Opth., p. 352.

2845. ———, Un accident possible, mais remediable dans la keratotomie. Revue Generale d'Opth., X, 3.

2846. Schnabel, Entwickelung der staaroperationen. Allg. Wien. Med. Zeitg., XXXVI, S. 425.

2847. Serebrennikowa, E., Bericht uber 30 staaroperationen. (Ottschjot o 300 staaroperatij katarakti.) Wjestnik Opth., VIII, 1, p. 82.

2848. Smith, E., Staar. Wie sollen wir uns zur kapsel verhalten? Neue Cystotompincette. Journ. Amer. Med. Assoc., November 5.

2849. Suarez de Mendoza, La suture de la cornee dans l'extraction de la cataracte. Recueil d'Opth., p. 577.

2850. ———, Nouveaux faits a l'appui des avantages de la suture de la cornee, dans l'operation de la cataracte. (Societe Francaise d'Opthalmologie.) Arch. d'Opth., XI, p. 463, 545, et XII, p. 323, et Annal. d'Oculist, T. CV, p. 265.

2851. Thomas, A report of 50 cases of cataract extraction. Journ. Opth. Otol. and Laryngol., p. 8.

2852. Valude, L'operation de la cataracte et son pansement. Ann. de Therap. Med. Chir., VI, p. 269. Paris, 1890.

2853. VanDuyse, De l'hemorrhagie choroidienne grave dans l'extraction du cristallin cataracte. Annal. d'Oculist, T. CV, p. 112.

2854. Vignes, Algunas palabras sobre las cataractas secundarias. Rev. Esp. de Oftal., Dermat., Sif., etc., XV, p. 289. Madrid, 1891.

2855. ———, Quelques mots sur les cataractes secondaires. Recueil d'Opth., p. 05.

2856. Wagenmann, A., Zur anatomie des dunnhautigen nachstaars, nebst bemerkungen uber die heilung von Wunden der Descemet'schen Membran. V. Graefe's Arch. f. Opth., XXXVII, 2, S. 21.

2857. Wahlfors, K. R., Bericht uber 150 staarextraktionen. Finska Lakaresallsk. Handl., XXXIII, p. 333.

2858. Webster, D., Notes of a case of diabetic cataract operated upon by Dr. C. R. Agnew. Amer. Journ. of Opth., p. 131.

2859. ———, Report of 136 cases of cataract extraction. Trans. of the Amer. Opth. Soc., 27th Meeting, p. 75.

1891. 2860. ———, Improved eye-pads for the after dressing in cataract operations. Med. News, March 28.

2861. DeWecker, Ablation de la capsule anterieure. Paris, Lecrosnier et Babe.

2862. ———, Nouveau procede operatoire de cataracte secondaire. (Societe Francaise d'Opthalmologie.) Arch. d'Opth., XI, p. 463, 545, et XII. 323, et Annal. d'Ocullst, T. CV, p. 227.

2863. Wickerkiewicz, Ein ungewohnliches ereignis bei einer normal ausgefuhrten alterstaar extraktion. (Polnisch.) S. A. aus Przeglada Lekarsk, Nr. 38.

2864. Wolkow, M., Zur frage der staarextraktion ohne iridektomie. (Kwoprosu ob extraktii katarakti bes iridektomii.) Wjestnik Opth., VIII, 2, p. 99, und Tagebl., d. IV, Kongresses d. Russ. Aerzte, Nr. 10.

2864a. Knaggs, On lenticomus. Lancet, 1891.

1892. 2865. Abadie, Nouvelle methode de traitement des luxations completes du cristallin. Soc. d'Opth. de Paris, July 5.

2866. Alt, A., A case of acquired anterior polar cataract. Amer. Journ. of Opth., IX, 11, p. 357.

2867. Arnold, Th., Mittheilungen uber 4000 staaroperationen, ausgefuhrt von Prof. O. Haab. Arch. f. Augenheilk., XXV, 1-2, S. 41.

2868. Audibert, Procede nouveau pour l'aspiration, en un seul temps, des cataractes liquides et demi-molles; description d'une aiguille keratotome creuse speciale. Ann. d'Ocul., CVIII, 2, p. 100.

2869. Ausin, Johann, Das eisen in der linse. Dorpat, 1891.

2870. Baker, A. R., The pathology and treatment of infantile cataract. Amer. Med. Assoc., Detroit, June, 7-10.

2871. Baker, A., Infantile cataract. Amer. Journ. of Opth., IX, 11, p. 350.

2872. Barsanti, Cataracte traumatique developpe soudainement a la suite d'une commotion du cristallin. Rec. d'Opth., No. 1, p. 1.

2873. Beaumont, W. M., Aphakial erythropsia. Opth. Rev. No. 125, p. 72.

2874. Bettman, B., A new operation for the speedy ripening of immature cataract. Chicago Medical Recorder, April.

2875. Bribosia, Guerison d'un aveugle de naissance; operation de cataracte congenitale double; chez un sujet de 15 ans. Arch. d'Opth., XII, 2, p. 88.

2876. Cant, W. J., On the management of prolapse of the iris after simple cataract extraction. Brit. Med. Journ., No. 1659, p. 834.

2877. Chisholm, J., The dislocation of an opaque lens. Amer. Journ. of Opth., IX, 4, p. 101.

2878. Colline, E. T., On the minute anatomy of pyramidal cataract. Trans. Opth. Soc., XII, p. 89.

2879. Colline, E. T., and Richardson Cross, Two cases of epithelial implantation cysts in the anterior chamber after extraction of cataract. Trans. Opth. Soc., XII, p. 175.

1892. 2880. Deschamps, A prospos d'un cas de luxation spontanee des deux cristallins. Annal. d'Ocul., CVIII, 5, p. 347.

2881. Dimmer, J., Noch einmal die glasercorrection bei aphakie. Klin. Mon. Bl., XXX, S. 73.

2882. Dittmer, J., Beitrag zur statistik der modificirten linear extraction. In. Diss. Kiel.

2883. Dolschenkow, W., Bericht uber einhundert cataract operationen. Wjestnik Opth., IX, 1, S. 26.

2884. Dor, Sur le traitement de la cataracte congenitale. Congr. Franc. d'Opth., May 2. Rapport sur le traitement de la cataracte congenitale. Compte Rend. de la Soc. Franc. d'Opth., May 2.

2885. Eiseck, Ein fall von lenticonus posterior. Klin. Mon. Bl., XXX, S. 116.

2886. Erwin, Treatment of incipient cataract. Amer. Med. Assoc., Detroit, June 7-10.

2887. Friebis, G., A case of congenital ectopia lentis. Ebenda.

2888. Galezowski, Sur un nouveau procede operatoire d'extraction des cataractes incompletes. Congr. Franc. d'Opth., May 2.

2889. ———, Nouveau procede operatoire d'extraction de cataractes incompletes par incision semielliptique de la cornee avec sphincterotomie. Rec. d'Opth., No. 5, p. 262.

2890. Gardner, C. R., Absorption of opacities in a case of senile cataract. Opth. Rec., I, 12, p. 111.

2891. Gayet. Un cas de luxation double du cristallin. La Province Med., No. 31.

2892. Hansell, H. J., The extraction of double congenital cataract; sympathetic inflammation after second operation; recovery. Ann. of Opth. and Otol., I, 2, p. 137.

2893. Higgens, Ch., Spontaneous cure of cataract. Opth. Soc. of the United Kingdom. Case of spontaneous disappearance of cataract. Trans. Soc., XII, p. 107.

2894. Hilbert R., Zur geschichte der kyanopie. Arch. f. Augenheilk. XXIV, 3, S. 240.

2895. Hirschberg, Ueber kernstaar—Ausziehung. Berlin. Klin. Woch., No. 26.

2896. Knapp, The methods and results of simple cataract extraction. Amer. Med. Assoc., Detroit, June 7-10.

2897. Kortnew, A., Ueber die rachitische cataract. Wjestnik Opth., IX, 2, S. 114.

2898. Landolt, L'operation de la cataracte de nos jours. Arch. d'Opth., XII, 9, p. 529.

2899. Lapersonne, De l'opportunite de l'intervention dans les cataractes traumatiques. Congr. Franc. d'Opth., May 2.

2900. Logetschnikow, S., Einige bemerkungen uber die cataract extractionen nach Dr. Wolkow. Wjestnik Opth., IX, 4, S. 358.

1892. 2901. Magnus, H., Die entwickelung des alterstaares. Augenarztliche unterrichtstafeln fur den academischen und selbstuntericht. Heft. II. Breslau.

2902. Milliken, Injury of the lens, with cases. Amer. Med. Assoc., Detroit, June 7-10.

2903. Mitvalsky, J., Ein neuer fall von lenticonus posterior mit theilweiser persistenz der arteria hyaloidea. Centralbl. f. Prakt. Augenheilk., S. 65.

2904. ———, Zur kentniss der spontanheilung des senilen totalstaars vermittelst der intracapsularen resorption nebs.

2905. ———, Bemerkungen uber cataracta Morgagniana. Centralbl. f. Prakt. Augenheilk., S. 289.

2906. Nicati, A la recherche d'un procede d'extraction de la cataracte capable d'eviter les enclavements et les hernies, ou d'en attenuer les effets. Arch. d'Opth., XI, 12, p. 731.

2907. Nuel, Troubles corneens consecutifs a l'extraction de la cataracte. Bull. de la Soc. Franc. d'Opth., p. 37.

2908. ———, De certain troubles corneens consecutifs a l'extraction de la cataracte. Bull. de la Soc. Franc. d'Opth., p. 37.

2909. Pfluger, Bemerkungen zum gegenwartigen stand der frage der staaroperation. Ebenda. S. 155.

2910. Pomeroy, O. D., A report of fifty cases of extraction of cataract without iridectomy. New York Med. Journ., LVI, 20, p. 535.

2911. Pooley, Th., Operation for secondary cataract, followed by iridiocyclitis and consecutive glaucoma. Amer. Journ. of Opth., VIII, 12, p. 377.

2912. Randolph, R. L., A series of fifty consecutive operations for cataract. John Hopkins Hosp. Bull., III, 20, p. 19.

2913. Raschewski, Einfluss des chinins auf die eiterung der wunde bei cataract extractionen. Wjestnik. Opth., IX, 3, S. 216.

2914. Richardson, Cross and Treacher Collins, Implanation cyst in the anterior chamber after cataract extraction. Opth. Soc. of the United Kingdom, July 8.

2915. Schanz, J., Ueber den einfluss der pupillaroffung auf das sehen aphakischer. Verhandl. d. Ges. Deutscher Naturforscher und Aerzte. Halle.

2916. Schulek, W., Ueber eine neue methode der cataract extraction. Szemeszet, No. 2.

2917. Snellen, Hansen Grut, Critchett, Secondi, Sur l'operation de la cataracte. Ann. d'Ocul., CVII, p. 74.

2918. Spicer, W. T. H., Lamellar cataract. Trans. Opth. Soc., XII, p. 74.

2919. Ryerson, Sterling, Miscellaneous facts regarding extraction of cataract. Opth. Rec., I. 7-8, p. 258.

2920. Suarez de Mendoza, Nouveaux faits de suture de la cornee dans l'extraction de la cataracte. Cong. Franc. d'Opth., May 2.

1892. 2921. Terson, Des corps estrangers du cristallin; indications de l'intervention operatoire. Arch. d'Opth., XII, 3, p. 156.

2922. Topolanski, A., Linsenranderhebungen. Klin. Mon. Bl., XXX, S. 89.

2923. Treacher Collins, The minute anatomy of pyramidal cataract. Brit. Med. Journ., No. 1692, p. 606.

2924. Trousseau, Quelques accidents des operations secondaires. Ann. d'Ocul., CVII, p. 338.

2925. Wagner, Bericht uber ein tausend cataract extractionen nach A. v. Graefe's tmethode. Wjestnik Opth., IX, 1, S. 1.

2926. Webster, F., Preliminary and after treatment in cataract operations. Annal. of Opth. and Otol., April. The preliminary and after treatment in cataract operations. Annal. of Opth. and Otol., I, 2, p. 88.

2927. Wecker, L. de, Quel progres reste a realiser pour l'extraction de la cataracte? Arch. d'Opth., XII, 6, p. 250. Extraction simple et extraction combinee. Arch. d'Opth., XII, 11, p. 657.

2928. White, J., Immature cataract and the best way of hastening maturity. Amer. Med. Soc., Detroit, June 7-10.

2829. Wickerkiewicz, Zur entstehung bleibender hornhaut trubungen nach cataract extractionen. Deutsche Med. Wochenschr., No. 7.

2930. Widmark, J., Om staarsmittels utveckling itter A. v. Graefe's Dod. Hygiea. September.

2931. Wray, Charles, Etiology, prognosis and treatment of disseminated cataract. Opth. Soc. of the United Kingdom, January 28. Aetiology, prognosis and treatment of disseminated cataract. Trans. Opth. Soc., XII, p. 109.

2932. Zirm, E., Doppelseitiger kernstaar. Klin. Mon. Bl., XXX, S. 5. Beiderseitige ectopia lentis bei zwei geschwistern. Wiener Klin. Wochenschr., No. 21.

1893. 2933. Abadie, Nouvelle methode de traitement des luxations completes du cristallin. Progres Med., XVI, p. 259.

2934. Albrand, W., Bericht uber 549 staar operationen der Prof. Scholer's chen Augenklinik in Berlin. Arch. f. Augenheilkunde, XXVI, Heft. 3 and 4.

2935. Audibert, Considerations pratiques sur deux operations de cataracte choroideenne avec issue considerable d'humeur vitree suivies de succes definitif. Gaz. Med. Chir. de Toulouse, XXV, p. 18.

2936. Baas, K. L., Ein fall von coloboma lentis congenitum durch persistierendes fotalgewebe. Klin. Monatsbl. f. Augenheilk., S. 297.

2937. Bauerlein, A., Meine erfahrungen uber staar und staar operationen in 25 jahren. Wiesbaden. J. F. Bergmann.

2938. Bajardi, P., Sul grado d'A. corneale negli operati di cataratta specialemente in rapporto col metodo operativo e con le complicazioni avvenute durante e dopo l'estrazione. (Rend. del. XIII. Congresso della Assoc. Ottalm. Ital.) Annali di Ottalm., XXII p. 552.

1893. 2939. Bates, Notes on cataract extraction. Virginia Med. Month., Richmond, XX, p. 217.

2940. Beaumont, W. M., The progress and prognosis of incipient senile cataract. Provincial Med. Journ., February 1. •

2941. Beccaria, J., Sul glaucoma secondario consecutivo a lussazione del cristalino. Annali di Ottalm., XXII, p. 115.

2942. Bettmann, Ripening of immature cataracts by direct trituration. Ann. Opth. and Otol., p. 26. St. Louis.

2943. Black, G. M., A successful cataract operation performed without the observance of the usual rules. Denver Med. Times, 1892, p. 380.

2944. Blancoeur, Cataracte consecutive a une contusion violente du globe de l'oeil. Annal. de la Policlinique de Bordeaux, No. 15.

2945. Blood, On a series of 282 extractions. Liverpool Med. Chir. Journ. July.

2946. Bourgeois, Intervention dans les luxations pathologiques du cristallin. Union Med. du Nord-ant. Reims, XVII, p. 172.

2947. Brainer, J. N., A cataract operation in a much mutilated eye. Trans. Michigan Med. Soc., XVII, p. 202. Detroit.

2948. Cereseto, Un operations di cataratta pres estrazione complicata a rilevantissima perdita di vitreo, che termina tuttavia sulla guarigione lasciando l'occhio con V2-3. Gaz. d'osp. Milano, XIV, p. 450.

2949. Chauvel, Etudes opthalmologiques. Affections du cristallin. Recueil d'Opth., March et April.

2950. Chisholm, Anteror dislocation of the lens in a child with ectopic pupils, and how it was reduced. Maryland Med. Journ., XXIX, p. 353. Baltimore.

2951. Claiborne. J. H., Blunt hook and book knife for facilitating the operation for secondary cataract. Med. Record, New York, p. 575.

2952. Dahlerup, S., Die behandlung des grauen staars (dan). Hospitalstidende, p. 885 u. 905.

2953. Dannich, Paul, Beitrag zur lehre von den staar operationen. Inaug. Diss. Halle a. S.

2954. Darier, A., Behandlung und prophylaxe der infektosen processe nach staar operation. Bericht uber die opth. Gesellschaft zu Heidelberg, S. 99.

2955. Dennotkin, S., Ueber verminderung des traumatismus bei der staar extraktion (Ob ummenschennii traumatisma dri iswletschenii katarakti). Chirurgitschesnaja Letopis, III, No. 5, p. 750.

2956. DeSchweinitz, G. E., Nuclear cataract; artificial ripening by direct trituration; extraction, followed by prolonged and at times violent dementia; recovery of reason and good vision. Annal. Opth. and Otol., II, p. 145. St. Louis.

2957. Dujardin, L'extraction de la cataracte selon la derniere methode de Daviel. Journ. des Sciences Med. de Lille, p. 1.

1893. 2958. Dunn, J., Three cases of dislocation of the lens occurring in cataract extraction; showing three of the positions the lens may assume; question as to the regeneration of the vitreous. Ann. Opth. and Otol. II, p. 250. St. Louis.

2959. ———. The cataract knife. New York Med. Record, p. 600.

2960. ———, Extraction of part of the capsule as an operative procedure in certain cases of secondary cataract. Arch. Opth., XXII, p. 344. New York.

2961. Eversbusch, Ein fall von ektopia lentis congenita binocularis bei einem 17 jahre alte manne. Versammelung Deutscher Naturforscher u. Aerzte. Nurnberg. 1893.

2962. Fage, Hemorrhagie intra-oculaire grave apres une extraction de cataracte. Annal. d'Oculist, T. CIX, p. 266.

2963. Faravelli, Sulla cataratta naftalinica. Annali di Ottalm., XXII, p. 8.

2964. Freeland, Fergus, On ten years' experience of cataract operations. Brit. Med. Journ., May 13.

2965. Fromaget, Cataractes congenitales hereditaires pendant six generations. Ibid., No. 31.

2966. Fuchs, Die neuen methoden der staar operationen. Vortrag Gehalten in der sitzung der k. k. Gesellschaft der Aerzte in Wien, December 2, 1892. Wien. Klin. Wochenschrift, No. 2.

2967. Galezowski, Extraction de la cataracte sans iridectomie. Ses avantages et ses eguells. Recueil d'Opth. May.

2968. Gillet de Grandmont, Observations de cataracte noire. Extraction. Analyze spectroscopique. Progres Medical, No. 17.

2969. Grosz, E., A szurke halyog operalasarol. (Operation des grauen staars.) Szemeszet, p. 29.

2970. Gullstrand, A., Ein fall von lenticonus posterior. Nordisk Opthalmologisch Tidsschrift. Vol I. (Typischer Fall von linksseitigem lenticonus posterior bei einem 30 jahringen Mann.)

2971. Heucke, A., Beitrag zur lehre von der aetiologie und behandlung der luxationen der krystallinse. Inaug. Diss. Strassburg.

2972. Higgens, C., Extraction of cataract. Lancet, II, p. 1180.

2973. Hippel, E. v. sen., Ueber den gegenwartigen stand der staar operation. Munch. Med. Wochenschr., S. 669.

2974. Hirschberg, J., Ueber schichtstaar bei alteren menschen. Centralbl. f. Prakt. Augenheilk., August. S. 225.

2975. ———, Heilung der kurzsichtigen netzhautablosung nach auszeihung der getrubten linse. Ebd. Marz.

2976. Howe, L., On the removal of hard cataract by section. Trans. of the Amer. Opth. Soc., 29th Meeting, p. 594.

2977. Jackson, E., When cataract is ready for operative treatment. Trans. Med. Soc. Pennsylvania, XXIV. p. 97. Philadelphia.

1893. 2978. Jackson, E., Indirect massage of the lens for the artificial ripening of cataract. Trans. of the Amer. Opth. Soc., 29th Meeting, p. 523.

2979. Kayser, Fritz, Iridectomy necessary twelve and fourteen days after normal extraction of cataract. Opth. Record, Nashville, 1892-93, p. 353.

2970a. Hess, Zur Pathologie und Pathologischen Anat. verschieden Staar formen. Graefe Hich. f. Opth., XXXIX, 1. 1893.

2980. Korschenewsky, S., Kurzer bericht uber das zweite hundert von katarakt extractionen in der land praxis. (Kratkij ottschott o wtoroj sotne iswletschenij katarakti w semskoj praktike.) Ibid., XL, p. 483.

2981. Krukow, A., Ein fall von pyramidal katarakt. Sitzungsberichte des Moskauer Opth. Vereines. 1892.

2982. Kuschew, N., Kurzer bericht uber das zweite hundert von kata-extraktionen (Kratkij ottschott o perwoj totne iswletschenij katarakti). Wjestnik Opth., X, p. 510.

2983. Landolt, Un couteau destine a la discission. Arch. d'Opth., XIII, p. 529.

2984. Logetschnikow, S., Eine eigenartige katarakt mit sequester. Sitzungsberichte des Moskauer Opth. Vereins. 1892.

2985. ——, Eine seltene anomalie von linsenstaar (Redkaja anomalia katarakti). Chirurgitscheskaja Lepotis, III, No. 4.

2986. Maschek, O operacyi zacmy bez woyciecia teczowki. (Uber staar operation ohne iridektomie.) S. A. aus Przeglad Lekarski.

2987. Magnus, H., Ueber das verhalten von fremdkorpern in der linse. Centralbl. f. Prakt. Augenheilk., November S. 327.

2988. Manolescu, A propos de l'extraction simple de la cataracte. Roumanie Med. Mars.

2989. Mastrocinque, Massagio diretto sul cristallino per la maturazzione artificiale della cataratta con un nuovo instrumento. (Rend. del XIII. Congr. della Assoc. Oftalm. Ital.) Annali di Ottalm., XXII. p. 45. (Empfehlung der direkten linsen massage mit einem eigenen sondenartigen instrument.)

2990. McCoy, T. J., A new shield for the protection of eyes after cataract operations. Med. Record, New York, 1892, XII, p. 664, and South. Californa Pract., Los Angeles, 1892, VII, p. 8.

2991. Meyer, E., Malformation du cristallin. Revue Generale d'Opth., p. 1.

2992. Mitvalsky, Microphakie und deren klinische bedeutung. Klin. Monatsbl. f. Augenheilk., S. 823.

2993. Moerner, C. Th., Untersuchung der proteinsubstanzen in den lichtbrechenden medien des auges. (3) Mitt. Zeitschr. f. Phys. Chem., XVIII, S. 61.

1893. 2994. Moore, W. O., The after treatment of cataract extraction. Med. News, Philadelphia, p. 253.

2995. Mooren, Die indikationsgrenzen der cataract discission. Deutsche Med. Wochenschr., S. 857.

2996. Moorehead, G. C., Cataract operations. Journ. Amer. Med. Assoc., Chicago, XX, p. 437.

2997. Mules, Pyramidal cataract. (Opth. Soc. of the United Kingdom.) Opth. Review, p. 159.

2998. Murell, T. E., The simple dressing after cataract extraction. Opth. Record, Nashville, 1893-4, III, p. 121.

2999. Neuburger, Ueber die haufigkeit der staarbildung in den vehschiedenen lebensaltern. Centralbl. f. Prakt. Augenheilk., September, S. 263. Beitrag zur entwickelung der katarakt. Ebd., S. 165.

3000. Nicati, La pointe conteaux a cataracte. Facheuse routine a deraciner. Arch. d'Opth., XVII, p. 136.

3001. Nickelsburg, Leopold, Weitere beitrage zur aetiologie der cataracta senilis. Inaug. Diss. Wurzburg, 1892.

3002. Panas, Prophylaxie des accidents infectieux consecutifs a l'operation de la cataracte. Arch. dOpth., XIII, p. 593.

3003. ———, L'operation des cataractes congenitales. Progres Med., No. 7.

3004. Parinaud, Le prolapsus de l'iris dans l'extraction simple de la cataracte. Soc. d'Opth. de Paris. April, 1893.

3005. Peters, A., Ueber die entstehung des schichtstaars und verwandter staarformen. V. Graefe's Arch., XXXIX, 1, S. 221.

3006. Piechaud, A., Cataracte congenitale demi-pierreuse. Recueil d'Opth. p. 552.

3007. Reche, A., Ein beitrag zur entwickelung der katarakt. Centralbl. fur Prakt. Augenheilk., May. S. 129.

3008. ———, Ein fernerer beitrag zur entwickelung der katarakt. Ebd. December. S. 963.

3009. Rivers, E. C., Cataract extraction. New York Med. Journ., p. 301.

3010. Roethlisberger, P., Ueber die ausspulungen der vorderen kammer bei der staarextraktion an der Basler Opth. Klinik. Inaug. Diss. Basel.

3011. Roosa, John, A series of cataract operations. Post Graduate, New York, VIII, p. 271.

3012. Rudall, J. T., Spontaneous rupture of capsule after iridectomy preliminary to cataract extraction. (Opth. Soc. of the United Kingdom.) Opth. Review, p. 347.

3013. Santos Fernandez, J., Conducta que debe observarse con las cataractas invalidas de glaucoma. Cron. Med. Quir. de la Habana, 1892, XVIII, p. 740.

3014. ———, Hernia voluminosa del iris despues de la extraccion simple de la cataracta. Ibid., p. 6.

556

1898. 3015. Sbordone, Osservazioni pratiche sulla operazione della cataratta col processo a lembo seuza iridectomia. (Rend. del XIII. Congresso della Assoc. Oftalm. Ital.) Annali di Ottalm., XXII, p. 539. (Siehe diesen Ber. pro 1892.)

3016. Schantz, Fritz-Jena, Ueber den einfluss der pupillaröffnung auf das sehen aphakischer. Verhandlungen der Gesellschaft Deutscher Naturforscher u. Aerzte. Halle, 1891.

3017. Schlosser, Ueber akkommodation aphakischer augen. (Gesellsch. f. Morphol. und Physiol.) Munch. Med. Wochenschr., S. 291.

3018. Schoen, W., Die anfange und ursachen der stare. Deutsche Revue. Breslau u. Berlin, XVIII, S. 115.

3019. ———Die funktionskrankheiten d. auges. Wiesbaden. J. F. Bergman.

3020. Schreiber, P., Elfter jahresbericht meiner augenklinik. Jahrg. 1893.

3021. Schweigger, Operative beseitigung hochgradigre myopie. Deutsche Med. Wochenschr., No. 20.

3022. Smith, and Travis, B. F., Report of a case of extraction of cataract in a negro said to be 116 years old. Journ. Amer. Assoc., Chicago, XXI, p. 684.

3023. Snell, S., Case presenting unusual appearances after extraction; simulating cyst, but really due to a distended capsule. Opth. Review, p. 345. Die ausgedehnte eine cyste vortauschende linsen kapsel bei einer vor 7 jahre staaroperierten. Frau entheilt Zerfallsprodukte der linse selbs.

3024. Sous, De l'uree apres les operations de cataracte. Journ. de Med. de Bordeaux, September 17.

3025. Stafford, H. E., Extraction of senile cataract. New York Polyclinic, I, p. 142.

3026. Swanzy, On the combined method of cataract extraction. (Opth. Soc. of the United Kingdom.) Opth. Review, p. 213.

3027. Teale, T. P., Bowman lecture on the abandonment of iridectomy in the extraction of hard cataract. Journ. Amer. Med. Assoc., Chicago, XXI, p. 684.

3028. Theobald, S., Exhibition of patient with zonular cataracts. John Hopkins Hospital Bull., Baltimore, IV, p. 55.

3029. Thier, Die operative behandlung hochstgradiger myopie durch discission der linse. Deutsche Med. Wochenschr., XIX, S. 717.

3030. Trousseau, Le pterygion et l'operation de la cataracte. Annal d'Oculist., T. CIX, p. 146. (Verf. glaubt versichern zu mussen, dass ein vorhandenes pterygium nicht die Gefahr der Eiterung nach einer staaroperation erhohe.)

3031. Vacher, M., Nouvelle technique operatoire de la capsulotomie dans l'operation, de la cataracte. Societe d'Opth. de Paris. Seance du 7 Novembre, 1893.

1893   3032. Velhagen, C., Ein seltene form von entwicklungsstorung und Gewebswicherung im Innern eines Tierauges. V. Graefe's Arch. f. Opth., XXXIX, 4, S. 224.

3033. Valk, Tr., Cataract extraction with the iris retractor. (Read before the section of opthalmology of the first Pan-American Medical Congress.) Amer. Journ. of Opth., p. 390.

3034. Vossius, A., Zur kasuistik der angeboren anomalien des auges.

3035. Deutschmann's Beitrage zur Augenheilkunde, IX, Heft.

3036. Warner, A. G., Dislocation of the lens and subsequent cataract by a shot from an air gun. Journ. Opth. Otol. and Laryngol., V, p. 88.

3037. Webster, D., A case of congenital cataract; both lenses removed by operation. Arch. Pediat., New York, X, p. 929.

3038. DeWecker, Reminiscences historiques concernant l'extraction de la cataracte. Arch. d'Opth., XIII, p. 212.

3039. ———, La section de Daviel. Ibid, p. 261.

3040. ———, Modifications apportees par Daviel a la section. Ibid, p. 401.

3041. ———, L'extraction a lambeau triangulaire ou ogival. Ibid, p. 412.

3042. Wescott, An unusual case of dislocation of the lens. Annal. of Opth. and Otol., January.

3043. Wintersteiner, Ein fall von einseitigen, doppelten schichstaar. Klin. Monatsbl. f. Augenheilkunde, S. 300.

3044. ———, Angularer aequatorialstaar. Ebd., S. 333.

3045. White, J. A., Cataract; report of 100 operations. Virginia Medical Monthly, Richmond, 1892-93, XIX, p. 731.

3046. Zimmermann, C., Dislocation of the lens into the anterior chamber with iridodialysis; extraction; recovery. Congenital unilateral anopthalmus. Arch. of Opth., XXII, No. 3.

1894.   3047. Adelheim, Ein fall von colobomallentis. Wjest. Opth., XI, 2, S. 191.

3048. Ahlstrom, G., Redogonelse for 100 staaroperationer. Goteborg's Lakar. Forh., N. I.

3049. Birnbacher, Ein neues verfahren der kapselentfernung bei staaroperationen. C. f. Pr., A., S. 65.

3050. Bitzos, G., Le point noir de l'operation de la cataracte par l'extraction. Ann. d'Ocul., CXI, 4, p. 247.

3051. Brose, L. D., Two cases of double-sided ectopia lentis. Opth. Rec., IV, 1, p. 24.

3052. Cheatham, W., Cataract extraction an office extraction. Ibid, IV, 2, p. 62.

3053. Chisolm, J. J., How cataract patients eyes are dressed at the Presbyterian Eye, Ear and Throat Charity Hospital of Baltimore. Ann. of Opth. and Otol., III, 1, p. 5.

3054. Chodin, Ueber eine merkwurdige complication bei der cataract extraction. Wjest. Opth., XI, S. 78.

3055. Christen, Th., Drei falle von angeborenem linsen colobom. Arch. f. Augenheilk., XXIX, S. 233.

1894. 3056. Clark, C. F., A case of binocular coloboma of the lens with accommodative power retained. Trans. of the Amer. Opth. Soc., p. 909. Dislocation of both crystalline lenses. Ibid, p. 239.

3057. Collins, Treacher, The association of lamellar cataracts and rickets. Opth. Soc. of the United Kingdom, November 4.

3058. Czermak, W., Ueber druckende verbande und wundsprengung nach staar extraction. Wiener Klin. Wochenschr., VII, No. 27, S. 506. Ueber extraction ohne iridectomie. Ibid, No. 27.

3059. Dalganow, Ueber den astigmatismus der hornhaut nach cataract extraction. Wjest. Opth., XI, 1, S. 78.

3060. Dehn, E., Ein beitrag zur kentniss der luxatio lentis. A. f. O., XL, S. 237.

3061. Derby, Hasket, Hints concerning the performance of the operation for the extraction of senile cataract, being a record of personal experience. Boston Med. and Surg. Journ., CXXXII, No. 5, p. 97.

3062. Dimmer, Das opthalmoscopische aussehen des linsenrandes. Wien. Klin. Wochenschr., No. 46-47.

3063. Dolard, Considerations generales sur l'operation de la cataracte ches enfants. Rec. d'Opth., No. 8, p. 468.

8064. Dolganoff, W., Ueber die veranderungen des wudastigmatismus der hornhaut nach der cataract extraction. Arch. f. Augenheilkunde, XXIX, S. 13.

3065. Dolganow, Ueber corneal astigmatismus nach staar operation. Wjest. Opth., No. 4, S. 388.

3066. Erwin, A. J., Two lenses extracted from one eye at the same sitting. Opth. Rec., III, 11, p. 433.

3067. Fage, Le, Le nettoyage secondaire de la pupille dans les operations de la cataracte traumatique. Inter. Med. Congr., XI. L'extraction simple de la cataracte sur les yeux atropinisees. Soc. Franc. d'Opth.

3068. Field le Mond, R., Cataract operation and office operation. Opth. Rec., IV, 2, p. 72.

3069. Fox, L. W., Immediate capsulotomy following the removal of cataract. Journ. Amer. Med. Assoc., June 2.

3070. Gasperini, E., Emmoragia consecutiva ad ablazione di cataratta e successiva guarigione sponatanea di ambo gli occhi. Annal. di Ottal, XXIII, p. 270.

3071. Gifford, H., The shield dressing for cataract extraction. Ann. of Opth. and Otol., III, 2, p. 141.

3072. Goerlitz, M., Beitrage zur pathologischen anatomie der cataracta diabetica. In. Diss. Freiburg.

3073. Graddy, L. B., The prevention or modification of astigmatism after cataract extraction. Opth. Rec., IV, 1, p. 1.

3074. Haltenhoff, Traitement de cataractes traumatiques. Soc. Franc. d'Opth.

1894. 3075. McHardy, The artificial maturation of immature senile cataract by trituration, after the method of Foerster. Trans. Internat. Opth. Congr., p. 270.

3076. Harlan, H., The plaster strip cataract dressing, new and yet old. Opth. Rec., III, 11, p. 431.

3077. Hocquart, E., Deformations mechaniques du cristallin dans les yeux pathologiques. Arch. d'Opth., XIV, 4, p. 209.

3078. Jackson, E., Astigmatism following cataract extraction and other sections of the cornea. Opth. Rec., III, 11, p. 409. Destruction of the eye by hemorrhage, following cataract extraction. Ann. of Opth. and Otol., III, 1, p. 9.

3079. Jelks, L. B., Report of cataract operation in the case of three sisters. Opth. Rec., IV, 2, p. 68.

3080. Kalt, De la suture corneenne apres l'extraction de la cataracte. Arch. of Opth., XIV, 10, p. 639. Die cornealnaht nach extraction des cataract. Arch. f. Augenh., XXX, S. 15.

3081. Kessler, H. M. C., Traumatische splijting der lens. Oogh. Versl. Utrecht.

3082. Knapp, H., Remarks on the extraction of cataract, based on the results of the operations of 600 consecutive cases. Trans. Intern. Opth. Congr., p. 14.

3083. Lawford, J. B., Peculiar cataracts of lamellar types. Trans. Opth. Soc., XIV, p. 138.

3084. Lippencott. J. A., Unusually large loss of vitreous in cataract extraction; recovery with useful vision. Trans. of the Amer. Opth. Soc., p. 252.

3085. Little, D., Extraction of senile cataract, with and without iridectomy; five years' hospital experience. Trans. Internat. Opth. Congr., p. 25.

3086. Logetschnikow, Ueber die einfache extraction des cataract auf dem atropinisirten auge. Wjest. Opth. XI, 2, p. 193.

3087. Lowe, J. W. C., Cataract extraction an office operation. Opth. Rec., IV, 6, p. 213.

3088. Marple, W. B., Coloboma lentis. New York Eye and Ear Infirmary Rep., Vol. II, p. 39.

3089. Millingen, van, Neue versuche uber die keratoplastik und uber die massregeln, um den irisvorfall nach der einfachen cataract operation zu vermeiden. Intern. Med. Congr., XI.

3090. Mitchell, S., Cataract extraction an office operation. Opth. Rec., IV, 1, p. 7.

3091. Mooren, A., Die operative behandlung der naturich und kunstlich gereiften staarformen. Wiesbaden. Bergmann.

3092. Moores Ball, J., Two cases of traumatic cataract in children. Ther. Gazette. XVIII, 10, p. 613.

1894. 3093. Muller, L., Hat der lenticonus seinen grund in einer anomalie der hinteren linsenflache? Klin. Mon. Bl., XXXII, S. 173.

3094. Nicati, M., Discissions cristaliniennes et iritomies ou couteau. Ann. d'Ocul., CXII, p. 398.

3095. Nicolukin, Bericht uber 204 cataract operationen in der land praxis. Wjest. Opth., XI, 3, p. 245.

3096. Pagenstecher, H., Practische rathschlage zur staar operation fur angehende augenarzte. Klin. Mon. f. Augenh.. XXXII, S. 339.

3097. Peters, A., Ueber die entstehung des schichtstaares. A. f. O., LXX, 3, p. 283.

3098. Purtscher, O.. Casuistischer beitrag zur lehre vom schichtstaar. C. f. Pr., A., February, S. 33.

3099. Risley, S. D., Destructive hemorrhage during extraction of cataract. Ann. of Opth. and Otol., III, 1, p. 16.

3100. Schramm. F.. Spontane aufsaugung eines alterstaares bei unverletzter linsenkapsel. Wiener Klin. Wochenschr., No. 37.

3101. Schweinitz, Jackson, Risley, Complications of cataract extractions and subsequent healing. Opth. Rec., III, 1, p. 421.

3102. Schweinitz, G. E., A case of intraocular hemorrhage after extraction of cataract. Ann. of Opth., January, April.

3103. Snell, S.. Case presenting unusual appearances after extraction of cataract. Trans. Opth. Soc., XIV, p. 135.

3104. Tenant, F., L'operation de la cataracte simplifiee procede du Dr. A. Trousseaux. These. de Paris.

3105. Theobald, S., A case of panopthalmitis suppurativa following discission of a capsular opacity. Amer. Journ. of Opth., XI, 7, p. 193.

3106. Terson, A., Sur la pathogenie et la prophylaxie de l'hemorrhagie expulsive apres l'extraction de la cataracte. Arch. d'Opth.. XIV, 2, p. 110.

3107. Thompson, L., Observations on some phases of opacity and luxation of the crystalline lens. Brit. Med. Journ.. No. 1759, p. 589.

3108. Vullers. H., Angeborene cataract beider augen mit perforation der linsenkapsel beim kaninchem. A. f. O., XL, 5, S. 190.

3109. Weeks, J. E., A case of lenticonus posterior, with remarks. Arch. of Opth., XX, 2. p. 260.

3110. Wicherkiewicz, Uebfier die behandlung intraocularer eiterung nach staar operationen. Wiener Klin. Wochenschr., No. 46-47.

3111. Wolkow, Ist die kapsulotomie bei der extraction seniler cataracte nothwendig? Ibid., No. 4, S. 366.

3112. Abadie, Rapport sur un travail de M. le Dr. Bistis (de Constantinople), intitule de la cataracte par rapport aux convulsions. Un cas de tetanie avec cataracte molle. Societe d'Opth. de Paris. March.

1894. 3113. Albrand, W., Report of 549 cataracts operated at Prof. Schoeler's eye clinic in Berlin. Arch. of Opth., XXIII, p. 153. Okt. (siehe diesen), Ber., 1893, S. 292.

3114. Ball, J. M., Two cases of traumatic cataract in children; successful results. Therap. Gaz., Detroit, X, p. 661.

3115. Barrett, J. W., Foreign body in lens; traumatic cataract; extraction of foreign body and lens in globe. Austral. Med. Journ., Melbourne, XVI, p. 157.

3116. ———, A case of couching for cataract; perfect vision thirteen years afterwards. Ibid, p. 381.

3117. Berceot, H., Quelques considerations sur le traitement des cataractes secondaires. These. de Paris. (Bringt Bekanntes.)

3118. ———, A propos de l'operation de Daviel. Ibid, p. 257.

3119. Bourgeois, Lunettes pour operes de cataracte. (Societe Francaise d'Opth.) Recueil d'Opth., p. 396.

3120. ———, Procede simple pour certaines extractions dans la chambre anterieure. Ibid, p. 286.

3121. Chand, M., Spontaneous falling down of cataract into the posterior chamber; restoration of sight. Med. Reporter, Calcutta, IV, p. 140.

3122. Chibret, Un cas de correction astigmatique du cristallin. Arch. d'Opth., XIV, p. 275.

3123. ———, On the good effects of dressing one eye only after cataract extractions. Brit. Med. Assoc., 62d Meeting. Bristol.

3124. Cirincione, Cataratta lussata nella camera anteriore e glaucoma consecutivo. Riforma Med., Napoli, II, p. 220.

3125. Collins, W. J., Note on non-pathological cataracts. Lancet, I, p. 1498.

3126. ———, Ueber druckende verbande und wundsprengung nach staar-extraktion. Ebd., p. 506.

3127. Schweinitz, de, A case of intraocular hemorrhage after extraction of cataract. Amer. Opth. and Otol., St. Louis, III, p. 12.

3128. ———, The treatment of immature cataract, and when to operate for cataract. Journ. Amer. Med. Assoc., Chicago, XXII, p. 105.

3129. Danesi, G., La medicatura antisettica nella chirurgia oculare. Boll. d'Ocul., XVI, 13.

3130. Dolard, De la cataracte chez les jeunes sujets. These. de Paris.

3131. Donberg, G., Ueber aseptik bei augen operationen. (Ob aseptike pri glasnich operatijach.) (V. Kongr. d. Russ. Aerzte in St. Petersburg.) Wjestnik Opth., XI, p. 73.

3132. Dujardin, A propos de l'operation de Daviel. Annal. d'Oculist, T. CXI, p. 258.

3133. Dunn, Vacuoles de cristallin. Virginia Med. Monthly, August.

3134. Egappa, T. A., A modified operation for extraction of cataract senilis. Indian Med. Record, Calcutta, 1893, V, p. 313.

1894. 3135. Egbert, J. H., The absorption of immature cataract with restoration of vision. Pacific Med. and Surg. Record, San Francisco. 1893-94, VIII, p. 147.

3136. Erwin, Two lenses extracted from the same eye at the same sitting. Opth. Record, May.

3137. ——, Soixante-dix extractions de cataracte; operations secondaires. Gaz. Med. de Picardie, Amiens, XII, p. 43.

3138. Fergus, Patients upon whom the operations of extraction of the lens had been performed for high degrees of myopia. Glasgow Med. Journal, XII, p. 146.

3139. Ferguson, Lindo H., A new form of capsular scissors. Opth. Review, p. 58.

3140. Fukala, Beitrag zur geschichte des operativen behandlung der myopie. Arch. f. Augenheilk., XXIX, S. 42.

3141. ——, Correction hochgrider myopie durch aphakie. Wahl des operations verfahrens, mit rucksicht auf die path. anatomischen veranderungen der choroidea. Trans. of the Seventh Internat. Opth. Congress, Edinburgh, p. 181.

3142. Heflebower, Foreign bodies in the crystalline lens. Cincinnati Lancet-Clinic, February 10.1

3143. Heuse, Einiges uber die ausziehung des alterstaares. Festschr. z. Feier des 50 jahr. Jubilaums des Vereins d. Aerzte des Reg. Bezirkes Dusseldorf, S. 302.

3144. Hippel, A. v., Ueber die operative behandlung hochgradiger kurzsichtigkeit. (Naturhistor. Med. Verein zu Heidelberg.) Munch. Med. Wochenschr., S. 157 u. 660.

3145. Hirschberg, Remarques sur l'historique de l'operation de Daviel. Arch. d'Opth., XIV, p. 208.

3146. ——, Ueber den staarstich der Inder. Centralbl. f. Prakt. Augenh., February, S. 48.

3147. ——, On the cataract pricking of the Hindus. Indian Med. Gaz., Calcutta, XXIX, p. 211.

3148. Hori, M., Beitrag zur operativen behandlung der hochgradigen myopie. Arch. f. Augenheilk., XXIX, S. 142.

3149. ——, Indirect massage of the lens for the artificial ripening of cataract. Therap. Gaz., January.

3150. Jackson, E., and Risley, S. D., Complication of cataract extraction and subsequent healing. Opth. Record, Nashville. 1893-94. III, p. 421.

3151. Jennings, L. B., Report of a cataract operation in the case of three sisters. Opth. Record, Nashville, 1894-95, IV, p. 68.

3152. Jennings, J. E., Remarks on the treatment of two cases of lamellar cataract. Med. Review, St. Louis, XXIX, p. 285.

1894. 3153. ——, On the corneal suture in cataract extraction. Translated by H. Knapp. Arch. of Opth.. XXIII, p. 421.

3154. Keiper, G. F., Immediate capsulotomy following the removal of cataract. Annal. Opth. and Otol., St. Louis, III, p. 420.

3155. Kirk, R., Extraction of a cataract in a myxoedematous subject aged 72 years. Lancet, II, p. 794.

3156. Knapp, Ueber glaucom nach discission des nachstaars und seine heilung. Arch. f. Augenheilk., XXX, S. 1.

3157. Lang, Krystallbildung in der linse. Opth. Soc. of the United Kingdom, November.

3158. Langenecker, D. F., Hemorrhage after cataract extraction, and some thoughts as to cause. Proceedings Kansas Med. Soc., Topeka, p. 291.

3159. Ljubornudrow, 14 augenoperationen, im lokallazareth zu Lurzk, in den Jahren 1892-93 ausgefuhrt. Wojenno. Med. Journ., April. (14 extraktionen. 1 Verlust durch Panopthalmie.)

3160. Manz, Ueber operative behandlung hochgradiger myopie. (Verein Freiburger Aerzte.) Munch. Med. Wochenschr., S. 1044.

3161. Martin, G., Sur le delire consecutif a l'operation de la cataracte. Communication faite a la Societe de Medicine de Bordeaux, April 15, 22, 29, et May 6.

3162. Meigham, T. S., Extraction of the lens for high degrees of myopie. Glasgow Med. Journal, p. 168.

3163. Milanitsch, P., Zwei hundert katarakt operationen im krankenhause der Stadt Cetinje (Dwe sotni operatij katarakti w bolnitze goroda Zetinje). Medizinskoje, LXII, p. 583.

3164. Neve, E. F., An analysis of two hundred cases of cataract extraction. Edinb. Med. Journ., 1894-95, p. 438.

3165. Noyes, The formation of a central pupil by excision in cases of occlusion with aphakia. Trans. of the Seventh Internat. Opth. Congress, Edinburgh, p. 190.

3166. ——, Clinical contributions. New York Eye and Ear Infirmary Reports, Vol. II, January.

3167. Pinckhard, C. P., Congenital ectopia lentis. Medical Standard, Chicago, XV, p. 33.

3168. Pfluger, Die behandlung der myopie durch discission der durchsichtigen linse. Internat. Congress zu Rom., XI.

3169. Raineri, A., Cataratta capsulare traumatica con estese aderenze iridee; corilisi con un nuova sinechiotoma e consecutiva esportazione della capsula; guargione con visione distinta. Gaz. Med. Cremonese, Cremona, XIV, p. 14.

3170. Ripault et A. Guepin, Diagnostic des cataractes. Gaz. Med. de Paris, XVII, p. 73.

1894. 3171. Rohmer, Les cataractes traumatiques. Revue Med. de l'Est., April 1. (Nichts Neues.)

3172. Roy, D., Detachment of retina following a simple extraction of cataract. Refractionist, Boston, I, p. 90.

3173. Schiotz, H., Vorbereitende behandlung bei staaroperationen. Norsk. Magaz., No. 4, und Verhandl. d. Med. Gesellisch., S. 36.

3174. Schneideman, T. B., Spontaneous resorption of cataract. Phila. Polyclinic, III, p. 384.

3175. Schneideman, T. B., A case of spontaneous resorption of a cataract lens. Amer. Journ. of Opth., p. 152.

3176. Schroder, Dr. Th. v., Ueber die bisherigen resultate der operativen behandlung der hochgradigen myopie nebst bemerkungen uber die antiseptik bei augenoperatione. St. Petersburg Med. Wochenschr., S. 34.

3177. Schroder, Ueber die resultate der operativen behandlung hochgradiger myopie durch extraktion der durchsichtigen linse (O resultatach operationawo letschenja wisokich stepenej blisorukosti posredstwom iswletschenja prosratschnawo chrustallka). Westnik Opth., XI, S. 101.

3178. ——, Die operative behandlung der hochgradigen Kurzsichtigkeit mittels entfornung der linse. Aerztl. Centr. Anzeig. Wien., VI, S. 37, 54.

3179. Simi, A., Discorso intorno 'all operazione della cataratta. Boll. d'Ocul., XVI, 1, 2, 3, 5. (Die einfache extraktion ist als methode vorzuziehen.)

3180. Smith, E., Cataract; morphine hypodermically, as a means to prevent prolapse of the iris in simple extraction. Arch. Opth., XXIII, p. 85.

3181. Snellen (senior), Traitement post-operatoire de la cataracte. (Societe Nederl. d'Opth.) Annal. d'Oculist, T. CXI, p. 137.

3182. Stafford, H. E., The extraction of clear lenses for myopia; report of five cases. South. Med. Record, Atlanta, XXIV, p. 296, and New York Polyclinic, III, p. 172.

3183. Swett, N. M., Delirium and death following cataract extraction. Occidental Med. Times, Sacramento, VIII, p. 655.

3184. Tenant, L'operation de la cataracte simplifiee. Procede du Dr. Trousseau. These. de Paris.

3185. Terson, A., Sur la pathogenie et la prophylaxie de l'hemorrhagie expulsive apres l'extraction de la cataracte. Arch. d'Opth., XIV, p. 110.

3186. Theobald, An unusual anomaly of the crystalline lens, coloboma lentis. Johns Hopkins Hosp. Bullet., Baltimore, V, p. 52.

3187. ——, A case of panopthalmitis suppurative, following discission of a capsular opacity. Amer. Journ. of Opth., p. 193. (Opthalmia suppurativa nach discission einer kapselkatarakt.)

1894. 3188. Thier, Beobachtungen uber operative korrektion der myopie. Trans. of the Internat. Opth. Congress, Edinburgh, p. 173.

3189. ——, Zur operativen korrektion der hochstgradigen myopie durch discission der linse. Wien. Klin. Wochenschr., VII, S. 399.

3190. Thompson, L. L., Observations on some phases of opacity and on luxation of the crystalline lens. Opth. Review, p. 313, and Brit. Med. Journ., II, p. 589.

3191. Tiffany, F. B., Cataract. Internat. Clin., Phila.. III, s. IV, p. 276.

3192. Treacher, Collins, Lamellar cataract and rickets. (Opth. Soc. of the United Kingdom.) Opth. Review. p. 373.

3193. Tyner, Austin, Praliminatorische capsulotomie bei der staaroperation. Internat. Med. Congress zu Rom.. XI. (Eroffnet die kapsel mit dem linsenmesser.)

3194. Vacher, De l'extraction du cristallin transparent comme moyen prophylactique de la myopie forte progressive et du decollement de la retine. Recueil d'Opth.. p. 271.

3195. Valk, Fr., Cataract extraction with iris retractor. Therapeut. Gazette. January.

3196. Valude, E., Les dyscrasies (diabete, albuminurie) et l'operation de la cataracte. Union Med., VII, p. 457.

3197. Vanderbergh, Un cas de l'operation de cataracte congenitale. Presse Med. Belge., October 28.

3198. Verghese, V.. Further observations on the modified operation for extraction of senile cataract. Indian Med. Gaz., Calcutta, XXIX. p. 87.

3199. Viguier, Contribution al'etude de l'anatomie pathologique de la capsule du cristallin. These. de Bordeaux. 1893-94.

3200. Wallace, J., The microscopical anatomy of the crystalline lens. University Med. Magazine, p. 797.

3201. Walter, O., Ueber die gegenwartige lage der frage uber die extraktion der kataraktosen und normalen linse (O sowremennom poloshenii woprosa ob extraktii kataraktosnawo 1 normalnawo chrustalika). Jushno-russkajamedizinskaja Gazeta. No. 11 u. 12, p. 149 u. 168.

3202. Weeks, C. J., An unusual case of extraction of the crystalline lens. Med. Record, New York, XIV. p. 494.

3203. Wicherkiewicz, Zur nachbehundlung staaroperierter bei eingetretener infektion. Bericht der Gesellschaft der Naturforscher und Aerzte. Wien.

3204. Widmark, J., Ueber correction von myopie excessiva durch extraktion der linse. Hygiea. p. 23.

3205. ——, Ueber extraktion des staares mit der kapsel (Ob iswletschenii katarakti wmeste s sumkoju). V. Kongress d. Russ. Aerzte in St. Petersburg. Ibid, p. 79.

1895. 3206. Burnett, Swan, Some exceptional features in cataract extraction. Virginia Med. Monthly, July, 1895.

3207. Ball, J. M., Treatment of traumatic cataract attended by rapid swelling of the lens. Annals of Opthal. and Otol., Vol. IV, No. 1, p. 16.

3208. Bettman. B.. Ripening of immature cataract by direct trituration. Annals of Opthal. and Otol., Vol. IV. No. 1, p. 29.

3209. Bettman. Boerne. Simple cataract extraction and some thoughts on prolapse of the iris. The Chicago Med. Reporter. August. 1895.

3210. Burnett. Swan. M., Some exceptional features in cataract extraction. Virginia Medical Monthly. Amer. Journ. of Opthal., Vol. XII, No. 8, p. 248.

3211. Clark, C. F., A case of binocular coloboma of the lens with accommodative power retained. Trans. of the Amer. Opth. Soc., 30th Annual Meeting. Washington, 1894, p. 199. Dislocation of both crystalline lenses. Trans. of the Amer. Opth. Soc., 30th Annual Meeting, 1894, p. 239.

3212. Darier, A., Vascularisation de la cristalloide anterieure dans un cas d'iridochoidite chronique. Ann. d'Oculist, T. CXIII, Livr. 1, p. 34.

3213. Derby, Hasket, Hints concerning the performance of the operation for the extraction of senile cataract, being a record of personal experience. Boston Med. and Surg. Journ., Vol. CXXXII, No. 5, p. 97.

3213a. Elsching, Lenticomus posterior. Klin. Monatsbl., 1895, p. 239.

3214. Ewetzky, Ein fall von bacillarer panopthalmitis nach katarakt extraction. Moskau. Moskauer Opthalmologischer Kreis im Jahre 1894, Marz, April, p. 222.

3215. Elschnig, Glaukom nach staar operationen. Klin. Monatsbl. fur Augenheilkunde, XXXIII, p. 233. Lenticonus posterior. Klin. Monatsbl. fur Augenheilkunde, XXXIII, p. 239.

3216. Francisco, H. A., Summary of cataract operations. New York Eye and Ear Infirmary Reports, Vol. III, 1, p. 49.

3217. Fuchs, E., On erythropsia. (Read at the annual meeting of the British Medical Association, held in London, July, 1895.) Opthal. Review, XIV, No. 166, p. 242.

3218. Knapp, H., Ueber glaukom nach discission des nachstaars und seine heilung. Arch. f. Augenheilkunde, Bd. XXX, Heft. 1, p. 1.

3219. Knapp, Hermann, Remarks on the extraction of cataract, based on the results of the operations of 600 consecutive cases. Trans. of the 8th Internat. Opth. Congr., held in Edinburgh, August, 1894.

1895.　3220. Kaijser, Fritz, Om det enkla stansimidet jemte en sammactallning af de under aren, 1891-94, a kongl. Serafimer lazarettet utsonda staaroperationer na a senil staar. (Ueber die einfache staarextraction nebst einer Zusammenstellung der wahrend, 1891 bis 1894, am konigl. Serafimer Lazarethe ausgefuhrten extractionen seniler staare.) Hyglea, Juli, August, 1895. Ueber die einfache staarextraction nebst einer Zusammenstellung der in den Jahren 1891 bis 1894 im konigl. Serafirmer Lazarethe ausgefuhrten operationen von senilem staar. Serafirmerlasarettets Ogon-Klin. Rapport, f. 1894.

3221. Esberg, Dr. Hermann, Zur operation des nachstaars. Monatsbl. f. Augenheilkunde, 1895.

3222. Grossmann, Karl, Entoptic perception of the retinal vessels. Opth. Review, Vol. VII, No. 85, p. 335. November, 1888.

3223. ——, Iridocyklitis nach kataract operation, secundair glaukom, sympathische affection des zweiten auges und ebenfalls secundair glaukom. Von Cand. Med. H. Merz. (Mit Figur.)

3224. Pagenstecher, Dr. Hermann, Ueber glaukom nach staaroperationen. Monatsbl. f. Augenheilkunde, 1895.

3225. Ring, Frank W., The combined versus the simple extraction of cataract. A study of over 2,000 cases. Medical Record, February 23, 1895.

3226. Zenker, Dr. Heinrich, Tausent staar operationen bericht aus der augenarztlichen Praxis Sr. Konigl. Hoheit des Herrn Herzogs Dr. Carl in Bayern. Wiesbaden. Verlag von J. F. Bergmann, 1895. (Autoreferat.)

3227. Lowe, J. W. C., Cataract extraction an office operation. Sometimes (and most of the time). Opthal. Record, Vol. IV, No. 6, p. 213.

3228. Little, David, Extraction of senile cataract, with and without iridectomy; five years' hospital experience. Trans. of the 8th Inter. Opthal. Congr., held in Edinburgh, August, 1894, p. 25.

3229. Liebrecht, Ueber isolirte linsen kapsel verletzungen. Ein geheilter fall von isolirtem gressen linsen kapselriss ohne kataraktbildung. Beitrage zur Augenheilkunde, Heft. XVIII.

3230. Lessing, Richard, Schichtstaar und schichtstaar operationen. Inaug. Dissert. Berlin, 1895.

3231. Lutz, Ernst, Ueber die pathologischen anatomischen veranderungen der linsen kapsel. Inaug. Dissert. Wurzburg, 1895.

3232. Lippincott, J. A., Unusually large loss of vitreous in cataract extraction; recovery with useful vision. Trans. of the Amer. Opth. Society, 30th Annual Meeting. Washington, 1894. P. 129.

3233. McHardy, The artificial maturation of immature senile cataract by trituration after the method of Foerster. Trans. of the 8th Inter. Opth. Congr., held in Edinburgh, August, 1894, p. 270.

568

1895. 3234. Merz, H., Iridocyklitis nach katarakt operation, secundair glaucom, sympathische affection des zweiten auges und ebenfalls
secundair glaucom. Klin. Monatsbl. f. Augenh., XXXIII, p. 50.

3235. Nicati, M., Discissions cristalliniennes et iritomies au couteau. Ann.
d'Oculist. T. CXII, p. 398. December.

3236. Neve, Ernst F., An analysis of 200 cases of cataract extraction.
Edinburgh Med. Journ., No. 1572, p. 438. November, 1894.

3237. Oger de Speville, Complication rare apres l'extraction de la cataracte. Progres Med., No. 19, p. 316.

3238. Poliacow, Ph., Zwei hundert ambulatorisch gemachte katarakt extractionen, No. 2, p. 46. January, February, 1895.

3239. Ring, Frank W., The combined versus the simple extraction of
cataract; a study of over 2,000 cases. Med. Rec., February 23,1895.

3240. Taylor, Bell, L'extraction de la cataracte a notre epoque. Ann.
d'Oculist, T. CXIII, Livr. 2, p. 106.

3241. Riedel, Max, Ein fall von traumatischer linsen luxation in die pupille mit umdrehung der linse. Inaug. Dissert. Greifswald, 1894.

3242. Rothschild, H. de O., Observations cliniques. Cataracte traumatique partielle a la suite de la penetration d'un eclat de fer
visible dans la partie du cristallin restee transparente. Revue
Gen. d'Opthal., No. 3, p. 99.

3243. Randolph, Robert, Two successful cataract operations on a dog.
John Hopkins Hospital Bulletin. Amer. Journ. of Opthal., Vol.
XII, No. 6, p. 174.

3244. Sym, William George, A case of lenticonus posterior. Opth. Rev.,
No. 161, p. 76.

3245. Schneideman, T. B., Note upon a condition of the pupil following
extraction of cataract. Opthal. Review, No. 165, p. 209.

3246. Speville, de, Complication rare apres l'extraction du cristallin. Ann.
d'Oculist, T. CXIV, p. 215. September.

3247. Tennant, Frederic, L'operation de la cataracte simplifiee procede
du Dr. A. Trousseau. These. de Paris, 1894.

3248. Truc, Des manifestations generales et refringentes du globe de
l'oeil, consecutives a l'extraction du cristallin. Frankreich. Societe Francaise d'Opthalmologie. May 9, 1895.

3249. Wicherkiewicz, Bol., Zur nachbehandlung staaroperirter nach eingetretener infection. (Nach einem auf der 66. Naturforscher
versammlung in Wien gehaltenen vortrag.) Therapeutische Wochenschrift, No. 6, 1895. Sur l'operation de la cataracte secondaire.
Frankreich. Societe Francaise d'Opthalmologie, May 6-9, 1895.

3250. Webster, David, Report of 118 cataract extractions, with remarks.
Manhattan Eye and Ear Hospital Reports, January, 1895.

3251. Weeks, John E., A report of 100 consecutive cases of cataract extraction, with remarks. New York Med. Journ., No. 5 (870), p. 137.

1895. 3252. Zenker, Heinrich, Tausent staar operationen. Bericht aus der augenarztlichen Praxis Sr. k. Hoheit des Herzogs Dr. Carl in Bayern. Wiesbaden, 1895. J. F. Bergmann.

3253. Vitali, Operazioni delle cataratte incomplete. Italia, XIV. Congresso dell' associazione oftalmologica Italiana, tenuto in Venezia dal 26 al 29 Agosto, 1895. Ann. di Ottalm., anno XXIV, supplemento al fasc., 4.

3254. Dimmer, Das opthalmoskopische aussehen des linsenrandes. 1Wen. Versammlung Deutscher Naturforscher und Aerzte in Wien. Abtheilung. Opthalmologie.

3255. Pagenstecher, Herman, Ueber glaukom nach staar operationen. Klin. Monatsbl. f. Augenheilkunde, XXXIII, p. 139.

1896. 3256. Allport, Frank, An unusual case of cataract. American Jaurnal of Opthal., Vol. XIII, No. 2, p. 52.

3257. Alt, Adolf, A case of probable spontaneous absorption of part of a cataractous lens. Dislocation of the small nucleus into the anterior chamber. Glaucoma. American Journal of Opthal., Vol. XIII, No. 2, p. 53.

3258. Bach, Ludwig, Anatomischer beitrag zur genese der angeborenen colobome des bulbus. Arch. f. Augenheilk., Bd. XXXII, 4, p. 277.

3259. Cerillo, Operation de la cataracte et methode pour l'extraction des couches corticales. Recueil d'Opthal., No. 10, p. 596.

3260. Collins, E. Treacher, Lamellar cataract and rickets. Trans. of the Opthal.mological Society of the United Kingdom, Vol. XV. London, 1895. J. and U. Churchill, p. 104.

3261. Cartwright, Posterior lental opacity; remains of hyaloid artery and coloboma lentis. England. Opthalmological Society of the United Kingdom, May 7, 1896.

3262. Cramer, Ein fall von lenticonus posterior. Klin. Monatsbl. fur Augenheilkunde, XXXIV, p. 278.

3263. Cramer, Dr., Ein fall von lenticonus posterior. Klin. Monatsbl. f. Augenheilkunde, 1894, p. 178.

3264. Hennicke, Dr., Ein fall von katarakt veranlasst durch entozoen (?) (mit 4 figuren).

3265. Hallauer, Otto, Uebersicht uber 400 staar extractionen. Augenheilanstalt in Basel, XXXII. Jahresbericht, 1896, p. 63.

3266. Pinto, J. daGama, Ein beitrag zur nachstaar operation. Klinische Monatsblatter f. Augenheilkunde, July, 1896.

3267. Webster, David, Report of 118 cataract extractions. Manhattan Eye and Ear Hospital Reports, p. 21. January, 1895.

3268. Weeks, John E., A report of 100 consecutive cases of cataract extractions. New York Med. Journ., Vol. LXII. No. 5 (whole No. 870), p. 137.

1896. 3269. Wilson, F. M., A third table of 10,000 cataract extractions. Trans. of the Amer. Opthal. Soc., 31st Meeting, 1896, p. 403.

3270. Albrand, Walter, Bericht uber 295 staar operationen in der Schoeler'schen Augenklinik. Arch. f. Augenh., Bd. XXXII, p. 71.

3271. Dickey, John L., A cataractous family. New York Med. Journ., No. 6 (897), p. 181.

3272. Darier, Des traumatismes du systeme cristallinien. Paris. Societe d'Opthalmologie de Paris. Seance du 4 Fevr., 1896.

3273. Duyse, van, Tuberculose attenuee des glandes lacrymales. Guerison spontanee. Arch. d'Ópthal.. No. 9, p. 573.

3274. Egner, Rudolf, Ueber contusionstaare, speciell die durch kapsel ruptur bedingten. Inaug. Dissert. Griefswald, 1896.

3275. Fromaget et Cabannes, De l'hemorrhagie intraoculaire expulsive consecutive a l'extraction de la cataracte. Ann. d'Oculist, T. CXVI, Livr. 2, p. 118.

3276. Gunn, R. Marcus, Peculiar corraliform cataract with crystals (? of cholesterine) in the lens, and peculiar variety of cataract. Trans. of the Opthalmological Society of the United Kingdom, Vol. XV. London, 1895. J. and A. Churchill. P. 119. Traumatic subluxation of lens of old standing; secondary zonular cataract and coloboma lentis. Trans. of the Opthalmological Society of the United Kingdom, Vol. XV, p. 121. London, 1895. J. and A. Churchill. Spontaneous symmetrical dislocation of both crystalline lenses. Transactions of the Opthalmological Society of the United Kingdom, Vol. XV, p. 122. London, 1895. J. and A. Churchill. Extreme congestion of opeic disc in a case of hypermetropia. Transactions of the Opthalmological Society of the United Kingdom, Vol. XV, p. 136. London, 1895. J. and A. Churchill.

3277. Gradenigo, Pietro, Sull' estrazione capsulo-lenticolare della cataratta. Ann. di Ottalm., XXV, Fasc. 1, p. 77. Siehe auch Italia, XIV. Congresso dell' Associazione Oftalmologica Italiana, tenuto in Venesia dal 26 al 29 Agosto, 1895. Ann. di Ottalm., anno XXIV, supplemento al fasc. 4.

3278. Ginsberg, Ueber die angeborenen colobome des augapfels. (Nach einem am 25. Juni in der Berliner opthalmologischen Gesellschaft Gehaltenen Vortrag.) Centralbl. f. Prakt. Augenheilkunde, p. 225. August.

3279. Grosser, Paul, Ueber ectopie lentis. Inaug. Dissert. Berlin, 1896.

3280. Galezowski, De l'operation des cataractes secondaires adherents par l'incision d'arriere en avant. (Suite et nn.) Recueil d'Opth., No. 10, p. 587.

3281. Hippel, Eugene, v., Zur pathologischen anatomie der centralen und perinuclearen katarakt. A. v. Graefe's Arch. f. Opthal., XLI, 3, p. 1. Ueber spontane resorption seniler katarakte. Bericht uber d. 24 Versammlung der Opthal., Ges., p. 97.

1896. 3282. Hess, C., Ueber linsentrubungen in ihren beziehungen zu Allgemeinerkrankungen. Sammlung zwangloser hefte aus dem gebiete der Augenheilkunde, Bd. 1, Heft. 2.

3283. Howe, Lucien, Note concerning the lens in the eyes of rodents. Transactions of the American Opthalmological Society, 31st Annual Meeting, p. 432. New London, Conn., 1895.

3284. Hallauer, Otto, Uebersicht uber 400 staar extractionen, ausgefuhrt in der Basler Opthalmologischen Klinik, vom 5 Januar, 1889, bis 11 April, 1895. XXXII Jahresber. d. Augenheilanstalt in Basel, p. 63.

3285. Hess, C., Pathologisch anatomische studien uber einige seltene angeborene missbildungen des auges. (Orbitalcyste linsen colobom und schichtstaar, lenticonus.) A. v. Graefe's Arch. f. Opthalm., Bd. XLII, 8, p. 249.

3286. Janowski, A., Aus der arzlichen opthalmologischen land praxis. Katarakt extraction 70 falle. Bd. XIII, 4 u. 5, p. 367.

3287. Knapp, Hermann, Beitrag zur casuistik der spontanen glaskorper blutungen. Inaug. Dissert. Freiburg, I, Br. 1896.

3288. Lang, W., Cholesterine crystals in the lens. Transactions of the Opthalmological Society of the United Kingdom, Vol. IV, p. 117. London, 1895. J. and A. Churchill. Cholesterine crystals found in a cataractous lens. Transactions of the Opthalmological Society of the United Kingdom, Vol. XV, p. 118. London, 1895. J. and A. Churchill. Right lenticonus posterior. Transactions of the Opthalmological Society of the United Kingdom, Vol. XV, p. 122. London, 1895. J. and A. Churchill.

3289. Lawford, J. B., Peculiar colored lenticular opacities, probably congenital. Transactions of the Opthalmological Society of the United Kingdom, Vol. XV, p. 197. London, 1895. J. and A. Churchill.

3290. Marshall, C. Devereux, On the immediate and remote results of cataract extraction. Opthalm. Hosp. Reports, Vol. XIV, part 1, p. 56.

3291. Mitchell, S., A cataractous family. New York Med. Journ., No. 9 (900), p. 289.

3292. Noyes, Henry D., Severe hemorrhage following extraction of cataract. America. Transactions of the American Opthalmological Society, 31st Annual Meeting. New London, Conn, 1895. P. 448 und 454.

3293. Nicolukin, J., Bericht uber 160 katarakt operationen in land krankenhause, fur 1894-95. Bd. XIII, Heft. 2, p. 143. March, April.

3294. Oliver, Charles A., History of a case of successful iridectomy and extraction of lens capsule and lens debris, with discovery of vision, in an eye that had been considered useless for more than ten years. Pennsylvania University Magazine, November, 1895.

1896. 3295. Prefontaine, L. A., Summary of operations for cataract done at the New York Eye and Ear Infirmary from October 1, 1894, to October 1, 1895. New York Eye and Ear Infirmary Reports, Vol. IV, part I, p. 55.

3296. Plettinck-Bauchau, Des inconvenients de l'operation de la cataracte avec iridectomie compares aux advantages de l'extraction simple avec le lambeau semielliptique de Galezowski pratiquee a l'institut opthalmique de Bruges. Recueil d'Opthalm., 18, annee, No. 8, p. 449.

3297. Puech. Cataractes traumatiques. Recueil d'Opthalm., 18, annee. No. 8, p. 466.

3298. Pinto, J. da Gama. Ein beitrag zur nachstaar operationen. Klin. Monatsbl. f. Augenheilk., XXXIV, p. 295.

3299. Rumschewitsch, K., Zur casuistik des glaukoms nach staar operationen. Klin. Monatsbl. f. Augenheilk., XXXIV, p. 191.

3300. Steiner, L., Persistence du canal de Cloquet et cataracte polaire posterieure compliquee de chorioretinite specifique; depots de pigment dans les parois du canal. Ann. d'Oculist, T. CXV, Livr. 1, p. 41.

3201. Story, John B., One hundred consecutive operations for senile cataract, complicated and uncomplicated. Transactions of the Royal Academy of Medicine in Ireland, Vol. XIII.

3302. Segal, L., Opthalmologische beobachtungen. Zur frage der pupillen bildung bei occlusio pupillae nach katarakt extraction. Bd. XIII. Heft. 1, p. 31. 1896.

3303. Schreiber, Julius, Zur lehre vom schichtstaar. Inaug. Dissert. Kiel, 1896.

3304. Sanford, Arthur, England. Opthalmological Society of the United Kingdom. October 15, 1896. Cataract extraction in an Albino. Brit. Med. Journ., No. 1869, p. 1231.

3305. Schoen, Wilhelm, Die staarkrankheit, ihre ursache und verhutung. Wiener Klin. Rundschau, 1896, Nos. 19, 20, 21, 23, 24, 25, 26, 28, 29, 30, 31.

3306. Topolanski, Alfred, Ueber kapselabhebungen. A. v. Graefe's Arch. f. Opthalm., XLI, 3, p. 198.

3307. Thomas, Wilhelm, Beitrag zur lehre von der cataracta diabetica. Inaug. Dissert. Kiel, 1896.

3308. Tretow, Otto, Operazione delle cataratte incomplete. Ann. di Ottalm., XXIV, fasc. 6, p. 580. Siehe auch Italia, XIV. Congresso dell' Associazione Oftalmologica Italiana, tenuto in Venezia, dal 26 al 29 Agosto, 1895. Ann. di Ottalm., anno XXIV, supplemento al fasc. 4.

1896. 3310. Vacher. Frankreich. Congress de la Societe Francaise d'Opthalmologie. Section tenue a Paris du 4 au 7 Mai, 1896. De l'extraction du cristallin transparent comme moyen prophylactique de la myopie forte, progressive et du decollement de la retine.

3311. Watson, W. Spencer, and W. J. Collins, A case of traumatic cataract with a foreign body imbedded in the lens successfully treated by operation. Transactions of the Opthalmological Society of the United Kingdom, Vol. XV, p. 115. London, 1895. J. and A. Churchill.

3312. Wood, Casey A., The after treatment of normal cataract extraction; a lecture delivered at the post-graduate medical school. Therap. Gaz., Vol. XX, No. 2, p. 77

3313. Wecker, L. de, L'extraction de la cataracte en 1952. Ann. d'Oculist, T. CXV, Livr. 4, p. 275.

3314. Weill, George, Aiguilles lancettes pour les operations de cataracte secondaire. Revue Gen. d'Opthal., No. 8, p. 338.

3315. Abadie, Ch., Etude clinique et pathogenique d'une complication peu connue consecutive a l'extraction de la cataracte avec iridectomie. Ann. d'Oculist, T. CXVI, Livr. 1, p. 45.

3316. Albrand, Walter, Bericht uber 295 staar operationen der Scholer'schen Augenklinik in Berlin. Arch. f. Augenheilk., Bd. XXXIII, Heft. 1, p. 71.

3317. Darier, Frankreich. Congres de la Societe Francaise d'Opthalmologie. Section tenue a Paris du 4 au 7 Mai, 1896. Nouveau procede de keratotomie pour pratiquer l'iridectomie ou 'extraction de la cataracte dans les cas d'effacement complet de la chambre anterieure.

3318. Davis, A. Edward, The report of a case of double senile cataract, with leucoma as a complication in each eye. Extractions after preliminary iridectomies. New York. Manhattan Eye and Ear Hospital Reports, Vol. III, p. 37. January, 1896.

3319. Hennicke, Ein fall von katarakt, veranlasst durch entozoen (?). Klin. Monatsbl. f. Augenheilkunde, XXXIV, p. 423.

3320. Schweinitz, G. de, Concerning the extraction of immature cataract, with the report of cases. Phila. Polyclinic, Vol. V. April, 1896.

3321. Stadfeldt, A. E., Die veranderung der linse bei traction der zonula. Klin. Monatsbl. f. Augenheilk., XXXIV, p. 429.

3322. Vignes, Frankreich. Societe d'Opthalmologie, November, 1896. Retard de cicatrisation chez les operes de cataracte.

1897. 3323. Augstein und Ginsberg, Ueber die resorption der linse und der linsenkapsel bei luxation in den glaskorper. Centralbl. f. Prakt. Augenheilk., p. 356. November.

3324. Antonelli, Albert, Le croissant lineaire du cristallin, dans certaines formes de cataracte; confirmation anatomo-pathologique. Ann. d'Oculist, T. CXVIII, Livr. 2, p. 17.

574

1897. 3325. Angelucci, A.. Una modificazione al processo di estrazione sempli-
              ficata della cataratta. Arch. di Ottalm., Vol. V, fasc. 3 u. 4, p. 71.

       3326. Bert, Ellis, Penetrating wounds of the lens; report of four cases.
              Opthalm. Record, Vol. VI, No. 3, p. 131.

       3327. Bach, L., Histologische und klinische mittheilungen uber spindel-
              staar und kapselstaar, nebst bemerkungen zur Genese dieser
              staarformen. A. v. Graefe's Arch. f. Opthalm., Bd. XLIII, abth.
              3, p. 663.

       3328. Barck, Carl, On retarded closure of the wound, and some rare acci-
              dents and sequelae of cataract extraction. Amer. Journ. of Opth.,
              Vol. XIV, No. 9, p. 281.

       3329. Bullard, W. L., A case of sympathetic opthalmia following a suc-
              cessful cataract extraction. Opthalm. Record, Vol. VI, No. 10,
              p. 518. October.

       3330. Crzellitzer, Zonularspannung und linsenform. Heidelberg. Bericht
              uber die XXV. Versammlung der opthalmologischen Gesellschaft
              Heidelberg, 1896. Unter mitwirkung von E. V. Hippel und A.
              Wagenmann, redigirt durch W. Hess und Th. Leber. Wiesbaden,
              1897. J. F. Bergmann. Page 48.

       3331. Cartwright, E. H., Congenital post-lental opacity with remains of
              hyaloid artery; irregular development of suspensory ligament and
              coloboma lentis. Transactions of the Opthalmological Society of
              the United Kingdom, Session 1895-96, Vol. XVI, p. 186. London,
              1896. J. and A. Churchill.

       3332. Critchett, Anderson, Extraction of dislocated lens with good result.
              Transactions of the Opthalmological Society of the United King-
              dom, Session 1895-96, Vol. XVI, p. 62. London, 1896. J. and A.
              Churchill.

       3333. Coover, David, An interesting but disastrous termination of a cata-
              ract operation. Opthalm. Record, Vol. VI, No. 3, p. 126.

       3334. Coleman, W. Franklin, Preliminary iridectomy in the extraction of
              senile cataract. Ann. of Opthalm., Vol. VI, No. 2, p. 218.

       3335. Dimmer, F., Beitrage zur opthalmoskopie. Der Rand geschrumpter
              oder theilweise getrubter linsen. A. v. Graefe's Arch. f. Opthal.,
              Bd. XLIII, abth. 1, p. 1.

       3336. DuBarry, Operation de cataracte suivie de suppuration guerie par
              les injections sous-conjunctivales de sublime a 1-1000. Clinique
              Opthalm., No. 13, p. 154.

       3337. Damianos, Nikolaus, Zwei falle von extopia pupillae et lentis. Bei-
              trage z. Augenheilkunde, heft. XXIX, p. 812.

       3338. Elschnig, Anton, Ueber die discission. Wiener Klin.. Wochenschr.,
              1896, No. 53.

1897. 8339. Ebner, Mittheilung uber 400 extractionen des alterstaars, ausgefuhrt durch Herrn Geheimrath Prof. v. Rothmund an kranken der Universitats Augenklinik zu Munchen. Munchener Med. Wochenschrift, No. 11, p. 275.

3340. Fryer, B. E., The technique of cataract extraction. (Read at the annual meeting of the Western Opth. Association, held in St. Louis, April 8-9, 1897.) American Journal of Opthalm., Vol. XIV, No. 7, p. 210.

3341. Grosjean, Ectopie cristallinienne bilaterale. Clinique Opthalm., No. 15, p. 179.

3342. Hess, C., Ueber excentrische bildung des linsenkernes und die histologie des lenticonus posterior. Heidelberg. Bericht uber die XXV. Versammlung der Opthalmologischen Gesellschaft. Heidelberg, 1896. Unter mitwirkung von E. v. Hippel und A. Wagenmann redigirt durch W. Hess und Th. Leber. Wiesbaden, 1897. J. F. Bergmann. Page 301.

3343. Hirschberg, J., Angeborener grauen staar als familienubel. (Vergl. No. 875.) Centralbl. f. Prakt. Augenheilkunde, p. 271. September.

3344. Inouye, Tatzushichiro, Ueber einem fall von Augenverletzung durch stumpfe Gewalt und insbesondere uber linsenkapsel-abhebung. Centralbl. f. Prakt. Augenheilk. Mai—Heft. Page 147.

3345. Ingoni, Cassiani, Dell' estrazione capsulo-lenticolare della cataratta. Ann. di Ottalm., anno XXVI, fasc. 5, p. 460.

3346. Jocqs, Frankreich. Societe d'Opthalmologie, Decembre, 1896. Extraction du cristallin dans un cas de tache circonscrite de la lentille. Progres Med., 1897, No. 1, p. 9.

3347. Jackson, Edward, The location of opacities near the posterior pole of the lens by means of the corneal reflex. Opthalm. Record, Vol. VI, No. 2. p. 58.

3348. Jenckel, Adolf, Ein fall von luxatio lentis mit acutem glaukom. Inaug. Dissert. Kiel, 1897.

8349. Lenz, A., Ein fall von contusionstaar. Centralbl. f. Prakt. Augenheilkunde, p. 15.

3350. Lauge, O., Zur frage der spontanen intracapsularen resorption der cataracta senilis. Beitrage zur wissenschaftl. Medicin. Festschr. zur 69. Versammlung Deutscher Naturf. u. Aerzte. Braunschweig, 1897.

3351. Mancae, Ovio, Studi intorno alla cataratta artificiale. Arch. di Ottalm., Vol. IV, fasc. 5 u. 6, p. 167.

3352. Moulton, H., A case of cataract extraction under discouraging conditions, but with especially gratifying results. Opthalm. Record, Vol. VI, No. 4, p. 180.

3353. Mulder, Dr. M. E., Ein fall von lenticonus posterior, anatomisch untersucht. Graefe-Saemisch, Bd. V. p. 236. Arch. f. Opthalm., Bd. XL, abth. III, p. 243.

1897. 3354. Pfluger, Dr., Der irisvorfall bei der extraction des alterstaares und seine verhutung. Monatsbl. f. Augenheilkunde. 1897.

3355. Mulder, M. E., Bijdragen, uitgegeven door het Nederlandsch Oogheelkundig Geselschap. Derde II. Aflevering, Haarlem, 1897. Cataracta polaris posterior en lenticonus.

3356. Manca, G. et G. Ovio, Studi intorno alla cataratta artificiale. II. Esperienze intorno alla proprieta osmotische della lente cristallina. Archivio di Ottalm., Vol. V, fasc. 3 u. 4, p. 112.

3357. Norris, W. F., Cases of persistent pupillary membrane, in which there was a firm attachment to the lens capsule, with partial opacity of this membrane, and of a thin layer of underlying lens substances. Transactions of the American Opthalmological Society, 32d Annual Meeting New London, Conn., 1896. Vol. VII, 1894-96. Hartford: Published by the Society. 1897. Page 580.

3358. Oliver, Chas., A case of traumatic subconjunctival dislocation of the lens. Philadelphia. College of Physicians of Philadelphia. Section of Opthalmology, March 16, 1897. Reported by Howard Hansell.

3359. Pinto, J. da Gama, Contribution a l'operation de la cataracte secondaire. Ann. d'Oculist. T. CXVII, Livr. 1. p. 22.

3360. Puech, A., A propos de la cataracte de Morgagni. Clinique Opthal., No. 4, p. 38.

3361. Peltesohn, Zwei falle angeborener missbildung am auge. Beiderseitige congenitale hereditare (familiare), ectopia lentis. Central. f. Prakt. Augenh., p. 112. April, 1897.

3362. Pergens, Ed., Bupthalmus mit lenticonus posterior. Arch. f. Augenheilkunde, Bd. XXXV, 1, p. 1.

3363. Purtscher, Aderhautblutung nach alterstaar ausziehung. Aderhautblutung nach geschwursbildung. Angeborener grauen staar als familien ubel. Centralbl. f. Prakt. Augen., p. 193 u. 198. July.

3364. Pansier, P., L'extraction du cristallin dans la myopie forte chez les vieillards. Clinique Opthalm., No. 14, p. 169.

3365. Pfluger, Der irisvorfall bei der extraction des alterstaares und seine verhutung. Klin. Monatsbl. f. Augenh., Bd. XXXIV, p. 332.

3366. Rumschewitsch, K., Zur pathologischen anatomie der spontanen linsen luxationen in die vordere kammer. Arch. f. Augenheilk., Bd. XXIV, heft. 3, p. 139.

3367. Rogman, Nouvelle contribution a l'etude des anamolies lenticulaires congenitales. Colobomes situes dans une direction differente a la fente foetale. Conclusions generales sur la genese des colobomes lenticulaires. Arch. d'Opthalm., T. XVII, No. 7, p. 427.

3368. Salzmann, Maximilian, Die brechungsverminderung durch verlust der linse. Arch. f. Augenh., Bd. XXIV, heft. 3, p. 152.

1997. 3369. Shumway, Edward A., Summary of operations for cataract done at the New York Eye and Ear Infirmary, from October 1, 1895, to October 1, 1896. New York Eye and Ear Infirmary Reports, Vol. V, p. 64.

3370. Schlodtmann, Walter, Ueber einem fall von luxation der linse in den Tenon'schen Raum bei aquatorial gelegenem skleralriss. A. v. Graefe's Arch. f. Opthalm., Bd. XLIV, 1, p. 127.

3371. Snellen, H., Erythropsie. A. v. Graefe's Arch. f. Opthalm., Bd. XLIV, 1, p. 19.

3372. Schanz, Fritz, Eine familie mit juveniler katarakt. Centralbl. f. Prakt. Augenheilk., p. 264. September.

3373. Thomson, Philadelphia. Section of Opthalmology, College of Physicians of Philadelphia, February 16, 1897. Case of foreign body in the lens.

3374. Vertiz, America. Report of the Section of Opthalmology, Pan-American Medical Congress, held at Mexico City, November, 1896. A new operation for cataract. American Journal of Opthalm., Vol. XIV, No. 1, p. 17.

3375. Walter, O., Zur casuistik der operirten angeborenen staare. Klinische Beobachtung.) Centralbl. f. Prakt. Augen., p. 364. December

3376. Wolff, Ueber regeneration der exstirpirten linse beim Triton. Sitzungsber. d. Wurzburger Phys. Med. Gesellschaft, p. 59. 1896.

3377. White, Joseph A., So-called accommodation in the lenseless eye. Opthalm. Record, Vol. VI, No. 9, p. 487.

3378. Chibret, Paul, Le lavage de la chambre posterieure apres l'operation de la cataracte. Arch. d'Opthalm., T. XVII, No. 9, p. 545.

3379. Demicheri, L., Anneaux d'interference du cristallin cataracte. Arch. d'Opthalm., T. XVII, No. 1, p. 38.

1898. 3380. Coover, D. H., An interesting but disastrous termination of a cataract operation. Opth. Record, March, 1897.

3381. Chibret, Lavage of the posterior chamber after cataract extraction. Arch. d'Opth., XVII, p. 545.

3382. Bach, L., A contribution to the histology and genesis of lenticonus posterior. Arch. f. Augenh., XXXVI, p. 161. Pathologisch anatomische studien uber verschiedene missbildungen des auges. Graefe's Arch., Bd. XLV, Part I.

3383. Bloom, S., Uber die retro-choroideal blutungen nach staar extractionen. Graefe's Arch., Bd. XLVI, Part I, p. 184.

3384. Baeck, S., Experimentelle histologische untersuchungen uber contusio bulbi. Bd. XLVII, Part I, p. 82.

3385. Baquis, On the spontaneous intracapsular absorption of cataract. Ann. di Ottalm., XXXVI, 1-2, p. 76.

3386. Bates, W. H., Suture of the cornea after removal of the lens. Arch. of Opthalm., Vol. XXVII, No. 2. p. 181.

578

1898. 3387. Back, Histology and development of lenticonus posterior. Arch.
f. Augenheilk., XXXVI, 1-2.

3388. Borthen, Johann, The open wound treatment for cataract operation. Klin. Monatsbl. f. Augenheilkunde. August, 1898.

3389. Demicheri, Posterior polar cataract and lenticonus. Nederlandische Ooghselk. Bydragen. Afl., 3, 41. 1897.

3390. DeSchweinitz, Glaucoma three years after extraction of cataract .by combined method. Opth. Record. December, 1897.

3391. Distler, Contribution to operations on senile cataract. Festschrift d. Stuttgarter Aerztl. Vereins. 1897.

3392. Dunn, A case of ossification of the lens. Pathology by Ward Holden. Arch. f. Opth., Vol XXVII, 5, p. 500.

3393. Freyer, The technique of cataract extraction. Amer. Journal of Opth., July, 1897.

3394. Fernandez, Santos, Cataract operations. Ann. d'Opth., Vol. I, No. 1. July, 1898.

3395. Frenkel, Henri, Researches into the renal permeability in the case of those suffering from senile cataract. Arch. d'Opthal. July,1898.

3396. Gayet, On the temporary folding back of the cornea for the purpose of operating a ciel onvert on the iris and the capsule of the lens. Ann. d'Ocul., XVIII, p. 346.

3396. Harlan, Geo., On delayed union after cataract extraction. Report of Trans. of Amer. Opth. Soc., 1898. Arch. of Opth., Vol. XVII. 'p. 455.

3398. Heine, L., Beitrage zur physiologie und pathologie der linse. Graef Arch., Bd. XLVI, Part III, p. 525.

3399. Hippel, E. v., Uber das normale auge des neugeborenen. Graefe's Arch., Bd. XLV, Part II, p. 286.

3400. Hippel, E. v., Uber anopthalmus congenitus. Graefe's Arch., Bd. XLVII, Part I, p. 227.

3401. Hidaka, Takashi, Tokyo. A contribution to statistics on cataract operation. Inaug. Dissert. Halle. 1897.

3402. Hirschberg, Congenital cataract as a family affection. Centralbl. fur Augen., Vol. XXI, p. 271. Cataract in glass blowers. Berlin. Klin. Woch., February 7, 1898. Ann. of Opth., No. 2, p. 247.

3403. Krautschneider, A case of crystal formation in the lens. Beitrag zur Augenh., XXVI.

3404. Knapp, (1) Recent experiences with cataract operations. Proceedings of the Moscow Internat. Congress. Arch. Opth., Vol. XXVII, No. 1, p. 94. (2) On operation for secondary cataract. Report of Trans. Amer. Opth. Society. Arch. of Opth., Vol. XXVII, 4, p. 447. (3) Recent experiences in operations for secondary cataract. Arch. of Opth., XXVII, No. 5, p. 467. (4) Remarks on cataract extraction, based on a large number of cases. Opth. Section, 12th Inter. Congress in Moscow. Wjest. Opth. (5) Complicated cataracts, their nature and results. Journ. Amer. Med. Assoc., Jan. 8, 1898.

1898. 8405. Kreiwitz, Corneal astygmatism after iridectomy and simple linear extraction. Inaug. Dissert. St. Petersburg, 1897.

3406. Lopez, Fernando, Expulsive hemorrhage after cataract extraction. Ann. d'Opth., No. 1, p. 2. 1898.

3407. Meyer, O., Beitrag zur pathologie und pathologische anatomie des schicht und kapsel staars. Bd. XLV, Part III, p. 540.

3408. Muttermilch, Notes on cataract operation. Ann. d'Ocul., XVIII, p. 408.

3409. Milbury, Report on 76 cases of cataract extraction. Journal of Amer. Med. Assoc., April 17, 1897.

3410. Mitvalsky, Remarks on subconjunctival luxation of the lens. Arch. d'Opthal., XVII, p. 337.

3411. Mittendorf, W. F., Some of the earlier symptoms of senile cataract. Report of Trans. Amer. Opth. Soc., 1898. Arch. of Opthal., Vol. XXVII, 4, p. 447.

3412. Mulder, Anatomical examination of a case of lenticonus posterior. Zehender's Klin. Monatsbl., XXXV, p. 409.

3413. Oliver, Clinical history of a case of subconjunctival dislocation of the lens. Opth. Record, June, 1897.

3414. Puccioni, A case of spontaneous luxation of both lenses. Boll. d'Ocul., XVIII, 14-15, p. 108.

3415. Pfluger, Prevention of prolapse of the iris in extraction of the senile cataract. Proceedings of Moscow International Congress. Arch. of Opthal., Vol. XXVII, Part I, p. 95. Zehender's Klin. Monatsbl., XXXV, p. 332.

3416. Purtscher, Congenital cataract as a family affection. Centralbl. fur Augenh., Vol. XXI, p. 198.

3417. Purtscher, Choroidal hemorrhage after extraction. Centralbl. fur Augenh., XXI, p. 193.

3418. Rogmann, A new contribution to the study of the congenital anomalies of the lens. Colobomas situated in direction not corresponding to the foetal cleft. General conclusions on the genesis of lenticular colobomas. Arch. fur Opth., XVII, p. 427.

3419. Rauschenbach, A contribution to the pathology and therapy of traumatic cataract. Inaug. Dissert. Basle, 1897.

3420. Sattler, H., Zuzatz zur Bloom'schen Arbeit. Uber die retro-choroideal blutungen nach staar extractionen. Graefe's Arch., Bd. XLVI, Part I, p. 184.

3421. Schweigger, C., Simple extraction downward. Arch. of Opth., Vol. XXVII, No. 3, p. 255. Ann. of Opth., Vol. VII, No. 2, p. 240.

3422. Schantz, A family with juvenile cataract. Centralbl. fur Augenh., Vol. XXI, p. 264.

3423. Schoen, Cataract following convulsions. Wiener Med. Wochenschr., No. 17. 1897.

580

1898. 3424. Sattler, On the operative treatment of ectopia lentis. Arch. fur Augenh., XXXV, 4, p. 355.

3425. Sourdille, Daviel's section, according to authoritative texts. Arch. f. Opth., XVII, p. 657.

3426. Schiotz, Cataract statistics. Nord. Mag. f. Lageridsk. Forhandl. Christiana, 1897, p. 159.

3427. Schumway, E. A., Summary of operations for cataract, done at New York Eye and Ear Infirmary, October, 1895, to October, 1896. January, 1897.

3428. Trousseau, Treatment of hemorrhage after extraction of cataract by corneal suture. Arch. f. Opth., XVII, 2, p. 106.

3429. Trocavo, Uribe, Delay in the past operative formation of the anterior chamber. Ann. d'Opth., Vol. I, No. 1. July, 1898.

3430. Valois, G., Delay in cicatrization after cataract operation. Recueil d'Opth., January, 1898.

3431. Velhagen, A case of pseudo-neoplasm in the interior of the eye after cataract extraction. Centralbl. fur Augenh., XXI, p. 363.

3432. Wettendorfer, A contribution of the aetiology of juvenile total cataract. Wiener Med. Wochenschrift, 1897, Nos. 11 and 12.

3433. Wilson, F. M., Senile cataract. Trans. Conn. Med. Soc. 1895.

INDEX.

INDEX—Continued.

INDEX—Continued.

INDEX—Continued.

INDEX—CONTINUED.

INDEX—Continued.

INDEX—Continued.